Chaucer's Fame in Britannia
1641–1700

Medieval and Renaissance
Texts and Studies

Volume 572

Chaucer's Fame in Britannia
1641–1700

By
Jackson Campbell Boswell

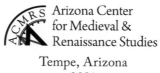
Arizona Center
for Medieval &
Renaissance Studies

Tempe, Arizona
2021

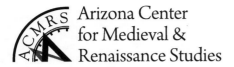
Arizona Center
for Medieval &
Renaissance Studies

Published by ACMRS (Arizona Center for Medieval and Renaissance Studies)
Tempe, Arizona
©2021 Arizona Board of Regents for Arizona State University.
All Rights Reserved.

978-0-86698-630-4

∞
Printed in the United States of America

TABLE OF CONTENTS

Acknowledgments

First and foremost, I thank the Folger Shakespeare Library's reading room staff whose patience and kindness sustained me through many happy years of research there; moreover, I thank Folger directors past and present, particularly Gail Kern Paster, Werner Gundersheimer, and Michael Whitmore. Special thanks to Georgianna Ziegler, reference librarian, and James Kuhn, electronic wizard and guru.

Heartfelt gratitude to other custodians of rare books in the British Library, the National Library of Scotland, and the university libraries of London, Oxford, Cambridge, Edinburgh, Glasgow, Chicago, Columbia, Harvard, Rutgers, UCLA, Yale, Library of Congress, and the Huntington Library.

More thanks for generous financial contributions from the Faculty Senate of the University of the District of Columbia, the Fulbright Commission, the Nannie Byrd Foundation, and the National Endowment for Humanities.

Yet more thanks to Gordon Braden for writing a such a fine introduction to this little book, and to Elizabeth Hageman, Peter Castle Molin, Lois Schwoerer, Marie Barnett, James Niessen, and Sylvia Holton Peterson, and William Peterson for sustained encouragement and support.

And finally to my late wife Ann and my stepsons Ted, Peter, and John my everlasting love and appreciation for indulging my passion for philology.

Editorial Note

Entries in this compilation are arranged chronologically and, within individual years, alphabetically by authors' surnames or initials. If neither of the latter is known, the entry is listed alphabetically by title.

Entry titles that have been shortened generally conform to those in the *STC* (*Short-title Catalogue of Books Printed in England, Scotland and Ireland and of English Books Printed Abroad, 1475–1640*) and Wing (*Short-title Catalogue of Books Printed in England, Scotland, Ireland, Wales and British America, 1641–1700*). Original spelling (but not capitalization) in the titles has been retained, and, unless noted otherwise, the place of publication of seventeenth-century volumes may be assumed to be London.

Many titles appear only once, but others are also recorded among entries in subsequent years, later editions being considered valid signs of either continuing or recurring interest in the work at hand.

Within the entries themselves, a few typographical errors have been corrected, but for the most part original spellings are retained, sometimes occasioning a *sic*.

Many of the passages quoted here were originally printed in a mixture of type fonts and with various combinations of capital and lowercase letters. Though it is assumed that readers will be more interested in substance than form, and that attempting to duplicate the original appearance of passages would be counter-productive (if not impossible), an effort has been made to preserve not only occasional eruptions of black letter and small capitals but also shifts from roman to italic characters. On the other hand, i/j, v/u, and vv/w have been regularized according to modern usage.

Because of the nature of this volume (a book not likely to be read from cover to cover), it has seemed advisable occasionally to explain or define something or other more than once. An attempt has been made, however, to keep repetition to a reasonable minimum.

Finally, as in most studies nowadays, calendar years are here taken to have begun on 1 January rather than 25 March.

BIBLIOGRAPHY
with Abbreviations Used Herein

Alderson, William L., and Arnold C. Henderson. *Chaucer and Augustan Scholarship*. UCPES, 35. Berkeley: U of California P, 1970. [A&H]

Atkinson, Dorothy F. "Chaucer Allusions." *Notes and Queries* 170 (1936): 207. [Atkinson, *N&Q* 1936]

———. "Some Notes on Heraldry and Chaucer." *Modern Language Notes* 51 (1936): 328–31. [Atkinson, *MLN* 1936]

———. "Some Further Chaucer Allusions." *Modern Language Notes* 55 (1940): 361–62. [Atkinson, *MLN* 1940]

———. "Some Further Chaucer Allusions." *Modern Language Notes* 59 (1944): 568–70. [Atkinson, *MLN* 1944]

Bond, Richmond P., John W. Bowyer, C. B. Millican, and G. Hubert Smith. "A Collection of Chaucer Allusions," *Studies in Philology* 28 (1931): 481–512. [*SP* 28]

Boswell, Jackson Campbell, and Sylvia Wallace Holton. *Chaucer's Fame in England*. New York: Modern Language Association of America, 2004. [Boswell & Holton]

Capp, Bernard. *English Almanacs, 1500–1800: Astrology and the Popular Press*. Ithaca, NY: Cornell University Press, 1979.

Dictionary of National Biography. [*DNB*]

Dobbins, Austin C. "Chaucer Allusions: 1619–1732." *Modern Language Quarterly* 18 (1957), 309–12. [Dobbins, *MLQ*]

———. "More Seventeenth-Century Chaucer Allusions." *Modern Language Notes* 68 (1953), 33–34. [Dobbins, *MLN*]

Frank, Joseph. "An Early Newspaper Reference to Chaucer." *Notes and Queries* 3 (1956), 298. [Frank]

Graves, Thornton S. "Some Chaucer Allusions." *Studies in Philology* 20 (1923): 469–78. [Graves]

Harris, Brice. "Some Seventeenth Century Chaucer Allusions." *Philological Quarterly* 18 (1939): 395–405. [Harris]

Jeayes, I. H., ed. *The Academy of Armory*. London: for the Roxburghe Club, 1905.

Klemp, P. J., ed. *The Faerie King (c. 1650) by Samuel Sheppard*. Salzburg Studies in English Literature. Elizabethan & Renaissance Studies (107:2). Salzburg,

Austria: Institut fur Anglistik und Amerikanistik, Universitat Salzburg, 1984.

Langston, Beach. "William Penn and Chaucer." *Notes and Queries* 1 (1954): 49–50. [Langston]

MacKerness, E. D. "Two Chaucer Allusions of 1659." *Notes and Queries* 5 (1958): 197–98. [MacKerness]

Malone, Edmund, ed. *The Critical and Miscellaneous Prose of Works of John Dryden.* London: H. Baldwin and Son, 1800. vol. 1 (of 3 vols.), pt. 1.

Mitchell, P. Beattie. "An Allusion to Chaucer" and "A Chaucer Allusion." *Modern Language Notes* 51 (1936): 435–37. [Mitchell]

Nelson, Carolyn, and Matthew Seccombe. *British Newspapers and Periodicals 1641–1700.* New York: Modern Language Association, 1987. [Nelson and Seccombe]

Oxford Dictionary of National Biography. [*Oxford DNB*]

Pierce, Marvin. "Another Chaucer Allusion: 1672." *Notes and Queries* 4 (1957): 2–3. [Pierce]

Short-title Catalogue of Books Printed in England, Scotland and Ireland and of English Books Printed Abroad, 1475–1640. Second edition revised and enlarged. London: The Bibliographical Society, 1976–1991. [*STC*]

Spurgeon, Caroline. *Five Hundred Years of Chaucer Criticism and Allusion 1357–1900.* London: 1923–1924. [Spurgeon]

Tatlock, John S. P., and Arthur G. Kennedy. *A Concordance of the Complete Works of Geoffrey Chaucer.* Washington: Carnegie Institution, 1927. [Tatlock & Kennedy]

Vaughan, Thomas. *The Works.* Ed. Alan Rudrum, with the assistance of Jennifer Drake-Brockman. Oxford: Oxford University Press, 1984. [Rudrum]

University Microfilms. [UMI]

Williams, Franklin B., Jr. "Unnoted Chaucer Allusions, 1550–1650," *Philological Quarterly* 16 (1937): 67–71. [Williams]

Wing, Donald. *Short-title Catalogue of Books Printed in England, Scotland, Ireland, Wales and British America, 1641–1700.* 2nd ed. New York: Modern Language Association, 1972_1998. [Wing]

Wright, Louis B. "A 'Character' from Chaucer." *Modern Language Notes* 44 (1929): 364–68. [Wright]

INTRODUCTION

GORDON BRADEN

Famously, Geoffrey Chaucer's life records, laboriously assembled by two generations of modern scholarship over a period of forty years, make no mention of his
literary work.[1] Strictly speaking, it is something of an act of faith to assume that
the Geoffrey Chaucer mentioned in them is the same Geoffrey Chaucer who
wrote the poems we still read, though nobody seriously doubts that he is. The
poetry itself floats a theory as to why in a brief glimpse of Chaucer's very mun-
dane and time-consuming day job. From 1374 he was controller (auditor) of the
collection of custom duties, primarily those on wool, in the port of London; in
House of Fame, a first-person poem probably composed a few years after he took
up that task, a concerned interlocutor worries about the way it has compartmen-
talized the poor man's life:

> when thy labour doon al ys
> And hast ymad thy rekenynges,
> Instede of reste and newe thynges,
> Thou goost hom to thy house anoon
> And, also dombe as any stoon,
> Thou sittest at another book . . . (652–57)[2]

The relentless bean-counting (Chaucer was required to write out his accounts
manu sua propria, [in his own handwriting]) has not kept him from working
devotedly after hours writing about love and lovers:

> bookes, songes, dytees
> In ryme or elles in cadence,
> As thou best canst, in reverence

---

[1] *Chaucer Life-Records*, ed. Martin M. Crow and Clair C. Olson from materials
compiled by John M. Manly, Edith Rickert, Lilian J. Redstone *et al* (Oxford: Clarendon,
1966).

[2] Quotations from Chaucer are from *The Complete Poetry and Prose*, ed. John H.
Fisher (New York: Holt, Rinehart and Winston, 1977).

> Of Love and of hys servantes eke
> That have hys servyse soght, and seke. (622–26)

But he has done so "Withoute guerdon ever yitte" (619): precious little to show for it in the way of reward or recognition. It could not of course have been as bad as all that; the serious courtly connections that secured Chaucer his employment would also have guaranteed an audience and readership, and even some payment for what he wrote. Still, the poem's speaker knows all too well in his heart that this is not what true literary success feels like. He can already guess how those life records—if anyone ever bothers to look at them—are going to read.

The poem, however, is about the search for an escape from this fate. It is from the start an escape from the reality in which accountants work their trade. The conversation just quoted takes place in mid-air; Chaucer's interlocutor is a glittering, talkative gold eagle—showing a pedantic streak when he gets on his favorite topic of acoustical physics ("Geffrey, thou wost ryght wel this . . ."; 729) —who swoops the forlorn writer up in his talons ("Me caryinge in his clawes starke / As lyghtly as I were a larke"; 545–46) on orders from the king of the pagan gods:

> Joves, thorgh hys grace,
> Wol that I bere the to a place
> Which that hight the Hous of Fame,
> To do the somme disport and game,
> In somme recompensacion
> Of labour and devocion
> That thou has had, loo causeles,
> To Cupido the rechcheles.
> And thus this god, thorgh his merite,
> Wol with somme maner thing the quyte,
> So that thou wolt be of good chere. (661–71)

It is not clear from the tone of things, but the eagle is also a visitor from Dante's *Divine Comedy*. His credentials include quite specific textual quotations, from Dante's dream while being lifted to the first terrace in Purgatory ("in sogno mi parea veder sospesa / un'aguglia nel ciel con penne d'or"; *Purgatorio* 9.19–20 [in a dream I seemed to see hovering an eagle with feathers of gold]) and from the passage at the start of the *Paradiso* (1.13–36) where Dante prays to Apollo for the power to win the laurel crown awarded to victorious Caesars and poets.[3] This is a message to England from Italy, Europe's cultural *avant garde*, "the one part of medieval Europe where fame was recognized as an incentive and a reward sur-

---

[3] On this second quotation, see Alice S. Miskimin, *The Renaissance Chaucer* (New Haven, CT: Yale University Press, 1975), 72–80.

passing even political power and material wealth,"[4] and where the ancient symbolism of the laurel was revived and took its modern form. Dante hoped to have his achievement recognized with a literal laurel crown, though he was unwilling to receive it until his exile was lifted and he could do so in Florence (*Paradiso* 25.1–2). In 1315 Albertino Mussato was laureated in Padua in a public ceremony in honor of his neo-Senecan tragedy *Ecerinis*. And most momentously, in 1341 — about the time Chaucer was born — Petrarch was crowned in Rome, and made a speech calling for a reborn civilization in which the prospect of undying fame is once again the noble spur to poetic ambition. It was on that point an astonishingly successful call, still powerful three centuries later:

> *Fame* is no plant that grows on mortal soil,
> Nor in the glistering foil
> Set off to th' world, nor in broad rumour lies,
> But lives and spreds aloft by those pure eyes,
> And perfet witness of all-judging *Jove*;
> As he pronounces lastly on each deed,
> Of so much fame in Heav'n expect thy meed. (*Lycidas* 78–84)

So wrote the young John Milton, nurturing the talent that would finally give English literature the epic poem that would match those of classical Greek and Rome; the lineage of that self-encouragement descends directly from Petrarch's manifesto. Chaucer may in fact have met Petrarch during a mission to Italy in 1368, or at least seen him from across the room at a princely wedding.[5] Back in England a few years later, a tour of Fame's house might have been just what he needed as he came to terms with what life was offering him. Chaucer's poem as we have it breaks off without a conclusion, but Renaissance texts include some final lines, authored by William Caxton, Chaucer's first editor, in which the dreamer awakens and seemingly rededicates himself to his literary efforts (B&H15). That is not an unreasonable conjecture, since even before this, Chaucer is so grateful for what he sees that he promises Apollo: "Thou shalt se me go as blyve / Unto the nexte laure y see, / And kysse yt, for hyt is thy tree" (1106–8). There is no Accountants' Hall of Fame (if there is, nobody's heard of it), but at least at certain times it can be the opposite for poets.

Among other things, Jackson Boswell's work — the present volume and its predecessor[6] that the current book both extends and deepens — documents with

---

[4] George Williams, *A New View of Chaucer* (Durham, NC: Duke University Press, 1965), 118.

[5] A possibility reported by Thomas Speght in his 1598 edition of Chaucer (B&H600, under "His Service"). See Donald R. Howard, *Chaucer: His Life, His Works, His World* (New York: Dutton, 1987), 120–22.

[6] Jackson Campbell Boswell and Sylvia Wallace Holton, *Chaucer's Fame in England: STC Chauceriana 1475–1640* (New York: MLA, 2004). I preface references to item num-

new fullness and rigor the uncanny accuracy of the prophecy implicit in Chaucer's poem. The life records say nothing about his poetry, but the records that follow begin his spectacular induction into the House of Fame. Petrarch himself was clear that the fame that counted was the fame that comes after you die: "the end of life is the beginning of glory."[7] Both the spectacle and the uncanniness are powerfully enhanced by a technological development neither Petrarch nor Chaucer could have foreseen: the invention of printing, which made it possible for an author's fame to be promulgated far more quickly, widely, and reliably than ever before. In Chaucer's case, there was also the happenstance that England's first printer had a particular interest in his work. Caxton interpolates references to Chaucer and *Troilus and Criseyde* into his translation of a French history of the Trojan war that he published in Bruges in 1475 (B&H1), and among his first publications after relocating to Westminster in 1477 are an edition of *The Canterbury Tales* (B&H3) and a *Book of Curtesye* that includes an extravagant tribute to

> fader and founder of ornate eloquence
> That enlumened hast alle our bretayne . . .
> I mene fader chaucer / maiser galfryde
> Alas the whyle / that ever he from us dyde (B&H2)

In an edition of Chaucer's translation of Boethius (B&H10), Caxton reiterates his praise of "the worshipful fader & first foundeur & embellissher of ornate eloquence in our english," and prints a Latin elegy on Chaucer by Stefano Surigone,

---

bers in this volume with B&H, those to the present volume with B or, for the Appendix, B&HA. Boswell's monumental predecessor here is Caroline F. E. Spurgeon, *Five Hundred Years of Chaucer Criticism and Allusion 1357–1900*, 3 vols. (Cambridge: Cambridge University Press, 1925). Her work remains impressive, and her substantial introduction (144 pages) is still unsurpassed as a survey of the subject. Almost a century later, though, Boswell has had the advantage not only of intervening scholarship but also of dramatically improved resources for conducting this kind of research systematically. Even though he has for practical reasons limited his search more narrowly than Spurgeon, to works appearing in print, he has significantly added to her list. For the years covered in this volume, Spurgeon presents 162 entries, Boswell 1062, an almost tenfold increase that invites reconsideration of Spurgeon's claim that the period represents an anomalous time of "gloom and neglect" in Chaucer's literary fortunes (1:xxxvii). Derek Brewer's *Geoffrey Chaucer: The Critical Heritage*, 2 vols. (London: Routledge, 1978), by design highly selective in its coverage (seven entries for the period 1641–1700), is valuable for the generosity of its quotations and an economical but excellent introduction.

    [7] Francesco Petrarca, *Rerum familiarum libri* I-VIII, trans. Aldo S. Bernardo (Albany: SUNY Press, 1975), 15 (1.2).

a Milanese humanist teaching in England in the later fifteenth century.[8] Surigone is called "Poete laureate," probably one of the honorifics widely bestowed by municipalities, courts, and especially universities in western Europe in imitation of Petrarch's coronation; John Skelton would boast of being laureated by both Oxford and Cambridge, and seems to have received a crown from Louvain as well. (There are universities that still provide a literal laurel crown along with an honorary degree.) Chaucer could lay no official claim to such a title, but Surigone's poem — that Caxton says he found hanging on a pillar near Chaucer's tomb in Westminster Abbey — calls him not just *poeta* but *vates*, compares him to Virgil, and awards him the full Petrarchan hyperbole of posthumous fame: "Non tamen extincto corpore fama perit / Vivet in eternum" (yet even when the body is dead fame does not perish; it will live forever). John Lydgate had written that Chaucer "worthy was the lawrer to have / Of poetrye" (B&H19), and Caxton in his second edition of *The Canterbury Tales* seconds that judgment: "we ought to gyve a singuler laude unto that noble & grete philosopher Gefferey chaucer the whiche for his ornate wrytyng in our tongue maye wel have the name of a laureate poete" (B&H16). A greater power than state or academia — or church for that matter — is disposing things here. Two centuries later the title can pass without challenge or comment, even when teamed with another one that its bearer never enjoyed when he was alive: "Sir *Geoffry Chaucer*, Poet-*Lawreat*" (B560).[9]

Part of what is at work here is a predictable appetite for some English poet to be standard-bearer for an emergent national literature, an English name to hold its own with the acknowledged classics of earlier literature in established languages:

> Dant in Itaile, Virgil in Rome towne,
> Petrark in Florence, had at his pleasaunce,
> And prudent Chaucer in Brutes Albion
> like his desyre found vertuous suffisaunce (B&H191)

---

[8] On this epitaph, with particular reference to its role in developing Chaucer's claim to laureateship, see Seth Lerer, *Chaucer and his Readers: Imagining the Author in Late-Medieval England* (Princeton: Princeton University Press, 1993), 152–66; the fifteenth-century process by which England gradually becomes conscious of itself as a nation "in need of a laureate poet" (3) is carefully traced by Lerer on 22–56.

[9] Likewise B881. Chaucer was a "knight of the shire" from Kent in the 1386 parliament (*Life-Records*, 364–69), but that was the traditional name for an elective post that did not in itself confer the title of knight. Chaucer's imagined knighthood is at least as old as 1548, when John Bale calls him *eques auratus* (B&H161). Boswell's collection does include one seventeenth-century proposal to defrock Chaucer for writing an unworthy poem: "That Poet *Laureat* forfeited his wreath of Bayes and Ivy-twine, who made his prayers to his Purse, to keep him out of debt" (B31). The context of this, though, is a paradoxical praise of owing other people money.

Up to a point any English writer of sufficient fecundity might do for such propaganda, and for a while Chaucer is often one of a ready Middle English triumvirate: "Chaucer Goweir and Lidgate laureate" (B&H146). But Chaucer's is the name with staying power; Lydgate and then Gower tend to slip off such lists, while Chaucer continues with remarkable consistency to anchor them as newer possibilities are floated: "Howe shuld I hit in *Chausers* vayn / Or toutche the typ, of *Surries* brayn / O dip my pen, in *Petrarkes* stiell . . ." (B&H327). This from an aspiring Thomas Churchyard in 1575, about the time George Gascoigne is recommending himself to Queen Elizabeth as "*Chaucers* boye and *Petrarks* jorneyman."[10] The modern end of the canon is of course continually evolving, through to the end of the next century:

> All Poets (as adition to their fames)
> Have by their Works eternized their names,
> As Chaucer, Spencer, and that noble earle,
> Of Surrie . . .
> *Sydney* and *Shakspire, Drayton, Withers* and
> Renowned *Jonson* glory of our Land:
> *Deker,* Learn'd *Chapman, Haywood* although good . . .
> And that sweet Seraph of our Nation, *Quarles* . . . (B15)

> And now come we to the first and last best Poets of the *English* Nation *Geffrey Chaucer,* and *Abraham Cowley,* the one being the Sun just rising, and shewing its self on the *English Horizon,* and so by degrees increasing and growing in strength till it came to its full *Glory* and *Meridian* in the incomparable *Cowley.* (B609)

> *Chaucer.* | *Spenser.* | *Shakespear.* | *Johnson.* | *Beaumont* and *Fletcher.* | *Draiton.* *Daniel.* | Sr. *John Suckling.* | Sr. *John Denham.* | *Crashaw.* | *Cowley.* | Sr. *William Davenant.* | Dr. *Donn.* | Mr. *Dryden.* | Mr. *Otway.* | Mr. *Lee.* | Mrs. *Behn.* | Mrs. *Phillips.* (B830)

In 1556 Chaucer's remains were moved to a more impressive tomb, which became the focus of a Poets' Corner in Westminster Abbey; imagined competition for a place there becomes a recurrent trope in the literature of praise: "Renowned *Spenser,* lye a thought more nigh / To learned *Chaucer,* and rare *Beaumont* lye, / A little nearer *Spenser,* to make room for *Shakespear*" (B671). At the very end of the period treated here, John Dryden, in a critical essay that considers Chaucer's achievement with some care and complexity, nevertheless grandly affirms his place as the patriarch of English poetry's great epic line: "*Milton* was the Poetical

---

[10] From a poetic sequence presented to the monarch in a manuscript book; see *The Complete Works of George Gascoigne,* ed. John W. Cunliffe (Cambridge: Cambridge University Press, 1907–10), 2: 517.

Son of *Spencer*, and . . . *Spencer* more than once insinuates, that the Soul of *Chaucer* was transfus'd into his Body; and that he was begotten by him Two hundred years after his Decease" (B1031). Less than two months after this is published, Dryden himself is buried in the Poets' Corner.[11]

Chaucer stays at the head of the list of English poets despite the fact that he writes in what can be and sometimes is called a dead language. As early as 1549 we find complaints that "Chaucers wordes . . . by reason of antiquitie be almost out of use" (B&H159). The difficulties that their obsolescence presents are acknowledged with increasing force as time goes on, and sometimes they are presented as fatal—"*Chaucers* Poems, which are in plain and old-fashion'd garments, which is Language, is to be despised, and his Wit condemned." But dismissals have a way of being accompanied, as in this case, by stirringly contrary affirmations: "certainly *Chaucers* Witty Poems, and Lively Descriptions, in despight of their Old Language, as they have lasted in great Esteem and Admiration these three hundred years, so they may do Eternally amongst the Wise in every Age" (B276, from a play by Margaret Cavendish). Spot quotations from Chaucer often quietly update his language. Wholescale translation of individual works into contemporary English may be as old as 1525, when what appears to be an updated version of *The Man of Law's Tale* is printed (B&H88). In 1630 Jonathan Sidnam composed (though he did not publish) a version of the first three books of *Troilus and Criseyde* "Translated into our Moderne English," which pursues interesting agendas beyond the strictly linguistic.[12] The essay by

---

[11] By some accounts he is actually buried in Chaucer's own grave, a misunderstanding (probably) whose life extended into the nineteenth century; on the complicated motives in play here, see Thomas A. Prendergast, *Chaucer's Dead Body: From Corpse to Corpus* (New York: Routledge, 2004), 57–69. Prendergast considers the whole phenomenon of the Poets' Corner in *Poetical Dust: Poets' Corner and the Making of Britain* (Philadelphia: University of Pennsylvania Press, 2015).

[12] *A Seventeenth Century Modernisation of the First Three Books of Chaucer's "Troilus and Criseyde,"* ed. Herbert G. Wright (Bern: Francke, 1960); see Clare Kinney, "Lost in Translation: The Vicissitudes of the Heroine and the Immasculation of the Reader in a Seventeenth-Century Paraphrase of *Troilus and Creseyde,*" *Exemplaria* 5 (1993): 343–63. Sidnam stands with almost all early modern readers in taking Chaucer's Criseyde as a straightforward examplar of female weakness and treachery: "The inconstancie of *Cressid* is so readie in every mans mouth," as George Whetstone puts it in 1577 (B&H350). Even for Dryden Chaucer's poem, like all other tellings of the story, was "intended I suppose a Satyr on the Inconstancy of Women" (B553). A rare reader with a different take does not dissent from this reading of Chaucer's poem but reproaches the poet for his misogyny: "Are all women evil? . . . *Chauser*, how chance thy golden pen so miscarryed?" (B607). An "Anglo-Latin" translation of the first two books of Chaucer's poem is published in 1635 (B&H1265), with the other three surviving in manuscript; see Tim William Machan, "Kynaston's *Troilus*, Textual Criticism and the Renaissance Reading of Chaucer," *Exemplaria* 5 (1993): 161–83.

Dryden quoted above prefaces a selection of Chaucerian texts in Augustan dress, together with similar translations from Latin, Greek, and Italian. Their appearance prompts celebrations of the rescue effort—"*Chaucer* shall again with Joy be Read, / Whose Language with its Master lay for Dead" (B1040)—but Dryden's own attitude toward the original Middle English texts lacks the condescension of those who see Chaucer as the English Ennius, that is the honored but obsolete predecessor of the language's true literary greatness (B&H248, etc.). Rather: "I hold him in the same Degree of Veneration as the Grecians held Homer, or the Romans Virgil" (B1031). The Middle English originals accompany Dryden's versions into print; Chaucer's language is not thought so alien from contemporary usage as to be of only specialized interest. The glossing of Chaucer's "hard words" is an ongoing activity in the entries Boswell collects, and not without alertness to their contemporary usefulness. "Obsolete Words may . . . be laudably reviv'd," writes Dryden, taking note of some retrievals by the most imposing figures in House of Fame of modern English: "As for Mr. *Milton* . . . His Antiquated words were his Choice, not his Necessity; for therein he imitated *Spencer*, as *Spencer* did *Chaucer*" (B857). Some of these revivals are sufficiently successful that we no longer register the words in question as archaic: "grisly," for example (B922).

During the period covered here, Chaucer's standing also receives a boost that now seems eccentric but was powerful and impressively durable at the time. He is seen as an early voice for ecclesiastical reform, a Protestant in all but name. The honorific reburial of Chaucer's body during Mary's reign may have been an attempt to secure his identity as an orthodox Catholic, but if so the effort had little long-term effect.[13] John Foxe, in his immensely influential *Acts and Monuments*, is only the first to link Chaucer's name in print with his polemical contemporary John Wycliffe ("a right Wiclevian," Foxe calls him; B&H285). The main reason for doing so is the characterization of most of the churchmen in *The Canterbury Tales*; in Elizabethan England, beset by Catholic menace, the satire in Chaucer's clerical portraits gains a sharp topical edge. The same context conditioned English interest in some of Chaucer's main continental predecessors: Dante, Boccaccio, and especially Petrarch, whose savage denunciations of the fourteenth-century Avignon papacy were for a time more popular in England than his love poems.[14] Chaucer's name is repeatedly linked to theirs, with literary and sectarian merit often mingling inseparably. So the prominent Protestant academic (and former Marian exile) Laurence Humphrey wrote in an attack on the Jesuits:

---

[13] See Prendergast, *Chaucer's Dead Body*, 45–57.

[14] The documentation here is set out more thoroughly than before in my own collaboration with Boswell: *Petrarch's English Laurels, 1475–1700* (Farnham, Surrey: Ashgate, 2012).

> From Oxford came Geoffrey Chaucer, the like of another Dante or Petrarch with regard to his elegant and free-flowing diction. Chaucer even translated them into our language, writers in whom the Church of Rome has been depicted as the seat of Antichrist and thus been completely exposed. Chaucer took every opportunity to unmask adroitly the petty friars, monks, mass-makers, episcopal ceremonies, and pilgrimages; he acknowledged true and spiritual food in the Sacrament of Christ; he reproached the foul practice of virginity under compulsion; and he approved of freedom to marry in the Lord. (B&H407)

Reading Chaucer this way is greatly facilitated by the proximity of what now seem clearly, even crudely non-canonical works—especially *The Ploughman's Tale*, an octosyllabic rant from the Parson's brother, which appeared (out of nowhere) in collections of Chaucer's poems from 1542 until W. W. Skeat's edition in 1894 (and even Skeat includes it in a volume of apocrypha).[15] It is a poem that leaves no ambiguity about its author's opinion on the Catholic Church: "Peter was never so great a foole / To leave his kaye with such a lorell" (373–74, as quoted in B&H695; the passage it is from is quoted several times elsewhere). Put next to this, the other Canterbury tales become angrier works, their author a more aggressive and uncompromising moralist: "such was his bolde spyrit, that what enormities he saw in any, he would not spare to pay them home" (B&H445). *The Ploughman's Tale* is one of the most cited of the individual tales and continues to be so throughout this period. It is there at both ends of the present volume: Milton gleefully uses it when denouncing the Anglican episcopacy in *Of Reformation* in 1641 (B14), and William Winstanley quotes it in *The Protestant Almanac, for the Year 1700* (B1048).

With *The loughman's Tale* removed from the canon, the combatively Protestant Chaucer becomes a fainter presence in his work; nor is it particularly congruent with his self-presentation in *House of Fame*, Chaucer's own most overt comment on his literary career. Neither, however, is the laureate national hero who *"Founded* the *Muses* Empire in *our* Soyl" (B648), for that is not exactly the future which the speaker of that poem forecasts for himself. The House of Fame as such, when he gets there, proves an intimidatingly grand place—"Ful of the fynest stones faire / That men rede in the Lapidaire / As grasses growen in a mede" (1351–53)—and he spends a while taking in the statues of the great

---

[15] A different, shorter *Ploughman's Tale*, actually lifted from a poem by Thomas Hoccleve, is entered into the Christ Church manuscript of *The Canterbury Tales*, but does not make it into printed editions; the references that Boswell gathers may be presumed to be to the other one. This and some other Chaucerian supplements that did not see print until our time can be found in John M. Bowers, ed., *The Canterbury Tales: Fifteenth-Century Continuations and Additions* (Kalamazoo, MI: Medieval Institute, 1992). On the complicated history of Chaucerian apocrypha and their equally complicated role in Chaucer's early modern fortunes, see Miskimin, 226–61.

poets who have been inducted and witnessing the unnerving and, one might even think, whimsical procedures by which Lady Fame processes new applications. When a stranger approaches and asks, "Frend, what is thy name? / Artow come hider to han fame?" (1871–72) Chaucer is quickly defensive:

"Nay, for sothe, frend," quod y.
"I cam noght hyder, graunt mercy,
For no such cause, by my hede.
Sufficeth me, as I were dede,
That no wight have my name in honde.
I wot myself best how y stonde." (1873–78)

What he seeks is not the memorialization of his own name, but just "Somme newe tydynges for to lere, / Somme newe thinges, y not what, / Tydynges other this or that" (1886–88)—and as luck would have it, the stranger knows just where those are to be had. They leave the House of Fame for another kind of house. The eagle is waiting for them when they get there.

Chaucer calls the new place "Domus Dedaly / That Laboryntus cleped ys" (1920–21); modern critics often refer to it as the House of Rumor. It is not in any usual sense a house, but a huge wicker cage, an astonishing "sixty myle of lengthe" (1979), spinning "swyft as thought" (1924), noisy as hell (if you put it in France, they'd hear it in Rome), and, as promised, filled with "tydynges." For a twenty-first-century reader, it is an uncanny prefiguring of the Internet. That garrulous eagle had earlier explained how anything ever said by anyone anywhere in the world makes a permanent impression on the air, and apparently this is where all those recordings are archived: in a windstorm of truths and lies buzzing around together. The destination of Chaucer's Dantescan journey turns out to be a vision of "the afterlife of words, not souls."[16] But this also appears to be where those words are generated, and the wicker structure leaves many holes through which these utterances strive to escape out into the world. The press to do so is so great that truths and lies jam up at the same exit (insufficient bandwidth) and become, as Chaucer puts it, sworn brothers that no one can tell apart anymore.[17] It is in his vision of the speakers of this endlessly dubious chatter that he seems to predict the actual source of his future fame:

Lord, this hous in alle tymes,
Was ful of shipmen and pilgrimes,
With scrippes bret-ful of lesynges [lies],

---

[16] Lisa J. Kiser, *Truth and Textuality in Chaucer's Poetry* (Hanover, NH: University Press of New England, 1991), 27.

[17] They make D. Vance Smith think of the Three Stooges: "Chaucer as an English Writer," in Seth Lerer, ed., *The Yale Companion to Chaucer* (New Haven, CT: Yale University Press, 2006), 110.

Entremedled with tydynges.
And eke allone be hemselve,
O many a thousand tymes twelve
Saugh I eke of these pardoners,
Currours, and eke messangers,
With boystes [boxes] crammed ful of lyes
As ever vessel was with lyes [lees]. (2121–30)

He is not going to write the English *Aeneid*; he is going to write, well, *The Canterbury Tales*—a work of far more uncertain *gravitas*.

Matthew Arnold, who thought Chaucer lacked "high seriousness," was not the first person to think that. A significant part of Chaucer's legacy, repeatedly on view in Boswell's catalogue, is a brand name for foolishness and unreliability: "for remedie of this disease, some do advise to open the vain of the leg, a thing not only frivolous to talke of, and a verie olde womans fable, or Cantorburie tale, but also verie perillous to be put in practise" (B&H339). One Protestant polemicist equates "Canturburies tales" with "lyes of Robin hoode, and many goodly myracles wrought by reliques" (B&H414); even for less angry writers, Chaucer's signature genre keeps some unimpressive company: "dreames & fantacies, introductions to pleasure, familier fruiteles talkinges, eloquent, formall orations, little material, of pleasant metinges & fables amonge women, of Caunterbury, or courser tales, with divers jestes, & vaine devises" (B&H367). The nice way of saying that Chaucer runs with this crowd is to call him "a facetious poet" (B170), "a merry Bard" (B879, from the young Joseph Addison), or a "joking bard" (B1028), though not everyone is comfortable with this aspect of his talent. John Hilton publishes a song (scored for three voices) about a woman who declines "to take a jape, a jape, a jape, as *Chaucer* meant" but only "allowes it, allowes it of the new translation," i.e., after delicate rephrasing (B105). He is referring of course to Chaucer's "salacity," often displayed "in plain, down right and homely termes, with wanton naturall Expressions" that may rate a trigger warning for "the squeamish Reder" (B222). Standards of taste regarding what words and expressions will do had changed along with the rest of the language since Chaucer's time; Shakespeare certainly has his bawdy side, but you will not find the word "fart" in his surviving works, or any reference to sexual intercourse as briskly graphic as the sex scene in *The Merchant's Tale*: "Damyan / Gan pullen up the smok and in he throng" (2352–53). A current of disapproval for what used to be acceptable seems quietly widespread in references to Chaucer, and occasionally comes to the surface. John Earle's *Micro-cosmographie* includes a satirical sketch of a "*vulgar-spirited Man*" whose taste in literature gives him away: he "is taken onely with broad and obscene wit, and hisses anything too deepe for him [and] cryes *Chaucer* for his money above all our English Poets" (B&H1117). Usually, though, acknowledgment of Chaucer's shady side does not eclipse his reputation, but how exactly it relates to that reputation is not much discussed.

The only really thoughtful attempt to assess the seriousness of an unserious poet comes at the end of the seventeenth century from Dryden, when the labor of translation occasions a comparison with Ovid: "it came into my mind, that our old *English* Poet *Chaucer* in many Things resembled him, and that with no disadvantage on the on the Side of the Modern Author" (B1031). The mere juxtaposition of Chaucer with the great classical poet of *nequitia* — a juxtaposition first made in passing by Chaucer's contemporary Eustace Deschamps, and very important in modern discussions of Chaucer — is already half an answer to the question.[18] Mostly, though, the disreputable Chaucer just sits incongruously alongside his more respectable relatives, as at an uncomfortable family dinner: "an acute Logician, a sweet Rhetorician, a facetious Poet, a grave Philosopher, and a holy Devine" (B170; the list, here freshly translated from Latin, goes back to John Leland, quoted in B&H600).

If we look for what writers took from Chaucer on a practical level, we find a modest run of direct imitation. Thomas Randolph slips a first-person rewriting of the description of the Franklin into his *Aristippus*, where it is attributed to "Ennius": "For I was *Epicurus* his owne sonne . . ." (B&H1162). The ecclesiastical portraits in the *General Prologue* inspire further examples in the mid-seventeenth century; there are two of them in an anthology called *Musarum Deliciae*:

> He had a liquorous tooth over all;
> Ne was there any Wight in all this Town,
> That tasted better a Pasty of Venisoun,
> Ybaked with Gravy Gods plenty,
> It relished better then *Austin*'s works or *Gregory*,
> Yet politick he was, and worldly wise,
> And purchac'd hath, a double Benefice. (B148)

The pamphlet that Alexander Brome publishes as *A Canterbury Tale, Translated out of Chaucers Old English into Our Now Usuall Language* is actually a pair of anti-Laudian satires, a tale and the Pardoner-like sales pitch of "The Scots Pedler" (B4). *The Ploughman's Tale* is in a line of what we would now call fan fiction, the most distinguished example being Robert Henryson's bitter *Testament of Cresseid*. In William Thynne's edition (B&H124) it is printed immediately after Book 5 of *Troilus and Criseyde*, without any indication that it is not by Chaucer. Speght, his successor, leaves almost the same impression, and generations of readers may well have found the *Testament* the entirely satisfactory conclusion to the story. An almost unique alternative is provided in Richard Edwards's *The Paradise of*

---

[18] For Deschamps (from a poem unpublished until the nineteenth century), see Brewer, 1: 39–41. Programmatic modern studies include Richard L. Hoffman, *Ovid and the Canterbury Tales* (Philadelphia: University of Pennsylvania Press, 1966), and especially John M. Fyler, *Chaucer and Ovid* (New Haven, CT: Yale University Press, 1979).

Dainty Devices, one of the lyric anthologies so popular in the Elizabethan age, where Cressida gets to respond to her former lover's now stereotyped complaint with righteous annoyance:

> You say in Troy I woulde not bee,
> With gadding minde you charge me still:
> When well you knowe that hie decree,
> Did send me forth against my will. (B&H390)

Just tell the whole story, she says (it wasn't God who made honky-tonk angels) and gets to have the last word. Other Chaucerian accounts get settled in an anonymous ballad of uncertain date (it may have run afoul of the authorities) in which the Wife of Bath dies and heads for heaven. A succession of biblical figures tries to shoo her away, but she will not take *No* for an answer: "The womans mad, said *Solomon,* / That thus doth taunt a King. / Not half so mad as you, she said . . ." (B20). Eventually Christ comes to see what all the fuss is about, and, as she always knew would happen, lets her in: "Come therefore into my joy, / I will not the deny." Two writers describe spectral visits from Chaucer's spirit: Robert Greene to give literary career advice (that Greene rejects in favor of advice from the spirit of Gower, B&H503), and Richard Brathwait to deplore the new popularity of tobacco (B&H934). Milton in *Il Penseroso* toys with the idea of conjuring Chaucer up to finish *The Squire's Tale* (B37).

The most widely dispersed influence in evidence here is of a less accountable kind, to which it is hard to assign any particular agenda. Detached bits and pieces of what Chaucer wrote — aphorisms, sentences, phrases, single words — can be tracked widely over the landscape: the precipitate, if you will, of some great cloud of verbal confetti thrown out by that whirling wicker cage. There is usually some uncertainty about spotting them. Enthusiastic early praise of Chaucer can make him sound like a virtuoso of the ostentatious high style, "Our ornate Chaucer" (B&H105) with his "frech anamalit termes celicall" (B&H56, from William Dunbar in *The Golden Targe*). Skelton is closer to the mark in *Philip Sparrow*: "His termes were not darke / But plesaunt / easy / and playne" (B&H157). Characteristically, they almost blend in with what becomes common wisdom and usage. Some instances rise to the level of what might be called proverbs. By far the most popular (for the period covered here. Chaucer's "to be or not to be") is for some reason an observation from *The Reeve's Tale* about the learned: "The gretteste clerkes been noght wisest men" (4054). We find it quoted as early as 1481 (B&H13) and as late as 1700 (B1038). Most of those who quote it seem to think of it as anonymously proverbial, though the connection to Chaucer is ready to hand: "I was reading to'ther day in Old *Chaucer* and there I met with an Old Saw, *That the greatest Clerks are not the wisest men*" (B590). Chaucer may indeed have been quoting a common saying — its precedents reach back to

Heraclitus ("Knowledge is not intelligence")[19] — but the operations of the wicker
cage tend to make these things undecidable and anyway beside the point. The
great majority of people who quote the saying here do quote it in iambic pentam-
eter, or something very close; if Chaucer was not the one who shaped it, some
other English poet of his time and manner likely did. This ambiguity about
pedigree does not really present itself with a downmarket metaphor from *The
Reeve's Prologue* for being an old man in heat: "To have an hoor heed and a grene
tayl, / As hath a leek" (3878–79). Citations of it begin in 1555 (B&H196), but
take on life in the seventeenth century when the dramatists discover it: "I am
thine Leeke, thou *Chaucer* eloquent; / Mine head is white, but o mine taile is
green" (B91, from an amorous antiquarian in William Cartwright's *The Ordinary*). Boswell's work also displays the afterlife for some striking phrases that
might theoretically have come to any practitioner of the language, but have
Chaucerian authority and not uncommonly carry with them the memory of his
name: "Unknowne, unkist" (*Troilus and Criseyde* 1. 809; morphed into "uncouth,
unkissed," which preserves the alliteration as the first "k" becomes silent), "I am
. . . At dulcarnon" (*Troilus and Criseyde* 3. 930–31), "Dun is in the myre" (*The
Manciple's Prologue* 5), "spiced conscience" (*The General Prologue* 526, *The Wife of
Bath's Prologue* 435; plucked by Ben Jonson and Philip Massinger for the stage,
B&HA 75 and B&H1209), "swyved for hir sustenance" (*The Cook's Tale* 4422;
"swyved," one of those problematic words, represented in B1018 as "S——"). It
has been the novelty of Boswell's approach to pursue such possibilities vigor-
ously, erring if necessary on the side of generosity; the appendix to the present
volume includes previously ungathered examples from 1475–1640. Particulars
are debatable, but the cumulative picture I think is not.

Two examples have particularly long resonance. One is the opening of *The
General Prologue*, now by a fair margin Chaucer's best known lines: "Whan that
Aprill with his shoures soote / The droghte of March hath perced to the roote
. . ." Descriptions of spring are no novelty in medieval literature, but Lydgate's
very specific imitation of this one — three times — is unmistakable:

Whan bryght phebus passed was the Ram
Myd of Aprell & in to the Bole cam (B&H34)

Whan Phebus in the crabbe had ner his cours ronne
And toward the lyon his jorney take (B&H37)

In may quhen flora the fresche lusty quene
the snyl hath cladde in redde quhyte grene aright
And phebus gan to shedde his stremes shene (B&H59)

---

[19] Frag. 40 (Diels-Kranz), from Diogenes Laertius 9.1; trans. Guy Davenport, *The
Guy Davenport Reader*, ed. Erik Reece (Berkeley, CA: Counterpoint, 2013), 367.

Chaucer's spring will continue to inhabit invocations of the season into the seventeenth century: "Aprill having with his sweete showers moystened the drought of March, bathing every veine of the rootes of trees and ingendring floures" (B&H670); "*Zephyrus* now with his sweet breath cools and perfumes the parching beams of Titan" (B263). But the same original underpins accounts of different seasons, to deliberately different effect:

> In Septembre in fallyinge of the lite
> Whan phebus made his declynacyon
> And all the whete gadred was in the shefe (Stephen Hawes, B&H47)

> Amyddes November that moneth mysty
> Whan the sonne fulle lowe his course did ron
> As I suspecte in the sygne of Sagyttary
> Without pleasaunce to man/ or confortacyon (B&H113)

The change of season can be an amiable business, a signal that it's time to go fishing (B&H866); but it also has graver potential. Henryson keeps a certain distance from Chaucer's specific wording, but his opening for *The Testament of Cresseid* is self-conscious about being a replacement for Chaucer's season, and of a piece with the poem's stern revision of the moral world of *Troilus and Criseyde*:

> Ane doolie sessoun to ane cairfull dyte
> Suld correspond and be equivalent:
> Richt sa it wes quhen I began to wryte
> This tragedie — the wedder richt fervent,
> Quhen Aries, in middis of the Lent,
> Schouris of haill can fra the north discend,
> That scantlie fra the cauld I micht defend.

In Thomas Sackville's somber "Induction" to *A Mirror for Magistrates* a vivid inversion of spring is the starting point for a Dantescan journey to the underworld to meet the dead and hear their stories:

> The wrathfull winter prochinge on a pace,
> With blustring blastes had all ybared the treen,
> And old Saturnus with his frosty face
> With chilling colde had pearst the tender green. (B&H234)

Three and a half centuries later a circle closes when a potential here — merging Chaucer's season and the affect of death — is harvested to inaugurate one of the defining poems of our own time, T. S. Eliot's *The Waste Land*: "April is the cruelest month . . . "

The other example, its path forward documented by Boswell more thoroughly than anyone else, comes at the conclusion of the most important work
Chaucer, never good at closure, actually completed:

> Go, litel bok, go litel myn tragedye,
> Ther God thi makere yet, er that he dye,
> So sende myght to make yn som comedye.
> But litel bok, no makyng thow n'envye,
> But subgit be to alle poesye,
> And kys the steppes where as thow seest pace
> Virgile, Ovyde, Omer, Lukan, and Stace. (*Troilus and Criseyde* 5. 1786–92)

The House of Fame is once again the focus of the speaker's attention; the steps
are in effect those up which the poets named walk to receive their reward. Presumably the speaker hopes—not, as it happens, unreasonably—to join their
number, but his posture is one of abasement so extreme as to hover on the edge
of being (for the suspicious) a joke. The kissing of the architecture (like the earlier promise to kiss Apollo's tree) is the worst of it, but what you remember, what
generations of readers did remember, is the adjective the speaker attaches to what
is now his book. He likely took that adjective from Boccaccio, specifically from
his *Filocolo* ("O piccolo mio libretto," followed soon by instructions not to try to
equal Virgil, Lucan, Statius, Ovid, or Dante),[20] but he catches on it, repeating it
twice more. It is a diminutive of modesty and affection, as in the paternal words
with which Chaucer opens his *Treatise on the Astrolabe*: "Litell Lowys my sone."
Once more the record of homage begins with Lydgate:

> Go lytell byll / with out tytle or date
> And of hole herte / recommaunde me
> Whiche that am called Johan Lydgate (B&H66)

From there the trail is long:

> Goe foorthe my little Booke,
> That all on thee may looke (B&HA24)

---

[20] On the background here, see John S. P. Tatlock, "The Epilog of Chaucer's *Troilus*," *Modern Philology* 18 (1921): 113–20; the lineage traces back to Ovid's address to his
parvus liber on sending the *Tristia* back to Rome (1.1.1). Ovid, however, is writing from
the disgrace of exile and hoping not for fame but just pardon. When he takes up the possibility of poetic immortality at the end of the *Metamorphoses*, he is anything but modest;
and the classical Roman treatments of that ambition to which medieval and Renaissance
poets were heir tend to be pretty brassy, even from a retiring poet such as Horace: "Exegi
monumentum aere perennius" (*Odes* 3.30.1; I have fashioned a monument more lasting
than bronze).

> Goe forth my little Booke,
> Thou art no longer mine (B&HA93)

> Goe litle Booke, (my unlick't Poetry) (B6)

> Go little Book, I envy not thy hap,
> Mayst thou be dandled in the Ladies lap (B397)

> Go, little *Book*, abroad, and tell mankind,
> What *graces* lodged in a *Virgins* mind. (B624)

So also John Bunyan in the second part of *Pilgrim's Progress*, by way of transition from the first: "Go, now my little Book, to every Place, / Where my first *Pilgrim* has but shewn his Face" (B647). The phrasing is sufficiently recognizable that it is possible to change the key adjective without breaking the line: "Go now plaine booke, where thou maist welcom find" (B&H551; Churchyard again).

The modesty in the *topos* can of course be a feint, a tactical move in the service of serious aggression. One of the earliest examples accompanies a savage satire on Thomas Wolsey:

> Go forthe lytell treatous nothynge afraide.
>   To the Cardinall of Yorcke dedicate
> And though he threaten the be not dismayde
> To pupplysshe his adhominable estate (B&H104; rephrased as "lytle boke" in B&H158)

One deceptive *captatio benevolentiae*—"Go little Creature, in thy poor Attire, / And crave a Kiss at every Hand thou meets" (B69)—introduces an intemperate attack on parliament from Mercurius Melancholicus. Righteousness and humility can make a belligerent pair: "Goe little Book, thine aid afford / Unto the Battailes of the Lord" (B38). But Chaucer's "little" is part of a genuine but sophisticated, often devious diffidence that pervades his work, and is used to similar effect by one of sixteenth-century England's most ambitious poets. Edmund Spenser keeps his name off the title page of his first book, *The Shepherd's Calendar* (B&H384); the first thing a reader encounters after that title page is an adaptation of the envoi to *Troilus and Criseyde* that simultaneously announces the author's anonymity and seeks to link him to Philip Sidney, by 1579 already one of the aristocratic lights of Elizabethan literature:

> Goe little booke: thy selfe present,
> As child whose parent is unkent:
> To him that is the president
> Of noblesse and of chevalree . . .

The homage is repeated in the "Envoy" at the end of the book: "Go lyttle Calender . . ." There is no question that Chaucer is on Spenser's mind. The letter of
Gabriel Harvey that immediately follows the dedication to Sidney begins as an
explication of "uncouthe unkiste," with appropriate reference to "the olde famous
Poete Chaucer"; mentions of Chaucer run throughout E. K.'s notes, including
the claim—that no one disputes—that the "Tityrus" referred to in the poems
(as in the "Envoy": "Dare not to match thy pype with Tityrus hys style") is meant
to be understood as Chaucer. References to Chaucer recur throughout Spenser's
work; the last thing he published during his lifetime contains his famous salute
to "Dan *Chaucer*, well of English undefyled" (B&H575)—among other things
a sharp defense of Chaucer's supposedly obsolete language, which Spenser emu-
lated in his own way. Spenserean scholars have come to take Spenser's engagement with Chaucer very seriously; to the shared sensibility of this engagement,
the "self-deprecation and put-on naivete" of "Go, little book" is a particularly
good window.[21]

Over the following centuries the address to one's own work comes to seem
more and more of a mannerism, and writers have less and less use for it. Yet a
fresh and intense sensitivity to literary history brings it alive again in a key mod-
ernist poem, one that makes indeed an important pair with *The Waste Land*:
"Go, dumb-born book, / Tell her that sang me once that song of Lawes . . ."
This "Envoi" from Ezra Pound's *Hugh Selwyn Mauberley*, the poem sequence
that Pound said constituted "a farewell to London"—England no longer the site
for poetry—and effectively concluded the first major phase of his work; after it,
based on the continent, he would devote himself almost exclusively to his *Cantos*.
The "Envoi" does not exactly conclude *Mauberley*, but sections its two parts, the
first sharply satiric, the shorter second part more humiliated and despairing. To
both parts it offers an unexpected momentary contrast, an interval of unleashed
lyricism about beauty and time. The proximate inspiration for that deliberately
old-fashioned lyricism is unambiguously signalled: Pound is recasting Edmund
Waller's famous "Go, lovely rose," which had been set to music by Henry Lawes.
But changing "rose" to "book" restores the specific genre that Chaucer is adopt-
ing, and the closeness of the phrasing is such that we understand "dumb-born"
(like Churchyard's "plaine") as the substitute for "little": the poem not so much
modest as, in the modern environment, incapable of being heard. As in *The Waste
Land*, something that had its birth with Chaucer now seems to be ending. The

---

[21] See Anthony M. Esolen, "The Disingenuous Poet Laureate: Spenser's Adoption
of Chaucer," *Studies in Philology* 87 (1990): 285–311; the quoted phrase is from 311. A
substantial chapter on "Chaucer and Spenser" is the climax of Miskimin's study, 262–99;
four of the ten essays in Theresa M. Krier, ed., *Refiguring Chaucer in the Renaissance*
(Gainesville: University Press of Florida, 1998), concern Spenser. For a recent overview,
see Andrew King, "Spenser, Chaucer, and Medieval Romance," in Richard A. McCabe,
ed., *The Oxford Handbook of Spenser* (Oxford: Oxford University Press, 2010), 553–61.

complicated shyness with which Chaucer launched what became the great and imperious enterprise of English literature, and which is one of his founding gifts to that literature, also shapes a gesture for its retirement.

CATALOGUE OF PRINTED REFERENCES
AND ALLUSIONS 1641–1700

Post-1640

1.   STOW, JOHN. *A Survey of London.* S5773A. UMI Early English Books 1825: 1.

For references to Chaucer's London associations, including his burial in Westminster Abbey, to his *Works* "lately printed," to the Tabard Inn in Southwark (with a quotation from *The General Prologue*), see STOW (1598) in Boswell & Holton No. 618; in this edition, the passages are found on sig. A8r, 151, 256, 267, 416, 456, 517.

For a reference to John Shirley, a collector of Chaucer's works, see STOW (1603) in Boswell & Holton No. 694; in this edition, the passage is found on 416.

For references to Chaucer's tomb in Westminster Abbey and Spenser's tomb nearby, see STOW (1618) in Boswell & Holton No. 966; in this edition, the passage is found on 517.

For references to Chaucer in the "Catalogue of Authors" and indexes, see STOW (1633) in Boswell & Holton No. 1238; in this edition, the passages are found on sigs. A8r, L1112r, Nnnn2r.

1641

2.   B., E. "The Life and Death of Mr. Bolton" in *The Workes of the Learned Robert Bolton.* B3512. UMI 976: 1

For an echo of a line in *The Reeve's Tale*, see B., E. (1632) in the Appendix; in this edition, the passage is found on sig. a8v.

3.   BRATHWAIT, RICHARD. *The English Gentleman*; and *The English Gentlewoman.* B4262. UMI 680: 24.

For a reference to Richard II's benevolent patronage of Chaucer, see BRATHWAIT (1630) in Boswell & Holton No. 1149; in this collection, the passage is found in a section headed "The English Gentleman" on 106–7.

Also found in *Times Treasury: or, Academy for Gentry*, B4276 (1652), 106–7.

4.   BROME, ALEXANDER. *A Canterbury Tale, Translated out of Chaucers Old English into Our Now Usuall Language. Whereunto Is Added the Scots Pedler.* B4847. UMI Thomason Tracts 29: E.168 (5).

Brome (1620–1666) is identified on the title page as "A. B." As Spurgeon notes (1: 219), he writes these satirical verses against Archbishop Laud and other prelates; *The Scots Pedler* is an imitation of Chaucer's *Pardoner's Tale.* Spurgeon calls special attention to parallels from *The General Prologue,* lines 671–716, and *Prologue to the Pardoner's Tale,* lines 329–462.

5.   CAVENDISH, GEORGE. *The Negotiations of Thomas Woolsey, the Great Cardinal of England.* C1619aA. UMI Thomason Tracts 29: E.166 (14).

George Cavendish (1495–1562?) is identified on the title page as Woolsey's "gentleman-usher." Although it was not printed until long after Cavendish's death, this popular biography of Woolsey survives in more than thirty manuscripts. Cavendish may allude to *The Clerk's Tale* with a reference to "patient Grissell" in chapter 10, "Of Mistris Anne Bullen her favour with the King." He writes:

> Queene *Katherine* . . . seemed neither to Mistris *Anne Bullen,* nor the King to carry any sparke of discontent, or displeasure, but accepted all things in good part, and with great wisdome, and much patience, dissembled the same, having Mistris *Anne Bullen* in more estimation for the Kings sake, then when she was with her before, declaring herselfe indeed to be a very patient *Grissell,* as by her long patience in all her troubles shall hereafter more plainly appeare. (27)

Another edition in 1641: C1619, same pagination.
    Other editions: C1619A (1650?), 22–23; and *The Life and Death of Thomas Woolsey, Cardinal,* C1618 (1667), 34–35.

6.   E., A. B. C. D. *Novembris monstrum: or, Rome Brought to Bed in England. With the Whores Miscarying. Made Long Since for the Anniversary Solemnity on the Fift Day of November, in a Private Colledge in Cambridge.* E3. UMI 1590: 36.

The author begins "The Dedicatory," with an echo of Chaucer's line, "Go, litel bok, go litel myn tragedye" (*Troilus and Criseyde* 5: 1786).

> *Goe litle Booke, (my unlick't Poetry)*
> *And be a Patron to thy selfe and mee,*
> *Shift it among the crowd, and never stay*
> *To dresse thy selfe, like other trim and gay,*
> *With borrow'd Titles.* (sig. *A*3r)

7.   HEYWOOD, THOMAS. *The Life of Merlin.* H1786. UMI 148: 1.

Heywood (d. 1641) is not named on the title page. He may allude to *The Squire's Tale* (lines 81, 115) when he writes of a steed of brass in one of Merlin's prophecies:

> *[A] brazen man shall come to passe,*
> *Who likewise mounted on his Steed of brasse,*
> *Both night and day will Londons prime Gate keep,*
> *Whether the carelesse people wake or sleepe.* (52–53)

8.   JONSON, BENJAMIN. *The Sad Shepherd: or, A Tale of Robin-Hood.* UMI 2008: 8.

Although frequently found bound with *The Workes of Benjamin Jonson*, STC 14754 (1631), the title page of this piece is dated 1641.

As Spurgeon notes (1: 220), Jonson (1573?–1637) appears to echo a line from Chaucer's description of the Cook in *The General Prologue*: "That on his shyne a mormal hadde he" (line 386). In act 2, scene 6, Mauldin, the envious witch of Papplewicke, intones:

> *The Swill and Dropsie enter in*
> *The Lazie* Cuke, *and swell his skin;*
> *And the old Mort-mal on his shin*
> *Now prick, and itch, withouten blin.* (147; sig. T4r)

Also found in Jonson's *Works* (1692): J1006, 539 (sig. Zzz3r).

9.   MARMION, SHAKERLEY. *The Antiquary. A Comedy.* M703. UMI 216: 11.

The playwright is identified on the title page as "Shackerly Mermion, Gent." As Spurgeon notes (1: 220), Marmion (1603–1639) echoes *The Merchant's Tale*: "But one thing warn I you, my friendis dere, | I wol no old wife have in no manere. | She shall not passin sixtene yere certeine | Old fish, and young flesh woll I haue full faine" (lines 1415–18) in this comedy "acted by Her Majesties servants at the Cock-pit" (title page). In the first act, Moccinigo, "an old Gentleman that would appear young," says:

> Yet this I resolve on,
> To have a Maid tender of age, and fair:
> Old fish, and yong flesh, that's still my dyet. (sig. C2r)

10.   PRYNNE, WILLIAM. *A Catalogue of Such Testimonies in All Ages as Plainly Evidence Bishops and Presbyters to Be Both One, Equall and the Same.* P3922. UMI 222: 17.

For references to the spurious work known as Chaucer's *Ploughman's Tale*, see *A Breviate of the Prelates Intollerable Usurpations*, PRYNNE (1637), Boswell & Holton No. 1314; in this issue, the passages are found on 26–27, 123.

11.   TWISSE, WILLIAM, in Joseph Mede's *The Apostasy of the Latter Times.* M1590. UMI Thomason Tracts 28: E.162 (3).

In a "Preface to the Reader," Twisse (1578?–1646) praises Mede (1586–1638), cites Chaucer, and quotes a couplet from Chaucer's description of the Clerk of Oxford in *The General Prologue* (lines 307–8):

> *A cup of good wine will be knowne where it is without an Ivy bush; such is the following discourse. . . . Many yeers agoe I was acquainted with it, by the Authors owne hand: for such was his scholasticall ingenuity; I found him most free in communicating his studies; right like unto the description of the Scholar in* Chaucer:

> Sounding in morall bertue was his speech,
> And gladly would Learne, and gladly teach. (sig. A2r)

Other editions: M1591 (1642), sig. A2r; M1592 (1644), sig. A2r; M1593 (1654), sig. A2r; M1593A (1655), sig. A2r.

12.   MENNES, JOHN. *Wits Recreations.* M1720. UMI 1531: 13.

As Spurgeon notes (1: 219), there is a reference to Chaucer in this edition that is not found in the 1640 edition (see Boswell & Holton No. 1377). In "Epitaph 140. On our prime English Poet, *Geffrey Chaucer* an ancient Epitaph":

> My Master Chaucer, with his fresh Comedies
> Is dead alas chiefe Poet of Brittaine,
> That whilome made full piteous Tragedies.
> The fault also of Princes he did complaine,
> As he that was of making Soberaigne;
> Whom all this land should of right preferre
> Sith of our language he was the Load-starre. (sig. R7r)

The epitaph is originally from Lydgate's prologue to his translation of Boccaccio's *The Falle of Princes*; see BOCCACCIO (1494) in Boswell & Holton No. 27.

For a reference to Chaucer in "Epitaph 144. On William Shake-speare," see *Wits Recreations* (1640) in Boswell & Holton No. 1377; in this edition, the passage is found on sig. R7v–8r.

Other editions with a different title, *Recreation for Ingenious Head-peeces*: M1712 (1645), sig. Q7r–v, Q8r; M1713 (1650), sig. O4r, O5r; M1714 (1654), sig. F11v, F12r; M1715 (1663), sig. O4r, O5r; M1715a (1665), sig. O4r, O5r; M1716 (1667), sig. O4r, O5r; M1717 (1667), sig. O4r, O5r; M1718 (1683), sig. O4r, O5r.

13. **MILTON, JOHN.** *Animadversions upon the Remonstrants Defence, against Smectymnuus.* M2089. UMI 155: 4.

Milton (1608–1674) is not named on the title page. As Spurgeon notes (1: 221), Milton cites Chaucer and appears to allude to *The Man of Law's Tale*, or *The Parliament of Fowls*, or *The Legend of Good Women* (for Chaucer's use of *Semyramus*): *The Book of the Duchess* (for Chaucer's use of *Sejes*); and *The Wife of Bath's Prologue*, or *The Complaint of Fair Anelida and False Arcite*, or *Troilus and Criseyde* (for Chaucer's use of *Amphiorax*). In a section about outlandish names and English usage, Milton writes:

> Remember how they mangle our Brittish names abroad; what trespasse were it, if wee in requitall should as much neglect theirs? and our learned *Chaucer* did not stick to doe so, writing *Semyramus* for *Semiramis*, *Amphiorax* for *Amphiaraus*, K. *Sejes* for K. *Ceyx* the husband of *Alcyone*, with many other names strangely metamorphis'd from true *Orthography*, if he had made any account of that in these kind of words. (6)

Also found in *The Works of Mr. John Milton* (1697), M2086, 297.

14. **MILTON, JOHN.** *Of Reformation Touching Church-Discipline in England.* M2134. UMI Thomason Tracts 37: E.208 (3).

As Spurgeon notes (1: 220–21), Milton (1608–1674) refers to Chaucer in this work. After citing Dante, Petrarch, and Ariosto's censure of Constantine's donation's to the Church, Milton alludes to the spurious work known as Chaucer's *Ploughman's Tale*. In book 1, Milton writes:

> And this was a truth well knowne in *England* before this *Poet* [i.e., Ariosto] was borne, as our *Chaucer's* Plowman shall tell you by and by upon another occasion. (31)

In a passage about those who hinder reformation, Milton cites Chaucer and quotes from the description of the Friar in *The General Prologue* (lines 221–23):

[T]he second sort of those that may be justly number'd among the hinderers of *Reformation*, are Libertines, these suggest that the Discipline sought would be intolerable: . . . 'Tis only the merry Frier in *Chaucer* can disple [*sic*] them.

> *Full sweetly heard he confession*
> *And pleasant was his absolution,*
> *He was an easie man to give pennance.*

And so I leave them. (40–41)

In book 2, in a passage about the Donation of Constantine, Milton again cites Chaucer and quotes from the spurious work known as Chaucer's *Ploughman's Tale*:

[B]esides *Petrarch*, whom I have cited, our *Chaucer* also hath observ'd, and gives from hence a caution to *England* to beware of her *Bishops* in time, for that their ends, and aymes are no more freindly [*sic*] *Monarchy* then the Popes.
  Thus hee brings in the Plow-man speaking, *2 Part. Stanz.* 28.

> *The Emperour Yafe the Pope sometime*
> *So high Lordship him above*
> *That at last the silly Kime,*
> *The Proud Pope put him out,*
> *So of this Realme is no doubt,*
> *But Lords beware, and them defend,*
> *For now these folks be wonders stout*
> *The King and Lords now this amend*

And in the next *Stanza* which begins the third part of the tale he argues that they ought not to bee Lords.

> *Moses Law forbode it tho*
> *That Preists should no Lordships welde*
> *Christs Gospell biddeth also,*
> *That they should no Lordships held*
> *Ne Christs Apostles were never so bold*
> *No such Lordships to hem embrace*
> *But smeren her Sheep, and keep her Fold.*

And so forward. Whether the Bishops of *England* have deserv'd thus to bee fear'd by men so wise as our *Chaucer* is esteem'd. (50–51)

In a passage about the conflict between popes and temporal rulers, Milton cites "our renowned Chaucer" as one who wrote of such matters:

> A good while the *Pope* suttl'y acted the *Lamb* . . . but hee threw off his Sheepes clothing, and started up a Wolfe, laying his pawes upon the Emperours right, as forfeited to *Peter.* Why may not wee as well, having been forewarn'd at home by our renowned *Chaucer.* . . . (67)

Also found in *The Works of Mr. John Milton* (1697), M2086, 181, 184–85, 188, 194.

15.   PARKER, MARTIN. *The Poet's Blind Mans Bough: or, Have among You My Blind Harpers.* **P443. UMI Thomason Tracts 30: E.172 (6).**

Parker (d. 1656?) is identified on the title page as "Martine Parker." As Spurgeon notes (1: 221), Parker places Chaucer among writers whose names will live forever. Parker's title page goes on to inform readers that his work is:

> "A pretty medicine to cure the Dimme, Double, Envious, Partial, and Diabolicall eyesight and Judgement of Those Dogmaticall, Schismaticall, Aenigmaticall, and nou [*sic*] Gramaticall Authors who Lycentiously, without eyther Name, Lycence, Wit or Charity, have raylingly, falsely, and foolishly written a numerous rable of pesteferous Pamphlets in this present (and the precedent yeare, justly observed and charitable censured."

He is particularly incensed at authors who publish without subscribing their names to their works. As Spurgeon notes, Parker links Chaucer with Spenser and the Earl of Surrey and places them in a constellation of English poets:

> All Poets (as adition [*sic*] to their fames)
> Have by their Works eternized their names,
> As Chaucer, Spencer, and that noble earle, [*sic,* no italics]
> Of Surrie ought [i.e., thought] it the most precious pearle,
> That dick'd his honour, to Subscribe to what
> His high engenue ever amed at
> *Sydney* and *Shakspire* [*sic*], *Drayton, Withers* and
> Renowned *Jonson* glory of our Land:
> *Deker,* Learn'd *Chapman, Haywood* althought [*sic*] good,
> To have their names in publike understood,
> And that sweet Seraph of our Nation, *Quarles*
> (In spight of each planatick cur that snarles)
> Subscribes to his Celestiall harmony,
> While Angels chant his Dulcit melodie. (sig. [A]4r–v)

16.   PRYNNE, WILLIAM. *The Antipathie of the English Lordly Prelacie, Both to Regall Monarchy and Civill Unity.* P3891. UMI 192: 2.

Prynne (1600–1669) is identified on the title page as "William Prynne, late (and now againe) an utter-barester of Lincolnes Inne." As Dobbins notes (*MLQ*), Prynne cites Chaucer and refers to the spurious work known as Chaucer's *Ploughman's Tale.* In a section about the "Lordlinesse and wealth of Bishops and Priests," he writes:

> *Sir* Geoffrey Chaucer [in a shoulder note: "The Plowman's Tale"] *our renowned Poet, writes much to the same effect.* [Here Prynne quotes 15 lines.]
>
>   *This Booke of* Chaucer *was authorised to be printed by Act of Parliament, in the* 34. *and* 35. *Hen.* 8. *C.2. When the Prelates by the same Act prohibited both the printing and reading of the Bible in English, such was their piety.* (337; sig. Vu*4r, pagination irregular)

Another edition in 1641: P3891A, same pagination.

17.   PRYNNE, WILLIAM. *A Catalogue of Such Testimonies in All Ages.* P3922. UMI 222: 17.

For a reference to the spurious work known as Chaucer's *Ploughman's Tale,* see PRYNNE, *A Breviate of the Prelates Intollerable Usurpations* (1637) in Boswell & Holton No. 1314; in this issue of that work, the passages are found on 26–27, 123.

18.   VAUGHAN, WILLIAM. *The Soules Exercise in the Daily Contemplation of Our Saviours Birth, Life, Passion, and Resurrection.* V156. UMI 1433: 2.

Sir William Vaughan (1577–1641) is identified on the title page as "William Vaughan, knight." In this work, he presents devotional readings for each day of the week. Tuesday's reading focuses on the miracle of the birth of the Savior. In a passage about John the Evangelist's vision "In *Pathmos,* where he saw by *Revelation,* | The *Churches State,* and *Babells Fornication,*" he alludes to the spurious work known as Chaucer's *Ploughman's Tale.* Vaughan writes:

> To feele *Remorse,* some feede their *Ravishments*
> *With Herods Sword unsheath'd on Innocents,*
> "That *bloody Sword,* wherewith the *Eagles Peeres*
> "Did persecute neere for *Three hundred yeeres*
> "The *Christians Race;* And which lay then suspended,
> "Till *Satan* it *to Babells Whore* Commended,
> "As witnessed old *Chaucers Pellican*
> "Against the *Griffon,* and his *Vatican;*

"Which *Berengarius*[1] long before discry'd,
"Which the *Waldenses* and *Albigians* try'd;
"And which as yet our Mother *Christendome*,
"*Like Rachel, feeles in her seedes Martyrdome.* (69)

19. WALKER, HENRY. *A Terrible Out-Cry Against the Loytering Exalted Prelates.* W389. UMI 649: 13.

The title page attributes authorship to "Mr. Prinne, a faithfull witnesse of Jesus Christ, and a Sufferer under them [i.e., the prelates]," but Wing says otherwise. Whoever the author is, he attributes a quotation to Chaucer in order to show the danger and impropriety of conferring any temporal office or dignity upon any prelate:

Oh all ye unpreaching Prelates, learne of the Devill, if you will not learn of God; he will give you example of diligence in your Office.
Verses written by our renowned Poet, Sir *Geffry Chaucer* many years ago, authorised to be printed by Act of *Parliament*, in the 34. and 35. *H.*8.c.I.
[Here the author quotes the same 15 lines from the spurious work known as Chaucer's *Ploughman's Tale* that Prynne did in *The Antipathie of the English Lordly Prelacie, q.v., supra*]
Learne to be diligent for shame, ye Prelates; But God be thanked, there is good hopes; that the King and Parliament will order you, which that they may, God grant. *Amen.* (5–6)

20. *The Wanton Wife of Bath.* W719B. UMI 2712: 18.

The date of this broadside ballad is uncertain; Wing places it somewhere between 1641–1681. As Spurgeon notes (3: 4.54), it dates back to 1600 when copies of "a Disorderly ballad of the wife of Bathe" was recalled by the authorities and ordered burnt and the printers fined.

In the poem, the Wife of Bath dies and goes to the pearly gates and asks for admission to heaven. Various biblical characters respond, usually reminding her of her sinful sojourn on earth. Eventually Christ comes forth, forgives her, and admits her into paradise. The work begins with a somewhat garbled reference to Chaucer:

In Bath a wanton wife did dwell
as Caucer [*sic*] she [*sic*] doth write,

---

[1] Berengarians, followers of Berengar of Tours, were a sect opposed to the doctrine of transubstantiation.

𝔚ho did in pleasure spend her days
   in many a fond delight.
𝔘pon a time sore sick she was,
   and at the length did dye:
ℌer soul at last at ℌeavens gate,
   did knock most mightily.

𝔗hen Adam came unto the gate,
   who knocketh there, quoth he,
𝔍 am the wife of 𝔅ath she said,
   and fain would come to thee.

A variant imprint (1641) is also identified as W719B.

    Other editions: M3151 (ca. 1665), verso of M3151; W721A (ca. 1684), Pepys Ballads (vol. 2, 29); W722 (ca. 1692); W723 (1690?); W723A (1698?), here Chaucer's name spelled correctly; W723B (1700?).

    Also found in Thomas Jevon's *The Devil of a Wife* (1686) J731, 26; J731A (1693), 26; J732 (1695), 21–22.

1642

21.   HALL, JOSEPH. *A Modest Confutation of a Slanderous and Scurrilous Libell.* H393. UMI Thomason Tracts 24: E.134 (1); UMI 249: E.134 (1).

As Spurgeon notes (1: 222), but does not transcribe, Bishop Hall (1575–1656) quotes modernized lines from *The Prologue of the Pardoner's Tale* (lines 413–22), *The Book of the Duchess* (lines 62–65), *Parliament of Fowls* (lines 288–89), and attributes Lydgate's *Complaint of the Black Knight* to Chaucer—all in response to Milton's *Animadversions upon the Remonstrants Defense against Smectymnuus* (1641), q.v. In section 6, in a passage about satires, Hall writes that what is forbidden to be spoken on the stage is frequently heard in church:

Though what was, and is denied the stage, is got up into the Pulpit: much as the manner was with Chaucers Pardoner.

𝔗hen woll 𝔍 sting hem with my tonge smert
𝔍n preaching, so that he shall not assert
𝔗o been disfamed falsely, if that he
ℌath trespassed to my brethren or me:
𝔉or though 𝔍 tell not his proper name,
𝔐en shall well know it is the same
𝔅y signes or by other circumstances,

Thus quite I folk that doth us displeasances,
Thus put I out my benym under hiew
Of holinesse, to semen holy and true.

As you have censured the Remonstrants Poesie, so in like manner you have justified a slip in the Smectymnuans Philology. . . . Every Country, I know, takes and gives that leave in the use of forraign words, to fit them to their own easiest pronunciation and best liking: sometimes out of necessity, sometimes of choice and pleasure onely. . . . [*Our learned* Chaucer *did not sticke to doe so.*] True.

—There was a King
That hyght Ceys, and had a wyfe,
The beste tha myght beare lyfe,
And this Queene hyght Alcione. Fol. 267.

Semiramus, Candace and Hercules,
Byblys, Dido, Tyche and Piramus. Fol. 275.

Ne like the pytte of Pegace
Under Pernaso where the Poets slept. (Fol. 301. [*sic*])

What is all this to the purpose? Chaucer hath mollifyed a termination [in a shoulder note: "*Ceys* for *Ceyx*"] . . . he hath not metamorphosed the name of a place into the name of a man: or if he had, it were one of those faults which ought to be forgiven (not imitated) in so revered antiquity. [In a shoulder note: "*Sir* Ph. Sidney *Defense of Poes.*"] (11–13)

This work is not collected in Hall's *Works*.

22.   KYNASTON, FRANCIS. *Leoline and Sydanis.* K759. UMI 109: 8.

Kynaston (1587–1642) is identified on the title page as "Sir Fr: Kinnaston, Knight." As Spurgeon notes (1: 222), Kynaston refers to "the fairy Cresseid" and "faithfull Troilus," probably alludes to *Troilus and Criseyde*:

'Mongst other stories did he call to minde
That of the fairy *Creseid*, who insteed
Of faithfull *Troilus* lov'd false *Diomed*. (89)

Another edition: K760 (1646), 89.

23.   Twisse, William, in Joseph Mede's *The Apostasy of the Latter Times.*
M1591. UMI 1016: 10.

For an allusion to the Clerk and a quotation from *The General Prologue*, see
Twisse (1641), M1590; in this edition, the passage is found on sig. A2r.

1643

24.   Baker, Richard. *A Chronicle of the Kings of England.* **B501. UMI 81: 3.**

Baker (1568–1645) is identified on the title page as "Sr R. Barker, Knight." As
Spurgeon notes (1: 222–23), Baker praises Chaucer as "the Homer of our nation,"
associates him with Woodstock, notes his translation of *The Romaunt of the Rose*
and burial place in Westminster. There is, moreover, another in his account of
the children of Edward III. In a passage about John of Gaunt, Baker notes the
Chaucerian connection:

> *John* of *Gaunts* third wife was *Katherine*, the Widow of Sir *Hugh Swin-*
> *ford*, a knight of *Lincolnshire*, eldest daughter and Coheire of *Payn Roet*,
> a *Gascoyne*, called Guien King of Armes for that Countrey; his younger
> daughter being married to Sir *Geofrey Chawcer*, our Laureat Poet. (179;
> sig. Y6r)

In his account of the life and reign of Edward III, in a section headed "Of Men
of Note in his time," Baker concludes with a reference to "the Homer of our
Nation":

> [A]nd lastly two other, worthy perhaps to have beene placed first; *John*
> *Mandevill* the great Tyravellour . . . and Sir *Geoffrey Chawcer*, the *Homer*
> of our Nation; and who found as sweete a Muse in the Groves of *Wood-*
> *stocke*, as the Antients did upon the banks of *Helicon*. (181; sig. Z1r)

In a section about men of note who flourished in the reign of Richard II, Baker
writes of Chaucer's translation of *The Romaunt of the Rose*:

> *John Moone*, an English man, but a Student in *Paris*; who compiled in
> the French tongue, *The Romant of the Rose*; translated into English by
> *Geoffry Chawcer*, and divers others. (229; sig. Dd3r)

In a section about men of note that throve in the reign of Henry IV, Baker links
Chaucer and Gower:

The next place after these, is justly due to *Geoffry Chaucer*, and *John Gower*, two famous Poets in this time, and the Fathers of *English* Poets in all the times after: *Chaucer* dyed in the fourth yeare of this king, and lyeth buried in *Westminster*: *Gower*, in this kings ninth yeare, and was buried in St. *Mary Overys* Church in *Southwarke*. (²45; sig. Ff3r)

Another edition in 1643:B502 (UMI 2417: 9), same pagination.

Other editions: B503 (1653), augmented, 191, 193–94, 224, 240, and in the index (sig. Iii1r); B503A (1653), 191, 193–94, 224, 240, and sig. Iii1r; B504 (1660), 144, 145–46, 168, 180, and sig. Mmm2r; B504A (1665); B505 (1665), 144, 145–46, 168, 180, and sig. Bbbb2r; B505A (1665), 144, 145–46, 168, 180, and sig. Bbbb2r; B506 (1670), 136, 138, 159, 171, and sig. Iiiii1r; B507 (1674), 136, 138, 159, 171, and sig. Iiiii1r; B507A (1679); B508 (1679), 132, 134, 155, 167, and sig. Hhhh4r; B508A (1679), 132, 134, 155, 167, and sig. Hhh4r; B509 (1684), 132, 134, 155, 167, and sig. Hhhh4r; B510 (1696), 132, 134, 155, 167, and sig. L11113v.

25. **BRAMHALL, JOHN.** *The Serpent Salve: or, A Remedie for the Biting of an Aspe.* B4236. UMI 15: 19.

Bramhall (1594–1663), eventually the Archbishop of Armagh in the Church of Ireland, published this work anonymously. In his first published composition, Bramhall writes in response to *Observations upon His Majesty's Late Papers and Expresses* (1642) and, on the title page, informs readers that his purpose is to lead "such of His Majesties well-meaning Subjects into the right Way who have been mis-led by that *Ignis fatuus*." In "The Epistle to the Reader," in a passage about the dangers of Presbyterian doctrines, he alludes to Chaucer's description of the Friar in *The General Prologue* and echoes lines 223–24. Bramhall writes:

> [T]hese men ["the Rabble"] make Kings and Nobles, but as Counters which stand sometimes for a pound, sometimes for a penny *pro arbitrio supputantis*, just like *Chawcers* Frier, he knew how to impose an easy Pennance, where he looked for a good Pittance. (sig. B3r)

Another edition in 1643: B4236A (no UMI).

26. *The Cities Warning-Peece.* C4336. UMI Thomason Tracts 266: E.246 (28).

The printer of this piece writes that it was "Written long since, but Printed in the Yeere | That every knave and foole turn'd Cavaleere." As Spurgeon notes (1: 223), Thomason records the date of 27 February 1643. The author, writing in response to John Taylor's *The Conversion, Confession, Contrition, Comming to*

Himselfe & Advice of a Misled, Ill-bred Round-head, refers to the decline of England since Chaucer's death:

> The Spanish Fleete in the Downs.
> Twixt our Religions, *Rome* and *Spaine*, and we
> Put all together, make but one of three:
> And shall you feare us, or shall we feare you?
> Tush, *Spain* is *England*, *England* is *Spain* now.
> . . . .
> *Pauls* for your sakes is almost newly built,
> And 'tis not long since *Cheapside-crosse* was guilt,
> Old *Charing* shall be now re-edified
> That lost his glory when old *Chaucer* died. (5–6)

27.   *The Cony-Catching Bride*. C5992. UMI 177: 11.

This anonymously published cautionary tale includes a reference to "poore patient Grissel," perhaps a faint allusion to *The Clerk's Tale*. A rich father pressures his fair daughter to marry a religious zealot, not in the customary fashion, in church, but in a private chamber with friends gathered to witness. A pragmatical cobbler, having preached a windy wedding sermon, hungrily partakes of the feast:

> After the Cobler had ended his Sermon, Dinner was sent in, and a long Grace said, so they fell to their cheere: but now the *Coblers* teeth walkt as fast as his tongue, and all the Guests fed apace; only the Bride being inwardly discontent, stood like a poore patient *Grissel*, sorry for what she had formerly done. (3)

28.   *The Pindar of Wakefield*. P2251A. UMI 2367: 7.

The title page of this eight-page pamphlet goes on to inform readers that the work at hand is *"A True Narration of the Unparalell'd victory obtained against the Popish army at the taking in of Wakefield in Yorkshire, by the Lord Fairfaxe his forces, May 20. 1643 As it was sent in a letter from one in that army, to his friend here in London, not altering it from his native tone, more like Chaucers English, then ours here."*

29.   *Powers to Be Resisted: or, A Dialogue Arguing the Parliaments Lawfull Resistance of the Powers Now in Armes Against Them*. P3111. UMI Thomason Tracts 241: E.79 (15); and UMI Thomason Tracts 14: E.79 (15).

As Spurgeon notes (3: 4.70), the anonymous author alludes to *The Summoner's Tale* and faintly echoes a line: "But that I nolde no beest for me were deed" (line 1842):

This is like old *Chaucer's* tale of a Fryar, whose belly was his god, he would feed upon the sweetest, Mutton, Goose, and Pig, but a pitifull man! he would have no creature killed for him, not he. (39–40)

1644

30.   CLEVELAND, JOHN. *The Character of a London-Diurnal with Severall Select Poems.* C4666. UMI 22: 2

In "The Authours Mock-Song to Marke Anthony," Cleveland (1613–1658) echoes a line from *The Manciple's Prologue*: "Sires, what! Dun is in the myre!" (line 5). He writes, "My spirits were duller than Dun in the mire" (11).

Other editions in 1644: C4660, 11; C4661, 11.

Also found in *The Character of a London-Diurnall: With Several Select Poems*: C4662 (1647), 11; C4663 (1647), 11; C4663aA (1647); C4663A (1647), 11; C4663B (1647), 11; C4664 (1647), 11; C4665 (1647), a ghost; C4666 (1647), 11.

Also found in *Poems by J. C.*, C4684 (1651), 54.

Also found in Cleveland's *Poems*: C4686 (1651), 55.

Also found in *Clevelandi vindiciæ*: C4669 (1677), 67; C4670 (1677), 67; C4671 (1677), 67.

Also found in Cleveland's *Works*: C4654 (1687), 67; C4655 (1699), 67.

31.   JORDAN, THOMAS. *The Debtors Apologie: or, A Quaint Paradox.* J1025. UMI 459: 31.

Thomas Jordan (1612?–1685?) is identified on the title page as "T. J." He was a boy actor (King's Revels Company), poet, and playwright. As Mitchell notes (*MLN*), he quotes a passage from the 1602 edition of Chaucer to buttress his point—that it is good to be in debt. In a passage that may allude to his experiences in debtor's prison, Jordan writes that he pities Seneca's weakness (i.e., he "blushed to borrow"), and he goes on to quote *The Compleynt of Chaucer to his Purse*:

That Poet *Laureat* forfeited his wreath of Bayes and Ivy-twine, who made his prayers to his Purse, to keep him out of debt, in this manner.

> *To you my Purse, and to none other wight*
> *Complain I, for you to be my Lady deer:*
> *I am sorry now that you be light,*
> *For certes yee now make me heavy cheer,*
> . . . .
> *But I pray unto your courtesie*
> *Be heavy again or else mote I dye.* (9–11)

The passage is marked with a shoulder note: "Ocleve in Chaucer" (9), probably because it was ascribed to Hoccleve by Speght in his 1602 edition.

32.   KNOX, JOHN. *A Historie of the Reformation of the Church of Scotland.* K738. UMI 280: 11.

For an echo a line from *The Reeve's Tale*, see KNOX (1587) in Appendix. In this edition, the passage is found on 17.

33.   TWISSE, WILLIAM, in Joseph Mede's *The Apostasy of the Latter Times.* M1592. UMI 642: 11.

For an allusion to the Clerk of Oxford and a quotation from *The General Prologue*, see TWISSE (1641), M1590; in this edition, the passage is found on sig. A2r.

34.   WILLIS, JOHN. *The Art of Stenography.* W2809. UMI 2203: 11

For quotations from *Troilus and Criseyde* and from the spurious work known as "Chaucer's Prophecy," see WILLIS (1602) in Boswell & Holton No. 682; in this edition, the passages are found in book 2, chapter 1.
  Another edition: W2810 (1647).

1645

35.   JOHNSON, EDMUND, in John Gower's *The Cow-ragious Castle-combat.* G1460. UMI Thomason Tracts 47: E284 (3).

For a commendatory poem in which Edmund Johnson notes the connection between Gower and Chaucer, see GOWER, *Pyrgomachia* (1635) in Boswell & Holton No. 1268; in this edition, the passage is found on sig. F4r.

36.   MENNES, JOHN. *Recreation for Ingenious Head-peeces.* M1712. UMI 2467: 4.

For an epitaph "On our prime English Poet, *Geffrey Chaucer*," see MENNES (1641). The epitaph is originally from Lydgate's prologue to his translation of Boccaccio's *The Falle of Princes*; see BOCCACCIO (1494) in Boswell & Holton No. 27. In this edition, the passage is found on sig. Q7r–v.

  For a reference to Chaucer in an epitaph "On William Shake-speare," see *Wits Recreations* (1640) in Boswell & Holton No. 1377; in this edition, the passage is found on sig. Q8r.

37.   MILTON, JOHN. *Poems of Mr. John Milton, Both English and Latin.* M2160. UMI Thomason Tracts 164: E.1126 (1) and UMI 2431: 15 (imperfect; no Latin Poems).

As Spurgeon notes (3: 4.71), near the beginning of "Il Penseroso" Milton echoes a line from *The Wife of Bath's Tale*, "As thikke as motes in the sonne-beem" (line 868). Milton writes:

> Hence vain deluding joyes,
>> The brood of folly without father bred,
> How little you bested,
>> Of fill the fixed mind with all your toyes;
> Dwell in som idle brain,
>> And fancies fond with gaudy shapes possess,
> As thick and numberless
>> As the gay motes that people the Sun Beams. (37)

As Spurgeon also notes (1: 204), Milton also alludes to Chaucer and *The Squire's Tale* in "Il Penseroso":

> O sad Virgin, that thy power
> Might. . . . .
> . . . . . . call up him that left half told
> The story of *Cambuscan* bold,
> Of *Camball*, and of *Algarsife*,
> And who had *Canace* to wife,
> That own'd the vertuous Ring and Glass,
> And of the wondrous Hors of Brass,
> On which the *Tartar* King did ride. (41)

In a separate section with its own title page (*Joannis Miltoni Londinensis Poemata. Quoirum pleraque intra annum ætatis vigesimum conscripsis. Nunc primum edita*), Milton alludes to Chaucer in a poem headed "Mansus." As Spurgeon notes (1: 219), Milton writes:

> Nos etiam in nostro modulantes flumine cygnos
> Credimus obscuras noctis sensisse per umbras,
> Quà Thamesis latè puris argenteus urnis
> Oceani glaucos perfundit gurgite crines;
> Quin & in has quondam pervenit Tityrus oras.[2] (273–74)

---

[2] "*We* also think that *we* have heard the swans in our river | Making music at night through all the shadowy darkness, | Where our silver Thames, at breadth of her

Also found in *Poems, &c. upon Several Occasions*, M2161A (1673), 41, 45–46; and 275; M2161 (1673), 41, 45–46; and 275; and in *Poems upon Several Occasions*: M2162 (1695), 4, 5, 54.

Also collected in *The Poetical Works*: M2163 (1695), 44, 45, and 454.

38.   Stone, Nicholas. *Enchiridion of Fortification: or, A Handfull of Knowledge in Martial Affaires.* S5732. UMI 550: 11.

In a commendatory poem headed "The Author, to his Book," Stone (1586–1647) faintly echoes Chaucer's line, "Go, litel bok, go litel myn tragedye" (*Troilus and Criseyde* 5: 1786):

> Goe little Book, thine aid afford
> Unto the Battailes of the Lord.
> Thy Commission (understood)
> Is onely to assist the Good. (sig. A3r)

Another edition: S5733 (1669), sig. A3r.

1646

39.   "Chaucer Junior." "A Character" in James Strong's *Joanereidos: or, Feminine Valour: Eminently Discovered in Westerne Women.* S5990. UMI Thomason Tracts 47: E.287 (1).

James Strong (1618/1619–1694) wrote a poem in praise of the Puritan women who had fought in defense of Lyme (Dorset) against Royalist troops led by Prince Maurice, "sometimes carrying stones, anon tumbling of stones over the Works of the Enemy, when they have been scaling them, some carrying powder, other charging of Peeces to ease the souldiers, constantly resolved for generality, not to think any ones life deare, to maintaine that Christian quarrell for the Parliament" (title page). Unfortunately for the author, the manuscript fell into the hands of Royalist sympathizers, and it was printed with an elaborate critical apparatus that was merciless in its satirical portrayal of Strong.

"A Character of the Author," signed "J. Chaucer *junior*," is written in pseudo-Chaucerian language, printed in black letter, and refers to "A Clerke of Oxenford." Moreover, as Louis B. Wright notes, this "belated son of Chaucer pieced together sentences and phrases from the Prologue of the *Canterbury Tales* and

---

pure-gushing current, | Bathes with tidal whirl the yellow locks of the Ocean: | Nay, and our Chaucer once came here [Italy] as a stranger before me." The translation is from Manson (1. 313). *Tityrus* was Spenser's nickname for Chaucer.

filled in where necessary with his own devices to make a ludicrous picture of Strong." He writes:

Me thynk it, Sirs, accordaunt to reason,
To tell you now all the condycion
Of thilke on, so as it semed me,
And what hem were, and of what degre,
And eke in what aray that he were in,
And all for forward by Saint Runnyon.
      A Clerke of Oxenford he was tho,
That unto Logicke had long ygoe,
Of his complexion nothing sanguyne
He is, but all swa swart; and of Latyne
A few termes hath he, two or thre,
That he han learned out of some degre:
His face is bald, and shines as any glas,
His mouth as great as is a furnas,
With scaled browes, blacke and pylled berde,
Of his bisage children are sore afferde;
His boyce as smale as is a Gotes fare,
I trow he was a Geldyng or a Mare;
His here is by his eeres round yshorne,
His top is docked like a Priest beforne;
He is short sholdered, a thicke gnarre,
There nis no doore but he wol heve the bar,
Or breke it at a renning with his heed,
Dares none one wyle him but he wol be deed,
Aye by his belt he bares a long Pavade
And, of a sword full trenchaunt is the blade,
To rage as twere a whelpe he is sayde,
Yet of his porte, as meeke as is a Mayde:
Full longe he lokes, and thereto soberly,
Full thred-bare is his over Court py;
For he han yet getten him no benefice
He is nought worthy to have none office,
And yet Saynt Julyan is in's countre,
And the best begger of his house truly:
Full longe are his legges and full lene,
I lyke a staffe, there is no calfe ysene,
Of yedding he batres utterly the price,
Well loveth he garlike, onyons, and eke lekes,
He holden a syde wemme for the none,
Full oft tyme he han the bourde begon,

No Crysten man soe oft in his degree,
And in Lyme at the siege had he be,
But soth to say he is somwhat squaimus
Of fartyng, and of speche dangerous.
Now is it not of God a ful fayre grace,
That such a lewde mans wit shal pace
The wisdome of an heape of learned men?
But I must sayne as that I farther thwyn,
I weene he fares as doth an open erse,
That ylke frute is ever lenger the wers,
Til it be rotten in molloke or in fire,
And so God save us al that here be. (sig. D3r–v)

Another edition: S5991 (1674), D3r–v.

40.   KYNASTON, FRANCIS. *Leoline & Sydanis*. K760. UMI 2033: 6.

For references to "the fairy Cresseid" and "faithful Troilus," probably allusions to *Troilus and Criseyde*, see KYNASTON (1642); in this edition, the passage is found on 89.

41.   *Mercurius Britanicus: Communicating the Affaires of Great Britaine*. Nelson and Seccombe 286.103.

As Mitchell (*MLN*) notes, in "Numb. 103," the issue covering events from 27 Oct – 3 Nov 1645, in an account of the conflict between Royalist and Parliamentarian forces in the north of England, a journalist (probably Robert White) calls on Chaucer's genius for inspiration:

> *Once upon a time*, in the moneth of October, 1645. The *King* having lost his *Newcastle-Coate* in the *North*, his chief Commanders would needs *fall by the eares* to catch themselves a heat in his presence at *Newark*; and they were (O *Chaucer*, and thy *Genius* come help on my *Tale!*) ycleped Rupert and Maurice. (913–14)

42.   MILL, HENRY. *A Funeral Elegy*. M2056. UMI Thomason Tracts 264: 669.f.10 (95).

In an elegiac poem for Robert Devereaux, Earl of Essex and Ewe, Henry Mill echoes the title of *The House of Fame*:

> What do our sighs and tears when Essex dyes,
> They are for him but petty Obsequies
> . . . .

Thy birth was Noble, but thy vertue more,
Which in the house of fame hath layd a store
That will endure whilst that a pen can run,
Or mortall threads of life by fate be spun. (broadside)

43.   PRYNNE, WILLIAM. *Canterburies Doome: or, The First Part of a Compleat History of the Commitment, Charge, Tryall, Condemnation, Execution of William Laud, Late Arch-Bishop of Canterbury.* P3917. UMI 288: 3.

Prynne (1600–1669), described on the title page as being "Of Lincolns Inn, Esquire," writes that Archbishop Laud, "without any other suggestion but his owne Romish Genius and good affection to the Pope," tried "to induce a more easie reconciliation with him" (276) despite the fact that such a reconciliation was against statute law. In addition to other authorities, Prynne cites the spurious work known as Chaucer's *Ploughman's Tale*:

[T]he whole torrent of our Protestant Martyrs, Writers . . . define the *Pope to be Antichrist, yea the great Antichrist, prophesied of in Scripture.* This was the direct position of our . . . Sir *Geofry Chaucer,* in his Ploughmans Tale. . . . (277)

1646

44.   G., E. "To the Author," in Martin Llewellyn's *Men Miracles.* L2625. UMI 1657: 2; UMI Thomason Tracts 251: E.1163 (1).

As Spurgeon notes (1: 224–25), E. G. mentions Chaucer's influence on Spenser in a commendatory poem headed "To the Author":

If ever I believ'd *Pythagoras,*
(My dearest friend) even now it was
While the grosse Bodies of the *Poets* die
Their Souls doe onely shift. And *Poesie*
Transmigrates, not by chance or lucke
So *Chaucers* learned soule in *Spencer* sung,
(*Edmund* the quaintest of the Fairy throng)
And when that doubled Spirit quitted place
It fill'd up *Ben*[3]. . . . (sig. A5r)

Other editions: L2626 (1656), sig. A5r; L2627 (1679), sig. A4r.
    Also found in *The Marrow of the Muses* (1661), L2624, sig. A4r.

---

[3] Ben Jonson, of course.

45.   LORT, ROGER. *Epigrammatum.* L3076. UMI 1993: 2.

Lort (1607/8–1663) is described on the title page as "Cambro-Britanni, Oxoniensis; Collegii olim Wadhamensis, nuper de Societate Medii Templi." As Williams notes, he mentions "Gulielmus Chaucer" in an epigram headed "Ad Robertum Rud Theologum doctissimum."[4] Lort writes:

> Qu d [*sic*] sint grata tibi juvenilia metra, Roberte,
>   Candor causa tuus, non meruere modi:
> Judicii vestri reverentur Musa tribunal,
>   Non te quod pungat carmen acumen habet:
> Est tamen hic vester juvenis respectus amici,
>   Ut fateare nihil displicuisse tibi.
> Sed cur me sacro cupis assimilare Poetæ
>   Pone Poëtrastros qui numerandus eram?
> A nemesi invisa est tantæ mihi gloria famæ,
>   Et me laude tua non sinit illa frui.
> Non equidem invedeo Gulielmus Chaucer haberi,
>   Quod Sidney me vis, invidet ille mihi. (8–9)

46.   SELDEN, JOHN. *Uxor Ebraica: seu, De nuptis & divortiis ex jure civili, id est, divino & Talmudico, veterum Ebræorum, libri tres.* S2443. UMI 294: 7.

The learned Selden (1584–1654) is identified on the title page as "Ioannis Seldeni." As Spurgeon notes (1: 225), in book 2, chapter 27, he refers to Chaucer and the Wife of Bath and quotes a couplet from *The General Prologue* (lines 459–60):

> [U]nde Galfredus Chaucerus qui sub Edwardo tertio floruit, de uxore sua Bathoniensi
>   She was a worthy woman all hir live
>   Husbands at the Church dore had she five
> Id est; fœmina erat quamdiu vixit celebris, & ad ostium Ecclesiæ quinque maritos acceperat. (285)

Although Spurgeon cites an edition of 1695 (203), Wing lists none such.

---

[4] Rud, i.e., Robert Rudd, archdeacon of Carmathen.

1647

47.   CLEVELAND, JOHN. *The Character of a London-Diurnal with Severall Select Poems.* C4662. UMI 21: 17.

For an echo of a line from *The Maniple's Prologue*, see CLEVELAND (1644); in this edition, the passage is found on 11.

    Other editions in 1647: C4663, 11; C4663aA; C4663A, 11; C4663B, 11; C4664, 11; C4665, a ghost; C4666, 11.

48.   CORBET, RICHARD. *Certain Elegant Poems.* C6270. UMI 89: 1.

Corbet (1582–1635) is identified on the title page as "Dr. Corbet, Bishop of Norwich." In "Iter Boreale," he notes that Chaucer wrote *The Romaunt of the Rose* near Bosworth Field:

> Loe yonder *Bosworth* stands, . . .
> Where the two Roses joyned, you would suppose,
> *Chaucer* nere writ the Romant of the Rose,
> Heare him: see yee yond' woods? (11–12)

Also found in *Poëtica Stromata: or, A Collection of Sundry Peices [sic] in Poetry*, C6272 (1648), 57; and in *Poems*, C6271 (1672), 18.

49.   *Doomes-Day: or, The Great Day of the Lords Judgement, Provd by Scripture; and Two Other Prophecies.* D1907. UMI 92: 9 and UMI Thomason Tracts 61: E.383 (23).

As Harris notes (*PQ*), the anonymous author of this pamphlet is much impressed with a spurious work known as "Chaucer's Prophecy." In a passage about prophecies in the *Book of Revelations* allegedly about the Church of Rome, he writes:

> This bringeth a Prophecy into my minde, which I once saw in the study
> of a great Schollar, and no meane Antiquary who deceased some few
> years since, which I copied out, and having this opportune occasion,
> will present it to publike view.
>> *When* Chawcers *Prophesie shall be*
>> *Found true by folk of* Britanie,
>> *When* Englands *walls, and* Scotlands *shall*
>> *Have pure religion 'mongst them all,*
>> *Then loe the Pope shall tumble downe,*
>> *And* F. *shall weare his triple crowne.*

Now the Prophesie of *Geofrey Chawcer*, who flourished in the dayes of King *Richard the second*, ran thus:

When faith failes in Priests Sawes,
And Lords hests are taken for Lawes,
Then shall the Isle of Brittanie
Be brought into great miserie.
Now let us compare and examine these two Prophecies:

The first saith, when Chawcers Prophecie shall be fulfilled, when troubles and miseries shall come upon great Britaine, occasioned through the wickednesse of the Pastors, who (themselves erring from the way) cause the people to walk astray with them; for so he certainly meant when he said,

When faith failes in Priests Sawes.

The fulfilling of the Prophesie wee all know before our present distractions: Was not the most part of the Clergy of this Kingdome given over to vice, and Epicurisme? when arbitrary power shall be endeavoured to be set up, and the Subjects of the Kingdome brought into bondage: for so he no doubt meant when he said,

When Lords hests are taken for Lawes.

Do we not know, that before the breaking forth of our present distractions, the power of the King was divulged to be over the people both body and goods, that a few persons in favour with his Majesty, imposed upon the Subjects of this Kingdome the great loane of Ship-money; and that the Earle of Strafford proposed, that the tyrannicall power of the Kings of France might warrantably be exercised by the Kings of England; therefore when things should bee thus carried, he prophesied:

Then shall the Isle of Brittanie
Be brought into great miserie.

And have not our eyes seen the same fulfilled? What greater miserie can come to a nation, then to be at variance among themselves, mutually to sheath their swords in each others bowells, to batter downe Cities ore one anothers heads, to have their Soveraigne in armes against them, and in a word, to have all the calamities of war at once heavy upon them; and this hath this poore Kingdome of England, till of late undergone; therefore the fulfilling of *Chawcers* Prophecie none but a mad man will denie. [In a shoulder note:

"His Prophesie began to bee effected in the yeare 1640. and was fulfilled in the year 1644."] (3–4)

50.   FANSHAWE, RICHARD, trans. *Il pastor fido*: *The Faithful Shepherd*. G2174. UMI Thomason Tracts 81: E.517 (1).

Fanshawe (1608–1666) is identified on the title page as "Richard Fanshawe, Esq." In this translation of Battista Guarini's *Il pastor fido*, Fanshawe may allude to *The House of Fame*. In the first scene of the fifth act, he writes:

> There saw I that lov'd *Egon*, first with Bayes,
> With Purple then, with Vertue deckt alwayes:
> That he on earth *Apollo*'s self did seem:
> Therefore my heart and Harp I unto him
> Did consecrate, devoted to his name.
> And in his house (which was the house of Fame)
> I should have set up my perpetually rest,
> There to admire and imitate the best [etc.] (168)

Another edition: G2175 (1648), 168.

51.   *The Kingdom's Weekly Intelligencer*: *Sent Abroad to Prevent Mis-information*. No. 241. Nelson and Seccombe 214.241.

As Frank notes (*N&Q*), in the issue covering events from 28 December 1647 – 4 January 1648, there is a reference to Chaucer in the opening lines of an account of a pro-Royalist riot in Canterbury. A journalist writes:

> It hath been the Custome heretofore to passe away the sloth of these Winter nights with a *Canterbury* tale or two out of *Chaucer*, but the Gravity of these Times not admitting of such vanities, *Canterbury* hath been at this season so unhappy as to make a tale of her self.

52.   LEIGH, EDWARD. *Analecta Caesarum Romanorum*: *or, Select Observations. Also Certain Choice French Proverbs*. L983. UMI 605: 3.

Leigh (1602–1671) is described on the title page as being "Of Magdalen-Hall in Oxford." In translating the French proverb *Qui veut jeune chair & vieux poisson, se trovere pugner la raison* as "*He that loves young flesh and old fish, loves contrary to reason*" (424), Leigh appears to echo a line from *The Merchant's Tale*: "Old fish, and young flesh woll I haue full faine" (line 1418).

   Other editions with different titles: *Select and Choyce Observations*, L1003 (1657), 274; *Select and Choice Observations*, L1004 (1663), 424; *Analecta Caesarum Romanorum*, L984 (1664), 424; *Select and Choice Observations*, L1005 (1670), 424.

53.   *Match Me These Two: or, The Conviction and Arraignment of Britannicus and Lilburne.* M1077. UMI Thomason Tracts 63: E.400 (9).

As Spurgeon notes (3: 4.71), this satirical pamphlet was written in reply (in part) to things written by Marchamont Nedham and Thomas Audley who had, the author claims, "made the Natives of *great Britaine* a mockery, and a word of reproach to all Nations." The author imagines the miscreants (known collectively as *Britannicus*, a name derived from their newspaper, *Mercurius Britannicus*) are brought to trial; there Britannicus responds to the charges brought against him and invokes the spirit of Chaucer to assist him:

> My worthy and learned Judges, it doth not the least affright me to ren-
> der an account to you, whom I know to have drank deep of the *Pierian
> fount,* & to be conversant with the Muses. . . . O *Chaucer* and thy *Genius,*
> help on my tale: I confesse I was bold and invective; he that undertakes
> to encounter Majesty, must not be shaken with Pannick fear; I esteem
> it my chief glory, that I shall be the sole wonder of the next Age, and be
> stiled THE PRINCE OF LIBELERS. (9)

54.   TOOKE, GEORGE. *The Belides: or, Eulogie and Elegie of John Lord Har-rington.* T1893. UMI 2115: 15.

Tooke (1595–1675) is identified on the title page as "G. T." As Spurgeon notes (1: 225), *The Belides or Eulogie of Major William Fairefax* is included in this edi-tion. In a passage about poetry, Tooke, an army officer himself, notes a criticism of Chaucer. Tooke writes:

> A Poet also has the perogative freely to follow the propensitude of his
> *Genius*; and our language as supplyed from abroad, is of richer variety
> for the cadence of either Prose or Verse. *Verstegan* will indeed upbraid
> *Chauc*[er] with it as prejudicial;[5] and another Netherlander has objected
> our English to me, for made of several shreds like a Beggars Cloake.
> (sig. A2v)

Another edition with different title: *The Belides: or, Eulogie of Major William Faire-fax*: T1893A (1660), sig. A2v.

55.   TRAPP, JOHN. *A Commentary or Exposition upon All the Epistles and the Revelation of John the Divine.* T2040. UMI 677: 5.

Trapp (1601–1669) is identified on the title page as "Pastour of Weston upon Avon in Gloucestershire." Under the running head "A Commentary upon the Revelation," in his notes for chapter 20: 5, he cites John Foxe on Chaucer's books:

---

[5] See Boswell & Holton No. 723.

M. *Fox* tels us, that by the reading of *Chaucers* books, some were brought to the knowledge of the truth.[6] (584)

Also found in *A Commentary or Exposition upon All the Books of the New Testament*: T2039 (1656), 1023.

56.　　TRAPP, JOHN. *A Commentary or Exposition upon the Four Evangelists, and the Acts of the Apostles.* T2042. UMI Thomason Tracts 60: E.376 (1).

In his commentary on Matthew 9:20, "And behold a woman . . ." Trapp alludes to *The Knight's Tale*: "Farewel phisik! Go ber the man to chirche!" (line 2760). He writes:

> [She] *had lavished money out of the bag* for help, but had none. Nay *she had suffered many things of the Physitians*, who had well night officiously killed her, and had utterly exhausted her. This made *Chaucer* take for his Motto, *Farewell physick.* . . . (322).

Also found in *A Commentary or Exposition upon All the Books of the New Testament*: T2039 (1656), 174.

57.　　WEBSTER, WILLIAM. *Webster's Tables. Fifth Edition.* W1233. UMI 2280: 4.

For a commendatory poem that begins with a faint echo of Chaucer's line, "Go, litel bok, go litel myn tragedye" (*Troilus and Criseyde* 5: 1786), see WEBSTER (1625); in this edition, the passage is found on sig. A4v.

58.　　WILLIS, JOHN. *The Art of Stenography.* W2810. No UMI.

For quotations from *Troilus and Criseyde* and from the spurious work known as "Chaucer's Prophecy," see WILLIS (1602) in Boswell & Holton No. 682.

59.　　WILSON, THOMAS. *A Christian Dictionarie. The Fifth Edition.* W2940. UMI 2163: 8.

For an echo of a line from *Troilus and Criseyde*, see WILSON (1612) in the Appendix; in this edition, the passage is found on sig. A4v.

---

[6] For Foxe's comment, see FOXE in Boswell & Holton No. 285.

1648

60. BEAUMONT, FRANCIS, and JOHN FLETCHER. *The Woman Hater.* B1618. UMI 374: 22.

For an echo of a line from *The Manciple's Prologue*, see BEAUMONT and FLETCHER (1607) in the Appendix; in this edition (where authorship is credited to "John Fletcher, Gent."), the passage is found on sig. D3v.

61. CORBET, RICHARD. *Poëtica Stromata: or, A Collection of Sundry Peices* [sic] *in Poetry.* C6272. UMI 1203: 14.

For a reference to Chaucer's having written *Romaunt of the Rose* near Bosworth Field, see CORBET (1647); in this edition, the passage is found on 57.

62. *England's New-yeares Gift: or, A Pearle for a Prince: With Such Grapes from Thornes, and Fruits from Foes, to the Whole Land, as None Shall Be Worse for Wrongs, nor Hurt by Any But Themselves, Though the Times Should Prove Worse and Worse.* E3004. UMI Thomason Tracts 67: E.424 (4).

The unnamed author of this tract exhorts all good Englishmen to eschew heresy and treason, mentions Troilus and Cressida, perhaps alludes to *Troilus and Criseyde*:

> I say all those Hydra-headed errours, different from truth, and from themselves, will no more gain or retain any peace, with one true Orthodox and Uniforme Religion, then there was peace amongst the diversified Lovers of one *Penelope*, all hating *Ulysses* her legall husband, as well as one another; or there was peace betwixt *Agamemnon* and *Achilles*, about *Briseis*; *Troilus* and *Diomedes* about one *Cressida.* (30)

63. FANSHAWE, RICHARD, trans. Guarini's *Il pastor fido: The Faithful Shepherd.* G2175. UMI 868: 9.

For a possible allusion to *The House of Fame*, see FANSHAWE (1647); in this edition, the passage is found on 168.

64. *A Fraction in the Assembly: or, The Synod in Armes.* F2050. UMI Thomason Tracts 71: E.447 (17).

This work purports to be a record of a meeting of "reverend Fathers" held in a tavern on 25 April 1648. As Spurgeon notes (1: 225), the author mentions Chaucer and alludes to *The Canterbury Tales*. In a passage describing the reaction of the daughter of the "fatt Mistress of the House" to the wanton language of the assembled gentlemen, the author seems to allude to the leisurely pace of the stories told by the pilgrims on their way to Canterbury:

[S]he retorted like another *Venus*, till her Tongue travel'd tantivie,[7] and
more then a *Canterbury* pace, and never Stopt till Mr.—Assaulted the
Chairman. . . . (7)

The assembly grew so high flown with wine that they were willing to take anything written by Chaucer as holy writ:

A black fellow . . . taking up a weighty Boll, brim-full of *Sack*, offered
to drink to any man in the Company that would pledge him, and be
of his opinion; his challenge was received immediatly [*sic*] by another:
what replied a third, that they say, seldome spake a true word, but in his
Drink, is not this in the Devills name, a trick of the beast, to tell the
people of a *Cock* and a *Bull*, and bind them to beleeve all the stories in
Chawcer for Articles of Faith: pray what's this, but *Implicita fides*: the
very bumbaste father of Ignorance. (10)

65.   LANE, JOHN. *Alarum to Poets.* L337. UMI 360: 6.

As Harris notes (*PQ*), Lane (*fl.* 1600–1630) places Chaucer in a bright constellation of English poets and refers to the "lost tale" of Chaucer's Squire. In this
poem, the daughter of Jove poses a tricky question to a group of poets, but they
prove somewhat inept in their answer. Lane writes:

Wherefor yee swans of *Thamesis*, what say?
Which of you hath this anagogick key?
For *Chaucer, Lidgate, Sydney, Spencer*, dead,
Have left this riddle harder to be read;
But if yee deigne this scandall to remove,
Your fame 'bove prose-arts quill-men, all will rove:
Then swans of *Olbion*, sing these strains of peace,
That shall make froggish crokers tongues surcease
. . . .
But first, ought sing a song of twelve monthes long,
Next, noblest *Guy*, (righted on others wrong)
Then *Chaucers Squires* lost tale, on his conditions,
The second last part of Poetick visions. (sig. B4r–v)

---

[7] *Tantivie*: top speed.

66.   LINDSAY, DAVID. *The Workes of the Famous and Worthie Knight, S^r. David Lindsay of the Mount, Alias, Lyon, King at Armes.* L2313. UMI 216: 3.

For a reference to Chaucer's skill as a poet in the prologue of *The Testament of Papingo*, see LINDSAY (1538) in Boswell & Holton No. 146; in this edition, the passage is found on sig. M4r.

For a passage that mentions the fable of *Troilus and Criseyde* in an epistle to the king that is set before the prologue to "The Dreme of Sir David Lindsay," see LINDSAY (1558) in Boswell & Holton No. 209; in this edition, the passage is found on sig. O6v.

Other editions: L2314 (1656?), sigs. G7v, H11r; L2315 (1665), sigs. H9r, K3r; L2316 (1670), sigs. G10v, I3r; L2317 (1672), sigs. G3r, H6r; L2318 (1683), sigs. G4v, H6v; L2319 (1686); L2320 (1696), sigs. G7v, H11r.

67.   LLOYD, DAVID. *The Legend of Captain Jones: Continued from His First Part to His End.* L2635. UMI Thomason Tracts 71: E.447 (16).

Lloyd (1597–1663), a Church of England clergyman, rose to be dean of St. Asaph, but is best remembered as the author of this bawdy mock epic. As Spurgeon notes (3: 4.71), there is an allusion to Chaucer in this edition continuation of Lloyd's *Legend* that is not found in the edition of 1631. Lloyd writes of Captain Jones's love of "the ancient stories | Of our old English Worthies, and their glories." Even in a sea storm, he calls his "boy" to his cabin and makes him read them to him. Among them Lloyd alludes to *The Tale of Sir Thopas*:

> How our S. George did the fell Dragon gore:
> The like atchievement of Sr. Eglemore:
> Topas hard quest after th' Elfe Queen to Barwick:
> Sr. Bevis cow, and Guy's fierce boare of Warwick,
> These stories read, exalt his haughty minde
> Above the servil feare of sea or winde . . . (3)

Topas is marked for a shoulder note: "Sr. Topas rime in Chaucer."

Another edition in 1648: L2630.

Other editions: L2631 (1656), 27; L2632 (1659), 27; L2633 (1671), 27; L2634 (1671), 27.

68.   *Look to It London, Threatned to Be Fired by Wilde-fire-zeal, Schismatical-faction, & Militant-mamon.* L3010. UMI Thomason Tracts 73: E.457 (27); UMI 1530: 4.

In a discourse purportedly recorded on 15 July 1648, there is a reference to a generic Canterbury tale, possibly an allusion to *The Canterbury Tales*. In "The Preface to the Premonition," the author writes that when he came upon a publication by one John Dias, he was at first inclined to think of the piece as coined news, a feigned passage like the lying legends of monks and friars, concocted to squeeze money from the credulous:

> I conjectured this pay-squib to be of that nature: so giving no more credit to it then to Æsops Fables, or a *Canterbury* tale, I slighted it. (1)

69.   *The Parliament Arraigned, Convicted; Wants Nothing but Execution. By Tom Tyranno-Maxtix; alias Mercurius Melancholicus.* P498. UMI 470: 11.

In a commendatory poem, "To the Work," the author faintly echoes Chaucer's line, "Go, litel bok, go litel myn tragedye" (*Troilus and Criseyde* 5: 1786). Howsoever faint the echo of the words, the situational echo is identical:

> Go little Creature, in thy poor Attire,
> 　　And crave a Kiss at every Hand thou meets;
> Although thou hast no Merit to admire,
> 　　Yet be the bolder tho' thou beggest i'th'Streets.
> If th'ask, what art? bid them look in and see,
> Then Ten to One but thou shalt welcome be. (sig. A2v)

70.   Prideaux, Mathias. *An Easy and Compendious Introduction for Reading All Sorts of Histories.* P3439. UMI Thomason Tracts 74: E.466 (1).

Prideaux (1622–1646?) is described on the title page as "M[aste]r of Arts and sometime fellow of Exeter Colledge in Oxford." In a section headed "Concerning History of Professions, As also Natural, Various, and Vaine Narrations," he approves of most histories, but not romances. Romances are, Prideaux writes, "the *Bastard* sort of *Histories* . . . noted not for any great *uses* in them, but for manifold *abuses* by them" (343), for most of them are rude (Huon of Bordeaux), endless (Amadis de Gaule), depraved (Arthur and his knights), or superstitious (Abdias Babilonaius). He makes an exception for the "wandering knights" found in Homer, Spenser, and Sidney and those romances which point to policy (More's *Utopia* and Bacon's *Atlantis*) and satirical romances which wittily scourge the others (*Don Quixote*). Regarding those useful romances, he writes:

> The *wandering Knights* . . . with other peices [*sic*] of the like straine may passe with singular Commendations for morall *Romances*, being nothing else but Poeticall *Ethicks*, that with apt *contrivance*, and winning Language, informe *Morality*. . . . To Romances that poynt at Policy . . . The *Vocall Forrest*, *Raynard* the *Fox*, diverse passages in *Chaucer*, and many other in the same kind may be referred. (344)

Atkinson (*N&Q* 1936) cites the 1682 edition of this work.

Other editions: P3440 (1650), 349; P3441 (1654), 349; P3442 (1655), 349; P3442a (1664), 349; P3443 (1664), 349; P3444 (1672), 349; P3444a (1673), 349; P3445 (1682), 379.

71.   TAYLOR, JOHN. *A Brown Dozen of Drunkards*: (*Ali-ass Drink-hards*) *Whipt, and Shipt to the Isle of Gulls.* T435. UMI 2557: 12; UMI Thomason Tracts 73: E.451 (14).

Taylor (1578–1653), known widely as "the water poet," is described on the title page as "one that hath drunk at S. Patricks Well." Here he writes of drunkards who are punished "For their abusing of Mr. Malt the bearded son, and Barley-broth the brainlesse daughter of Sir John Barley-corne. All joco-seriously descanted to our Wine-drunk, Wrath-drunk, Zeale-drunk, staggering Times" (title page). As Spurgeon notes (3: 4.71), in a section headed "One drunken Tom Trouble-towne, or Troublesome," Taylor refers to Chaucer and alludes to *The Nun's Priest's Tale*:

> When he ["turbulent Tom"] drinks fluently, the shouts which the old wives in *Chaucer* gave, and Dame *Partlet* the Hen, when the Fox carried *Chanticleere* the Cock to the wood . . . scarce parallel the clamours. (6)

In a section headed "Drunken Don Quixot, ali-ass Wittypoll," Taylor alludes to Virgil's influence on Chaucer and Spenser. Taylor writes of himself, one who is no water-drinking "mushrump Poet":

> [H]e holds this Axiome above any Article in the Nicine or Apostolick Creed . . . that as good verses come from Rurall Skinker, as from our Hydro-Poets, water-drinkers, and he is verily perswaded that however *Tailour* row in the water,[8] yet when he shaped his best Poeticall shreds, his Muse drunk wine out of the old bottells of the Tower: in briefe, lapping out of old *Homers* bason, that *Vinum Cos*[9] which *Homer* drunk, though he doe not as exactly as *Virgil* imitate *Homer*, nor as our *Chaucer* and *Spenser Virgil* . . . yet as *Homers* raptures smell of wine, so doe his [i.e., Taylor's] Rapsodies. . . . (16)

---

    [8] *Row in the water*: an allusion to Taylor's vocation, rowing a water taxi.
    [9] *Vinum Cos*: wine of Kos. Kos, one of the Greek islands celebrated for its wine, is reportedly the birthplace of Dionysus.

72.   WARE, JAMES. *Librorum manuscriptorum.* W846. UMI Thomason Tracts 76: E447 (21).

Ware (1594–1666) is identified on the title page as "Jacobi Waræi equitis." In his catalog of manuscripts, under the heading "Libri poetici," he lists "Galfridi Chauceri Fabulæ, Anglicè, in fol." (21).

73.   WESTMORLAND, MILDMAY FANE. *Otia sacra optima fides.* W1476. UMI 480: 23.

In a commendatory poem, "To my Book," Fane (1601–1666), the second earl of Westmorland, faintly echoes Chaucer's line, "Go, litel bok, go litel myn tragedye" (*Troilus and Criseyde* 5: 1786). He writes:

> Goe, and my Blessing with Thee; then remain
> Secure, with such as kindly entertain:
> If sent to any Others, tell them this,
> The Author so takes but his Mark amis:
> Who's fearless of reproach from Criticks skill,
> Seing, t'look a given horse ith' mouth sounds ill:
> And what alone to Friends he would impart,
> Hath not at all to doe with Fair or Mart.
> Wherefore whoever shall peruse these Rimes,
> Must know, they were beguilers of spare times. (174)

74.   WILSON, THOMAS. *A Christian Dictionarie.* W2940A. UMI 2959: 19.

For an echo of a line from *Troilus and Criseyde*, see WILSON (1612) in the Appendix; in this edition, the passage is found on sig. A4v.

1649

75.   BEAUMONT, FRANCIS, and JOHN FLETCHER. *The Woman Hater.* B1619. UMI 1857: 21.

For an echo of a line from *The Manciple's Prologue*, see BEAUMONT and FLETCHER (1607) in the Appendix; in this edition, the passge is found on sig. D3v.

76.   CHARLES I, KING OF ENGLAND. *The Papers Which Passed at New-Castle Betwixt His Sacred Majestie and Mr Alex: Henderson Concerning the Change of Church Government.* C2535A. UMI 2347: 17.

Writing in response to a paper by Henderson, in "His Majesty's Second Paper" (dated Newcastle, 6 June 1646) the king concludes with an aphorism that he attributes to Chaucer (but may allude to *The Squire's Tale*, lines 220–24). The monarch writes:

[C]*oncerning the King* My Father,[10] *of Happy and Famous Memory both for his Piety and Learning, I must tell you, that I had the Happiness to know Him much better than you; wherefore I desire you not to be too confident in the knowledge of His Opinions.* . . .

   To conclude . . . I cannot but observe to you, that you have given Me no Answer to my last Quære. *It may be you are (as* Chaucer *says) like the People of* England, What they not like, they never understood. . . . (²166)

Also found in *The Works of King Charles the Martyr* (1662), C2075, ²166.

77.   PRYNNE, WILLIAM. *The Substance of a Speech Made in the House of Commons.* **P4093. UMI 1099: 6.**

Prynne (1600–1669) is identified on the title page as "Wil. Prynn of Lincolns-Inn, Esquire." He spoke in the House of Commons on 4 December 1648 about "the Kings answer to the propositions of both Houses" (title page). In a passage about abuses in the Church, he writes:

[F]or the Judgment of Divines, I could produce divers against the great *Possessions* of *Bishops* in all ages; as making them secular, proud, vitious, lasie, which I have *formerly* published at large: but I shall onely at present [cite a handfull, including] . . . *Pierce Plowman, Geffrey Chaucer,* Mr. *Tyndall.* . . . (70)

Another edition in 1649: P4092.

78.   SADLER, JOHN. *Rights of the Kingdom: or, Customs of our Ancestors Touching the Duty, Power, Election, or Succession of Our Kings and Parliaments.* **S278A. UMI Thomason Tracts 87: E.563 (11).**

Sadler (1615–1674) was a political theorist who advocated prison reform. In the anonymously published work at hand, after a passage in which he digresses on riddles of statecraft that poets of old veiled in fables, Sadler links Chaucer with the historian Richard Grafton and alludes to Chaucer's use of the word *commons* in *The Knight's Tale* (line 2509). He thus sets Chaucer up as an authority on the English language. Sadler writes:

But to return to our *British Ancestors.* . . . I shall only add, that *Proceres* and *Magnates,* Heer, are rendred *Estates, People,* or *Commons* in *Grafton* and *Chaucer,* or the old *Fructus,* by *Julian* of St. *Albans.* (49)

---

[10] James VI and I, king of Scotland and England.

After another digression about representation of all estates in parliaments of old, Sadler cites Chaucer as an authority:

> But to return to our *British* Kings, I cannot deny but some Authors, do record the Crown (as by Act of Parliament) setled [*sic*] on the Heirs of *Cassivelane*. But Themselves also, can shew us, the very next King, brought in by *Election* (not from *Cassivelane*) and That, both of *Lords* and *Commons* too; if we may believe *Chaucer*, or the old *Fructus Temporum*. (51)

After yet another digression about the Sybil's prophecy that three British princes should conquer Rome, Sadler returns to the reign of King Edgar and again cites Chaucer as a British historian:

> But of *Edgar*'s Parliaments: One was at *Salisbury*. So we read in *Chaucer*, or the Old *Fructus Temporum*. . . . (94)

Neither *Edgar* nor *Salisbury* is found in Tatlock & Kennedy's *Concordance*, so the reference appears to be spurious.
    Another edition in 1649: S278B.
    Another edition: S279 (1682), 45–46, 49, 177.

1650

79.   CAVENDISH, GEORGE. *The Negotiations of Thomas Woolsey, the Great Cardinal of England*. C1619A. UMI 2456: 2.

For a reference to Henry VIII's Queen Katherine as a "patient Grissell," perhaps an allusion to *The Clerk's Tale*, see CAVENDISH (1641); in this edition, the passage is found on 22–23.

80.   CLARKE, JOHN. *Phraseologia puerilis, Anglo-Latina, in usum tirocinii scholastici: or, Selected Latine and English Phrases. The Second Edition*. C4473. UMI 886: 27.

For an echo of a line from *The Manciple's Prologue*, see CLARKE (1638) in the Appendix; in this edition, the passage is found on sig. B1v.
    Other editions: C4474 (1655); C4474A (1670), sig. H2v.

81.   DONE, JOHN. *A Miscellania of Morall, Theologicall, and Philosophicall Sentances*; *Worthy Observation*. D1857. UMI 313: 10.

For an allusion to *The Wife of Bath's Prologue* (lines 143–46), see DONE, *Polydoron* (1631) in Boswell & Holton No. 1176; in this edition, the passage is found on 29–30.

82.   LE FÈVRE, RAOUL. *The Destruction of Troy*. L929. UMI 2266: 12; and UMI 2266: 14 (book 3 as L938).

For two references to *Troilus and Criseyde*, see LE FÈVRE (1475) in Boswell & Holton No. 1; in this edition, the first reference to Chaucer's renaming Breseyda is omitted, but the second passage commending *Troilus and Criseyde* to readers is found in book 3, chapter 15, on ²67.

    Other editions: L930 (1670), ²67; L931 (1676), ²67; L932 (1680), ²67; L933 (1684), ²64.

83.   MENNES, JOHN. *Recreation for Ingenious Head-Peeces*. M1713. UMI 284: 2.

For an epitaph "On our prime English Poet, *Geffrey Chaucer*," see MENNES (1641). The epitaph is originally from Lydgate's prologue to his translation of Boccaccio's *The Falle of Princes*; see BOCCACCIO (1494) in Boswell & Holton No. 27. In this edition, the passage is found on sig. O4r.

    For a reference to Chaucer in an epitaph headed "On William Shake-speare," see *Wits Recreations* (1640) in Boswell & Holton No. 1377; in this edition, the passage is found on sig. O5r.

84.   PRIDEAUX, MATHIAS. *An Easy and Compendious Introduction for Reading All Sorts of Histories*. P3440. UMI 1533: 26.

For a reference to "diverse passages" in Chaucer's works that are "useful" for students of history, see PRIDEAUX (1648); in this edition, the passage is found on 349.

85.   SIMPSON, JOHN. *Catalogus Bibliotheca Collegii Sionii*. S4959. UMI Thomason Tracts 98: E.636 (7).

As Spurgeon notes (1: 227), Simpson records that a volume of Chaucer's works was included in the collection. In the catalogue, under the heading "Galfrid. *Chawcer*" he lists "Opera Anglicè *Lond*. 1602. C 6. 8." (37).

86.   TOLL, THOMAS, JR. "To the Author," in Nicholas Murford's *Fragmenta Poetica*. M3100. UMI 1153: 8.

As Spurgeon notes (3: 4.72), Toll refers to Chaucer in a commendatory poem headed "To the Author." Murford was a merchant; hence, the language of commerce:

When whole-sale Men are bankrupt, & none left
To trade in wit, but those who do't by theft;
Such as retail rime weekly by a sheet,
To gain perhaps the Counter or the Fleet:
In such a Fancy-famin not to raise,
But make wit cheap; deserves a double Bayes

. . . .

Thy stock is verse, thy factors are the Muses
Thy returns Fame; thine is such Merchandize,
As feeds not Custom, and quite starves Excise:
Trade on wits Merchant, give the world to know
Chaucer was bred in *Lyn*, and so wert Thou. (sig. A5r)

Chaucer's association with Lynn is tenuous at best, but he does mention Nicholas of Lynn (i.e., formerly Bishop's Lynn in Norfolk, now King's Lynn) in *A Treatise on the Astrolabe.*

87.　VAUGHAN, THOMAS. *Anima magia abscondita: or, A Discourse of the Universall Spirit of Nature. By Eugenius Philalathes.* V142. UMI 749: 18.

As both Harris (*PQ*) and Rudrum (614) note, Vaughan (1621–1666) mentions "Roman Chaucer" and alludes to *Troilus and Criseyde* as if Chaucer had been wasting his time in writing it. In his epistle addressed "To the Reade," Vaughan writes:

NOW God defend! What will become of me? I have neither consulted with the *stars*, nor their *Urinals*, the Almanacks. . . . Reader, if I studied *these things*, I should think my self worst imployd then the *Roman Chaucer* was in his *Troilus.* (sig. A2v)

88.　VAUGHAN, THOMAS. *Magia Adamica: or, The Antiquitie of Magic, and the Descent Thereof from Adam Downwards, Proved. By Eugenius Philalethes.* V151. UMI Thomason Tracts 174: E.1299 (1).

As Rudrum notes (642), perhaps Vaughan echoes *The Monk's Tale*: "Loo Adam, in the feeld of Damyssene | With Goddes owene fynger wroght was he" (lines 2006–7) when he says:

This is the true *Damascen Earth*, out of which *God* made man. (45)

Another edition: V152 (1656), 45.

89.   WARD, NATHANIEL. "Commendatory verses" in Ann Bradstreet's *The Tenth Muse*. B4167. UMI Thomason Tracts 179: E.1365 (4).

As Smith notes (*SP* 28), there is a reference to Chaucer's boots in commendatory verses by Nathaniel Ward (1578–1652). Ward appears to pen a warning to men to work harder or women will soon be wearing the boots and will walk all over them. He writes:

> M*ercury* shew'd *Apollo, Bartas*[11] Book,
> *Minerva* this, and wisht him well to look,
> And tell uprightly, which did which excell;
> He view'd, and view'd, and vow'd he could not tell.
> . . . .
> They both 'gan laugh, and said, it was no mar'l
> The Auth'resse was a right *Du Bartas* Girle.
> Good sooth quoth the old *Don*, tel, ye me so,
> I muse whither at length these Girls wil go;
> It half revives my chil frost-bitten blood,
> To see a woman once do, ought, that's good;
> And chode [*sic*] by *Chaucers* Boots, and *Homers* Furrs,
> Let men look to't, least women weare the Spurs. (sig. A4r)

Another edition, corrected and enlarged, with a different title: *Several Poems*: B4166 (1678), sig. *a*4r.

1651

90.   CARTWRIGHT, WILLIAM. *The Lady-Errant, a Tragi-Comedy*. C710. UMI 2226: 2.

Cartwright (1611–1643) is identified on the title page of his collected works as "Mr William Cartwright, late student of Christ-Church, and proctor of the University." In the fourth act of the work at hand, Cartwright refers to a steed of brass and may allude to *The Squire's Tale* (lines 81, 115). Eumela (companion and confidant to the Princess) says to Machessa (a Lady-Errant for the times):

> Will you be
> Famous in History then? fill swelling Volumes
> With your sole Name? be read aloud, and high
> I'th' *Cyprian* Annals? and live fresh upon
> The Tongue of Fame for ever? will you stand

---

[11] Saluste, Guillaume de, Seigneur du Bartas, author of *Divine Weeks*.

High on your Steed in Brass, and be at once
The stop of Strangers, and Natives Worship
By one fair Peacefull Action? (51)

91.   CARTWRIGHT, WILLIAM. *The Ordinary, a Comedy.* C714. UMI 2226: 3.

In the first scene of the fourth act, Cartwright (1611–1643) refers to Chaucer and echoes a line in *The Reeve's Prologue*: "For in oure wyl ther striketh evere a nayl, | To have an hoor heed and a grene tayl, | As hath a leek" (3876–78). In the play, Robert Moth, an antiquary, uses Chaucerian language to woo Mrs. Potluck:

Harrow alas! I swelt here as I go
Brenning in fire of little *Cupido.*
I no where hoart yfeele, but on mine head.
Huh, huh, hunh, so; ycapred very wele.
I am thine Leeke, thou *Chaucer* eloquent;
Mine head is white, but o mine taile is green.
This is the Palyes where mine Lady wendeth. (36)

Moth continues and again echoes Chaucer, this time *The Miller's Tale*: "Jhesu Crist and seinte Benedight, | Blesse this hous from every wikked wight" (lines 3483–84).

Saint Francis, *and Saint* Benedight,
Blesse this house from wicked wight,
From the Night-mare and the Goblin,
That is hight good fellow Robin.
Keep it from all evill Spirits,
Fayries, Weezels, Rats and Ferrets,
From Curfew time
To the next prime. (36)

Having finished rhyming, Moth again echoes *The Miller's Tale*: "What do ye, hony-comb, sweet Alisoun, | My faire byrd, my sweete cynamome?" (lines 3698–99).

Come forth mine Duck, mine Byrd, mine honycomb.
Come forth mine Cinnamon. (36)

Moth invokes Chanticlere and Pertelote, an allusion to *The Nun's Priest's Tale*, as he pledges his love to Mrs. Potluck:

> I'll be as faithfull to thee,
> As Chaunticleere to Madam Partelot. (37–38)

Also collected in Cartwright's *Comedies Tragi-Comedies, with Other Poems* (1651): C709, 36–38.

92.   CARTWRIGHT, WILLIAM. *Comedies Tragi-Comedies, with Other Poems.* **C709. UMI Thomason Tracts 169: 3.1224 (1).**

In addition to references and allusions in *The Ordinary*, there is another in this collection. For references to Chaucer in a commendatory poem for Sir Francis Kynaston's translation of Chaucer's *Troilus and Creseide* into Latin, see CHAU- CER (1635) in Boswell & Holton No. 1265; in this work, the passage is found on 249–50.

93.   CLEVELAND, JOHN. *Poems. By J. C.* **C4686. UMI 2891: 20.**

For an echo of a line from *The Manciple's Prologue*, see CLEVELAND (1644); in this edition, the passage is found on 55.

Another edition in 1651: C4684, 54.

Other editions: C4688 (1653), 65; C4689 (1653), 90; C4689A (1654), 90; C4690 (1654), 90; C4691 (1656), 90; C4692 (1657), 90; C4692A (1658), 83; C4693 (1658), 87; C4694 (1659), 183; C4695 (1661), 182; C4696 (1662), 183; C4697 (1665), 183; C4698 (1669), 183; C4697 (1655), 183.

94.   GREVILLE, FULKE. *The Life of the Renowned Sr Philip Sidney.* **B4899. UMI Thomason Tracts 173: E. 1288 (1).**

Greville (1554–1528) is identified on the title page as "Sir Fulke Grevil Knight, Lord Brook, a servant to Queen Elizabeth, and his [i.e., Sidney's] companion & friend." In this biography Greville appears to allude to *The House of Fame*. In the sixteenth chapter, in a passage about Queen Elizabeth, Greville writes:

> [S]he preserved her Religion without waving, kept her Martiall, and Civill Goverment [*sic*] intire above neglect, or practice, by which, with a multitude of like instances, she manifested to the World, that the well governing of Princes own Inheritances, is (in the cleare house of Fame) superiour to all the far noised conquests of her over-griping Ances- tors. . . . (223)

95.   OGILBY, JOHN, trans. *The Fables of Æsop Paraphras'd in Verse.* **A689. UMI Thomason Tracts 121: E.792 (1).**

Ogilby (1600–1676) calls the cock *Chanticleere* throughout his translation of Æsop. In fable no. 1, "Of the Cock and Precious Stone," he writes:

Stout *Chanticleere* four times aloud
Day's signall victorie ore nights vanquish'd flames [etc.] (1)

In the second book, in fable no. 42, "Of the Fox and the Weesell," Ogilby alludes to *The Nun's Priest's Tale*. The crafty Reynard seeking an entryway into a poultry house is, uncharacteristically, briefly pricked by his conscience, but he quickly reverts to type and commences his slaughter of the innocents:

Seaven times the rockie passe with teeth and claws
He [the Fox] strives to open, and as oft did pause.
Then Conscience pricks, a melancholy fear
    Shews all his slaughters,
Sad *Partlet* following of a wofull beer,[12]
    Where lay bold *Chanticleer*,
    And his three Daughters;
Then jetting Turkies with blue snouts he spy'd,
And white fleec'd Lambs which he in Scarlet dy'd. (²53–54)

In a shoulder note, Ogilby annotates "Sad Partlet" as "The Hen" (²54). *Partlet* is, of course, a variant pronunciation of Chaucer's Pertelote.
    In book 3, in fable no. 49, "Of the Fox and the Cock," Ogilby again names the cock *Chanticleere*:

Soon as the *Fox* to *Pullein*-furnish'd Farms
    Approaches made,
Though valiant, *Chanticleere* not trusting Arms
    Nor humane aid,
    Ascends a tree,
    Where he
    Stood safe from harms. [Etc.] (³19–22).

Other editions: A693 (1665), 1, 103–4, 120; A697 (1668), 1, 103–4, 120; A700 (1673), 1, 123–24, 142; A702 (1675), 1, 123–24, 142.

96.   SCOTT, REGINALD. *Scot's Discovery of Witchcraft Proving the Common Opinions of Witches Contracting with Divels, Spirits, or Familiars to Be but Imaginary, Erronious Conceptions and Novelties.* S943. UMI 159: 5.

Scott (1538?–1599) is identified on the title page as "Reginald Scot, Esquire." For references to Chaucer and quotations from *The Wife of Bath's Tale*, and *The*

---

[12] *Beer*: i.e., bier.

Canon's Yeoman's Prologue and *Tale*, see SCOTT (1584) in Boswell & Holton No. 427; in this edition, the passages are found on 67–68, 249, 250–51, 253.

For an echo of a line from *The Reeve's Tale* and Chaucer listed in Scott's bibliography, see SCOTT (1584) in the Appendix; in this edition, the passages are found on 344 and sig. B4v.

Another edition in 1651: S943A, same pagination.

Other editions: S944 (1654), sig. B4v and 67–68, 249, 250–51, 253, 344; S945A (1665), sig. (b4)v and 49, 202, 203–4, 205; S945 (1665), sig. (b4)v and 49, 202, 203–4, 205.

97.   SHEPPARD, SAMUEL. *Epigrams Theological, Philosophical, and Romantick.* **S3161. UMI 1212: 19.**

As Spurgeon notes (3: 4.72), Sheppard (ca. 1624–1655?) refers to Chaucer's influence on Spencer in book 4, epigram 28, "On Mr. Spencer's inimitable Poem, the Faerie Queen":[13]

> Collin my Master, O Muse sound his praise,
> Extol his never to be qual'd Layes,
> Whom thou dost Imitate with all thy might,
> As he did once in *Chawcers* veine delight. (95)

In *The Third Pastoral* are other allusions to Chaucer, here called *Tytirus*, Spenser's nickname for him:

> But I to thee will now display
> What I have heard my Father say.
> Next unto *Tytirus* there came
> One that deservd a greater name,
> Then was bestowed; but when She swaid,
> Whom to this day some call a Maid,[14]
> Then *Collin Clout* his pipe did sound,
> Making both Heaven and Earth resound;
> . . . .
> O gentle Shepheard still pipe on,
> Stil take deep draughts of *Helicon*,
> And thou'lt be rankt I make no doubt
> With *Tytirus* and *Collin Clout*. (sig. S2v–5v)

---

[13] Sheppard's interesting and thoughtful verse epic with a Spenserian title *The Faerie King* was edited by P. J. Klemp and published in 1984.

[14] "She" is Queen Elizabeth, the virgin queen.

98.   TAYLOR, JOHN. *Nonsence upon Sence: or, Sence, upon Nonsence.* T491A. UMI 2241: 11.

In this nonsensical poem, "written by John Taylor at the Signe of the poore Poets Head, in Phenix Alley, neare the middle of Long Aker, or Covent Garden," Taylor (1580–1653 and often called "the water poet") mentions Chaucer's cypress gown.

> The Lake of Learna I did clarifie,
> My Verse the Æthiop Queen did beautifie,
> With rage my patience I would qualifie,
> I can both certifie and testifie
> How death did live, and Life did mortifie:
> Feare alwayes did my courage fortifie,
> He's crafty that his wits can rectifie:
> To villifie, make glad and terrifie,
> And with course words old debts to satisfie,
> That man, I'le ratifie and notifie:
> To be one that himselfe will justifie,
> And fie, fo, fum, concludes him with O fie.
> Thus from complexions I have Minerals drawn,
> Brave Captain Fumble layd his sword to pawn
> To ransome Jeffery Chaucers Cipresse Gown,[15]
> Thersites with a Rush knock'd Ajax down. (10)

99.   VAUGHAN, THOMAS. *Lumen de Lumine: or, A New Magicall Light Discovered. By Eugenius Philalethes.* V150. UMI 299: 20.

As Rudrum (675) notes, Vaughan's protagonist dreams he finds himself in a place that is reminiscent of one in *The Parliament of Fowls*: "Of braunches were here halles and here bowres | Inwrought" (lines 304–5).

> The *Texture* of the *Branches* was so even, the *Leaves* so *thick*, and in that conspiring *order*, it was not a *wood* but a *Building*. (3)

1652

100.   ASHMOLE, ELIAS. *Theatrum chemicum Britannicum.* A3987. UMI Thomason Tracts 100: E.653 (1).

Ashmole (1617–1692), lawyer, astrologer, and antiquary, is best remembered today as founder of Oxford's Ashmolean Museum; he is identified on the title page as

---

[15] *Cipresse*: various textile fabrics imported from or through the island of Cyprus.

"Elias Ashmole, Esq. Qui est Mercuriophilus Anglicus." The work at hand has been called "the most important of all English alchemical publications."[16] As Spurgeon notes (1: 227), he cites Chaucer several times. The first reference is found in the "Prolegomena," a commendatory epistle addressed to "All Ingeniously Elaborate Students, in the most Divine Mysteries of *Hermetique Learning*." There Ashmole quotes *The Man of Law's Tale*, lines 545–48:

> *Our* English Nation *hath ever beene happy for* Learning *and* Learned men, *and to illustrate this, I hope it will not prove distastfull.* . . . [T]he Bardi, *who celebrated the* Illustrious Deeds *of* Famous men, *which they ingeniously dispos'd in* Heroique Verse, *and sung them to the sweete* Melody *of the* Harpe: *Amongst other* Testimonies *hereof receive* Chaucer's;
>
> > The old gentle Brittons in her dayes
> > Of divers adventures maden Layes,
> > Rymed first in her Mother Tongue,
> > Whych Layes, with her Instruments they songe. (sig. A2v–3r)

In another passage, Ashmole continues with a quotation from *The Parliament of Fowls* (lines 22–25):

> [W]e *must needs say that of* Later Times (*since the* Conquest) *our Nation hath produced such* Famous *and* eminent learned Men, *as have equall'd* (*if not surpast*) *the greatest* Schollers *of other* Nations, *and happy were we if now we could but partake of those* Legacies *they left, and which* Envy *and* Ignorance *has defrauded us of*: (*Howsoever the small remainder which is left, we have good reason to prize,*
>
> > For out of olde Fields as Men saythe,
> > Cometh alle this new Corne fro yeare to yeare;
> > And out of olde Bokes in good faythe
> > Cometh alle this Seyence, that Men leare.)
>
> *That* England *hath beene successively enrich'd with such* Men, *our Country men* John Leland . . . *abundantly* Testifies. . . . (sig. A3v)

As Spurgeon notes, Ashmole reprints one of *The Canterbury Tales* under the heading "The Tale of the *Chanons Yeoman*. Written by our Ancient and famous English Poet, *Geoffry Chaucer*" (227–56). On the page preceding the text, there is an engraving of Chaucer's tomb.

---

[16] Michael Hunter, *Oxford DNB*.

In a verse treatise headed "Sir Edward Kelle's Worke," Ashmole appears to echo a line from *The Reeve's Tale*: "The gretteste clerkes been noght wisest men" (line 4054). He writes:

> Although to my one Booke you have red tenn,
>   Thats not inough, for I have heard it said,
> The greatest Clarkes ar not the wisest men [etc.] (324)

Under the heading "Annotations and Discourses upon Some part of the preceding Worke," Ashmole refers several times to Chaucer. Some of these references were mentioned by Spurgeon, and some not. One of those missed by Spurgeon is found in Ashmole's comments on the accomplishments of Sir Sampson Norton, Master of the Ordinance of War in the days of Henry VIII. Ashmole quotes *Chaucer's Wordes unto Adam, His Owne Scriveyn* as he writes of scribes who negligently or willfully altered their copy:

> Doubtlesse *Norton* was truly sensible of the high injuries done to *learned men* through the *Erronious Transcriptions* of their *Bookes*, and had shared in the unimaginable *misfortune* which thereby befell the then *Students in Philosophy*. . . . How ordinary a fault this was amongst the *Transcribers* of former times may appeare by *Chaucer*, who (I am confident) tooke as greate care as any man to be served with the best and heedefullest *Scribes*, and yet we find him complayning against *Adam* his *Scrivener* for the very same:
>
>> So ofte a daye J mote thy worke renew,
>> Jt to Correct and eke to rubbe and scrape,
>> And all is thorow thy neglegence and rape.

The passage is marked with a shoulder note: "*Chaucer to his Scrivener*" (439).

Ashmole quotes ten lines from the prologue to *The Tale of Melibee* in a section in which he writes of learned ancients who made their works less reader-friendly than they might have done:

> Their chiefest study was to wrap up their *Secrets* in *Fables*, and spin out their *Fancies* in *Vailes* and *shadows*, whose *Radii* seems to extend every way, yet so, that they all meete in a *Common Center*, and point onely at One thing.
>
>> And thus ye wote that every Ebangelist,
>> That telleth us the pains of Jesu Christ
>> . . . .

I meane of Mark Mathew Luike and John,
But doubtlesse her Sentence is all one.

The passage is marked with a shoulder note: "*Chauc. Prol.* To his owne *Tale*" (440).

In a passage about "Naturall Magick" being the gift of God, Ashmole again quotes eight lines from *The Cannon's Yeoman's Tale* and the passage is marked with a shoulder note, "Chan. Yeom Tale":

The Philosophers were y sworne eche one,
That they shulde discover it unto none [etc.] (447)

In a discussion of a work called *The Compounde of Alchymie* (also called *The Twelve Gates*), Ashmole notes that the author "gives an account of his own *Errenious Experiments*, therein following *Chaucer* . . . and divers other honest and Consciencious *Philosophers*" (456).

In a discussion of a work called *Liber patris Sapientie*, Ashmole closes with a couplet from "The Ten Commandments of Love" (which was, in Ashmole's day, in the Chaucerian canon):

I shall only adde Chaucers Councell which may prove of no litle advantage if they remember it.

Make privy to your dealing as few as you maie,
For three may keepe Councell if twaine be awaie.

The passage is marked with a shoulder note: "*Ten comman. of Love*" (465). This is a misattribution of the *Testament of Love* to Chaucer.

In an apologia for reprinting *The Canon's Yeoman's Tale*, Ashmole writes:

One Reason why I selected out of *Chaucer's Canterbury Tales*, that of the *Chanon's Yeoman* was, to let the *World* see what notorious *Cheating* there has beene ever used, under pretence of this true (though Injur'd) *Science*; Another is, to shew that *Chaucer* himselfe was a *Master* therein.

For, in this *Tale Chaucer* sets forth the deceipts in *Alchimy* to the life, and notably declaimes against all such villanous *Pretenders*, who being wholly ignorant of *Art*, have notwithstanding learnt the *Cunning*, to abuse the World; And this paines he tooke (as himselfe professeth) merely

To the intent that men maie beware thereby,
And for no other cause truly.

[The passage is marked with a shoulder note: *"Chan. Yeom. Tale."*]

Herein following the *President* of all sincere and conscientious *Philosophers*, then whom, the *Injur'd world* cannot more condemne the abuses of these *Impostors* that disgrace the *Art*, in that they are continually *advising* to shun them as spreading *Infection*. . . . This is the *Misery* . . . that there are a Generation of *People* that rush headlong into the acquaintance of such *Men*, there's nor staving them off, much like the doting *Idiotts* which so eagerly courted *Chaucer's Chanon*, after whom

> Men riden and gone full many a Myle
> Him for to seeke and have acquaintance,
> Not knowing of his false governance.

[In a shoulder note: "Chan. Yeom. Tale."]

Let *Philosophers* say whgat they can, and *wise men* give never so good Counsell, no warning will serve, they must be Couzened, nay they have a greedy appetite thereunto. . . .

Yet to those that have been Decoy'd into the *snare*, and would gladly for the future pursue a more hopefull Course, let them heare . . . Chaucer,

> If that your Eyne cannot seene right,
> Loketh that your Minde lack not his sight.

[In a shoulder note: "Chan. Yeom. Tale."]

And . . . If what hath been delivered be not of force to make men watch over their *undertakings* . . . Ile leave them with this incouragement,

> Who soe that lysteth to utter his folly,
> Let him come forth and learne to Multiplie;
> And every man that hath ought in his Cofer,
> Let him appeare and wexe a Philosopher.

[In a shoulder note: "Chan. Yeom. Tale."]

Now as Concerning *Chaucer* (the *Author* of this *Tale*) he is ranked amongst the *Hermetick Philosophers*, and his *Master* in this *Science* was Sir *John Gower*, whose familiar and neere acquaintance began at the *Inner Temple* upon *Chaucer's* return into *England*, for the Troubles of the *Times* towards the latter end of *Rich: the second's Raign* had caused him to retire out of their *Danger* into *Holland*, *Zeland*, and *France*.

He is cited by Norton for an Authentique Author, in these words;

> And Chaucer rehearseth how Tytans is the same.

Besides he that Reads the latter part of the *Chanon's Yeoman's Tale*, wil easily perceive him to be a *Judicious Philosopher*, and one that fully knew the *Mistery*.

Master *Speght* (in that commendable Account he gives of *Chaucer's* life,) is perswaded he was borne in *London*, from something intimated in his *Testament of love*. But *Bale* saith, He was *nobili loco natus*, and that neere unto *Oxford*, for (saith he) *Leland* had *Arguments* which made him believe he was borne either in *Oxford-shire* or *Bark-shire*. But what those *Arguments* were we now know not, yet may believe them to be of considerable *weight*. . . . But begging *Pardon* for this *Digression* . . . I return to *Chaucer*. *Pitts* Positively saies he was born in *Woodstock*, of *noble Parents*, and that . . . his *Father* was a *Knight*. And this may not be unlikely if we Consider, that not onely the *Name* is *Auncient* as *William* the *Conqueror's* time, but . . . our *Geffrey Chaucer* is written in the *Records* of *Ed*. 3. and *Rich. the second*. [In a shoulder note: "Speght in vit. Chaucer."]

But wheresoever he was *Borne*, his *Education* was chiefly in the *University* of *Oxford* in *Canterbury-Colledge* . . . though for some time he studied at *Cambridge*. . . . He quickly became a Witty *Logitian*, a sweet *Rhetoritian*, a pleasant *Poet*, and a grave *Philosopher*, a holy *Divine*, a skilfull *Mathematitian*, his Tutors therein were 𝔉𝔯𝔢𝔯𝔢 𝔍𝔬𝔥𝔫 𝔖𝔬𝔫, 𝔞𝔫𝔡 𝔉𝔯𝔢𝔯𝔢 𝔑. 𝔏𝔢𝔫𝔫𝔢 . . . remembered with honour in his *Treatise* of the *Astrolabe*) and moreover (I may safely adde) an able *Astrologian*, for almost in every Worke he inter-weaves most sound and perfect *Astrologie*. In Brief, he was *Universally learned*, and so affirmes his Scholar *Tho. Occleve*. . . .

Pitts stiles him . . . A Man that excelled in *Arts* both of *Warre* and *Peace* . . . For ere he came to *Mans Estate*, he was an *Elegant Poet*, and one, who illustrated *English Poesy*, that he might have been deservedly accounted the 𝔈𝔫𝔤𝔩𝔦𝔰𝔥 𝔥𝔬𝔪𝔢𝔯. *Lidgate* the *Monke* of *Bury* calls him the *Load star* of our *Language*. . . . For indeed in all his time all good Letters were laid asleep in most parts of the *World*, and in *England* our *Tongue* was exceeding wild and rude, yet (through his *refining* and *polishing*) it became more sweet and pleasant. . . . He spent many of his yeares in *France* and *Flanders*: severall *Preferences* he had at *Court* . . . With these he had several *Annuall pensions* during his Life granted from *R*. 2. and *H*. 4. His Abilities for *Forraigne Imployments* were so farre taken notice of, that he was twice or thrice sent abroad into other *Countries*, and thought fit to be one of the *Embassadors* into *France* to move a *Marriage* betweene *Richard* the second (while *Prince* of *Wales*) and the *Lady Mary*, *Daughter* to the *French King*. His *Revenue* was 10001. *per annum*. a very plentifull *Estate*, the times considered.

He dyed at *London* 25. *Octob. Ann.* 1400. as appeares by the *Inscription* upon his *Tombe* at Saint *Peters* in *Westminster Abby*, in an *Isle* on the *South* side of the *Church.*

Mr. *Nicholas Brigham* built this *Marble Monument* to his *Memory*, the true *Pourtraicture* whereof I have caused to be exactly graved in *Brasse*, and placed in page 226. There was formerly round the ledge of the *Tombe* these following *Verses*, but not no remainder of them left. . . .

The *Picture* of *Chaucer* is now somwhat decay'd, but the *Graver* has recovered it after a *Principall* left to *posterity* by his worthy Scholar *Tho. Occleve*, who hath also these *Verses* upon it
And though his life be queinte the resemblaunce

> Of him hath in me so fresshe listnesse,
> That to putte other men in remembraunce
> Of his persone, I have here the liknesse
> Do make, to this ende in forthfastnesse,
> That thei that have of hem lost thoute and mynde,
> By this Peintuyre, may ageine him fynde.

[In a shoulder note: "Occl. de Regem. Princ: *cap. de Concilio.* Upon the figure of *Chaucer*."]

Before Mr. *Brigham* built the aforesaid *Monument* it seems *Chaucer* had a *Stone* layd over his *Grave* upon which was ingraved this following *Epitaph.*

> *Galfridus Chaucer Vates & fama Poesis,*
> *Materna hac sacra sum tumulatus humo.* (467–72)

In a passage about John Gower, Ashmole writes of Gower's association with Chaucer:

[Gower] is placed in the *Register* of our *Hermetique Philosophers*: and one that adopted into the Inheritance of this *Mistery*, our famous *English Poet*, *Geoffry Chaucer*. . . . The first acquaintance betweene *Him* and *Chaucer* began at the *Inner Temple*, where Sir *John Gower* studied the *Lawes*, and whither *Chaucer* came to follow the like course of studies upon his returne out of *France*. He was (saith *Pitts*[17]) a noble and learned *Man* . . . resembling *Geoffry* almost in every thing, and who had surely the same proposed end of all their *Studies*; they soone perceived the similitude of their manners, quickly joyned in *Friendship* and *Labours*;

---

[17] Pitts, probably John Pitts, author of *De Illustribus Angliæ Scriptibus* (Paris, 1619).

they had dayly meetings and familiarity, and all their endeavour was
to refine and polish their *Mother Tongue*, that there might appeare the
expresse footesteps of the *Roman Eloquence* in our *English Speech*.

This appeares by *Chaucer*'s sending to *Gower* his *Troylus* and *Cressida* after he had finished it, for his perusal and amendments.

> 𝔒 𝔐𝔬𝔯𝔞𝔩𝔩 𝔊𝔬𝔴𝔢𝔯, 𝔱𝔥𝔦𝔰 𝔅𝔬𝔬𝔨𝔢 𝔍 𝔡𝔦𝔯𝔢𝔠𝔱
> 𝔗𝔬 𝔱𝔥𝔢, 𝔞𝔫𝔡 𝔱𝔬 𝔱𝔥𝔢 𝔓𝔥𝔦𝔩𝔬𝔰𝔬𝔭𝔥𝔦𝔠𝔞𝔩𝔩 𝔖𝔱𝔯𝔬𝔡𝔢
> 𝔗𝔬 𝔳𝔬𝔲𝔠𝔥𝔰𝔞𝔣𝔢, 𝔱𝔥𝔢𝔯 𝔫𝔢𝔢𝔡𝔢 𝔦𝔰, 𝔱𝔬 𝔠𝔬𝔯𝔯𝔢𝔠𝔱,
> 𝔒𝔣 𝔶𝔬𝔲𝔯 𝔅𝔢𝔫𝔦𝔤𝔫𝔦𝔱𝔢𝔢𝔰 𝔞𝔫𝔡 ℨ𝔢𝔩𝔢𝔰 𝔤𝔬𝔬𝔡.

[In a shoulder note: "See the end of Troylus and Cres."]

And surely these two added so much of splendour and ornament to
our *English ideome*, as never any the like before them: for they set foote
to foote, and lovingly contended, whether should bring most *honour* to
his *Country* both endeavouring to overcome, and to be overcome each
of other. . . . (484–85)

Ashmole's bibliography is headed "A Table of The severall Treatises, with their
Authors Names, contained in this Worke." There he lists "Chanon's Yeoman's
Tale. *Geoffry Chaucer*" (sig. Sss1r).

101.   BRATHWAIT, RICHARD. *Times Treasury: or, Academy for Gentry.* **B4276.
UMI 1399: 5.**

For a reference to Richard II's benevolent patronage of Chaucer, see BRATHWAIT
(1630) in Boswell & Holton No. 1149; in this edition, the passage is found in a
section headed "The English Gentleman," 106–7.

102.   CHAPMAN, GEORGE. *Caesar and Pompey: a Roman Tragedie.* **C1946.**

For an echo of a line from *The Reeve's Tale*, see CHAPMAN (1631) in Appendix; in
this edition, the passage is found on sig. C4v.

Another edition: C1947 (1653), sig. C4v.

103.   FISHER, PAYNE. *Veni; vidi; vici. The Triumph of the Most Excellent &
Illustrious Oliver Cromwell.* **F1044. UMI 938: 29**

In a poem translated from Fisher's Latin by Thomas Manley (1628–1690) and
addressed "To the Most Excellent, The Lord Generall of Great Brittayne, Oliver Cromwell," Fisher (1616–1693) echoes the title of *The House of Fame*. Manley
translates:

> Make me but happy by thy smile,
> If thou with favour dain my toile,

By that thy favourable breath
We are (as 'twere) redeem'd from death.
Thus rais'd by thee,
It shall our Triumph be,
In the eternal house of Fame
To register thy present name,
That future ages each succeeding hour
To thy blest name may new Encomiums powr. (sig. I1r–v)

104.   GRACIÁN Y MORALES, BALTASAR. *The Heroe of Lorenzo: or, The Way to Eminence and Perfection.* G1471. UMI 98: 2.

The translator of *Héroe* is identified on the title page as "Sir John Skeffington Kt. and Barronet"; he eventually was Viscount Massereene (d. 1695). In this "piece of serious Spanish wit" by Gracián (1601–1658) there may be an allusion to *The House of Fame.* Skeffington translates:

The ordinary speeches of a King are refin'd and crown'd subtilties: The great treasures of Monarchs have often perisht and come to nothing, but their sententious and wise speeches, are kept in the Cabinet and Jewell-house of Fame. (22–22, pagination is confused)

105.   HILTON, JOHN. *Catch That Catch Can: or, A Choice Collection of Catches, Rounds & Canons.* H2036. UMI 2124: 4 (3).

Hilton (1599–1657), composer and organist at St. Margaret's in Westminster, writes knowingly of the meaning of Chaucer's jape in a song scored for three voices:

My Mistresse will not be content to take a jape, a jape, a jape, as *Chaucer* meant, but following still the womans fashion, allowes it, allowes it of the new translation: Nor with the word she'l not dispence, and yet, and yet, and yet and yet I know she loves the sence. (49)

Other editions: H2037 (1658), 48; H2038 (1663); H2039 (1667), 65.
    Also found in *Westminster-Drollery*, W1457 (1671) *et seq.*, q.v.

106.   SELDEN, JOHN. *Of the Dominion or Ownership of the Sea.* Trans. Marchamont Nedham. S2430. UMI 294: 1.

This translation by Nedham (1620–1678) includes additions that do not appear in Selden's Latin edition published in 1635; see SELDEN (1635) in Boswell & Holton No. 1278.

In book 1, chapter 12, "The Testimonies of Edgar and Canutus," in a section devoted to writers later than the English Saxons, Selden (1584–1654) writes of *The Man of Law's Tale* and quotes modernized and amended lines (540–43):

> *Geoffrie Chaucer* (who was not onely the most famous Poët of his time, but, as Learning went in those daies, a very well accomplisht Scholar, in one of his *Canterburie* Tales, bring's [*sic*] in his *Man of Law* telling a storie which hee would have relate to the time of *Alla* King of *Northumberland*, who reigned thirtie years. . . . In this Tale there is brought in a Ladie, Called *Constantia*, the Daughter of I know not what Roman Emperor, married to the King of *Syria*; driven shee was by weather to a place which lay under the command of a Fortress upon the Shore of *Northumberland*, and there the Ship ran aground; shee was a Christian, banished for her Religion, and there taken Prisoner by the Commander of that Fortress. In this Relation of the sad adventures of *Constantia*, he saith (what indeed is true) that Christian Religion was not received into any part of that Territorie, but that *Pagans* had over-run and did hold those Northern Countries under their Dominion as well by Sea as Land. His words to this purpose are these,

> In all that lond dursten non Christen rout;
> All Christen folk been fled from the Countre
> Through Paynims that conquer'd all about
> The Plagues of Northunderland by land & See.

> He said discreetly, that the neighboring Sea fell to the Conquerers of this Isle as well as the Land, knowing what was the resolution and generally received opinion of his Ancestors concerning that matter[.] He lived two hundred and thirtie years ago in the time of *Richard* the Second. Nor is it any prejudice to this autoritie, that the other things there related are fabulous; For wee know that out of the Fables of *Heliodorus* . . . and such others, whether of an amorous or any other strain, sometimes many useful observations may bee gathered concerning the customs, manners, and received opinions, as well of the men among whom they are feigned to bee acted, as of the times to which they are related. (280–81)

In chapter 14, "That the Kings of England, since the coming in of the Normans, have petrually enjoied the Dominion of the Sea flowing about them," Selden again cites Chaucer, alludes to his description of the Merchant, and quotes modernized lines from *The General Prologue* (lines 274–77):

Geoffrie Chaucer (who lived in the time of *Richard* the Second, and was a man verie knowing in the affairs of his Countrie) among other most elegant and lively characters of several sorts of men, written in the *English* Tongue, describe's [*sic*] the humor of an *English* Merchant of that time, how that his desire above all things is, that the Sea bee well guarded, never left destitute of such protection as may keep it safe and quiet. Which hee speak's [*sic*] to set out the whole generation of Merchants in that age, whose custom it was to bee sollicitous for traffick above all things, and consequently about the Sea it self, which would not afford them safe Voyages, did not the Kings of *England*, as Sovereigns thereof, according to their Right and Custom, provide for the securitie of this, as a Province under their Protection. The words of *Chaucer* are these,

> His reasons spake hee full solemnely,
> Shewing alway the encreas of his winning;
> He would the See were kept for any thing
> Betwixe Middleborough and Orewel.

Orwel is an Haven upon the Coasts in *Suffolk. Middleborough* is in *Zealand.* (291)

Another edition in 1652 with title *Mare Clausum: The Right and Dominion of the Sea in Two Books*: S2432, same pagination.
  Another edition: S2431 (1663), UMI 333: 8, 280–81, 291.

107.   SAUL, ARTHUR. *The Famous Game of Chesse-Play.* S729A. UMI 1557: 11.

For an echo of Chaucer's line, "Go, litel bok, go litel myn tragedye" (*Troilus and Criseyde* 5: 1786) in Saul's commendatory poem "To his Booke," see SAUL (1614); in this edition, the passage is found on sig. A5v–6r.
  Other editions: S730 (1672), sig. A5v–6r; S730A (1673), sig. A5v–6r.

108.   SHAKESPEARE, WILLIAM. *The Most Excellent Historie of the Merchant of Venice: With the Extreame Cruelty of Shylocke the Jew towards the Said Merchant. As It Hath Been Diverse Times Acted by the Lord Chamberlaine His Servants.* S2938. UMI 297: 32.

For an allusion to *Troilus and Criseyde* and possible allusions and similarities to *The Legend of Good Women, The Wife of Bath's Tale*, and *The Canon's Yeoman's Tale*, see SHAKESPEARE (1600), Boswell & Holton No. 656.

109.   SHEPPARD, SAMUEL. *The Secretaries Studie: Containing New Familiar Epistles.* S3169. UMI 1240: 4.

Sheppard (ca. 1624–1655?) is identified on the title page as "S. S." As Williams notes, in a section headed "Requesting Letters," in a letter that is "A Request to requite a Discourtesie," he alludes to *The Merchant's Tale*:

> In those Poeticall fictions, such were the prerogatives of deity, that whatsoever one God confirmed, no other would disallow: . . . . So that if *Tiresias* were stricken blind, there was no restoring of his eyes, however hee might bee helped with the gift of Divination. If *Jupiter* give again the sight to *January*, (as in *Chaucers* tale) to discover his wives incontinency, *Juno* could quicken her spirits to find such a witty answer as might pacifie all indignation. (205–6)

110.   WHARTON, GEORGE. "To my Very Honoured Friend," in Gaultier de Coste, Seigneur de La Calprenède's *Hymen's Præludia: or, Love's Master-Piece. Being that So-Much-Admired Romance, Intituled, Cleopatra. In Twelve Parts. . . . Now rendred into English, by Robert Loveday.* L111. UMI Thomason Tracts 176: E1327 (1).

As Spurgeon notes (1: 228), Sir George Wharton (1617–1681) links Chaucer and Gower and notes their role in refining the English language. In a commendatory poem headed "To my very Honoured Friend Mr. Robert Loveday upon this His Matchless Version, Entituled Love's Master-piece," Wharton writes:

> S*ir*, there is nothing that offends Mee so
> (Next to my *Sins*) as these your *Lines*) must goe
> For a *Translation*, which no lesse exceed
> The *French*, than *Fertile-Nile* the *Barren Tweed*:
> . . . .
> *Chaucer* and *Gow'r* our *Language* but *Refin'd*,
> You (*SIR*) true *Chemist*-like, have it *Calcin'd*,
> *Hew'd* out the *Barbarous Knots*, and made it *Run*
> As *Smooth*, as doth the *Chariot* of the *Sun*;
> Whilst *French* is but the *Foyle*, to let us see
> The *Lustre* of our *Tongue's Propriety*.
>   And this *Choyce worke* more fitly styled is
>   (Not onely *LOVE'S*, but) *LOVE-DAYE'S* Master-piece. (sig. A6v)

Another edition in 1652: *Cleopatra* (L110A), has no commendatory poems.

Other editions: L112 (1654), sig. A4v; L112A (1657), sig. A4v; L112B (1663), sig. A4v; L122 (1665), sig. A4v; L122A (1668), sig. A4v; L123 (1674), sig. A4v; L124 (1687), sig. A4v; L124A (1698), sig. A4v.

111. WILLIAMS, ROGER. *The Bloody Tenent yet More Bloody.* W2760. UMI Thomason Tracts 101: E.661 (6).

Williams (1604–1683) is identified on the title page as a resident of "Providence in New-England." Writing a rejoinder to John Cotton's *The Bloudy Tenent, Washed, and Made White in the Bloud of the Lambe* (1644), Williams possibly alludes to *The General Prologue* (lines 208–11) where in his description of the Friar, Chaucer mentions the four orders of friars. Williams' work is cast as a dialogue between "Peace" and "Truth," and they debate the power of the clergy to enforce spiritual conformity. "Peace" says, "But Mr [John] Cotton will say, Gods people would live at peace in Godlinesse and Honestie." "Truth" replies:

> I remember when old *Chaucer* puts this *Querie* to the foure chiefe sorts of *Fryers* in his Time [which of the *foure sorts* is the best] he finds every sort applauding it selfe, whence in Conclusion he finds them all guilty of *Lying* (in a round) before *God*, for all profest themselves to be the only *godly* men.

> I may now ask, who among all the sorts of *Churches* and *Ministers* applaud not themselves (like the *Fryars* in *Chaucers* dayes) to be *Christs* onely *Churches, Chirsts Ministers,* &c. [In a shoulder note: "Fryars in *Chaucers* time and the *Clergie* in our time considered."] (252)

1653

112. BAKER, RICHARD. *A Chronicle of the Kings of England. The Second Edition with Divers Additions.* B503. UMI 1394: 48.

Baker (1568–1645) is identified on the title page as "Sir R. Baker Knight." For references to Chaucer as John of Gaunt's brother-in-law, "the Homer of our nation," his association with Woodstock, his translation of *The Romaunt of the Rose*, his burial place in Westminster, and his association with Gower, see BAKER, B501 (1643); in this edition, the passages are found on 191, 193–94, 224, 240.

In this edition, the passage regarding Chaucer as "the Homer of our nation" is marked with a shoulder note: "Sir *Geoffrey Chaucer* lived at this time" (194); and the passage for *The Romaunt of the Rose* is also marked: "The *Romant of the Rose*, translated into *English* by *Geoffry Chawcer*, by whom composed" (224). In the index, Chaucer is also featured in a glaring error: "Sir *Geoffry Chawcer*, our English *Homer*, and when he lived . . . he marryed the daughter of *John* of *Gaunt*" (sig. Iii1r).

Another edition in 1653: B503A, same pagination.

113.   CHAPMAN, GEORGE. *Caesar and Pompey: a Roman Tragedy.* C1947. UMI Thomason Tracts 110: E.714 (17).

For an echo of a line from *The Reeve's Tale*, see CHAPMAN (1631) in Appendix; in this edition, the passage is found on sig. C4v.

114.   CLEVELAND, JOHN. *Poems. By J. C.* C4688. UMI 734: 4.

For an echo of a line from *The Manciple's Prologue*, see CLEVELAND (1644); in this edition, the passage is found on 65.
   Another edition in 1653: C4689, 90.

115.   FLECKNOE, RICHARD. *Miscellanea: or, Poems of All Sorts.* F1231. UMI Thomason Tracts 174: E.1295 (1).

Flecknoe (d. 1678?) is identified on the title page a "Richard Fleckno." He was a poet and playwright, but he is best remembered today for his role in Dryden's *Mac Flecknoe.* As Spurgeon notes (3: 4.72), here Flecknoe quotes Chaucer's description of the Sergeant of Law from *The General Prologue* (lines 321–22). In "A Letter treating of Conversation, Acquaintance and freindship [*sic*], Written to a noble Freind [*sic*], during his Residence in Rome," in a passage about various types of men whose company and conversation he advises his friend to avoid, Flecknoe writes:

> One of whome is Chawcer's busy man, of whom it may well be sayd, *That a busier man nere was, and yet he seemed far busier than he was*, out of whose way ile [*sic*] timely get me gone, least whilst he observes only those above mee, for haste to get up to them, he tramples all below him underfoot. (126–27)

Another edition in 1653: F1231aA.

116.   GATAKER, THOMAS. *Vindication of the Annotations.* G328. UMI 531: 8.

Gataker (1574–1654) is identified on the title page as "Thomas Gataker B.D." In a passage about William Lilly's "prophetical skill," Gataker, a brilliant humanist scholar, suggests first that Lilly (1602–1681),[18] a well known astrologer and advocate of "judiciary astrologie," succeeds Tiresias "as his rightful heir, and a

---

[18] See Derek Parker, *Familiar to All: William Lilly and Astrology in the 17th Century* (London: Jonathan Cape, 1975), 236. Lilly was an authority on angels and fairies and a writer whose annual almanacs were known throughout the land (sales reached close to 30,000 in 1649). Patrick Curry writes that in the 1650s these almanacs were translated into Dutch, German, Swedish, and Danish. Popular as he was, however, Lilly found himself increasingly out of step with the Restoration world and was famously mocked as the astrologer Sidrophel in Samuel Butler's *Hudibras*. See *ODNB* 33.794–98.

genuine bird of that kind." Gataker continues with a reference to Chaucer and the *Canterbury Tales*, and echoes a line from *The Wife of Bath's Tale* (line 880):

> But it may wel be, as some other would have it, that *Incubus*, of which his *Ancester Merlin* was bred, was no other then such an one, as our old Poet Chaucer in his *Canterburie Tales* saith in his days were so rife and ready at hand in most places, that for loose creatures, such as belike Merlines mother was, *no other Incubus* then such then needed. (60)

Other editions in 1653: G329, 60; G330, 60; G331, 60; G331a, 60; G331b, 60; G331c, 60.

117.   HARRINGTON, JOHN. *A Briefe View of the State of the Church of England as It Stood in Q. Elizabeths and King James His Reigne.* H770. UMI 356: 6.

Harrington (1560–1612) is identified on the title page as "Sir John Harington, of Kelston neer Bath, Knight." In giving a "character and history of the bishops of those times" (title page), he appears to echo a line from *The Reeve's Tale*: "The gretteste clerkes been noght wisest men" (line 4054). In a section headed "Of St. Davids, and the present Bishop Dr. Anthony Rudd," he writes of Queen Elizabeth's visit to the cathedral and her reaction to Dr. Rudd's sermon in which he touched on "the infirmities of age." Harrington writes:

> The Queen as the manner was opened the window, but she was [so] farre from giving him thanks or good countenance, that she said plainly he should have kept his Arithmetick for himselfe, but I see said she the greatest Clerks are not the wisest men, and so went away for the time discontented. (162)

118.   LUPTON, DONALD. *England's Command on the Seas: or, The English Seas Guarded.* L3489. UMI 2592: 5.

Lupton (d. 1676) concludes a section headed "Of the English Soveraignty [*sic*] of the Seas," with a reference to Chaucer and attributes a quotation to him that echoes a line from his description of the Merchant in *The General Prologue* (line 277):

> [I]n the Reign of the same King [Henry VI], the Commons desired, and did think it fit that the seas be kept. . . . And no lesse appears by *Chaucer* who lived in the time of King *Richard* the second, a famous Poet, who sayes (*ut mare custodiretur*) that the sea might be guarded and kept, and he gives this reason.
> *Keep your seas 'twixt* Orwel *and Middleborough still,*
> *You'l be sure to have wealth Flow in at your will.* (50–51)

119.   PARTRIDGE, JOHN. *The Treasury of Hidden Secrets.* P628. UMI 1533: 12.

For a commendatory poem that appears to echo a line from *Troilus and Criseyde*, see PARTRIDGE (1582) in the Appendix; in this edition, the passage is found on sig. A2v.

120.   TWISSE, WILLIAM. *The Riches of Gods Love unto the Vessells of Mercy.* T3423. UMI 117: 1.

Twisse (1578?–1646), a clergyman and theologian, rose to be Prolocutor of the Westminster Assembly and thus was reckoned one of the most prominent churchmen of the Commonwealth; he is identified on the title page as "that great and famous light of Gods Church, William Twisse D.D." In a passage about the authority of the ancients (those who lived near the time of the apostles), Twisse declares that "soundnesse of faith is grounded upon the soundnesse of interpretation of Gods word" not on chronology. He continues with a reference to Chaucer:

> If only by relation from others, the same exceptions lye against this and over and above, this must be of somewhat farre lesse authority then the former: it being so difficult a matter to report from another without adding somewhat of his own, whether it be much or little, as *Chaucer* speaketh. (42)

121.   VERSTEGEN (OR ROWLANDS), RICHARD. *A Restitution of Decayed Intelligence in Antiquities.* V269. UMI 619: 6

For references to Chaucer's translation of *The Romaunt of the Rose*, to his contributions to the English language, and to his diction, see ROWLANDS (1605) in Boswell & Holton No. 723; in this edition, the passages are found on 156, 158, 164, 195, and sig. S8v.

Other editions: V270 (1655), 156, 158, 164, 195, and sig. S8v; V271 (1673), 218, 222, 231, 274, sig. Bb5r.

122.   WALLIS, JOHN. *Grammatica linguæ anglicanæ.* W584. UMI Thomason Tracts 174: E.1293 (2).

Although Spurgeon notes (1: 229) that there is a reference to Chaucer, she does not record it. In "Tractatus Prœmialis," section 3, "De Consonantibus," Wallis writes:

> 3 quam pro *y* consonâ perpetuò scribebant, quæ etiam in illis vocibus (ut dictum est) reperitur quæ nunc per *gh* scribuntur: Hunc autem characterem, prout tunc pingi solebat, nescienter forsan posteriores librarii, ipsus loco characterem literæ *z* fœdissimo errore substituderunt; unde monstra illa vocabulorum *thouzt, souzt*, &c. pro *thought, sought*, &c. seu potiùs pro *thouyt, souyt*, (prout tunc nempe per *y*consonam scribi sole-

bant) in impressis Chauceri aliorúnq[ue] veterum poetarum libris con-
spiciuntur. (34)

In the editions of 1674, the passage is amended to read: "unde monstra illa vocab-
ulorum thouƷt, souƷt, &c."
Another edition in 1653: W584a, same pagination.
Other editions: W585 (1664), 34; W586 (1674), 24; W586a (1674), 24.

123.   WATERHOUSE, EDWARD. *An Humble Apologie for Learning and Learned Men.* W1048. UMI 44: 4.

Waterhouse (1619–1670) is identified on the title page as "Edward Waterhous,
Esq." In a passage about "the great Masters of Learning, and the most notable
Advancers of it," Waterhouse cites the examples of Chaucer and Gower:

> Our Annals tell us of some of the Laity, that for their on pleasures have
> been versed in Books, and Writers of Books: . . . [including] *Chaucer* and
> *Gower* Poets, the refines of our Language *in anno* 1400. (70)

124.   WITHER, GEORGE. *The Modern States-man. By G. W. Esq.* W3172. UMI 1981: 13.

In an epistle addressed to the reader, Wither (1558–1667) claims that he gathered
"a few conceptions and observations hudled together during my confinement to
my Chamber by an arrest from Heaven." In chapter 21, "Of the Causes of Prudence, Natural parts, Experience, Learning, Travel, &c.," he echoes a line from
The Reeve's Tale: "The gretteste clerkes been noght wisest men" (line 4054). In a
section about experience, Wither writes:

> [N]atural abilities, and learning do often make men opiniative, and to
> presume themselves knowing and wise: but it is experience that brings
> solidity. The greatest Clerks are not alwaies the wisest men. (197)

Another edition: W3172A (1654), 197.

1654

125.   BAKER, R., in Guido Bentivoglio's *The Compleat History of the Warrs of Flanders.* Trans. by Henry Carey, Earl of Monmouth. B1910. UMI 83: 6.

There is a reference to "Squire Jeffrey," an allusion to Chaucer and the state of the
language in his time, in a commendatory poem by "R. Baker."

There are who *Languages* a *Mysterie*
Would make, that yet does undiscover'd lie;
Boasting the *Spaniard* lofty, *Toscan* sweet,
And *aery-French* to dance with gracefull feet;
Whose *well-turn'd-Layes*, in Times, then *Ours*, less rude,
By such, whose hasty *Vanity* t'intrude
Into the *Press*, having been rendered hoarse,
Sense, and Words massacred without remorse:
Those, by *Fantastick prejudice*, condemn,
Young *Travellers* infection, root and stem
Of all *Translations*; as implicitly,
As some damn all who on a *Scaffold* dy.
But 'tis not now as when *Squire-Jeffrey* liv'd,
The tongue's not cramp'd ere it can be repriev'd;
Words, here, are facil, apt, significant;
Such, as not make the *Sense* too wide, nor scant. (sig. B2r)

Another edition in 1654: B1911A, following title page.

126.   BLOUNT, THOMAS. *The Academie of Eloquence*. B3321. UMI 14: 20.

Blount (1618–1679) is identified on the title page as "Tho. Blount Gent." In a section headed "An English Rhetorique exemplified," he echoes the title of *The House of Fame*. In a segment about the proper use of rhetorical exclamation, Blount writes:

Exclamation is not lawful, but in the extremity of motion. . . . *Europe, how canst thou be famous?* . . . But Europe is the house of Fame, *because it is the Nursery of Arts, and Books, wherein reports are preserved. O weak imagination!* (29)

Other editions: B3322 (1656), 29; B3323 (1663), 29; B3324 (1664), 29; B3325 (1670), 29; B3326 (1683), 29.

127.   BRAMHALL, JOHN. *A Just Vindication of the Church of England from the Unjust Aspersion of Criminal Schisme*. B4226. UMI 976: 8.

Identified on the title page as "Dr. in Divinity, and Lord Bishop of Derry," Bramhall (1594–1663) ultimately became Archbishop of Armagh and Lord Primate of Ireland. In chapter 6, "That the King and Church of England had both sufficient authority and sufficient grounds to withdraw their obedience from Rome, and did it with due moderation," he commends Chaucer, alludes to *The Canterbury Tales* and refers to the spurious work known as Chaucer's *Ploughman's Tale*. Bramhall writes:

Those who desire to know what opinion the English had of the greedi-
nesse and extortion of the Court of *Rome*, may find them drawn out to
the life by Chaucer in sundry places. [In a shoulder note: "Plowmans
tale and else where."] (134)

Another edition: B4227 (1661), 134.
Also found in Bramhall's *Works*: B4210 (1676), 93.

128.   CLEVELAND, JOHN. *The Idol of the Clownes: or, Insurrection of Wat the
Tyler, with His Priests Baal and Straw.* C4673. UMI 310: 3.

Spurgeon (1: 235) cites this reference in Cleveland's *Works* (1687) rather than this
earlier edition. In his account of Wat Tyler's rebellion, Cleveland recall's Chaucer's reference to Jack Straw's riot in *The Nun's Priest's Tale*, quotes modernized
versions of lines 3389, 3393–96:

Our most famous *Chaucer* flourishing then, in his description of this
terrible fright, and noyse, at the carrying away of *Chanticlere* the Cock
by *Reinold* the Fox, reflects upon these cries, but in an Hyperbole of his
Poeticall feined ones, and much undervaluing the horrour of the *Kentish*
throats, as he will have it.

𝔗𝔥𝔢𝔶 𝔶𝔢𝔩𝔩𝔢𝔫 𝔞𝔰 𝔉𝔦𝔢𝔫𝔡𝔰 𝔟𝔢 𝔦𝔫 𝔥𝔢𝔩𝔩, &𝔠.
𝔖𝔬 𝔥𝔦𝔡𝔢𝔬𝔲𝔰 𝔴𝔞𝔰 𝔱𝔥𝔢 𝔫𝔬𝔶𝔰𝔢, A benedicte!
𝔠𝔢𝔯𝔱𝔢𝔰 𝔍𝔞𝔠𝔨-𝔖𝔱𝔯𝔞𝔴 𝔫𝔢 𝔥𝔦𝔰 𝔪𝔢𝔶𝔫𝔱𝔶
ℜ𝔢 𝔪𝔞𝔡𝔢 𝔰𝔥𝔬𝔲𝔱𝔰 𝔥𝔞𝔩𝔣𝔢 𝔰𝔬 𝔰𝔥𝔯𝔦𝔩𝔩,
𝔚𝔥𝔢𝔫 𝔱𝔥𝔢𝔶 𝔴𝔬𝔲𝔩𝔡 𝔞𝔫𝔶 𝔉𝔩𝔢𝔪𝔪𝔦𝔫𝔤 𝔨𝔦𝔩𝔩.

The *Lombards* scaped better, they were onely robbed of what they
had. . . . (36–37)

A reissue with new title: *The Rustick Rampant: or Rural Anarchy Affronting Monarchy* (1658), same pagination.
Also found in Cleveland's *Works*: C4654 (1687), 424; C4655 (1699), 424.

129.   CLEVELAND, JOHN. *Poems.* C4689A. UMI 734: 5.

For an echo of a line from *The Manciple's Prologue*, see CLEVELAND (1644); in this
edition, the passage is found on 90.
Another edition in 1654: C4690, 90.

130.   GAYTON, EDMUND. *Pleasant Notes upon Don Quixot.* G415. UMI 145: 6.

Gayton (1608–1666) is identified on the title page as "Edmund Gayton, Esq." As
Spurgeon notes (3: 4.72), Gayton refers to January and May, perhaps an allusion

to the *Merchant's Tale* in book 2. In a section about parents who arrange the marriages of their children without regard to their likes or dislikes:

> Miserable must needs be the condition of two so joyn'd, especially . . . unfortunate it is, when fifteen joines to seventy, there's old doings (as they say) the Man and Wife fitting together like *January* and *May* day, his Nose with *Isicles* dangling. (50)

As Spurgeon (1: 229) notes, in book 3, chapter 9, in a passage about English poets, Gayton begins with Chaucer:

> Our Nation also had its Poets, and they their wives: To pass the Bards: Sir *Jeffery Chaucer* liv'd very honestly at Woodstock, with his Lady, (the house yet remaining), and wrote against the vice most wittily, which Wedlocke restraines. (150)

131.   MENNES, JOHN. *Recreation for Ingenious Head-peeces, or, A Pleasant Grove for Their Wits to Walk In.* **M1714. UMI 1508: 9.**

For an epitaph "On our prime English Poet, *Geffrey Chaucer*," see MENNES (1641). The epitaph is originally from Lydgate's prologue to his translation of Boccaccio's *The Falle of Princes*; see BOCCACCIO (1494) in Boswell & Holton No. 27. In this edition, the passage is found on sig. F11v.

For a reference to Chaucer in an epitaph "On William Shake-speare," see *Wits Recreations* (1640) in Boswell & Holton No. 1377; in this edition, the passage is found on sig. F12r.

132.   PRIDEAUX, MATHIAS. *An Easy and Compendious Introduction for Reading All Sorts of Histories.* **P3441. UMI 1468: 7.**

For a reference to "diverse passages" in Chaucer's works that are "useful" for students of history, see PRIDEAUX, P3439 (1648); in this edition, the passage is found on 349.

133.   ROGERS, JOHN. *Sagrir: or, Doomes-day Drawing Nigh, with Thunder and Lightning to Lawyers.* **R1815. UMI 47: 11.**

Rogers (1627–1665?) is described on the title page as "an unfained Servant of Christ, and this Common-wealth." In a passage about oaths, he appears to echo the description of the shipman in *The General Prologue*: "Of nyce conscience took he no keep" (line 398). Rogers writes:

> [A] *Gentlewoman* . . . was left a *Widow* to some considerable *Estate* and *Goods*, but the *Court* requiring her to take *oath*, that the *Inventory* was true, she refused it, not *scrupelling* that *oath*, but any *oath*; the *Court*

perceiving her (out of *Conscience*) *inflexible*, up starts one of the *Lawyers* (who never saw her before; nor since) Ha! says he! this *Gentlewoman* hath a *nice conscience* truly. (80)

One might think that a term like *nice conscience* would be a commonplace; however, it turns up only eight times outside Chaucer's works.

134.   S., W., in John Bullokar's *An English Expositor: Teaching the Interpretation of the Hardest Words Used in Our Language.* **B5429A. UMI 2635: 6.**

In this revised, corrected, and augmented edition ("above a thousand words enlarged. By W. S.") of Bullokar's perennially popular work, W. S. introduces a definition that refers to Chaucer and *The Prologue to The Squire's Tale*:

> *Chivancy.* Chivalry; riding. So Chaucers Interpreter; but I conceive with
> a mistake for Chivancie, or Cheuancie. See the Squires Prologue. (sig.
> E4r)

Other editions: B5429 (1641), UMI 1417: 12, not present; B5430 (1656), sig. E4r; B5430A (1663), sig. D7r; B5431 (1667), sig. B12r; B5431A (1671), sig. B12r; B5432 (1676), sig. B12r; B5433 (1680), sig. B12r; B5434 (1684), sig. B12r; B5435 (1688), sig. B12r; B5435A (1695), sig. B12r; B5436 (1698), sig. B12r.

135.   SCOTT, REGINALD. *Scot's Discovery of Witchcraft.* **S944. UMI 822: 21**

For references to Chaucer in Scot's bibliography, for quotations from *The Cannon's Yeoman's Prologue and Tale* and *The Wife of Bath's Tale* and an echo of a line from *The Reeve's Tale*; in this edition, the passages are found on sig. B4v and 67–68, 249, 250–51, 253, 344.

136.   TWISSE, WILLIAM, in Joseph Mede's *The Apostasy of the Latter Times.* **M1593. UMI 1955: 1.**

For an allusion to the Clerk and a quotation from *The General Prologue*, see TWISSE (1641), M1590; in this edition, the passage is found on sig. A2r.

137.   WHARTON, GEORGE. "To my Very Honoured Friend," in Gaultier de Coste, Seigneur de La Calprenède's *Hymen's Præludia: or, Love's Master-Piece. Now Rendred into English by Robert Loveday.* **L112. UMI 569: 6.**

For a reference to Chaucer and Gower as a pair who refined the English language, see WHARTON (1652); in this edition, the passage is found on sig. A4v.

138.   WILSON, THOMAS. *A Complete Christian Dictionarie.* **W2942. No UMI.**

For an echo of a line from *Troilus and Criseyde*, see WILSON (1612) in the Appendix.

139.   WITHER, GEORGE. *The Modern States-man. By G. W. Esq.* W3172A.
UMI Thomason Tracts 195: E.1452(2).

See Wither (1653); in this edition, the passage is found on 197.

1655

140.   BRIAN, THOMAS. *The Pisse-Prophet: or, Certaine Pisse-Pot Lectures.* B4437.
UMI 1198: 7.

For an echo of a line in *The Manciple's Prologue*, see BRIAN (1637) in the Appendix; in this edition, the passage is found on 47.

141.   CARTER, MATTHEW. *Honor Rediviuus* [sic]: *or, An Analysis of Honor and Armory.* C658. UMI Thomason Tracts 186: E.1458(2).

Carter (*fl.* 1660) is identified on the title page as "Matt: Carter Esq." He uses Chaucer's escutcheon to illustrate a point:

> The second quarter bears party *per* pale, a bend counter-changed *Argent*
> & *Gules*, by Sir *Geofry Caucer* [sic]. (46; sig. C7v, pagination irregular)

Another edition in 1655: C658A (1655).
      Other editions: C659 (1660), 134 (Chaucer's name corrected); C659A (1660);
C661 (1673), 225, (+ 348); C661A (1692), 225, (+ 348).

142.   DAVENPORT, ROBERT. *King John and Matilda.* D370. UMI 312: 12.

Davenport is described on the title page as "Robert Davenport Gent." This tragedy "was acted with great applause by Her Majesties servants at the Cock-pit in Drury-Lane" (title page). Davenport includes an echo of the Wife of Bath's claim that "Women desiren have sovereyntee" (*The Wife of Bath's Tale*, line 1038). In 5.1, Fitzwater speaks to the Matilda:

> [W]omen naturally
> Do affect soveraignty. (sig. H1v)

Another edition: D371 (1662), sig. G1v.

143.   FULLER, THOMAS. *The Church-History of Britain.* F2416. UMI 1357: 16;
UMI 843: 9.

Fuller (1608–1661) cites Chaucer often. Spurgeon (1: 230–31) notes references to Chaucer in books 4 and 6, but there are many more.

In book 1, in a section headed "The Fifth Century," in a passage about life and learning in Saxon times, Fuller alludes to *The Wife of Bath's Tale* (line 880):

> This Age is assigned by Authors for that Famous *Ambrose Merlin* . . . though it be doubtfull whether ever such a man *in rerum natura*; it being suspicious, . . . Because it was said his Mother was a Nun, got with Child by a Devil in the form of an *Incubus*; perchance such a one as *Chaucer* describes. (38)

In book 2, "The Seventh Century," in a passage in commendation of the English language, Fuller comments on the difficulty of Chaucer's English for contemporaries:

> Other Tongues are daily disguised with forrain Words, so that in a Century of years, they grow Strangers to themselves: as now an *English*-man needs an Interpreter to understand *Chaucer*'s English. (65)

Following book 2, Fuller gives us "Severall Copies Battle-Abbey Roll," in which the name *Chaucer* appears in Stow's transcription (156). In another catalogue "late in the possession of *Thomas Scriven*," the name *Chaucer* again appears (166).

In book 3, in a section headed "Cent. XI," in a passage about Henry I's succession to the throne following William Rufus, Fuller appears to echo a line from *The Reeve's Tale*: "The gretteste clerkes been noght wisest men" (line 4054). He writes:

> *Henry Beauclarke*, his brother, succeeded him in the Throne, one that crossed the common proverb, *The greatest Clerks are not the wisest men*, being one of the most profoundest Scholars, and most politick Princes in his generation. (13)

In book 3, in the third section of century thirteen, in a passage about Merton College (Oxford), Fuller appears to allude to *The Reeve's Tale*:

> Amongst the many *Manors* which the first *Founder* [i.e., Walter de Merton, Bishop of Rochester and Chancellor of England] bestowed on this *Colledg* [*sic*], one lay in the *Parish* of St *Peters* and *West suburbe* of *Cambridg* [*sic*], beyond the *Bridg* [*sic*], anciently called *Pythagoras house*, since *Merton Hall*. To this belongeth much good Land thereabout (as also the *Mills* at *Grantchester* mentioned in *Chaucer*) those of *Merton Colledg* [*sic*] keeping yearly a *Court Baron* here. (275)

In book 3, in a section devoted to learned men of fourteenth-century England, in a passage about Thomas Bradwardine, Fuller quotes three slightly modernized lines from *The Nun's Priest's Tale* (lines 3230–33):

> *Thomas Bradwardine* [was] . . . in learning and piety (if not superiour) equal to any. . . . This *Bradwardine* was afterwards Arch-Bishop of Canterbury, and highly esteemed, let *Chaucer* tell you [in a shoulder note: "In the nuns Priests tale."].

> 𝕭ut 𝕴 ne cannot boult it to the bren,
> 𝕬s can the holy 𝕯octour 𝕾t 𝕬ustin,
> 𝕺r 𝕭oece, or the 𝕭ishop 𝕭radwardin.

> This testimony of *Chaucer* by the exact computation of time, written within forty years after *Bradwardines* death, which addeth much to his honour, that in so short a time his memory was in the peaceable possession of so general a veneration, as to be joyned in companhy with St *Augustine* and *Boethius*, two such eminent persons in their several capacities. (298)

In book 4, in a section about the life and literary works of John Wicklife, Fuller writes:

> We may couple with him, his contemporary *Geffery Chaucer*, born (some say) in *Berke-shire*, others in *Oxford-shire*, most and truest in *London*. If the Grecian *Homer* had seven, let our English have three places contest for his Nativity. Our *Homer* (I say) onely herein he differed . . . *Homer* himself did leave no pelf. Whereas our *Chaucer* left behind him a rich and worshipful estate. [In a shoulder note, Fuller writes that Wicklife managed to escape persecution, "As did his contemporary *Geoffery Chaucer*."]
>
> His Father was a Vintner in *London*; and I have heard his Armes quarell'd at, being *Argent* and *Gules* strangely contrived, and hard to be blazon'd. Some more wits have made it the dashing of white and red wine (the parents of our ordinary Claret) as nicking his fathers profession. But were *Chaucer* alive, he would justifie his own Armes in the face of all his opposers, being not so devoted to the Muses, but he was also a son of *Mars*. He was the Prince of English Poets; married the daughter of *Pain Roët*, King of Armes in *France*, and sister to the Wife of *John* of *Gaunt*, King of *Castile*. [In a shoulder note: "His parentage and armes."]
>
> He was a great *Refiner*, and *Illuminer* of our English tongue (and if he left it so bad, how much worse did he find it?) witness *Leland* thus

praising him . . . [Here Fuller quotes Leland's quatrain that praises
Chaucer and yokes him with Dante and Petrarch; see LELAND (1542),
Boswell & Holton No. 146).] Indeed *Versetgan* [in a shoulder note: "In
his restitution of the decaied intelligence, 203."], a learned Antiquary,
condemns him, for spoiling the purity of the English tongue, by the
mixture of so many French and Latin words. But, he who mingles wine
with water, though he destroies the nature of water, improves the quality thereof.

I finde this *Chaucer* fined in the Temple two shillings, for striking a Franciscan Frier in *Fleet-street*, and it seems his hands ever after
itched to be revenged, and have his penniworths out of them, so *tick-
ling* Religious-Orders with his *tales*, and yet so *pinching* them with his
truths, that Friers in reading his books, know not how to dispose their
faces betwixt *crying* and *laughing*. [In a shoulder note: "A great enemy
to Friers."] He lies buried in the South-Isle of *St Peters, Westminster,*
and since hath got the company of *Spencer* and *Drayton* (a pair-royal of
Poets) enough (almost) to make passengers feet to move metrically, who
go over the place, where so much *Poetical dust* is interred. (²151–52)

In book 6, "The History of Abbeys," in a passage about Augustinian monks,
Fuller quotes from the spurious work known as Chaucer's *Ploughman's Tale*:

These *Augustinians* were also called *Canons Regular,* where, by the way,
I meet with such a nice distinction, which disheartens me from pretend-
ing to exactnesse in reckoning up these Orders. For this I finde in our
English Ennius [in a shoulder note: "*Chaucer* in the Plow-mans Tale."]:

And all such other Counterfaitours
Chanons, Canons and such disguised
Been Goddes enemies and Traytours
His truye religion han foule despised. [*sic*]

It seems the *H* here amounteth to a letter so effectuall as to discriminate
Chanons from *Canons* . . . but what should be the difference betwixt
them, I dare not interpose my conjecture. (²268)

In book 10, in the fourth section of century seventeen, in a passage about Isaac
Causabon, the learned French cleric, Fuller notes Chaucer's burial place in Westminster Abbey:

[H]e lieth entombed in the South-Ile of *Westminster*-Abbey. Not on the East, or Poetical Side thereof, (where *Chaucer, Spencer, Draiton*,[19] are interred) but on the West or Historical Side of the Ile, next the Monument of Mr. *Camden*. (469)

In a section headed "The History of the University of Cambridge, Since the Conquest," in a passage about Clare Hall, Fuller quotes a pair of slightly modernized lines from *The Reeve's Tale* (lines 3989–90):

This CLARE-Hall was also called *Solere Hall* in the daies of *Chaucer*, as our Antiquary hath observed [in a shoulder note: "*Chaucer* in the *Reves* tale."].

And namely there was a great College
Men clepen it the Solers hall of Cambrege.

Some will say, And whence termed *Solere* Hal [*sic*]? (538)

In a passage about events that occurred during the reign of Edward III, Fuller cites lines from *The Court of Love*, attributed to Chaucer by John Stow in his edition of 1651 (see Boswell & Holton No. 210), and *The Astrolabe* (lines 1–5 or 20–25):

About this time [1373] GEFFREY CHAUCER studied in Cambridge, as the Writer of his Life (prefixed to the last and best Edition of his Works) hath well observed [in a shoulder note: "*Chaucer* a *Cambridge* Student."] For, being commanded to give an account of himself [in a shoulder note: "*In his Court of Love, fol.* 352."],

What is your name, reherse it here I pray,
Of whens and where, of what condition
That ye been of, let see, come off and say,
Faine would I know your disposicion:

He returned under the assumed name of PHILOGENET,

Of Cambridge Clerk.

Here *Clerk* is not taken in the restrictive sense, for one in Orders (CHAUCER being a militarie man) but for a Scholar, skill'd in Learn-

---

[19] Draiton, i.e., Michael Drayton.

ing; in which Contradistinction all men were divided (as *Time* into *Day & Night*) into *Clerks*, and *no Clerks*. I confesse this CHAUCER, living at *New-Elme* in *Oxfordshire*, *compowned his Astrolabye for the Orizont of Oxenford* [in a shoulder note: "*In his Astrolaby, fol.* 261], and probably studied also in that University, being one of that Merit, who may with Honour be acknowledged a Member of both Universities. (§52–53)

Another edition: F2417 (1656), 38, 65, 75, 98, ²151–52, ⁴69, ⁵38, §52–53.

144.   GUILD, WILLIAM. *Anti-Christ Pointed and Painted Out in His True Colours, or, The Popes of Rome Proven to Bee That Man of Sinne and Sonne of Perdition Fore-prophesied in Scripture.* G2203. UMI 1332: 26.

Guild (1586–1657) is identified on the title page as "William Guild, Doctor of Divinitie, and preacher of Gods word." In chapter 8, "Antichrists Seat, or his place in particular . . . proved to be Rome," Guild cites Chaucer and quotes from *The Ploughman's Tale*:

A worthie gentleman *Gefrey Chaucer*, of woodstok [*sic*] & *Elme* esquyre, Embassadour oftimes from king *Edward* the third to forraigne Princes, did plainlie expresse in his poeme of the plough-mans tale speaking first of the *Pope* himself thus;

> CHRIST sent the poore to preach,
> The royall rich Hee did not so,
> Now dare no poore the people teach,
> For Antichrist is all their foe.

And thereafter of his Clergie hee speaketh thus.

> CHRISTS Ministers clepen they beene
> And rule all in robberie,
> But *Antichrist* they serven cleane
> Attyred in all tyrrannie. (74)

In chapter 10, "Of Antichrists exorbitant & matchlesse Pride," Guild again cites Chaucer and quotes the spurious work known as Chaucer's *Ploughman's Tale*:

[Matthew of Paris says] That the Pope beyound all mortall men was the most ambitious and proudest. As likewise made that worshipfull Gentleman, and great poet in his time *Gefrey Chaucer*, of whom we spoke before [in a shoulder note: "anno 1340"], to say of the Pope, as head of the Roman Church, in his plow-mans tale.

Her head loveth all honour,
...... 7 lines ......
Such pride before God doth stink. (87–88)

In chapter 11, "Of Antichrists sitting in the Temple of GOD, as GOD, Showing himself that he is GOD," Guild again cites Chaucer and quotes from *The
Ploughman's Tale*:

[T]hat worshipfull Gentleman forenamed *Gefrey Chaucer* speaketh thus
of the Pope in his tyme, in his Plow-mans tale.

And to Popes hest's such take more heed
...... 2 lines ......
They hold him whole Omnipotent. (93–94)

In chapter 14, "Of the Popes or Antichrists bloodie crueltie," Guild again turns
to Chaucer and *The Ploughman's Tale*:

[T]hat forecited worshipfull Esquyre and famous Poët in his time *Chaucer* [in a shoulder note: "Chaucer in his ploughmans Tale"] to speak thus
of the Pope and his Cleargie.

Were CHRIST on the earth eftsoone,
These would damne Him to die,
...... 5 lines ......
GOD Almightie them amend. (127–28)

In chapter 15, "Of Antichrists, or the Popes spirituall Merchandise or Simonie,"
Guild cites Chaucer and *The Ploughman's Tale* yet once more:

As likewise the worthie English Esquyre *Gefrey Chaucer* of Woodstock,
in his plowe-mans tale, 400 yeares ago, saying of the Popes Clergie.

They Christs people proudlie curse,
With brad book and braying bell,
To put pennies in their purse
They will sell both Heaven and hell. (144–45)

And finally, in chapter 17, "Of Antichrists or the Pope and his Clergie their
fained Miracles & lyeing wonders," Guild cites Chaucer (among other learned
authorities) and the spurious work known as Chaucer's *Ploughman's Tale*:

Likewise in the 1300 yeare of God, *Marsilius Patavinus* . . . affirmeth
that the Pope was that foretold *Antichrist*. So likewise did that worthie
gentleman & famous Poet in his time, *Gefrey Chaucer* in his plow-mans
tale at large. (170)

145. HALL, GEORGE. *The Triumphs of Rome over Despised Protestancie.* H337.
UMI 629: 10.

Hall (1612?–1668), the son of a bishop, rose through the ranks of the Church of
England to become Bishop of Chester. In chapter 3, "The triumph of Holinesse,"
in a passage about wicked priests, Hall cites Chaucer, doubtlessly alludes to *The
Canterbury Tales*:

> Ill Prelates . . . commit soules to the Devils to keep, that is, to lewde
> Curates which destroy them more then the Devils themselves; for the
> very Devils would not commit such riotous outrages, nor give so many
> wicked examples as they: not to make any reckoning of our *Jeffry Chau-
> cer* or their Fryar *Mantuan*, whose tongues shall passe for no slander.
> (35)

In chapter 12, "The triumph of Peace and Unanimity," Hall quotes from *The
Romaunt of the Rose*:

> [I]f it were possible for ought under heaven to be more vile then . . . the
> authors and abetytors of that everlasting Gospel which was set on foot
> by the *Benedictines* and *Franciscans*, about the yeer 1255. whereof our
> *Chaucer* thus [in a shoulder note: "*Geffr. Caucer* [sic] in the Rom. of the
> Rose fol. 163"]:

> > *For they through wicked invention,*
> > *In the yeer of the Incarnation*
> > *A thousand and two hundred yeare,*
> > *Five and fifty, furder ne neer,*
> > *Broughten a book with sorry grace,*
> > *To your ensample in common place,*
> > *That said thus; though it were fable,*
> > *This is the Gospel per durable*
> > *That from the Holy Ghost was sent;*
> > *Well were it worthy to be brent.* (141)

Another edition: H338 (1667), 30, 134–35.

146.   HEYWOOD, THOMAS, and WILLIAM ROWLY. *Fortune by Land and Sea. A Tragi-comedy.* H1783. UMI 147: 10.

In this piece "Acted with great Applause by the Queens Servants," Heywood (d. 1641) and Rowly (1585?–1642?) appear to allude to *The Nun's Priest's Tale.* In the first scene of the third act, Mrs. Anne Harding, asks Clown what he is doing in her chicken house, a place she was not expecting him to be. He wittily replies:

> We are going, as they way, to remove, or according to the vulgar, make clean, where Chanticleer and Damepartlet the henne have had some doings . . . to make clean this hen-roost. . . . (22)

147.   MASSINGER, PHILIP. *Three New Playes.* M1050. UMI Thomason Tracts 197: E.1559 (2).

Massinger (1583–1640) is characterized on the title page as a "gent." In *The Guardian,* "often acted at the private-house in Black-Friers, by His Majesties Servants, with great applause," Massinger appears to echo the description of the Wife of Bath in *The General Prologue,* "For she koude of that art the olde daunce" (line 476). Massinger writes:

> My Nephew is an ass,
> What a devil hath he to do with Virgin-honor,
> Altars, or lawful flames? when he should tell her
> They are superstitious nothings, and speak to the purpose,
> Of the delight to meet in the old dance
> Between a pair of sheets; my Grandame call'd it
> The peopling of the world. (sig. H2v; 8, pagination is confused)

148.   MENNES, JOHN. *Musarum deliciæ: or, the Muses Recreation. By Sr J. M. and Ja: S.* M1710. UMI Thomason Tracts 209: E.1672 (1).

As Spurgeon notes (1: 231), Mennes (1599–1671) imitates Chaucer in verses headed "*Partus Chauceri Posthumus* Gulielmi Nelson":

> Listen you Lordlings to a noble game,
> Which I shall tell you, by thilk Lord S. Jame,
> Of a lewd Clerk, and of his haviour bold,
> He was, I trow, some threescore winters old.
> Of *Cambridge* was this Clerk, not *Oxenford,*
> Well known at *Stilton, Stewkey,* and *Stamford.*
> He haunted fenny Staunton, and Saint Ives,
> And fair could gloze among the Country Wives,
> A lusty Runnyon ware he in his hose,
> Lowd could he speak, and crackle in the Nose.

For Schollarship him card' him light or nought,
To serve his turn, he English Postills bought.
He us'd no colour, nor no Rhetorick,
But yet he couth some termes of art Logick,
He was full rude and hot in disputation,
And wondrous frequent in his predication.
For gravely couth he spit, fore he gan speak,
And in his mouth some Sugar-Candy break,
But yet his preaching was to small effect,
Though lowd he roar'd, inth' Northern Dialect.
He ware a Cassock deep, but of small cost,
His state was spent in Nutmeg, Ale and Toast.
A gauld back'd spittle Jade for travelling
He kept in summer, but the wintering
Too costly was, rode he early or later,
Nought was his provender but grass and water,
Well liquor'd were his Boots, & wondrous wide,
Ne Sword, ne Rapyer ware he by his side,
A long vast Cloak-bag was his Caryage
Ther nis the like from *Hull* unto *Carthage*.
But, sooth to say, he was for ay formall,
And ware a thred bare Cloak Canonicall.
He had a Deanship and a Parsonage,
Yet was in debt and danger all his age,
His greater summe he payes by borrowing,
And lesser scores, by often punishing.
If that a Problem, or a common place
Comes to his share, he is in jolly case;
Then to a Nape of Ling he would invite
Some Rascall Tapster, hardly worth a Mite.
    Well was he known in every Village Town,
The good Wives clep'd him Gossip up & down;
Oft was he Maudlin drunk, then would he weep,
Not for his sinnes, of them he took small keep:
It was the humour fell down from his eyn,
Distill'd from Ale, he drank but little wine;
And being asked why those teares did fall,
Soothly he preached at a Funerall.
And when with drinking he was some deal mellow,
His Motto was, *Faith Lad, I's halfe good fellow*.
Thus preach'd he often on an Ale-house Bench,
And, when the Spirit mov'd, cough'd for his Wench,
And Bastards got, which, if God send them grace,

They may succeed him in his Seniors place.
He was an idle Senior for the nonce,
Foul may befall his body, and his bones. (71–73)

These verses are followed by a quatrain, *"Upon the same"*:

Twice twenty Sermons, & twice five, I ween,
(And yet not one of them in print is seen)
He preach'd, God and St. *Mary's* witnesseth,
Where loud he roar'd, yet he had but little pith. (73)

Another poem, headed *"Imitatio Chauceri altera, In eundem,"* mentions January
and May and quotes at least one line of *The Merchant's Tale*, "Old fish, and young
flesh woll I haue full faine" (line 118):

Leave, *Jeffrey Chaucer*, to describen a Man
In thine old phrason, so well as I can.
I ken no glozing, for my wit is rude,
Nath'lesse I'le limb out his similitude.
Fierce was his look, 'twas danger him to meet,
He passed like a Tempest through the street.
Narrow his eyn, his Nose was Chamised,
Sawfleum his Face, forked his Beard and head.
Pardie I wot not what men doe him call,
Dan Thomas. ne Dan Richard, n'of what Hall
He is, ne Colledge; but, by th' holy Mattin,
He was a frequent guest at *John Port Lattin*;
And eke at all other dayes festivall,
He had a liquorous tooth over all;
Ne was there any Wight in all this Town,
That tasted better a Pasty of Venisoun,
Ybaked with Gravy Gods plenty,
It relished better then *Austin's* works or *Gregory*,
Yet politick he was, and worldly wise,
And purchac'd hath, a double Benefice.
Small was his Wage, and little was his hire,
He let his sheep accumber in the mire;
And solac'd at St. *Johns*, or at St. *Pauls*,
That was a Sanctuary for his Soules.
Sir *John* of them, must alwaies taken keep,
A shitten Sheepherd cannot make clean sheep.
Ne God *Mercurius*, ne *Melpomene*,
E're look'd upon him at's Nativity:

Or if they look'd, they looked all ascaunce,
So was he made a Priest by foule mischance.
Pardie he was of the worst clay y'maked,
That e're Dame Nature in her Furnace baked.
For in his youth he was a Serving man,
And busily on his Masters errand ran;
And fairely sore a Cloak-bag couth he ride,
Algates a rusty whinyard by his side;
And he that whilom could not change a groat,
Hath changed, for a Cassock, his blew Coat.
One cannot see the Body, nor the Bulke
That whilom did attend on aged Fulk;
A larger Gown hath all y'cover'd,
And a square Cap doth pent-house his sweynes head.
    Yet notes he got, when his Master disputed,
And when the learned Papists he confuted.
The Borel men sayn, he preach well ynough,
But others known, that he stoln all his stuffe.
    Lustfull he was, at Forty needs must wed,
Old *January* will have *May* in Bed,
And live in glee, for, as wise men have sayn,
Old Fish, and young Flesh, would I have fayn,
And thus he swinketh; but, to end my story,
Men sayn, he needs no other Purgatory. (74–75)

Another edition: M1711 (1656), 85–89.

149. **PLATTES, GABRIEL.** "A Caveat for Alchymists: or, A Warning to All Ingenious Gentlemen," in *Chymical, Medicial, and Chyrurgical Addresses Made to Samuel Hartlib*. UMI 2049: 35 (identified as H978); UMI Thomason Tracts: 193: E. 1509 (2).

The fourth address in this collection directed to Samuel Hartlib (ca. 1600, B1662) is described on the title page as "A Conference Concerning the Phylosophers Stone" and identified in the table of contents as *A Caveat for Alchymists* by "Gabriel Plats" (ca. 1600–1644). In a section headed "The fourth Cheat," Plattes summarizes the plot of *The Canon's Yeoman's Tale* from memory but admits that it has been twenty years since he read *The Canterbury Tales*. He also comments on the difficulty of readily finding a copy of Chaucer's *Tales*:

This Cheat is described in old *Chawcer*, in his *Canterbury* Tale; but because everyone hath not that book, I will relate it briefly, and those

that would see it more largely described, shall be referred to the said
book. . . . (81, really 79)

[T]he cheated found by experience, as he verily thought, and so was
earnest with the cheater to teach him his Art, but what bargain they
made I have for gotten, for it is twenty years since I read *Chawcers* book.

Now whereas I have received the reports of some of these Cheaters
in divers manners, yet I am sure that they being wrought according to
my prescription, will cheat almost any man that hath not read this book
of *Chawcers*, unless a man should happen upon one that knoweth the
great work, which is hardly to be found in ten Kingdoms . . . (80–81)

150.   PRIDEAUX, MATHIAS. *An Easy and Compendious Introduction for Reading All Sorts of Histories.* P3442. UMI 1512: 9.

For a reference to "diverse passages" in Chaucer's works that are "useful" for
students of history, see PRIDEAUX, P3439 (1648); in this edition, the passage is
found on 349.

151.   SHAKESPEARE, WILLIAM. *Mr. William Shake-speare, His True Chronicle History of the Life and Death of King Lear, and His Three Daughters.* S2957. UMI 297: 43.

The title page informs readers that the play "Was Plaid Before the Kings Majesty at Whit-Hall, upon S. Stephens Night, in Christmas Hollldaies [*sic*]. By His Majesties Servants, Playing Usually at the Globe on the Bankside."

For possible references and allusions to *The Monk's Tale*, to the spurious
"Merlin's Prophecy," and *Troilus and Criseyde*, see SHAKESPEARE (1608), Boswell
& Holton No. 783.

152.   SHAKESPEARE, WILLIAM. *Rape of Lucrece.* S2943. UMI 877: 24.

For possible contextual similarities, loose verbal parallels, Chaucerian names,
ideas, and images from *The Legend of Good Women*, *Troilus and Criseyde*, and *The
Canterbury Tales*, see SHAKESPEARE (1594), Boswell & Holton No. 546.

153.   SHAKESPEARE, WILLIAM. *The Tragœdy of Othello the Moore of Venice.* S2939. UMI 297: 33.

For possible similarities to *Troilus and Criseyde*, see SHAKESPEARE (1622), Boswell
& Holton No. 1035.

Other editions: S2940 (1681); S2941 (1687); S2942 (1695).

154.   Twisse, William, in Joseph Mede's *The Apostasy of the Latter Times.* M1593A. UMI 2051: 2.

For an allusion to the Clerk and a quotation from *The General Prologue,* see Twisse (1641), M1590; in this edition, the passage is found on sig. A2r.

155.   Verstegen (or Rowlands), Richard. *A Restitution of Decayed Intelligence in Antiquities.* V270. UMI 587: 8.

For references to Chaucer's translation of *The Romaunt of the Rose,* to his contributions to the English language, and to his diction, see Rowlands (1623) in Boswell & Holton No. 723; in this edition, the passages are found on 156, 158, 164, 195, and sig. S8v.

1656

156.   Blount, Thomas. *The Academy of Eloquence.* B3322. UMI 1398: 4.

For an echo of the title of *The House of Fame,* see Blount (1654); in this edition, the passage is found on 29.

157.   Blount, Thomas. *Glossographia: or, A Dictionary.* B3334. UMI 122: 16 and UMI Thomason Tracts 199: E.1573 (1).

Blount (1618–1679) is identified on the title page as "T. B. of the Inner-Temple, Barrester." In this dictionary "interpreting all such hard words . . . as are now used in our refined English tongue," Blount cites Chaucer frequently as an authority on the English language.

Spurgeon (1: 231) notes a reference to "old Chaucer" and a quotation from *Troilus and Criseyde* (2: 22–26) in the epistle to the reader (sig. A4r) and in the definition of *Dulcarnon* (sig. O1v).

> [W]*ords in Common Tongues, like leaves, must of necessity have their buddings, their blossomings, their ripenings, and their fallings: Which old* Chaucer *also thus remarks.*

> I know that in form the speech is change
> Within a hundred years and words tho
> That hadde price, now wonder nice and strange
> Think we then, and yet then speak them so,
> And sped as well in love, as men now do. (sig. A4v)

Atkinson notes (*MLN* 1940) references to Chaucer in the definitions of a dozen words: *Agrise, Alnath, Barbican, Cheve, Covent, Creance, Dissheviled, Lodemanage, Losener, Ouch, Pilgrim, Romance, Romant,* and *Taberd.* There are others:

Agrise . . . afraid. *Chaucer.* (sig. B7v) [Chaucer uses the term six times: *Nun's Priest Tale,* line 4083; *The Wife of Bath's Tale,* line 191; *Parliament of Fowles,* line 543; *Troilus and Criseyde,* 3: 862, 3: 1621, 4: 613.]

Agroted . . . cloy'd, made big, swelled. *Chaucer.* (sig. B7v) [*The Legend of Good Women,* line 2454.]

Algebra . . . the Art of figurative numbers or of equation. An Art consisting both of Arithmetick and Geometry; *Chaucer* calls it *Algrim.* (sig. B8v) [Neither *algrim* nor *algebra* is found in Tatlock & Kennedy.]

Alnath is a fixed star in the horns of *Aries,* from whence the first mansion of the Moon taketh his name, and is called *Alnath. Chaucer.* (sig. C2r) [*The Franklin's Tale,* line 1281.]

Amortize . . . to deaden, ill or slay. Lord *Bacon* and *Chaucer.* (sig. C4v) [*The Parson's Tale,* lines 245–50.]

Barbican . . . *Chaucer* useth the word of *Barbican,* for a Watch-Tower, hence *Barbican* by *Red-cross-street* in *London* is thought to take its denomination. (sig. F4v) [Not in Tatlock & Kennedy.]

Benison, blessing: *Chaucer.* (sig. F7r) [Chaucer uses the word at least three times: in *The Merchant's Tale,* line 1365, *The Tale of Melibee,* lines 2285–90, and *The Parson's Tale,* lines 440–45.]

Bordel (from the Ital. *Burdello*) a Brothel-house, or Bawdy-house. *Chau.* (sig. G2r) [*The Parson's Tale,* lines 975–80.]

Burlybrand (Sax.) A great sword. *Chaucer.* (sig. G4v) [Not in Tatlock & Kennedy.]

Callot . . . a lewd woman. *Chauc.* (sig. G6v) [Not in Tatlock & Kennedy.]

Cheve . . . to thrive. *Chaucer.* (sig. I1r) [Not found in Tatlock & Kennedy's *Concordance,* but *a-cheve* is: *The Romaunt of the Rose,* line 5883.]

Covent . . . The whole number of religious persons dwelling in one house together, which according to *Chaucer* in the *Sompners* Tale, is but thirteen, viz. twelve and the Confessor. (sig. L4r) [Chaucer uses this word sixteen times: *The Prioress' Tale,* lines 1827, 1867; *The Summoner's Tale,* lines 1863, 1959, 1963, 1964, 1975, 2130, 2183, 2250, 2259, 2261, 2285; *The Canon Yeoman's Tale,* line 1007, *The Romaunt of the Rose,* lines 4904, 7378.]

Creance (Fr.) Trust, faith belief, confidence; also credit, &c. *Chaucer.* (sig. L5v) [*The Man of Law's Tale,* 340, 915; *The Shipman's Tale,* 1479; *A.B.C.,* 61.]

Dissheviled or Discheveled . . . an old word used by *Chaucer,* and yet still in use (sig. N4v) [*The Legend of Good Women,* lines 1315, 1720, 1829; *The General Prologue,* line 683; *The Parliament of Fowls,* line 235.]

Dulcarron is a proportion in *Euclid* . . . which was found out by *Pythagoras* after a whole years study, and much beating his brain; in thankfulness whereof, he sacrificed an Oxe to the Gods; which sacrifice he called *Dulcarron*. . . . *Chaucer* aptly applies it to *Creseide*; shewing, that she was as much amazed how to answer *Troilus*, as *Pythagorus* was wearied in bringing his desire to effect. (sig. O1v)

Frith . . . a wood. *Chaucer.* (sig. R6v) [Not in Tatlock & Kennedy.]

Gossymeare or **Gossomor** . . . the white and cobweb-like exhalations, which fly abroad in hot sunny weather. *Chau.* (sig. S5r) [*The Squire's Tale*, line 259.]

Lodemanage, is the hire of a Pilot for conducting a Ship from one place to another. . . . *Chaucer* makes this word to signifie the skill or art of Navigation. (sig. Z7v) [*The General Prologue*, line 403.]

Losenger . . . a flatterer or lyar. *Chaucer.* (sig. Aa1r) [*The Nun's Priest's Tale*, line 4516; *The Legend of Good Women*, line 352; *The Romaunt of the Rose*, line 1050.]

Meritot, a sport used by children by swinging themselves in Bel-ropes, or such like, till they be giddy. . . . *Chauc.* (sig. Bb5r) [Not in Tatlock & Kennedy.]

Moiles . . . also used by *Chaucer*, for a dish made of Marrow and grated bread. (sig. Cc1r) [Not in Tatlock & Kennedy.]

Mortress, a meat made of boyled Hens, crums of bread, yolkes of eggs, and Saffron, all boyled together. *Chauc.* (sig. Cc3v) [*Mortreux*, in *The General Prologue*, line 384.]

Orfraies . . . frizled cloth of gold, made and used in *England* both before and since the Conquest . . . a damask garmet guarded with *Orfraies. Chauc.* (sig. Ee3v) [*The Romaunt of the Rose*, lines 52, 869, 1076.]

Ouch . . . a kind of collar of gold, or such like Ornament, which women did wear about their necks. . . . And is sometimes used for a Boss or button of gold. *Chauc.* (sig. Ee5r) [*The House of Fame*, line 360; *The Clerk's Tale*, line 382.]

Paraments, Robes of state, or the place where they are kept. *Chau.* (sig. Ff2r) [*Knight's Tale*, line 2501; *Squire's Tale*, line 269; *The Legend of Good Women*, line 1106.]

Pilgrim . . . one that travels into strange Countreys, commonly taken for him that goes in devotion to any holy place. . . . *Chauc.* (sig. Gg6v–7r) [*The Cook's Tale*, line 4349; *Troilus and Criseyde*, 5: 1577; *Truth*, line 18.]

Rebeck . . . a Fiddle, or certain Musical Instrument of three strings. *Chaucer* uses it for an old trot. (sig. Kk4r) [*Friar's Tale*, line 1573.]

Romance . . . a feigned History, either in Verse or Prose in the Vulgar Lanugage, the first news we heard of this word, was from a Poem writ in French by *John Clopinel* alias *Meung*, intituled *Le Romant de la Rose*, and afterward translated into English by *Geffery Chaucer*; but we now give the name Romance most commonly to a feigned History writ in Prose. (sig. L15r)

Romant, the most eloquent French, or any thing written eloquently, was in old time termed *Roman*, of the *Roman*, or most eloquent
Language. Hence *Le Roman de la Rose*, the *Romant* of the *Rose*. . . .
Chaucer useth it for a brief History. (sig. L15r) [Chaucer uses the term
in *The Merchant's Tale*, line 2032; *The Book of the Duchess*, lines 48, 334;
Troilus and Criseyde, 2: 100, 3: 980; *The Legend of Good Women*, line 329;
and *The Romaunt of the Rose*, lines 39, 2148, 2154, 2168, 2170, 3793.]

Strond . . . a shoar or bank; Hence the *Strand* a street in the Suburbs of *London*, so called because it lies by the River side. *Chau.* (sig.
Oo8v) [*The Miller's Tale*, lines 825, 864; *The Legend of Good Women*,
lines 1498, 2189, 2205.]

Superstition . . . an excess of Ceremonious worship . . . a vain
reverence or fear towards that thing wherein is no efficacy or force
but onely by illusion; spiced conscience in vain things. [Here Blount
appears to echo Chaucer's description of the poor Parson, "Ne maked
him a spiced conscience" (*The General Prologue*, line 526) and *The Wife of
Bath's Prologue*, "Ye sholde been al pacient and meke, | And han a sweete
spiced conscience" (lines 434–35).]

Taberd or Tabard . . . a jacket, jerkin, mandilion, or sleevelesse
coat. . . . It is now the name onely of an Heralds coat, and is called their
coat of armes in service. It is also the signe of an ancient Inne in *Southwark*. (sig. Qq1r) [*The General Prologue*, lines 20, 541, 719.]

Tailage . . . a tax, task, tribute or imposition. Hence also *Taulagiers*
in *Chaucer* for tax or toll gatherers. (sig. Qq2r) [*The Parson's Tale*, lines
565–70, 750–55.]

Other editions: B3334a (1659), epistle (A4v), *agrise* (B7v), *agroted* (B7v), *algebra*
(B8v), *alnath* (C2r), *amortize* (C4v), *barbicane* (F4v), *benison* (F7r), *bordel* (G2r),
burlybrand (G4v), *callot* (G6v), *cheve* (omitted), *covent* (L4r), *creance* (L5v), *dissheviled / disheviled* (N4v), *dulcarnon* (O1v), *fryth* (R6v), *gossymeare* (S5r), *lodemanage* (Z7v), *losender* (Aa1r), *meriot* (Bb5r), *moiles* (Cc1r), *mortress* (Cc3v), *Orfraies*
(Ee3v), *ouch* (Ee5r), *paraments* (Ff2r), *pilgrim* (Gg6v–7r), *rebeck* (Kk4r), *romance*
(L15r), *romant* (L15r), *strand / strond* (Oo8v), superstition (Pp4v), *taberd* (Qq1r),
tailage (Qq2r).

B3335 (1661), epistle (A4v), *agrise* (omitted), *agroted* (B8r), *algebra* (C1r),
alnath (C2v), *amortize* (C5r), *barbicane* (F5v), *benison* (F8r), [+ *boon*, G3v], *bordel*
(G3v), *burlybrand* (G6r), *callot* (G8r), *cheve* (omitted), *covent* (L7v), *creance* (L8v),
disheviled (N8r), *dulcarnon* (O5r–v), *frythe* (S2v), *gossymeare* (T1v), [+ *lectern*, Z7r],
lodemanage (Aa3v), *losender* (Aa5r), *meriot* (Bb8v), *moiles* (Cc4v), *mortress* (Cc7v),
Orfraies (definition altered, no Chaucer, Ee7r), *ouch* (Ee8v), *paraments* (FF5v),
pilgrim (Hh1v), *rebeck* (Kk6v), *romance* (L17v), *romant* (definition altered, no
Chaucer, L17v), *Strand / Strond* (definition altered, no Chaucer, Pp1v), *superstition* (Pp5v), *taberd* (Qq2v), *tailage* (Qq3r).

B3335A (1661?), epistle (A4v), *agrise* (omitted), *agroted* (B8r), *algebra* (C1r), *alnath* (C2v), *amortize* (C5r), *barbicane* (F5v), *benison* (F8r), [+ *boon*, G3v], *bordel* (G3v), *burlybrand* (G6r), *callot* (G8r), *cheve* (omitted), *covent* (L7v), *creance* (L8v), *disheviled* (N8r), *dulcarnon* (O5r–v), *frythe* (S2v), *gossymeare* (T1v), [+ *lectern*, Z7r], *lodemanage* (Aa3v), *losender* (Aa5r), *meriot* (Bb8v), *moiles* (Cc4v), *mortress* (Cc7v), *orfraies* (definition altered, no Chaucer, Ee7r), *ouch* (Ee8v), *paraments* (FF5v), *pilgrim* (Hh1v), *rebeck* (Kk6v), *romance* (L17v), *romant* (definition altered, no Chaucer, L17v), *strand / strond* (definition altered, no Chaucer, Pp1v), superstition (Pp5v), *taberd* (Qq2v), *tailage* (Qq3r).

B3336 (1670), epistle (A4v), *agrise* (omitted), *agroted* (B8r), *algebra* (C1r), *alnath* (C2v), *amortize* (definition altered, no Chaucer, C5r), *barbicane* (F64), *benison* (F8v), [+ *boon*, G4v], *bordel* (G4v), *callot* (H1v), *cheve* (omitted), *covent* (M1r), *creance* (M2r), *dissheviled / disheviled* (O2v), *dulcarnon* (O8r), [+ dwindle, O8v], *frythe* (S6v), *gossymeare* (T5v), [+ *lectern*, Aa4v], *lodemanage* (Bb1r), *losender* (Bb2v), *meriot* (Cc6v), *moiles* (Dd2v), *mortress* (Dd5v), *orfraies* (definition altered, no Chaucer, Ff5v), *ouch* (Ff7r), *paraments* (Gg4r), *pilgrim* (Hh8v), [+ *rap and ren*, L15v], *rebeck* (L16v), *romance* (Mm7v), *romant* (definition altered, no Chaucer, L17v), *strand / strond* (definition altered, no Chaucer, Qq2r), *superstition* (Qq6v–7r), *taberd* (+ definition expanded), Rr4r, *tailage* (Rr5r).

B3337 (1674), epistle (A4v), *agrise* (omitted), *agroted* (B8r), *algebra* (C1r–v), *alnath* (C3r), *amortize* (definition altered, no Chaucer, C5v), *barbican* (F6v), *benison* (G1v), [+ *boon*, G5v], *bordel* (G5v), *burlybrand* (G8v), *calot* (definition altered, no Chaucer) H3r, *cheve* (omitted), *covent* (M3r), *creance* (M4r), *disheviled* (O5r), [+ *divinistre*, sig. O6v], *dulcarnon* (P2v), [+ dwindle, P3r], *fryth* (T1v), *gossymear / gossomor* (definition altered, no Chaucer, V1r [*sic*; really U1r]), [+ lectern, Aa8v], *lodemanage* (Bb5v), *losenger* (Bb7r), *meriot* (Dd3v), *moiles* (Dd7v), *mortress* (Ee3r), *orfraies* (definition altered, no Chaucer, Gg3r), *ouch* (Gg4v), *paraments* (Hh1v), *pilgrim* (Ii6v), [+ *rap and ren*, Mm3v], *romance* (Nn6r), *romant* (definition altered, no Chaucer, Nn6r), *strand* (definition altered, no Chaucer, Rr1v), *superstition* (Rr6r), *taberd* [+ definition expanded], (Ss3v), *tailage* (Ss4v).

B3338 (1681), epistle (A4v), *agrise* (omitted), *agroted* (B8r), *algebra* (C1v), alnath (C3r), *amortize* (definition altered, no Chaucer, C5v), *barbican* (F6v), *benison* (G1v), [+ *boon*, G5v], *bordel* (G5v), *burlybrand* (G8v), *calot* (definition altered, no Chaucer) H3r, *cheve* (omitted), *covent* (M3v), *creance* (M4v), *disheviled* (O5v–O6r), [+ *divinistre*, O7r], *dulcarnon* (P3r), [+ *dwindle*, P3v], *fryth* (T2r), *gossymear / gossomor* (definition altered, no Chaucer, U2r), [+ *lectern*, Bb2r], *lodemanage* (Bb7r), *losenger* (Bb8r), *meriot* (Dd5v), *moiles* (Ee1v), *mortress* (Ee4v), *orfraies* (definition altered, no Chaucer, Gg4v–5r), *ouch* (Gg6v), *paraments* (Hh3v), *pilgrim* (Ii8v), [+ *rap and ren*, Mm5v], *romance* (Nn8r), *romant* (definition altered, no Chaucer, Nn8r), *strand* (definition altered, no Chaucer, Rr3v), *superstition* (Rr8r), *taberd* (+ definition expanded, Ss5v), *tailage* (Ss6v).

158.   CLEVELAND, JOHN. *Poems.* C4691. UMI 734: 6.

For an echo of a line from *The Manciple's Prologue*, see CLEVELAND (1644); in this edition, the passage is found on 90.

159.   COLLOP, JOHN. *Poesis rediviva: or, Poesie Reviv'd.* C5395. UMI 136: 2.

Collop is identified on the title page as "John Collop M. D." In a poem headed "On Marriage," he echoes lines from *The Reeve's Prologue*, "To have a hoor head and a green tayl, | As hath a leek" (lines 3878–79). Collop writes:

> A widows lust may live whose love is dead,
> The Leek hath a green tail with a grey head. (95)

160.   *Choyce Drollery*: Songs & Sonnets. C3916. UMI 486: 19.

This work is a collection of poems hitherto unpublished by several authors. In "On the Time-Poets," an unidentified author praises English poets, and Chaucer welcomes them to the fraternity of Apollo:

> One night the great *Apollo* pleas'd with *Ben*,
> Made the odde number of the Muses ten;
> . . . .
> Old *Chaucer* welcomes them unto the Green,
> And *Spencer* brings them to the fairy Queen;
> The finger they present, and she in grace
> Transform'd it to a May-pole, 'bout which trace
> Her skipping servants, that do nightly sing,
> And dance about the same a Fayrie ring. (5–7; sig. B3r–4r)

There is also a possible allusion to *The Tale of Sir Thopas* in a poem without a heading that was not noted by Spurgeon. The poet describes a knight called Cassimen who dwelt in the Forest of Arden:

> Fell he was and eager bent
> In battaile and in Turnament,
>   As was the good Sr. *Topas*. (73)

161.   COWLEY, ABRAHAM. *Poems.* C6683. UMI 487: 14.

Cowley (1618–1667) is identified on the title page as "A. Cowley." As Spurgeon notes (1: 232), Cowley refers to Chaucer in *Pindarique Odes*, in the "Notes" for his ode addressed "To Dr. Scarborough"[20] in a passage about the kind of rhymes in which the French delight:

> *Rich Rhymes . . .* are very frequent in *Chaucer*, and our old *Poets*, but that is not good authority for us now. There can be no *Musick* with only *one Note*. (37, n. 2)

Also collected in Cowley's *Works*: C6649 (1668), 37 (sig. Aa1r); C6650 (1669), 37 (sig. Aa2r); C6651 (1672), 37 (sig. Aa2r); C6652 (1674), 37 (sig. Aa2r); C6653 (1678), 37 (sig. Aa2r); C6654 (1680), 37 (sig. Aa2r); C6655 (1681), 37 (sig. Aa2r); C6656 (1681), 54 (sig. L6v); C6656A (1684), 37 (sig. Aa2); C6656B (1684); C6657 (1684), 37 (sig. Aa2r); C6658 (1688), 37 (sig. Aa2r); C6659 (1693), 37 (sig. Aa2r); C6660 (1700), 96 (sig. Q4v).

162. Du Bosc, Jacques. *The Accomplish'd Woman Written Originally in French; Since Made English by the Honourable Walter Montague, Esq.* D2407A. UMI 141: 7.

This work is a translation by Walter Montague (1603?–1677) of the first part of *L'honeste femme* by Du Bosc (d. 1660). In a section headed "Of Cloathes and Ornaments," Montague interpolates a reference to Chaucer's language being outdated:

> [T]he light and giddy invent fashions, but the wise and sober accommodate themselves to them, in stead of contradicting them. Habits and words should be suted to the time: and as one would think them mad, that should speak in the Court the language of *Chaucer*; so we could not judg better of such as would affect to be cloathed so too. (117)

Another edition: D2407AB (1671), 117.

163. Flecknoe, Richard. *The Diarium or Journall Divided into 12 Jornadas in Burlesque Rhime or Drolling Verse: With Other Pieces of the Same Author.* F1212. UMI Thomason Tracts 209: E.1669 (2); UMI 143: 8.

In the sixth "Jornada," Flecknoe (d. 1678?) may allude to *The Nun's Priest's Tale* as he indulges in what he calls "Poets language" to describe day-break. He writes:

> And now *Aurora* blushing red,
> Came stealing out of *Titans* bed,
> Whilst the *hours* that swiftly run,
> Harnass'd the horses of the *Sun*.

---

[20] Dr. Scarborough, physician to royalty, was Sir Charles Scarborough (1615–1694).

Now *Chantecleer* with stretcht-out wings,
The glad approach of *Phœbus* sings,
While *Bats* and *Owles*, and birds of night
Were all confounded, put to flight.
All which is onely for to say
In *Poets language*, that 'twas day . . . (28)

164.   FULLER, THOMAS. *The Church-History of Britain.* F2417. UMI 627: 6.

For numerous references to Chaucer and allusions to and quotations from *The Wife of Bath's Tale*, *The Reeve's Tale*, *The Nun's Priest's Tale*, *The Astrolabe*, and the spurious work known as *The Ploughman's Tale*, see FULLER (1656); in this edition, the passages are found on 38, 65, ²75, ²98, ²151-52, ⁴69. UMI film ends with Book XI, no "History of the University of Cambridge."

165.   G., E. "To the Author," in Martin Llewellyn's *Men Miracles*. L2626. UMI 606: 4.

For a reference to Chaucer's "learned soul" and his influence on Spenser, see a commendatory poem by E. G., L2625 (1646); in this edition, the passage is found on sig. A5r.

166.   GUILD, WILLIAM. *An Answer to a Popish Pamphlet.* G2202. UMI 2187: 7.

Guild (1586-1657) is identified on the title page as a doctor of divinity and "Preacher of Gods Word." In a section headed "That Priests and other religio[us] persons who have vowed chastitie to God, may frelie marrie notwithstanding of their vow," Guild cites *The Ploughman's Tale*, a spurious work that he attributes to Chaucer. In a passage about Pope Gregory VII's "decree of forced single life," Guild writes:

> [Opposition to the Pope's edict] made that noble poet in his time *Chaucer*, Esq. of *Woodstock* anno 1341. to say in his plowmans tale. *They live not in lecherie, but haunt Wenches, Widows & wives, and punisheth the poore for poultrie* [sic], *Themselves using it all their lives.* (292-93)

167.   HARRINGTON, JAMES. *The Common-wealth of Oceana.* H809. UMI 919: 2.

In a passage about the folly of mixing civil government with "popery," Harrington (1611-1677) appears to echo a line from *The Reeve's Tale*: "The gretteste clerkes been noght wisest men" (line 4054). He writes:

> An ounce of wisdom is worth a pound of Clergy: Your greatest Clerks are not your wisest men. (223)

Another edition: H810 (1658), 223

Also found in *The Oceana of James Harrington, and His Other Works* (1700),
H816, 181–82.

168.   HEYLYN, PETER. *Extraneus vapulans: or, The Observator Rescued.* H1708.
UMI Thomason Tracts 206: E.1641(1).

In his translation of a letter headed "Philip the 3. to the Conde of Olivarez,"
Heylyn (1600–1662) echoes a line from *The Manciple's Prologue*: "Sires, what!
Dun is in the myre!" (line 5). He writes:

> But Sir, a good Historian . . . must write both properly and plainly . . .
> and not trouble and torment the Reader, in drawing *dun out of the mire*,
> in a piece of *English.* (93)

169.   HOLLAND, SAMUEL. *Don Zara del Fogo.* H2437. UMI 148: 12.

This work is purportedly "written originally in the British tongue, and made
English by a person of much honor, Basilius Musophilus."

In book 1, chapter 1, Don Zara summons his squire and commands him to
read to him (for he could not read himself); among the options offered was "the
hard Quest of Sir *Topaz* after the Queen of *Elves* to *Barwick*" (2), an allusion to
The Tale of Sir Thopas.

As Spurgeon notes (1: 232), Holland refers to Chaucer as England's literary progenitor in book 2, chapter 4, in which the enchantress and Zara visit the
"Elizian Shades." Among the sublime souls who inhabit this thrice-happy place,
they find Chaucer in the middle of a dogfight:

> [T]he British Bards (forsooth) were also ingagd in quarrel for Superi-
> ority; and who think you, threw the Apple of Discord amongst them,
> but *Ben Johnson*, who had openly vaunted himself the first and best of
> English Poets; this Brave was resented by all with the highest indigna-
> tion, for *Chaucer* (by most there) was esteemed the Father of English
> Poesie, whose onely unhappines it was, that he was made for the time
> he lived in, but the time not for him . . . : *Chapman* was wondrously
> exasperated at *Bens* boldness . . . ; hereupon *Spencer* (who was very busie
> in finishing his *Fairy Queen*) thrust himself amid the throng, and was
> received with a showt . . . ; but behold *Shakespeare* and *Fletcher* (bring-
> ing with them a strong party) appeared, as if they meant to water their
> Bayes with blood, rather then part with their proper Right . . . ; *Skelton*,
> *Gower*, and the Monk of *Bury* were at Daggers-drawing for *Chawcer*;
> *Spencer* waited upon by a numerous Troup of the best Bookmen in the
> World; *Shakespear* and *Fletcher* surrounded with their Life-Guard . . . O
> ye *Pernassides*! what a curse have ye cast upon your Helliconian Water-
> Bailiffs? that those whose Names (both Sir and Christen) are filed on

Fames Trumpet, and whom Envy cannot wound, shall now perish by
intestine Discord, and home-bred Dissention? (101–2)

Another edition in 1656, with new title, *Wit and Fancy in a Maze: or, The Incompa-
rable Champion of Love and Beautie*: H2445, same pagination.
   Another edition, with a different title: *Romancio-mastrix: or, A Romance on
Romances*, H2443 (1660), 2, 101–2.

170.   LEIGH, EDWARD. *A Treatise of Religion & Learning.* L1013. UMI 35: 23.
Leigh (1602–1671) is identified on the title page as "Edward Leigh Master of
Arts of Magdalen-Hall in Oxford." As Spurgeon notes (1: 232–33), there is a
reference in an epistle addressed "To the Judicious and Candid Reader" where
Leigh cites Chaucer in a short list of old poets:

> I might here expatiate in the just praises of *England*, for the purity of its
> Doctrine in Religion, and also for the many learned Authors here bred
> and fostered. But because I speak somewhat of it in the Book, I shall be
> briefer here. . . . For Poets of old, *Chaucer, Spenser, Ockland* [*sic*].[21] (sig.
> A5v–6r)

In book 2, chapter 13, "Of the Universities of England," Chaucer is again listed
amongst England's poets:

> *England* hath been famous for Learned men, and for her Seminaries of
> Learning, as well as other things. . . . For Poetry, *Gower, Chaucer, Spen-
> cer,* Sir *Philip Sidnie* [sic], *Daniel* and *Draiton, Beaumont* and *Fletcher,
> Ben. Johnson.* (91; sig. N2r)

In book 3, chapter 11, under the running head "Of such as were Famous for Zeal
in the True Religion, or in Learning," in an alphabetical catalogue of religious or
learned men, Chaucer is again cited:

> *Galfridus Chaucerus. Jeffery Chaucer,* he was born in *Oxfordshire.*
>   He first of all so illustrated the English Poetry, that he may be
> esteemed our English *Homer.* He is our best English Poet, and *Spencer*
> the next.
>
> *Prædicat Algerum meriò Florentina Dantem,*
> *Italia & numeros tota Petrarcha tuos.*

---

[21] Ockland, presumably Hoccleve.

Anglia Chaucerum *veneratur nostra Poeta*
Cui Veneres debet patria lingua suas. Lel. *lib. Epig.*

He seems in his Works to be a right *Wiclevian*, as that of the Pellican and Griffin shews.

He was an acute Logician, a sweet Rhetorician, a facetious Poet, a grave Philosopher, and a holy Devine.

His Monument is in *Westminster* Abbey.

Chaucerus *linguam patriam magna ingenii solertia ac cultura plurimùm ornavit, itemque alia, cum* Joannis Mone *poema de arte amandi Gallicè tantùm legeretur, Anglico illud metro feliciter reddidit.* Voss. *De Histor. Lat.*1.3.c.2.

[In a shoulder note:] Vixit Anno Domini 1402. Propter docendi gratiam & libertatem quasi alter Dantes aut Petrarcha quos ille etiam in linguam nostram transtulit, in quibus Romana Ecclesia tanquam sedes Antichristi describitur, & ad vivum ex primitur. *Humphr.* Præfat. Ad lib de Jesuitisno. Fuere & in Britannorum idiomate & eorum vernaculo sermone aliqui poetæ ab eis summo pretio habiti inter quos *Galfredus Chaucerus* vetustior qui multa scripsit, & *Thomas Viatus*, ambo insignes equites. *Lil. Gyrald.* De Poet. noit. Temp. Dial. 2. (160; sig. X4v)

In book 4, chapter 2, in a passage about John Gower:

Joannes Goverus, sive *Gouerus*, a learned English Knight, and Poet *Laureate*.
Hic nomes suum extulit partim iis quæ & Gallicè & eleganter Anglicè elaboravit. Sane is & Gualterus Chaucerus primi Anglicam linguam expolire cœperunt. Vossius *de Histor: Lat:1.3.c.3.* (211)

In book 5, chapter 14, in a passage that Spurgeon missed, Leigh notes the Spenser-Chaucer connection:

Edmund Spencer, the Prince of Poets in his time. [In a shoulder note:] *Edmundus Spencer*, Londinensis, Anglicorum Poetarum nostri fæculi facile princeps, quod ejus Poemata faventibus musis, & victuro genio conscripta conprobant prope *Galfredum Chaucerum* conditur, qui fœlicssimè Poesin Anglicis literis primus illustravit. *Camd.* Monum Reg. Heromque Westm. Condit.

His Monument stands in *Westminster* Abbey, near *Chaucers*, with this Epitaph,

Hic prope Chaucerum
Situs est Spenserius, *illi*

> *Proximus ingenio*
> *Proximus ut tumulo,*
> *Hic prope* Chaucerum
> Spensere *Poeta Poetam*
> *Conderis, & versu,*
> *Quam tumulo propior,*
> *Anglica te vivo vixit,*
> *Plausitque Poesis;*
> *Nunc morituratimet,*
> *Te moriente, mori.* (328; sig. Tt4v)

In the index, Chaucer is listed under *C*: "*Jeffery Chaucer*, born in Oxfordshire, our English *Homer*," (sig. Ccc3r).

Another edition with title *Fœlix Consortium; or, A Fit Conjuncture of Religion and Learning*: L995 (1663), same pagination.

171.   LINDSAY, DAVID. *The Works of the Famous and Worthy Knight, Sir David Lindesay of the Mount, Alias.* L2314. UMI 1445: 12.

For a reference to Chaucer's skill as a poet in the prologue of *The Testament of Papingo*, see LINDSAY (1538) in Boswell & Holton No. 146; in this edition, the passage is found on sig. G7v.

For a passage that mentions the fable of *Troilus and Criseyde* in an epistle to the king that is set before the prologue to "The Dreme of Sir David Lindsay," see LINDSAY (1558) in Boswell & Holton No. 209; in this edition, the passage is found and appears on sig. H11r.

172.   LLOYD, DAVID. *The Legend of Captain Jones.* L2631. UMI 606: 5.

For a reference to Chaucer and *The Tale of Sir Thopas*, see LLOYD L2635 (1648); in this edition, the passage is found on 27.

173.   MASSINGER, PHILIP; MIDDLETON, THOMAS; ROWLEY, WILLIAM. *The Old Law: or, A New Way to Please You.* M1048. UMI 154: 15.

The title page advises readers that this "Excellent Comedy" was "Acted before the King and Queene at Salisbury House, and at severall other places, with great Applause." In 4.1, in which a Bayliff, a Clown, and a Taylor discuss whether Helen of Troy was known as Ellen, or Nel of Troy, or Bonny Nell while playing on an expression for measuring the weight of gold, i.e., "Troy ounces." The Taylor inquires, "Why did she grow shorer [sic] when she came to Troy?" The Clown responds with a faint allusion to *Troilus and Criseyde*:

> She grew longer if you marke the story, when shee grew to be an ell shee was deeper then any yard of Troy could reach by a quarter: there was

Cressid was Troy waight, and *Nell* was haberdepoyse, she held more by fowre ounces then *Cresida*. (48)

Clearly you had to be there to appreciate the humor.

At the end of the play appears "An Exact and perfect Catalogue of all the Plaies that were ever printed." The compiler (probably Edward Archer, bookseller at the Sign of Adam and Eve in Little Britain) records a tragedy called "Troilus and Cressida." Although Shakespeare is credited with authorship of some other plays listed there (including some not in the canon), he is not named here.

174. NEWCASTLE, MARGARET CAVENDISH. *Natures Pictures Drawn by Fancies Pencil to the Life.* **N855. UMI 1575: 38.**

Newcastle (1624?–1674) is identified on the title page as "the thrice noble, illustrious, and excellent princess, the lady Marchioness of Newcastle." In "The Preaching Lady," in a section about the "Land of Poetry," she appears to allude to *The House of Fame.* The lady preacher lays out her text in seven parts (in the manner of hair-splitting preachers who find deep meaning in every word—including *a, and,* and *the*—of scripture. She writes:

> *Dearly beloved Brethren,* I have called you together, to instruct, exhort, and admonish you. My Text I take out of Nature . . . [which] I will divide into seven parts.

> At first, *In the Land of Poetry.*
> Secondly, *there stands a Mount . . .*
> Sixthly, *there issues from the top a Flame.*
> Seventhly and Lastly, *the Flame ascends to Fames Mansion.* (159)

> *From the top of this Mount* Parnassus, *issues out a Flame:* . . . *This insensible Flame ascends to Fame's Mansion:* And though, dearly Beloved, Fame's Mansion is but an old Library, wherein lies ancient Records of Actions, Accidents, Chronologies, Moulds, Medals, Coins, and the like; yet Fame her self is a Goddess, and the Sister to Fortune; and she is not only a Goddess, but a powerful Goddess; and not only a powerful Goddess, but a terrible Goddess; for she can both damn and glorifie; and her Sentence of Damnation is, most commonly, of more force than her Sentence of Glorification; for those that she damns, she damns without Redemption; but she sets, many times, a period to those she Glorifies. (160)

Another edition: N856 (1671), 275, 278–79.

175.   PHILLIPS, JOHN. *Sportive Wit*: *The Muses Meriment*. P2113. UMI 1154: 19.

In the second part of this volume, under the running head "Wits Merriment: Or, Lusty Drollery," in a poem headed "To his Friend; A Censure of the Poets," Phillips (1631–1706) refers to Chaucer and Gower and their contributions to English poetry:

> Then to the matter that we took in hand,
> *Jove* and *Apollo* for the Muses stand,
> That noble *Chaucer* in those former times,
> That did enrich our English with his Rimes,
> And was the first of ours that ever brake
> Into the Muses treasure, and first spake
> In weighty number, delving in the Mine
> Of perfect knowledge, which he could refine
> And coyn for currant, and as much as then
> The English Language could express to men;
> He made to do onely his wondrous skill
> Gave us much light from his abundant quill.
> And honest *Gower*, who in respect of him,
> Had onely sipt at *Aganippe*'s brim;
> And though in yeares this last was him before,
> Yet fell he far short of the others store;
> When after those four ages, very near,
> They with the Muses which conversed were. (67–68)

176.   S., W., in John Bullokar's *An English Expositor*: *Teaching the Interpretation of the Hardest Words Used in Our Language*. B5430. UMI 1248: 7.

For a reference to Chaucer and *The Prologue to The Squire's Tale*, see S., W. (1654); in this edition, the passage is found on sig. E4r.

177.   SANDYS, GEORGE, trans. *Ovid's Metamorphosis Englished*. O684.

For an echo of the title of *The House of Fame*, see SANDYS (1628) in Appendix; in this edition, the passage is found on 232.

Other editions: 0686 (1664), 232; 0687 (1669), 232; 0688 (1678), 232; 0688A (1690), 232.

178.   SMITH, JAMES. "The Preface to That Most Elaborate Piece of Poetry Entituled Penelope and Ulysses," in *Wit and Drollery*. W3131. UMI Thomason Tracts 204: E. 1617(1).

As Spurgeon notes (1: 233–34), Smith refers to "ould" Chaucer in "The Preface to that most elaborate piece of Poetry Entituled Penelope [and] Ulysses." In recounting an incident at a tavern, Smith relates that an irate poet once dashed white-wine vinegar in his face because he had the temerity to say his muse was above Chaucer's. Smith chides his muse for having run away. He writes:

> Thou Slut quoth I, hadst thou not run away,
> I had made Verses all this Live-long Day.
> But in good sooth, o're much I durst not chide her,
> Lest she should run away again and hide her.
> But when my heat was o're, I spake thus to her,
> Why did'st thou play the wag? I'm very sure
> I have commended thee above ould *Chaucer*;
> And in a Tavern once I had a Sawcer
> Of Whit-wine Vinegar, dasht in my face,
> For saying thou deservest a better grace. . . . (2)

For another reference in this same volume, see *Wit and Drollery* (1656).
Other editions: W3132 (1661), 2; W3133 (1682), 212.
Also found in *Wit Restor'd* (1658), M1719, 149 (and another).

179.   SMITH, JOHN. *The Mysterie of Rhetorique Unvail'd.* S4116A. UMI Thomason Tracts 199: E.1579 (2).

In a section headed "English Examples of Onomatopeia," Smith (who is described on the title page as a "Gent.")[22] cites Spenser's imitation of Chaucer as an example:

> By reviving antiquity; touching this I refer the reader to *Chaucer*, and to the shepherds Kalendar. (64)

Other editions: S4116B (1665), 64; S4116C (1673), 64; S4166D (1683), 64; S4166E (1683), 64; S4166F (1688), 64.

180.   TRAPP, JOHN. *A Commentary or Exposition upon All the Books of the New Testament.* T2039. UMI 583: 8.

For a reference to John Foxe's commendation of Chaucer's books, see TRAPP, *A Commentary or Exposition upon All the Epistles* (1647); in this edition, the passage is found on 1023.

For another reference to Chaucer's motto, see TRAPP, *A Commentary or Exposition upon the Four Evangelists* (1647); in this edition, the passage is found on 174.

---

[22] Wing attributes authorship to John Sergeant (1622–1707).

181.   VAUGHAN, THOMAS. *Magia Adamica: or, The Antiquitie of Magic, and the Descent Thereof from Adam Downwards, Proved. By Eugenius Philalethes.* V152. UMI 1877: 3.

For a reference that may echo *The Monk's Tale*, see VAUGHAN, V151 (1650); in this edition, the passage is found on 45.

182.   *Wit and Drollery.* W3131. UMI Thomason Tracts 204: E. 1617(1).

As Spurgeon notes (1: 233–34), there are two references in this collection. The first is found in James Smith's "Preface," *q.v. supra.* The other is by an unknown poet.

   In "Verses Written Over the Chair of Ben: Johnson, now remaining at Robert Wilsons, at the signe of Johnson's head in the Strand":

> We ask not Ben, what's the design, did raise,
> This Mausoleum, to thy flesh or bayes?
> . . . .
> And though our Nation could afford no room,
> Near *Chaucer, Spencer, Draiton,* for thy tomb;
> What thou ordain'st, though for thy pleasures,
> Then Pyramids or Marbles guilded o're. (79)

Other editions: W3132 (1661), reference not present; W3133 (1682), reference not present.

1657

183.   BIRCKBECK, SIMON. *The Protestants Evidence. Second Edition Corrected and Much Enlarged.* B2945. UMI 270: 13.

In "A Catalogue of such Witnesses as are produced in this Treatise, for proof of the Protestants Religion, disposed according to the Times wherein they flourished," in a section from 1300–1400: "1400 *Sir* Geoffrey Chaucer" (sig. C1v).

   Other references in this work are noted in Dobbins (*MLQ*) and Boswell & Holton No. 1244. In this edition, in "The Fourteenth Century," in a section headed "Dante and Petrarch," Chaucer ("our English Laureat") is linked with these famous poets, 351; and in a section headed "Chaucer," there are references to his connection with John of Gaunt, and to the spurious *Ploughman's Tale, The General Prologue, The Prologue to the Pardoner's Tale, The Pardoner's Tale, The Summoner's Tale, The Romaunt of the Rose,* and the spurious *Tale of Jack Upland,* 355–57.

   Another edition in 1657: B2944a.

184.   CLEVELAND, JOHN. *Poems.* C4692. UMI 1438: 4.

For an echo of a line from *The Manciple's Prologue*, see CLEVELAND (1644); in this edition, the passage is found on 90.

185.   CROMPTON, HUGH. *Poems.* C7029. UMI 62: 5.

Crompton (fl. 1652–58) is identified on the title page as "the god-son of Bacchus, and god-son of Apollo," and his collection of poems is described as "a fardle of fancies or a medley of musick, stewed in four ounces of the oyle of epigrams."

In "A brave temper," Crompton echoes a line from *The Manciple's Prologue*: "Sires, what! Dun is in the myre!" (line 5). He writes:

> You lumps of the earth, will you never be wise?
> Go barter your plumbets for plumes, and arise.
> Your spirits you tire, like Dun in the mire. [etc.] (24)

In "Deformity" Crompton writes of Chaucer's "rustical" speech:

> Oh help, I am beset about
> With snakie-hair'd *Medusa*, and I doubt
> I shall be frantick: Heaven grant me aid
> To back my weakness, or I am berraid.
> Blesse me! What eyes be these? what flaming sawcers?
> What speech is this, more rustical then *Chaucers*? (57)

186.   DAVIES, JOHN, trans. Vincent Voiture's *Letters of Affaires, Love, and Courtship.* V683. UMI Thomason Tracts 203: E. 1607 (1).

In this translation of some letters by Voiture (1597–1648), Davies (1625–1693) uses a proverb that echoes a line from *The Merchant's Tale*: "Old fish, and young flesh woll I haue full faine" (line 1418). In Voiture's letter addressed "To my Lord Duke d'Anguien," Davies translates:

> Indeed Gossip, it must needs be confess'd, you have satisfy'd he Proverb
> that says, *young flesh, and old fish.* . . . . (235)

187.   GREENWOOD, WILLIAM. Ἀπογ ϛογης [Apograph' storg's]: *or, A Description of the Passion of Love.* G1869. UMI 1718: 27.

Greenwood may allude to *Troilus and Criseyde* in a passage under the running head "The Power and Effects of Love":

> Some are as inconstant as *Cressida*, that, be *Troylus* never so true, yet out
> of sight out of minde; and so soon as *Diomede* begins to *court*, she like

Venetian traffick, is for his penny currant, à currendo, sterling coyne; possable [*sic*] from man to man in way of exchange. (54)

188.   HOWELL, JAMES. *Londinopolis.* **H3090. UMI 384: 15 (incomplete and/ or confused pagination; skips from 124 to 301). Copy at LC.**

Howell (1594?–1666) is identified on the title page as "Jam Howel, Esq: Senesco, non Segnesco." As Graves notes (*SP*), Howell mentions Chaucer three times in this "historical discourse . . . of the city of London, the imperial chamber, and chief emporium of Great Britain" (title page). He attributes a quotation to Chaucer in a section about Aldgate Ward:

> At the North-West corner of this Ward, in the said High street, standeth the fair and beautiful Parish Church of St. *Andrew the Apostle*, with an Addition, to be known from other Churches of that Name, of the *Knape*, or *Undershaft* and so called St. *Andrew Undershaft*: because that of old time, every year (on *May-day* in the morning) it was used, that an high or long shaft, or May-pole, was set up there, in the midst of the street, before the South door of the said Church, which Shaft or Pole, when it was set on end, and fixed in the ground, was higher then the Church Steeple. *Jeffrey Chaucer*, writing of a vain boaster, hath these words, meaning of the said Shaft.
>
>> Right well aloft, and high ye bear your head,
>> The Weather-Cock, with flying, as ye would kill,
>> When ye be stuffed, bet of Wine, then bread,
>> Then look ye, when your wombe doth fill,
>> As ye would bear the great Shaft of *Corn-hill*.
>> Lord so merrily, crowdeth then your Croke,
>> That all the Street may bear your Body Cloke. (55)

Graves also notes a reference to Chaucer's father in a section about "the Fifteenth Ward, or Aldermanry [*sic*] of the City of London, called Cordwayner Ward":

> [O]n the . . . East side of *Cordwainer-street*, is one other fair Church, called *Aldermary Church*, because the same was very old, and elder then any Church of St. *Mary* in the City. . . . *Richard Chawcer* Vintner, thought to be the Father of *Jeffrey Chawcer* the Poet, was a great Benefactor of this Church. (108 — *not* 180 as in Graves *SP*)

In a section headed "Of Westminster Abbey," Howell notes Chaucer's burial place:

[T]here lie here buried . . . And (whom in no wise we must forget) the Prince of *English* Poets, *Geoffrey Chaucer*; as also he that for pregnant wit, and an excellent gift in Poetry, of all *English* Poets came nearest unto him, *Edmund Spencer.* (355, irregular pagination; sig. Gg2r)

Another edition in 1657: H3091, same pagination.

189. JACKSON, THOMAS. Μαραν αθα [Maran atha]: *or, Dominus veniet. Commentaries upon These Articles of the Creed.* J92. UMI 1852: 33.

Jackson (1579–1640) is identified on the title page as "President of Corpus Christi Coll. in Oxford." He was also dean of Peterborough cathedral. As Spurgeon notes (3: 4.71), he refers to Chaucer and alludes to *The Canterbury Tales* and comments on Chaucer's increasing marginalization. In chapter 42, a sermon or exposition of Matthew 23: 34–36, in a discussion of the ambiguity of ancient texts, Jackson writes:

[A]ll antient Satyrists, or such as tax the capital vices of their own times, are hardly understood by later Ages, without the Comments of such as lived with them or not long after them: as our Posterity in a few years will hardly understand some passages in the *Fairy Queen*, or in *Mother Hubbards*, or other Tales in *Chaucer*, better known at this day to old Courtiers than to young Students. (3732)

Also found in *The Works of the Reverend and Learned Divine, Thomas Jackson* (1673), J90, 3: 746.

190. JORDAN, THOMAS. *The Walks of Islington and Hogsdon.* J1071. UMI Thomason Tracts 137: E.910 (5).

Jordan (1612?–1685?) is characterized on the title page as a "Gent." As Spurgeon notes (3: 4.72), Jordan refers to Chaucer as a bawdy poet. In the first scene of act 4 of this comedy "as it was publikely acted 19. dayes together, with extraordinary applause" (title page), Jordan's Jack Wildwood speaks to his drinking companion Frank Rivers, who is not as jovial as usual:

Blood of the Rivers, thou beginst to droop,
Thy soul seems not so active as it was:
Where be those capering pieces of pure flash,
That made the genius of the place grow Comick?
By the wanton memory of *Chaucer* I could turn Poet,
And write in as Heathen English; and as bawdy. . . . (sig. E4v)

An issue with new title: *Tricks of Youth* (1663), J1067, same pagination.

191.   LEIGH, EDWARD. *Select and Choyce Observations*. L1003. UMI 672: 18.

For an echo of a line from *The Merchant's Tale*, see LEIGH (1647); in this edition, the passage is found on 274.

192.   MIDDLETON, THOMAS. *No Wit*, [and No] *Help Like a Womans*. M1985. UMI 111: 12.

Middleton (d. 1627) is characterized on the title page as a "Gent." In this comedy, he writes of a rich widow appropriately named Lady Goldenfleece. In the second act, she drops in to visit an acquaintance named Weatherwise who is entertaining a couple of gentlemen. They amuse themselves by introducing witty *double entendres* into the conversation, thus attempting a little "saucy courting" of the lady. In a discussion of the best diet for various months of the year, Sir Gilbert Lambston (one of the guests) quotes versified advice from an almanac regarding suitable foods for September. In Lady Goldenfleece's response, she alludes to the evolution of the meanings of words since Chaucer's day:

> [Lambston]. *Now may'st thou Physicks safely take,*
>   *And bleed, and bathe for thy healths sake.*
>   *Eat Figs and Grapes, and spicery,*
>   *For to refresh thy Members dry.*

> [The widow responds]. Thus it is still, when a mans simple meaning lights among wantons; how many honest words have suffered corruption, since *Chaucers* days? A Virgin would speak those words then, that a very Midwife[23] would blush to hear now. . . . And who is this long on, but such wags as you, that use your words like your wenches?[24] you cannot let 'em pass honestly by you, but you must still have a flirt at 'em. (36)

193.   MIDDLETON, THOMAS. *Two New Playes by Tho. Middleton, Gent.* M1989. UMI 111: 13.

In act 1.4 of *More Dissemblers Besides Women*, Dondolo asks a young page to sing a song, but the youngster says he cannot sing. To which Dondolo responds with a saying attributed to Chaucer. Middleton writes:

> Take heed, you may speak at such an hour, that your voice may be clean taken away from you: I have known many a good Gentlewoman say so much as you say now, and have presently gone to Bed, and lay speech-

---

[23] *Midwife*: midwives have seen everything and nothing can make them blush.
[24] *Wenches*: servant girls, usually single women, whose virtue was frequently tested by horny men.

less: 'Tis not good to jest, as old *Chaucer* was wont to say, that broad
famous English Poet. Cannot you sing say you? Oh that a Boy should so
keep cut with his Mother, and be given to dissembling. (17)

194. POOLE, JOSUA. *The English Parnassus: or, A Helpe to English Poesie.*
P2814. UMI 1237: 7.

Poole (*fl.* 1632–1646) is identified on the title page as "Josua Poole, M. A. Clare
Hall Camb." As Spurgeon notes (1: 234), he includes Chaucer in a list of "Books
principally made use of in the compiling of this work" (41).

  Other editions: P2815 (1677), 33; P2816 (1678), no UMI (unique copy at
Princeton).

195. PURCHAS, SAMUEL. *Theatre of Politicall Flying-Insects.* **P4224. UMI 472: 23.**

Purchas (d. ca. 1658) is described on the title page as "Master of Arts, and Pastor
at Sutton in Essex." In this work, "Wherein Especially the Nature, the Worth,
the Work, the Wonder, and the manner of the Right-ordering of the Bee Is Discovered and Described" (title page), he cites Chaucer under the letter "C" in "A
Catalogue of such Authors as are cited, and made use of in this Tractate" (sig.
*2v).

  As Harris notes (*PQ*), Purchas quotes lines from *The Prologue to The Legend
of Good Women* (lines 125–30) in chapter 13, "Of the Bees work." He writes:

> When the Earth begins to put on her new apparel, and the Sun runs
> a most even course between the night, and the day, then most com-
> mon ly, sometimes before in warmer seasons, the industrious Bee hat-
> ing idleness more than death, diligently visits every tree and flower that
> may affect her materials for her livelihood. Hear how an ancient Poet
> expresseth it.

> > *When forgot had the Earth his poor estate*
> > *Of Winter, that him naked made, and mate,*
> > *And with his sword of Cloud so sore grieved,*
> > *Now hath the attempre Sun all that relieved,*
> > *That naked was, and clad it new again,*
> > *The busie Bees of the season fain, &c.*

The passage is marked with a shoulder note: "Chawcer Prologue to the legend of
good women," (67).

  In chapter 20, "Of Bees, Enemies and Sicknesses," Purchas quotes modernized lines from *The Parliament of Fowls* (lines 353–54). In a passage about
enemies of bees, he writes:

The Swallow hath an ill-name, but I could never observe any great hurt done by them [to bees].

> *The Swallow murdresse of the Bees small,*
> *That maken hony of flowers fresh of hue.*

The passage is marked with a shoulder note: "Chaucer assembly of Fowles" (118).

In chapter 22, "Of Hony," Purchas quotes a modernized couplet from *The Knight's Tale* (lines 2907–8):

> *Chaucer* relating the burning of Arsite, tells what they used to cast into the Funeral flames.

> *With vessels in her hand of gold full fine,*
> *All full of Hony, Milk, Blood, and Wine.* (144–45)

The passage is marked with a shoulder note: "Chaucer in the Knights tale."

196.   SHIRLEY, JAMES. *Two Playes.* S3490. No UMI.

Shirley (1596–1666) is identified on the title page as a gentleman. For an echo of a line from *The Manciple's Prologue* in *St. Patrick for Ireland*, see SHIRLEY (1640) in the Appendix.

197.   WHARTON, GEORGE. "To my Very Honoured Friend," in Gaultier de Coste, Seigneur de La Calprenède's *Hymen's Præludia: or, Love's Master-Piece. Now Rendred into English by Robert Loveday.* L112A. UMI 1927: 7.

For a reference to the role of Chaucer and Gower in refining the English language, see WHARTON (1652); in this edition, the passage is found on sig. A4v.

1658

198.   ATKINS, JAMES. "Commendatory Poem" placed before James Smith's *The Innovation of Penelope and Ulysses, a Mock-Poem* in Sir John Mennes's *Wit Restor'd.* M1719. UMI 1036: 21.

As Spurgeon notes (1: 234), James Atkins mentions Chaucer in a commendatory poem addressed "To his Worthy Friend, Mr. J[ames] S[mith] Upon his happy Innovation of Penelope and Ulysses." Atkins writes:

> *It was no idle fancie, I beheld*
> *A reall object, that around did gild*
> *The neighbouring vallies and the mountaine tops,*

> *That sided to* Parnassus, *with the drops*
> *From her disheveld hayre. I sought the cause.*
> *And loe, she had her dwelling in the jawes*
> *Of pearly* Helicon, *assign'd to bee*
> *Guide ore the Comiock straynes of poetry.*
> *She* [Thalia] *lowr'd her flight, and soone assembled all*
> *That since old* Chaucer, *had tane leave to call*
> *Upon her name in print.* . . . (sig. K8r)

Thalia does not appear in Tatlock & Kennedy's *Concordance.*

199.   ATWELL, GEORGE. *The Faithfull Surveyor.* A4163. UMI 1221: 22.

In a commendatory poem headed "The Author to his Book," Atwell ("aliàs Wells, now teacher of the mathematicks in Cambridge") echoes Chaucer's line, "Go, litel bok, go litel myn tragedye" (*Troilus and Criseyde* 5: 1786):

> *Go,* little book, *and travel through the land*:
> *None will refuse to take thee in their hand.* (sig. *4v)

Other editions: A4164 (1662), no pagination, no signature; A4165 (1665), no pagination, no signature.

200.   AUSTIN, SAMUEL. Commendatory poem in *Naps upon Parnassus.* F1140. UMI Thomason Tracts 229: E.1840 (1).

As Spurgeon notes (1: 235), Samuel Austin (the younger) refers to Chaucer in a commendatory poem addressed "To his ingenuous Friend, the Author, on his incomparable Poem." Austin (*fl.* 1652–1671) writes that, compared to Thomas Flatman, Chaucer was worthless:

> If I may guess at Poets in our Land,
> *Thou beat'st* them all *above*, and *underhand*;
> . . . .
> To thee compar'd, our English Poets all stop,
> And vail their Bonnets, even *Shakespear's Falstop* [*sic*].
> *Chaucer* the first of all wasn't worth a farthing,
> *Lidgate*, and *Huntingdon*, with Gaffer *Harding*. (sig. B4v–5r).

201.   CLEVELAND, JOHN. *Poems, Characters, and Letters. By J. C. with Additions Never Before Printed.* C4692A. UMI 2493: 4.

For an echo of a line from *The Manciple's Prologue,* see CLEVELAND (1644); in this edition, the passage is found on 83.

Spurgeon (1: 224), citing Cleveland's *Works* (1687), rather than this earlier version, notes a reference to Chaucer and an allusion to *The Prologue of the Pardoner's Tale* in "A Letter sent from a Parliament Officer at Grantham." In this collection, Cleveland includes four letters that appear to have passed between himself and an officer in the Parliamentary forces: "A Letter to J. C.," "J. C. his Answer," "A Reply to J. C. his Answer," and "J. C. his second answer." In "A Reply to J. C. his Answer," in a passage about the Cleveland's misemployed rhetorical gifts, the officer writes:

> I'le allow you the gift in preaching . . . Pity it is such accomplish'd gifts, and prodigious parts, should be misimploy'd in secular affairs, such an holy Father might have begot as many babes for the Mother-Church of *Newark* as your party hath of late done Garrisons, and converted as many souls as *Chaucer's* Friar with the shoulderbone of the lost Sheep. (71)

Another edition in 1658: C4693 (UMI 1611: 70), 79, 87.

"Letters" are also found in *Clievelandi vindiciae: or, Cleveland's Genuine Poems, Orations, Epistles, &c.* C4671 (1677), 124.

"Letters" are also included in Cleveland's *Works*: C4654 (1687), 95–96; C4655 (1699), 95–96.

202.   CLEVELAND, JOHN. *The Rustick Rampant: or, Rurall Anarchy Affronting Monarchy in the Insurrection of Wat Tiler.* **C4699. UMI Thomason Tracts 243: E. 2133 (1).**

For a reference to Chaucer and a somewhat modernized quotation from *The Nun's Priest's Tale*, see CLEVELAND (1654); in this edition, the passage is found on 36–37.

203.   COCKAYNE, ASTON. *Small Poems of Divers Sorts.* **C4898. UMI 1280: 5.**

Cockayne (1608–1684) is identified on the title page as "Sir Aston Cokain." Spurgeon (1: 235–36) notes three references to Chaucer.

In "A Remedy for Love," in a passage about worthy sights in London, Cokayne refers first to London Bridge with its nineteen arches and then to Chaucer's tomb:

> There thou maist see the famous Monuments
> Of our *Heroes*, fram'd with large expence:
> There thou upon the Sepulchre maist look
> Of *Chaucer*, our true *Ennius*, whose old book
> Hath taught our Nation so to Poetize,
> That English rhthmes [*sic*] now any equalize;

That we no more need envy at the straine
Of *Tiber, Taugus*, or our neighbour *Seine*. (8)

In a commendatory poem addressed "To Mr. Humphry C. on his Poem entitled Loves Hawking-Boy," Cockayne alludes to *The Romaunt of the Rose* and he
compares "Humphry C." to Homer (and other ancient poets) and to Chaucer,
Lydgate, Gower, and Spenser:

Chaucer, we now commit thee to repose,
And care not for thy Romance of the *Rose*. (105)

In his first book of epigrams, number 36 is headed "Of Chaucer." Cockayne
writes:

Our good old *Chaucer* some despise: and why?
Because say they he writeth barbarously.
Blame him not (Ignorants) but your selves, that do
Not at these years your native language know. (155)

Spurgeon may have missed an allusion in a collection of Cockayne's songs. Number thirteen is headed "William the Conquerour to Emma the Miliners daughter of Manchester"; the reference to Cressida may be an allusion to *Troilus and
Criseyde*.

Hellen of Greece I should despise,
And *Cressida* unhandsome call;
Poppæa would not please mine eyes,
My *Emma* so exceeds them all. (267; sig. S6r)

Also collected in *A Chain of Golden Poems* (1658): C4894 (1658), 8, 60, 155, 267.

204.   HARRINGTON, JAMES. *The Commonwealth of Oceana.* H810. UMI 815: 21.

For an echo a line from *The Reeve's Tale*, see HARRINGTON (1656); in this edition,
the passage is found on 223.

205.   HILTON, JOHN. *Catch That Catch Can: or, A Choice Collection of Catches,
Rounds & Canons.* H2037. No UMI.

For a reference to Chaucer's jape in a song, see HILTON (1652); in this edition,
the passage is found on 48.

206.   MASSINGER, PHILIP. *The City-Madam.* M1046. (1658) UMI 324: 11.

Massinger (1583–1640) is characterized on the title page as a "gent." In this comedy "acted at the private house in Black Friers with great applause" (title page), Massinger appears to echo the Wife of Bath's claim that "Women desiren have sovereyntee" (*The Wife of Bath's Tale*, line 1038). In the second act, Stargaze (an astrologer) speaks to a group of London ladies:

> *Stargaze.* Now for the soverigntie of my future Ladies, your daughters after they are married.
> *Plenty.* Wearing the breeches you mean.
> *Lady.* Touch that point home,
> It is the principal one, and with London Ladies
> Of main consideration.
> *Stargaze.* This is infallible: . . . the Radix of the native in feminine figures, argue foretel, and declare preheminence, rule, preheminence and absolute soveraignity in women. (25)

Another edition: M1047 (1659), same pagination.

207.   MENNES, JOHN. *Wit Restor'd in Several Select Poems Not Formerly Publish't.* M1719. (1658) UMI 1036: 21.

For a commendatory poem addressed "To his Worthy Friend Mr. I. S. upon his happy Innovation of Penelope and Ulysses" that alludes to a spurious invocation of Thalia by Chaucer, see ATKINS (1658). The poem is found here on 75.

For a reference to "ould Chaucer" in "The Preface to that most elaborate piece of Poetry, entituled, Penelope and Ulysses," see JAMES SMITH (1656); in this edition, the passage is found on 149.

208.   OSBORNE, FRANCIS. *Historical Memoires on the Reigns of Queen Elizabeth and King James.* O515. UMI 218: 16.

Osborne (1593–1659) is not named or otherwise identified on the title page. As Bond notes (*SP* 28, but he cites the 1673 edition of Osborne's *Works*), in a section headed "Traditionall Memoyres on the Reigne of King James," Osborne mentions Chaucer. In a passage about the willful ignorance of Puritan divines, he writes of Chaucer's marginalization:

> [O]ur *Divines* for the generality did sacrifice more time to *Bacchus* than *Minerva* . . . scorning in their ordinary discourse at *Luther* and *Calvin*, but especially the last, so as I have heard a Bishop *thank God he never* (though a good Poet himself) *had read a line in him* [i.e., Calvin] *or* Chaucer. (247–48)

Another edition in 1658: 0515A, same pagination.

Also printed in Osborne's *Works*: 0505 (1673), 492; 0506 (1682), 441–42; 0507 (1689), 441–42; 0507A (1700), 396.

209.   PHILLIPS, EDWARD. *The Mysteries of Love and Eloquence.* **P2066. UMI 328: 15; UMI Thomason Tracts 216: E.1735 (1).**

As Spurgeon notes (1: 236), in a section headed "Miscelania. Fancy awakened: Natural, Amorous, Moral, Experimental Parasoxical, Enigmatical, Jesting, and Jovial Questions, with their several Answers and Solutions," Phillips (1630–1696?) attributes a couplet to Chaucer:

Q.   *What was old* Chaucers *Saw?*
A.   Lord be merciful unto us,
Fools or Knaves will else undo us. (180; sig. N2v)

Another edition: P2067 (1685), 196; and another with a different title: *The Beau's Academy*, P2064 (1699), 196.

210.   PHILLIPS, EDWARD. *The New World of English Words: or, A General Dictionary.* **P2068. UMI 286: 9.**

Phillips (1630–1696?) is identified on the title page as "E. P." As Spurgeon notes (1: 236), the engraved title page of this work is adorned with representations of learned writers. Chaucer is depicted in quarter length and is paired with Spenser; Lambard is paired with Camden; Selden with Spelman; and a scholar of Cambridge with a scholar of Oxford.

As Graves notes (*SP*), there is another reference in a dedicatory epistle addressed to "the most illustrious, and impartial sisters, the two universities." Phillips refers to Chaucer in a passage about his intention to make a better dictionary that had hitherto been produced:

[I]f the Grandeur of such an undertaking be rightly considered, no ordinary industry will be required, next the consulting with the Monuments of ancient Records and Manuscripts derived to us from reverend Authours, there will be occasion to peruse the Works of our ancient Poets, as *Geffry Chaucer* the greatest in his time, for the honour of our Nation; as also some of our modern Modern Poets, as *Spencer, Sidney, Draiton, Daniel*, with our Reformers of the Scene, *Johnson, Shakesphear* [*sic*], *Beaumont*, and *Fletcher* . . . and divers others. (sig. a3v)

Spurgeon (1: 236) also notes a reference in the preface:

[I]t is evident, that the Saxon, or German tongue is the ground-work upon which our language is founded, the mighty stream of forraigne words that hath since *Chaucers* time broke in upon it, having not yet wash't away the root. (sig. b4v)

Chaucer is also cited as the source of many definitions, yet some of them are not found in Tatlock & Kennedy's *Concordance*. For those that are, we have cited their usage:

Advenale, a Coat of defence, *Chaucer*. (sig. A4r)

An *Agiler*, a marker of men Chaucer. (sig. B1r)

Amalgaminge, an old word used by *Chaucer*, signifying a mixture of Quicksilver, with other metals. (sig. B3r) [*The Canon's Yeoman's Tale*, line 771]

Amortize, to kill, a word used by *Chaucer*. (sig. B4r) [*The Parson's Tale*, line 245–50]

Appeteth, desireth, a word used by *Chaucer*. (sig. C3r)

Apprentice, skill, *Chaucer*. (sig. C3r) [*The Romaunt of the Rose*, line 687]

Arblaster, a word used by *Chaucer*, signifying a Cros-bow. (sig. C3v) [*The Romaunt of the Rose*, line 4196]

Argoil, Clay, a word used by *Chaucer*. (sig. C3v) [*The Canon's Yeoman's Tale*, line 813]

Arretteth, layeth blame, an old word used by *Chaucer*. (sig. C4r) [*The Parson's Tale*, lines 580–85]

Arten, to constrain, an (old word) used by *Chaucer*. (sig. C4v) [*Troilus and Criseyde* 1: 388]

Assise, Order, *Chaucer*. (sig. D1r) [*The Romaunt of the Rose*, lines 900, 1237, 1392]

Assoyle, to acquit, to pardon, also to answer, *Chaucer*. (sig. D1r) [*The Pardoner's Prologue* and *Tale*, lines 387, 913, 933, 939; and elsewhere]

Asterlagour, a word used by *Chaucer*, signifying an Astrolabe. (sig. D1r)

Autremite, another attire, a word used by *Chaucer*. (sig. D3r)

Barm-cloth, an Apron, *Chaucer*. (sig. D4v) [*The Miller's Tale*, line 3236]

Baudon, custody, a word used by *Chaucer*. (sig. E1r) [*The Romaunt of the Rose*, line 1163]

Bay . . . *Chaucer* also useth it for a stake. (sig. E1r)

Beau Sir, fair sir, a word used by *Chaucer*. (sig. E1v) [*The Romaunt of the Rose*, line 6053]

Bend, used by *Chaucer* for a muffler, a caul, a kercher. (sig. E2r) [*The Romaunt of the Rose*, line 1079]

Burnet, . . . a word used by *Chauser* [*sic*], signifying woolen, also a hood, or attire for the head. (sig. F1v) [*The Romaunt of the Rose*, line 226]

Caitisned, chained, a word used by *Chaucer*. (sig. F2v)

Canceline, chamlet, a word used by *Chaucer*. (sig. F3v)

Chasteleyn, a word used by *Chaucer*, signifying a Gentle-woman of a great house. (sig. G4v) [*The Romaunt of the Rose*, lines 3740, 6327]

Chekelaton, a stuff like motly. *Chaucer*. (sig. H1r)

Chelandri, a Goldfinch, a word used by *Chaucer*. (sig. H1r) [*The Romaunt of the Rose*, lines 81, 914]

Chertes, merry people, *Chaucer*. (sig. H1r)

Chevesal, a Gorget. *Chaucer*. (sig. H1r) [*The Romaunt of the Rose*, line 1082]

Chimbe, the uttermost part of a barrel. *Chaucer*. (sig. H1v)

Chincherie, niggardlinesse, a word used by *Chaucer*. (sig. H1v) [*The Tale of Melibee*, lines 2790–95]

Cierges, wax candles, lamps. *Chaucer*. (sig. H2r) [*The Romaunt of the Rose*, line 6248]

Citriale, a Cittern, a word used by *Chaucer*. (sig. H3r)

Clergion, a Clark, *Chaucer*. (sig. H3r) [*The Prioress's Tale*, line 1693]

Clicket, a clapper of a door, *Chaucer* also useth it for a key. (sig. H3r) [*The Merchant's Tale*, lines 2046, 2117, 2121, 2123, 2151]

Curebulli, tann'd leather, a word used by *Chaucer*. (sig. H4v)

Dennington, a Castle in *Bark-shire*, built by Sir *Richard de Aberbury*, it was once the Residence of the Poet *Chaucer*, afterwards of *Charles Brandon* Duke of *Suffolk*. (sig. L4r)

Desidery, from the Latin *desiderium*, desire or lust. It is a word used by *Chaucer*. (sig. M1r)

Deslavy, leacherous beastly, a word used by *Chaucer*. (sig. M1r) [*The Parson's Tale*, lines 625–30, 830–35]

Digne, from the Latin word *dignus*, neat, gentyle, worthy. It is a word used by *Chaucer*. (sig. M2v) [*The General Prologue*, lines 141, 517; and elsewhere]

Discure, to discover, a word used by *Chaucer*. (sig. M3r) [*The Book of the Duchess*, line 548]

Divine, (lat.) Heavenly, also it is taken substantively for a professour of Theology, whom *Chaucer* calls a divinistre. (sig. M4r) [*The Knight's Tale*, line 2811]

Dowtremere, fair wearing, a word used by *Chaucer*. (sig. N1v) [*The Book of the Duchess*, line 253]

Ebrack, the Hebrew tongue; a word used by *Chaucer*. (sig. N2v) [*The Man of Law's Tale*, line 489; *The Prioress's Tale*, line 1750; *The House of Fame*, 3: 343]

Gibsere, a pouch, a word used by *Chaucer*. (sig. Q4r)

Giglet, or *Giglot*, a wanton woman or strumpet. *Chaucer*. (sig. Q4r)

Gourd, a kind of plant, somewhat like a coucumber, also used by *Chaucer* for a bottel. (sig. R1r) [*The Manciple's Tale*, lines 82, 91]

Haketon, a Jacket without sleeves. *Chaucer.* (sig. R3r)

Hanselines, upper slopes. *Chaucer.* (sig. R3v)

Losenger, a flatterer, a word used by *Chaucer.* (sig. Aa1r) [*The Nun's Priest's Tale*, line 4516; *The Legend of Good Women*, line 352; *The Romaunt of the Rose*, line 1050]

Magonel, according to *Chaucer*, is an instrument to cast stones with. (sig. Aa3v) [*The Romaunt of the Rose*, line 6279]

Rebeck, an old Trot, *Chaucer.* (sig. Kk2r) [*The Friar's Tale*, line 1573]

Woodstock. . . In this Town *Geffery Chaucer* a most famous English Poet was brought up (sig. Rr4r)

Other editions: P2069 (1662), Chaucer's "portrait" on engraved title page; references in dedication, sig. (a3)v; in preface, sig. (b4)v; in definitions *passim* (with additions).

P2070 (1663), no engraved title page for UMI copy; dedication, sig. (a3)v; preface, sig. (b4)v; in definitions *passim*.

P2071 (1671), engraved title page; no dedicatory epistle; preface, sig. (b)1v; in definitions *passim* (with an omission).

P2072 (1678), engraved title page, a different dedication (no Chaucer reference), preface (sig. a2v); in definitions *passim* (with omissions and additions).

P2072A (1678), engraved title page, preface (sig. a2v); in definitions *passim*.

P2073 (1696), engraved title page, no dedication, preface (sig. a2v), in definitions *passim* (with omissions and additions).

P2074 (1700), UMI 2729: 3, engraved title page, no dedication, preface (no pagination or signature), in definitions *passim*.

211.   SANDERSON, WILLIAM. *A Compleat History of the Life and Raigne of King Charles from His Cradle to His Grave.* **S646. UMI 226: 8.**

Sanderson (1586?–1676) is identified on the title page as "William Sanderson Esq." In a section about the king's relations with the Scots, he cites Chaucer's description of the Sergeant of Law in *The General Prologue* and quotes lines 321–22:

> The House of *Commons* intent upon Reformation of any thing any kinde of way, and to please the Presbyter, with little debate made an Order for taking away all scandalous Pictures, Crosses, and Figures within the Churches, and afterwards from without, suppressing the very Signs and Sign-posts; and this curiosity of Imployment was conferred upon such as had least to do, and could intend to be busied abroad. Sir *Robert Harloe* was found out to be the fittest person, which makes me remember *Chaucer's* Character of such another.

A busier man there never was,
Yet seemed busier than he was. (430)

212.   SPENCER, JOHN. Καινα και παλαια [Kaina kai palaia]. *Things New and Old: or, A Store-house of Similies.* S4960. UMI 549: 6.

Spencer (d. 1680) is characterized on the title page as "a lover of Learning and Learned Men." He appears to echo a line from *The Reeve's Tale*: "The gretteste clerkes been noght wisest men" (line 4054) in a section headed "Experimental Knowledge, the onely Knowledg [*sic*]." Spencer writes:

It is well known, that the *great Doctors* of the World by much reading and speculation attain unto a great *height of Knowledge*, but seldom to *sound Wisdome*, which hath given way to that common Proverb, *The greatest Clerks, are not alwaies the wisest Men.* (437)

213.   SMITH, JAMES. "The Preface to That Most Elaborate Piece of Poetry Entituled Penelope and Ulysses," in *Wit Restored.* M1719. UMI 1036: 21.

For a reference to a sharp disagreement about a poet's commendation of "ould" Chaucer, see SMITH (1656); in this edition, the passage is found on 149.

214.   TOPSELL, EDWARD. *The History of Four-footed Beasts and Serpents.* G624. UMI 70: 1.

For a passage in which Topsell quotes a modernized and amended description of the Franklin from *The General Prologue* (lines 352–54), see TOPSELL (1608), Boswell & Holton No. 785; in this edition, the passage is found in *The Historie of Serpents* on 780–81.

1659

215.   BLOUNT, THOMAS. *Glossographia: or, A Dictionary.* B3334a. UMI 2600: 6.

For a reference to "old Chaucer" and a quotation from *Troilus and Cryssede* and to Chaucer as an authority on language and word usage, see BLOUNT (1656); in this edition, the passages are found in the epistle (A4v), and in definitions for *agrise* (B7v), *agroted* (B7v), *algebra* (B8v), *alnath* (C2r), *amortize* (C4v), *barbicane* (F4v), *benison* (F7r), *bordel* (G2r), *burlybrand* (G4v), *callot* (G6v), *cheve* (omitted), *covent* (L4r), *creance* (L5v), *dissheviled / disheviled* (N4v), *dulcarnon* (O1r), *fryth* (R6v), *gossymeare* (S5r), *lodemanage* (Z7v), *losender* (Aa1r), *meriot* (Bb5r), *moiles* (Cc1r), *mortress* (Cc3v), *orfraies* (Ee3v), *ouch* (Ee5r), *paraments* (Ff2r), *pilgrim* (Gg6v–7r), *rebeck* (Kk4r), *romance* (L15r), *romant* (L15r), *strand / strond* (Oo8v), *superstition* (Pp4v), *taberd* (Qq1r), *tailage* (Qq2r).

216.   CLEVELAND, JOHN. *Poems.* C4694. UMI 1438: 5.

For an echo of a line from *The Manciple's Prologue*, see CLEVELAND (1644); in this edition, the passage is found on 183.

217.   DELONEY, THOMAS. *The Garland of Good-Will.* **This edition is not in Wing; unique copy is in a private collection.**

For what may be a faint allusion to *The Clerk's Tale*, see DELONEY (1628) in Boswell & Holton No. 1116.

    Other editions: D946 (1678), sigs. E7r–F2v; D947 (1685), sigs. E7r–F2v; D947A (before 1688), sig. D5v–10r; D948 (1688), sigs. E7r–F2v; D951 (1696?), sigs. D6–8v.

218.   GAYTON, EDMUND. *The Art of Longevity: or, A Diæteticall Institution.* G406. UMI 1207: 2.

Gayton (1608–1666) is identified on the title page as "Bachelor of Physick, of St. John Bapt. Coll. Oxford." He alludes faintly to Pertelote ("Mistresse of sir *Chanticler*") and *The Nun's Priest's Tale* in this treatise on the connection between diet and longevity. In chapter 19, "Of the members and parts of Creatures," Gayton writes:

> Livers of Beasts are hot and moist, and breed
> Much blood (they are congealed blood indeed)
> But hard and heavy: that of Lamb or Calf,
> Or of the sucking Pig, is diet safe:
> But *Isaak* saith that liver doth prefer,
> Of the sweet Mistresse of sir *Chanticler*. . . . (39)

In chapter 22, "Of Hens," Gayton again alludes to *The Nun's Priest's Tale*. According to "Rabbi Isaak," Gayton writes, for a healthy diet we should

>   the Chick before the Mother chuse,
> As being the tougher nourishment, enough,
> But for my meal give me a Hen tooth-proof,
> Not tough as buff, nor yet as whit-leather,
> But often humbled by Sir *Chanticler*;
> Then full of Embrion chick, let her appear
> In Claret-sawce throughout all *Janivere*. (44)

219.   HARRINGTON, JAMES. *Politicaster: or, A Comical Discourse.* H818a. UMI Thomason Tracts 241: E.2112 (2).

In this *Comical Discourse* Harrington (1611–1677) answers Matthew Wren's *Monarchy Asserted* which was written against Harrington's *Oceana*. In his "Prologue," written in answer to Wren's "Preface," which, Harrington says, dared his muse to answer, he says he will answer Wren's provocations some time in the future; in the meantime, he gives Wren a taste of his wares in Chaucerian language:

> [I will answer you with] some Poems not abhorring from your desires or
> or provocations, not in the Thunder-thumping way of Grandsire *Virgil*,
> but in the sugar'd speech of mine Uncle *Chaucer*. If you please by the
> way to take a lick of it, I shall at this distance from the *Opera*, insert the
> Prologue.

> What Chaucer ho, ye han the English Key
> Of the high Rock Parnas with the Tow'rs twey.
> Your sooten gab, so ken I well thus far,
> Of curtesie the Yate till me unspar.
> But here be Babins in the way I trow,
> All to be prickle like Urchin, hi ho.
> Forth come wi brond, gin ye no bren em green
> Ne Note they keepen out that nere wer in.

Pray, Sir, ha' me commended to them that say, Your book is unanswerable; and let them know, it is to them that the Prologue is spoken. (2–3)

220.   HEATH, ROBERT. *Paradoxical Assertions and Philosophical Problems Full of Delight and Recreation for All Ladies and Youthful Fancies.* H1341. UMI 601: 12.

In the second part, in a section headed "Why men talk most and loudest when they are drunk," Heath (*fl.* 1636–1659) refers to Chaucer's mill, perhaps alludes to *The Reeve's Tale*:

> [I]n a Deluge and Sea of Drink, where the Understanding is first shipwrackt, the troubled Sea-sick Sailors must with the Billows storm for company in this Confusion, or else they cannot hear: for understand one another either but seldom do, unless it be by signs.

> Or doth the continual pouring forth of their Liquors deafn them, like the by-dwellers to the Cataracts of *Nyle*? and so make them hoop and hollow to one another as they were all hunting the Fox in the *Wild* of *Kent*, or dwelt in *Chaucer's* Mill? Or doth the Drink make them wise . . .? (^{2} (12)

Another edition: H1341A (1664), ^{2}12.

221.   HEYLYN, PETER. *Certamen epistolare: or, The Letter-Combate. Managed by Peter Heylyn.* H1687. UMI Thomason Tracts 214: E. 1722 (1).

Heylyn (1600–1662) is identified on the title page as "Peter Heylyn, D.D." This work is composed of a series of letters by various hands addressed to Heylyn and his response to them. Dr. N. Barnard of Gray's Inn wrote to chide Heylyn for having publicly burned a book by an "eminent and pious Primate." Heylyn echoes Chaucer as he refers to Ovid's description of the home of Rumor as the "House of Fame." Heylyn writes:

> *Ovid*, in his *Metamorphosis* . . . lays down the Character of the House of *Fame*. . . . According to this Character of the House of *Fame*, the report of burning the Book aforesaid, being taken thence, flew far, and grew greater by the flying. (108–9)

222.   HOWELL, JAMES. Παροιμιογραφια [Paroimiographia]. *Proverbs: or, Old Sayed Sawes & Adages.* H3098. UMI 421: 16.

Howell (1594?–1666) is identified on the title page as "J. H. Esqr." As Harris notes (*PQ*), Howell mentions Chaucer's salty language in an epistle addressed to "The Knowingest Kind of Philologers":

> Now let the squeamish Reder [*sic*] take this Rule along with him, that Proverbs being Proleticall, and free familiar Countrey sayings do assume the Libertie to be sometimes in plain, down right and homely termes, with wanton naturall Expressions, that with their Salt forme some of them carry a kind of Salacity (which are very frequent in *Gower, Chaucer, Skelton, Jo. Heywood* and others) yet they cannot be taxt of beastlines, or bawdry. (sig. ¶1r)

In his collection of proverbs, Howell appears to echo a line from *The Reeve's Tale*: "The gretteste clerkes been noght wisest men" (line 4054). He writes:

> The greatest Clerks are not alwayes the wisest men. (2)
> The greatest Clerks are not alwayes the learnedest men. (18)

Howell also seems to echo the description of the Wife of Bath in *The General Prologue*, "For she koude of that art the olde daunce" (line 476). He writes:

> She knowes enough of the old dance. (17)

Also found in *Lexicon tetraglotton, An English-French-Italian-Spanish Dictionary*: H3087 (1660), H3088 (1660), H3089 (1660), all with the same pagination.

223. JONES, BASSETT. *Herm'ælogium: or, An Essay on the Rationality of the Art of Speaking. Offered by B. J.* J925. UMI Thomason Tracts 242: E.2122 (3).

As Spurgeon notes (1: 237), Jones quotes two modernized passages from Chaucer to buttress his argument in part 3, chapter 1, "Shewing the variations and affections of the word of Motion. And first of its distinguishment by number and person: Also of the Verb impersonal." The first is from *The Canon's Yeoman's Tale* (lines 1326–29), and the second is from *The Parliament of Fowls* (lines 22–25). Jones writes:

> [T]he first and seconde persons of the Verb be aswell digitally as vocally notified; but this third person never digitally, saving in order to contempt. So that it was not without reason that the old *English* usurped it for the heightning [*sic*] of perswasion. As Sir *Geoffery Chaucer* when representing the cheating Alchymist [in a shoulder note: "The Chanons yeomans tale"]

> —Thus said he in his game,
> Stoopeth a down in faith you be to blame.
> Helpeth me now, as I did you wylere,
> Put in your hond and looketh what is there. (42)

The Verb Impersonal of the of the Passive Voice I observe to vary from the sense of its personality only while it fixeth our observance to it self; just as the fore-quoted noble *Chaucer* doth by a personal Active, where he thus singeth [in a shoulder note: "In Assembly of fowls"]:

> As from awd ground MENSAIEH cometh Corn fro yeer to year.
> So from awd books, by my faith, commen all new Science that men lere.   (43)

In part 4, chapter 1, "Being a transient disquisition of the state of our Author's four undeclined parts of Speech; with their Concomitant Mutes; and lastly of the Pronoune," in a passage on the gravity of Italians, Jones again turns to Chaucer, this time to *The Squire's Tale* (lines 103–04):

> [O]bserve that, before the use of Bandstrings, this gravity hath been emulated by the English. The noble *Chaucer*, as he encomiat's the deportment of the Arabian Envoy in the Tartarian presence; thus singing [in a shoulder note: "The Squier Tale"]:

Accordant to his woords was his chere;
As teacheth art of speech hem that it lere. (69)

224. *Lady Alimony: or, The Alimony Lady. An Excellent Pleasant New Comedy Duly Authorized, Daily Acted, and Frequently Followed.* **L162A. UMI 152: 8.**

This anonymously published play features six "Cashiered Consorts," six "Alimony Ladies," and six gentlemen described as "The Ladies Platonick Confidents" (sig. A2r). In the second act, Madam Fricase, one of the Alimony Ladies, may allude to *The Clerk's Tale* as she asks in an aside:

Could the patience
Of *Grissel*, were she living, reap content
In such enjoyments? Could she suffer youth
Quickned with blooming fancy to expire
And quench her heat with such an useless snuff? (sig. C4v)

Later in the same scene, as Atkinson (*MLN* 1944), Graves (*SP*), and Harris (*PQ*) note, there is a reference to *The Wife of Bath's Tale*. Madam Caveare, another Alimony Lady, responds to Caranto, one of the Platonic companions:

[N]e're was woman matcht
To such a stupid, sottish animal;
One that's compos'd of Non-sense, and so weak
In Masculine abilities, he ne're read
The *Wife of Bathes Tale*, nor what thing might please
A woman best. . . . (sig. D1r)

225. **LEIGH, EDWARD.** *England Described.* **L994. UMI Thomason Tracts 224: E.1792 (2).**

Leigh (1602–1671) is identified on the title page as "Mr of Arts of Magdalen-Hall in Oxford." In a section headed "Middlesex," in a passage about famous men who were born there, Leigh writes:

Chaucer, Edmund Spenser the famous *English* Poets were born in *London.* (130) . . . [In Westminster] are buried the Prince of *English* Poets *Geffrey Chaucer*: as also he that for pregnant wit, and an excellent gift in Poetry of all *English* poets came neerest unto him *Edmund Spenser.* (134–35)

In a section headed "Oxfordshire," in a passage about Woodstock, Leigh adds:

The Town it self having nothing at all to shew, glorieth yet in this, that *Jeffrey Chaucer* our *English Homer* was there bred and brought up. (156)

226.   LLOYD, DAVID. *The Legend of Captain Jones.* L2632. UMI 2573: 3.

For a reference to Chaucer and *The Tale of Sir Thopas*, see LLOYD L2635 (1648); in this edition, the passage is found on 27.

227.   LOVEDAY, ROBERT. *Loveday's Letters Domestick and Forrein.* L3225. UMI Thomason Tracts 223: E.1784 (1).

Loveday (*fl.* 1655) is identified on the title page as a gentleman who was "the late Translator of the three first parts of *Cleopatra*." This collection of letters is addressed "to Several Persons, Occasionally distributed in Subjects Philosophicall, Historicall & Morall" (title page). As Harris notes (*PQ*), in letter No. 52, "To his Brother Mr. A. L.," Loveday refers to Chaucer as a prophet and poet. Perhaps Loveday alludes to the spurious work known as "Chaucer's Prophecy":

> *Dear Brother* . . . Nothing can come from you that shall not bit it self welcome; but your precepts that way will find an extraordinary entertainment. I fear the product of these uncivill wars will prove your *Chaucer* as much Prophet as Poet; but as it is not in our power to stay the hand that scourges us, so it is not in our knowledge how soon the Chirurgery of Heaven will drop balm into our wounds. (98–99)

Other editions: L3226 (1662), 98–99; L3227 (1663), 98–99; L3228 (1669), 98–99; L3228A (1669), 98–99; L3229 (1673), 98–99; L3229B (1677), 98–99; L3230 (1684), 98–99.

228.   MASSINGER, PHILIP. *The City-Madam.* M1047. UMI 698: 19.

See MASSINGER (1658); in this edition, the passage is found on 25.

229.   SOMNER, WILLIAM. *Dictionarium Saxonico-Latino-Anglicum.* S4663. UMI 194: 2.

Somner (1598–1669) is identified on the title page as "Guliel. Somneri Cantuariensis." In a Latin epistle addressed "Ad Lectorem," Somner notes his indebtedness to "*Chauceri*, & aliorum quorundam verendæ antiquitatis scriptorum, secerim mentionem" (sig. b1r).

As Alderson & Henderson note, Somner cites Chaucer as he traces the etymology of *Acolian, Aedwitan, Bode, Gatge-treow, Geare, Naes, Ohwater, Ord, Scathe, Scendan, Undern, Wissian, Wite.* There are more than a few other references. Some of Somner's citations appear in Tatlock & Kennedy's *Concordance*, but several others do not and appear to be attributions rather than true Chaucerisms. Citations found with the aid of Tatlock & Kennedy are noted in square brackets following Somner's reference. When there are unique citations (or a very few), I cite Chaucer's usage; otherwise, I note that there are many citations in

Tatlock & Kennedy. I have transliterated Old English words into their equivalents in the modern English alphabet and placed them in square brackets.

[Acolian] . . . Hinc nostratium acold, Chaucero acale, frigidus. (sig. A2r) [Chaucer uses *acoolde* in *The Romaunt of the Rose*.]

[Ædwitan] . . . twitted, mocked. Chaucero nostro, attwite. (sig. A3r) [Not found in Tatlock & Kennedy.]

[Agrisan] . . . to dread and fear greatly. Hinc *Chauceri* nostri agrise & agrisen. (sig. B2r) [Eight citations (with variants) in Tatlock & Kennedy.]

[Agyltan] . . . Hinc *Chauceri* nostri agilted . . . be offended. (sig. B2v) [Chaucer uses *a-gilt* (and variants) multiple times.]

[Aldor] . . . an Elder or Senator, a Chieftan, a Prince, a Dictator, a Magistrate. Chaucero nostro Aldor. (sig. B3r) [Tatlock & Kennedy cite *alder* and *elder*, but not *aldor*.]

[Algeats] . . . all manner of ways . . . altogether. Chaucero, algate. (sig. B3r) [Many citations in Tatlock & Kennedy.]

[Alotene] . . . groveling . . . Hinc *Chauceri* nostri loute (sig. B3v) [Many citations in Tatlock & Kennedy.]

[Bana] . . . the undoing or bane. *Chaucero* nostro bane. (sig. D1r) [Many citations in Tatlock & Kennedy.]

[Barme] . . . a bosome, a lappe. *Chaucero* nostro barme . . . barm-cloth. (sig. D1r-v) [Chaucer uses *barmeclooth* in *The Miller's Tale*.]

[Behat] . . . a vow, a promise. *Chaucero* nostro, behete, behote. (sig. D3r) [Many citations in Tatlock & Kennedy.]

[Bema] . . . a trumpet. *Chaucero* nostro bemes. (sig. D3v) [Chaucer uses *beme* and *bemes* in *The House of Fame*, *The Nun's Priest's Tale*, and *The Romaunt of the Rose*.]

[Bemænan] . . . to bewail, to bemoan . . . *Chauceri* bemeint. (sig. D3v) [Chaucer uses *bemene* in *The Romaunt of the Rose*.]

[Bene] . . . *Chaucero*, bone. (sig. D3v) [Many citations in Tatlock & Kennedy.]

[Benemde] . . . taken away. *Chaucero*, benimmeth, *pro* bereaveth. (sig. D3v) [Many citations in Tatlock & Kennedy.]

[Bilith] an image, a representation, resemblance, or likenesse. . . . Hoc *Chaucero* nostro, blee. Hence to know one by the blee. . . . (sig. E3r) [The phrase is not found in Tatlock & Kennedy.]

[Blinnan] . . . to cease, to give over . . . cease, Chaucero blin. (sig. E3v-4r) [Chaucer uses *blinne* (and variant spellings) in *The Canon's Yeoman's Tale*, *Troilus and Criseyde*, and *The Romaunt of the Rose*.]

[Bode] . . . a message, a charge or injunction . . . *Chaucero* nostro, bode. (sig. E4v) [Five citations in Tatlock & Kennedy.]

[Borhoe] . . . *Chaucero*, borrow, *Scotis*, borgh. (sig. F1r) [Many citations in Tatlock & Kennedy.]

[Bot. bote]. . . . our, to boote. *Chaucero*, boote. . . . (sig. F1r) [Many citations in Tatlock & Kennedy.]

[Bræde] . . . *Chaucero*, brede. (sig. F1v) [Many citations in Tatlock & Kennedy.]

[Bratt] . . . a cloak . . . cum *Chaucero*, paniculus, a ragge. (sig. F1v) [Chaucer uses *Ragges* twice in *The Romaunt of the Rose*.]

[Brice] . . . a breach. *Chaucero*, brecke. (sig. F2r) [Tatlock & Kennedy cite multiple uses of *breke* (and variant spellings).]

[Brid] . . . a spouse, a bride. *Chaucero*, brede. (sig. F2r) [Chaucer uses *bryde* and *bride* but not *brede* in this sense.]

[Brucan] . . . to profit . . . *Chaucero*, broke, & brouke (sig. F2v) [Many citations in Tatlock & Kennedy.]

[Buce] . . . the belly or paunch. *Chaucero*, bewke. (sig. F3r) [Chaucer uses *bouke* in *The Knight's Tale*.]

[Butan] . . . without punishment. *Chaucero* nostro, bout, sine, without. (sig. F3v) [Not found in Tatlock & Kennedy.]

[Cælan] . . . to coole or make cold, to refresh. *Chaucero*, kele. (sig. F4v) [Not found in Tatlock & Kennedy.]

[Cearcian] . . . to charke, or (as in *Chaucers* language) to chirke. . . . chattering teeth. . . . *Chaucero* nostro chirking. (sig. G1v) [Several citations in Tatlock & Kennedy.]

[Ceorl-boren] . . . a plebian, clown or churle by birth or place. Chaucero, churliche. (sig. G2r) [Chaucer uses *cherlyssh* and *cherlishly* in *The Franklin's Tale* and *The Romaunt of the Rose*.]

[Cleopian] . . . *Chaucero*, clepen. (sig. G3v) [Many citations in Tatlock & Kennedy.]

[Clumian] . . . to mutter or murmur . . . Hinc *Chauceri* nostri clum. (sig. G4r) [Chaucer uses *clom* twice in *The Miller's Tale*.]

[Cweman] . . . to please, to delight . . . *Chaucero*, queme, & quemen. (sig. H3r) [Chaucer uses *queme* in *Troilus and Criseyde*, *Gentilesse*, and *The Romaunt of the Rose*.]

[Cyththe] [*sic*, C&ððe] . . . acquaintance, kindred, alliance. *Chaucero* nostro, kith. (sig. H4v) [Chaucer uses *kith* twice in *Troilus and Criseyde*.]

[Dreori. dreorig] . . . sorrowfull, pensive, dreery. *Chaucero*, dreri. (sig. I3v) [Chaucer uses *drery* several times and *drerihede* once in *The Romaunt of the Rose*.]

[Dreorignysse] . . . sadnesse . . . *Chaucero*, drerienes. (sig. I3v) [Chaucer uses *drerinesse* twice in *Troilus and Criseyde*.]

[Dwinan] . . . to dwindle . . . *Chaucero*, dwined. (sig. K1r) [Chaucer uses *dwined* once, in *The Romaunt of the Rose*.]

[Dyrn] . . . secret, privie. *Chaucero*, derne. (sig. K1r) [Chaucer uses *deerne* three times in *The Miller's Tale*.]

[Eath] . . . soft ready. *Chaucero*, eth, eyth. (sig. K3r) [Chaucer uses *ethe* three times, in *The Parliament of Fowles*, *Troilus and Criseyde*, and *The Romaunt of the Rose*.]

[Elde] . . . age. *Chaucero*, elth, eld. (sig. L1r) [Tatlock & Kennedy cite multiple uses of *eld*, *elde*, and *eelde*.]

[Eode] . . . went out. *Chaucero*, yde, yeden, yode. (sig. L2r) [Many citations of *yede* and *yeden* in Tatlock & Kennedy.]

[Fela] . . . many. *Chaucero*, fele. (sig. M2r) [Many citations in Tatlock & Kennedy.]

[Feorrne] . . . *Chaucero*, ferne. (sig. M3r) [Several citations in Tatlock & Kennedy.]

[Feorth] . . . the fourth. *Chaucero*, ferth. (sig. M3r) [Many citations in Tatlock & Kennedy.]

[Fla] . . . an arrow, a shaft, a dart. *Chaucero*, flo. (sig. M4v) [Chaucer uses *flo* once, in *The Manciple's Tale*.]

[Flitan] . . . to contend, to strive, to brawle. *Chaucero*, flite & slight. (sig. M4v) [Not found in Tatlock & Kennedy.]

[For-lætan] . . . *Chaucero*, forlete, forleten. (sig. N4r) [Many citations in Tatlock & Kennedy.]

[Forthi] . . . wherefore, why. *Chaucer*, forthy. (sig. O1r) [Many citations in Tatlock & Kennedy.]

[Forword] . . . a bargain . . . an agreement. *Chaucero*, forward. (sig. O1v) [Many citations in Tatlock & Kennedy.]

[Fother] . . . *Chaucero*, fother. (sig. O2r) [Chaucer uses *fother* twice, in *The General Prologue* and *The Knight's Tale*.]

[Fremd] . . . forain, strange . . . a stranger . . . *Chaucero*, fremd, fremed. (sig. O2v) [Four citations in Tatlock & Kennedy.]

[Frith-splott] . . . Happily some consecrated grove. *Chaucer* useth the word *fryth* for a wood. (sig. O3v) [Not found in Tatlock & Kennedy.]

[Gate-treow] . . . *Chaucero* nostro, gaytere-berries. (sig. P3r) [Not found in Tatlock & Kennedy.]

[Geare] . . . of old. Hinc *Chauceri* & nostratium yore. . . . (sig. P3v) [Many citations in Tatlock & Kennedy.]

[Gearwe] . . . ready, quick, prepared . . . *Chauceri* yare . . . (sig. P3v) [Chaucer uses *yare* once, in *The Legend of Good Women*.]

[Ge-beaten] . . . beaten, stamped. *Chaucer* (changing the *ge* into *i*, as in many other words) hath it, ibet. (sig. P4r). [*Ibet* is not found in Tatlock & Kennedy.]

[Gemænced] . . . mixed, mingled. . . . *Chaucer* (with a change of the particle *ge* into *I*) hath it *imeint*. (sig. R2r) [Not found in Tatlock & Kennedy.]

[Georn] . . . studious . . . earnest . . . *Chaucero*, yerne. (sig. R4r) [Not found in Tatlock & Kennedy.]

[Gete] . . . a gate. *Chaucero*, yate. (sig. S2v) [Many citations in Tatlock & Kennedy.]

[Gewrigen] . . . covered, hid. iwri, & iwrien, *Chaucero*. (sig. S4v) [Not found in Tatlock & Kennedy.]

[Gif] . . . if . . . *Chaucero*, yif. (sig. T1v) [Chaucer uses *gif* several times, but *yif* is not found in Tatlock & Kennedy.]

[Gled] . . . a burning coal. *Chaucero*, glede. (sig. T2r) [Several citations in Tatlock & Kennedy.]

[Grani] . . . anger, fury. *Chaucero*, grame. (sig. T3v) [Chaucer uses *grame* in *The Canon's Yeoman's Tale*, *Anelida*, and *Troilus and Criseyda*.]

[Grith] . . . peace. *Chaucero*, grith. (sig. T4r) [Not found in Tatlock & Kennedy.]

[Hæl . . . health, safety, safe-guard . . . *Chaucero*, hele, heyle. (sig. V1v) [Many citations in Tatlock & Kennedy.]

[Hæwen] . . . rotten . . . gray of colour, or blew . . . *Chaucero*, hewen, hewed. (sig. V2v) [Chaucer uses *hewen* in *The Knight's Tale*.]

[Half] . . . the neck. *Chaucero*, halfe.(sig. V3r) [*Halfe* in this sense is not found in Tatlock & Kennedy.]

[Hamelan] . . . to cut asunder . . . *Chaucero*, hameled. (sig. V3v) [Chaucer uses *hameled* once, in *Troilus and Criseyde*.]

[Hentan] . . . to catch or snatch. *Chaucero* eodem sensu, henten ut henters ei pro raptores. (sig. X2v) [Chaucer uses *henters* once, in *Boethius*; he uses *hent* and variants many times.]

[Heom] . . . them. *Chaucero*, hem. (sig. X2v) [Many citations in Tatlock & Kennedy.]

[Here-berga] . . . a harbour, or harborow. *Chaucero*, herborow. (sig. X3r) [Chaucer uses *herbergage* four times, in *The Cook's Tale*, *The Man of Law's Tale*, *The Nun's Priest's Tale*, and *The Clerk's Tale*.]

[Herian] . . . to praise, to commend . . . *Chaucero* heried. (sig. X3v) [Several citations in Tatlock & Kennedy.]

[Hete] . . . promised, vowed . . . *Chaucero*, hete, hote. (sig. X3v) [Many citations in Tatlock & Kennedy.]

[Hine-man] . . . a husband-man, or plow-man. *Chaucero*, heyne, & hyne. (sig. X4r) [Chaucer uses *hyne* in *The General Prologue* and *The Pardoner's Tale*.]

[Hiora] . . . theirs. *Chaucero*, her. (sig. X4r) [Many citations in Tatlock & Kennedy]

[Horig] . . . hoary, mouldy, filthy. *Chaucero*, horrow. (sig. Y3r) [Chaucer uses *horwe* in *The Complaint of Mars*.]

[Leasung-full] . . . a liar . . . *Chaucero*, losenger. (sig. Aa3v) [Chaucer uses *losenger* (and variants) in *The Nun's Priest's Tale*, *The Parson's Tale*, *The Legend of Good Women*, and five times in *The Romaunt of the Rose*.]

[Masse-daeg] . . . a holiday, a festivall day. *Chaucero*, mass-day. (sig. Bb4r) [Chaucer uses *messe dayes* in *The Nun's Priest's Tale*.]

[Micel] . . . many, much, great. *Chaucero*, mikell, mokell. (sig. Cc2v) [Several references in Tatlock & Kennedy.]

[Micelnesse] . . . greatnesse, largenesse . . . *Chaucero*, mokell. (sig. Cc2v) [Not found in Tatlock & Kennedy.]

[Mist] . . . a mist. *Chaucero* nostro, mistihede, pro darknesse, mistery. (sig. Cc3v) [Chaucer uses *mistihede* once, in *The Complaint of Mars*.]

[Næddre] . . . a serpent, an aspe, a snake, a viper, a basilisk, an adder, a water snake or adder, a dragon. *Chaucero* nostro, neders pro adders. (sig. Dd2r) [Chaucer uses *naddre* and *naddres* in *The Merchant's Tale*, *The Parson's Tale*, *The Legend of Good Women*, and in *Boethius*.]

[Næs] . . . not . . . *Chaucero*, nas: cui etiam nat, & nere. (sig. Dd2v) [Many citations in Tatlock & Kennedy.]

[Natic] . . . I know not, I wot not. *Chaucer* hath *nist* for *wist not*. (sig. Dd2v) [Many citations in Tatlock & Kennedy.]

[Nehst] . . . *Chaucero*, nest. (sig. Dd3r) [Several citations in Tatlock & Kennedy.]

[Nesc] . . . soft, tender . . . gentle, mild. *Chaucero*, nesh. (sig. Dd3v) [Not found in Tatlock & Kennedy.]

[Niehst] . . . next, nighest. *Chaucero*, nest. (sig. Dd3v) [This usage of *nest* is not found in Tatlock & Kennedy.]

[Nillan] . . . to nill or be unwilling. *Chaucer* hath *nil*, for *ne wil*, or *will not*. (sig. Dd4r) [Many citations in Tatlock & Kennedy.]

[Not. Note. Notu] . . . use . . . ministery or function. *Chaucero*, note, busines. (sig. Dd4v) [Chaucer uses variants of *business* many times.]

[Ohwær] . . . any where. *Chaucero*, codem significatu, owhere. (sig. Ee3v) [Five citations of *o-where* in Tatlock & Kennedy.]

[Ord] . . . the point of any thing: and in that sence used of *Chaucer*. also an edge, the front of a battell. (sig. Ff2r) [Chaucer uses *orde* in this sense in *The Legend of Good Women*.]

[Pæl] . . . a covering. *Pale* in *Chaucer* for a robe. (sig. Ff4r) [*Pale* used in this sense is not found in Tatlock & Kennedy.]

[Raa] . . . *Chaucer* useth the word for a Roe. (sig. Gg1v) [Chaucer uses *raa* in *The Reeve's Tale*.]

[Ran] . . . *Ren* also is used of *Chaucer* for pull, get. (sig. Gg2v) [Many citations in Tatlock & Kennedy.]

[Reccan] . . . to care for, to esteem . . . *Chaucer* hath *recketh* for careth. (sig. Gg3r) [Many citations in Tatlock & Kennedy.]

[Sælignesse] . . . happinesse. *Chaucero* nostro, selinesse. (sig. Hh2r) [Chaucer uses the word three times in *Troilus and Criseyde*.]

[Salwig] . . . willow-coloured. Salow *Chaucero*, white. (sig. Hh2v) [Chaucer uses *sallow* twice in *The Romaunt of the Rose*.]

[Scæthan] . . . to hurt, to do harm or displeasure to . . . Scathlike *Chaucero*, harmfull. (sig. Hh3v) [Tatlock & Kennedy cite *scathe* but not *scathlike*.]

[Scathe] . . . harm, hurt, damage . . . scath. *Chaucero*, skath. (sig. Hh3v) [Chaucer uses *skathe* in *The Romaunt of the Rose*.]

[Sceal] . . . shall. *Chaucero*, schall. (sig. Hh4r) [Many citations in Tatlock & Kennedy.]

[Scendan] . . . shamed, shent. *Chaucer* hath *shenden* in the same sence, viz. to blame, to spoile, marre, hurt. (sig. Hh4v) [Chaucer uses *shenden* once in *Troilus and Criseyde* and variants of *shende* several times.]

[Seld] . . . seldome. *Chaucero*, seld. (sig. Ii4r) [Many citations in Tatlock & Kennedy.]

[Sithon] . . . courses, turns, times. *Chaucero*, sith eodem sensu. (sig. Kk2r) [Many citations in Tatlock & Kennedy.]

[Sped] . . . substance, riches, wealth . . . *Chaucero*, spedefull. (sig. Kk4v) [Chaucer uses *spedeful* in *The Man of Law's Tale*.]

[Stele] . . . a stalk, a stock or stump of a tree . . . *Chaucerus* . . . an handle: in which sence we yet retain it. (sig. L12v) [Chaucer uses *stele* twice, in *The Miller's Tale* and *The Wife of Bath's Tale*.]

[Stod-hors] . . . *Chaucer*, for a young horse useth *Stot*. (sig. L13v) [Chaucer uses *stot* twice, in *The General Prologue* and *The Friar's Tale*.]

[Swa] . . . so. *Chaucero*, swa. (sig. Mm1v) [Chaucer uses *swa* three times in *The Reeve's Tale*.]

[Swefen] . . . a dream, a vision in ones sleep. *Chaucero*, sweven.(sig. Mm2r) [Chaucer uses the word many times.]

[Swelgan] . . . to swallow. *Chaucero*, swelwen. (sig. Mm2v) [Tatlock & Kennedy cite numerous variants.]

[Swelgnysse] . . . a swallow or deep pit in a water, a gulf, a whirlpoole. *Chaucero*, swolow. (sig. Mm2v) [Chaucer uses *swolowe* in this sense in *The Legend of Good Women*.]

[Swincan] . . . to labour . . . Hence with *Chaucer*, swinker, for a labourer. (sig. Mm3v) [Chaucer uses *swinker* twice, in *The General Prologue* and *The Romaunt of the Rose*; and he uses variants of *swinke* Many times.]

[Swura] . . . *Chaucero*, swyre. (sig. Mm3v) [Chaucer uses *swire* once, in *Romaunt of the Rose*.]

[Swylce] . . . such. *Chaucero*, swilke. (sig. Mm4r) [Chaucer uses *swilke* once, in *The Reeve's Tale*; many citations of variants Tatlock & Kennedy.]

[Syb] . . . kindred, alliance, affinity. Quo sensu sib utitur *Chaucerus*. (sig. Mm4r) [Chaucer uses *syb* twice in *The Tale of Melibee* and *sibbe* in *Romaunt of the Rose*.]

[Tas] . . . a tasse or mow of corn. *Chaucero*, taas. (sig. Nn1v) [Chaucer uses *taas* three times in *The Knight's Tale*.]

[Thean] . . . to thrive . . . *Chaucer* useth *thedom* for thriving. (sig. Nn3r–v) [Not found in Tatlock & Kennedy.]

[Theaw] . . . a manner, custome . . . *Chaucero*, thewes. And hence, probablhy, [*sic*] the word *thewghes* or *thewes*, to wit, vertues, good qualityies or parts of the mind. (sig. Nn3v) [Tatlock & Kennedy cite *thewes* (and variants) several times.]

[Thirlian] . . . *Chaucero*, thirled. And hereof our *drill*. . . . (sig. Oo1r) [Chaucer uses *thirled* (and variants) in *The Knight's Tale*, *The Parson's Tale*, *Troilus and Criseyde*, *Romaunt of the Rose*, and twice in *The Complaint of Fair Anelida and False Arcite*.]

[Tholian] . . . *Chaucer* hath *tholed* for suffered. (sig. Oo1r) [Chaucer uses *tholed* once, in *The Friar's Tale*.]

[Thriccan] . . . to thrust . . . *Chaucero*, threke pro thrust. (sig. Oo1v) [Not found in Tatlock & Kennedy.]

[Thingan] . . . *Chaucer* useth *thringing*, for thrusting, clustering together. (sig. Oo2r) [Chaucer uses *thringing* once, in *Romaunt of the Rose*.]

[Undern] . . . the forenoon, the third houre of the day, that is nine of the clock with us. . . . Accordingly both *Chaucers* interpreter and *Verstegan* are to be corrected, who by *undern* & *underntide* understand afternoone. (sig. Qq1v) [Chaucer uses *undern* three times, once in *The Nun's Priest's Tale* and twice in *The Clerk's Tale*.]

[Un-eathe] . . . scarcely. *Chaucero*, unneath. (sig. Qq2r) [Many citations in Tatlock & Kennedy.]

[Wang] . . . the mandible or jaw wherein the teeth are set. Hence with *Chaucer*, we call the cheeke-teeth or grinders *wangs* and *wang treeth*. (sig. Ss2r) [Chaucer uses *wang-tooth* in *The Monk's Tale*.]

[Wed] . . . a pledge . . . *Chaucero*, wed. (sig. Ss3v) [Chaucer uses *wed* in this sense in *Lack of Steadfastness*.]

[Weda] . . . clothes, apparell . . . *Chaucero*, wede. (sig. Ss3v) [Chaucer uses *wede* several times.]

[Wem-leas] . . . immaculate, spotlesse, faultlesse, blamelesse. *Chaucero*, wemlesse. (sig. Ss4v) [Chaucer uses *wemmeless* once, in *The Second Nun's Tale*.]

[Weore] . . . a wile, deceit or crafty device . . . *Chaucero*, werch. (sig. Tt1r) [Several citations in Tatlock & Kennedy.]

[Wissian] . . . a guider, a governour, a ruler, a tutor. Hence *Chaucers* wisse, for instruct, direct. (sig. Tt4v) [Eight citations in Tatlock & Kennedy.]

[Wite] . . . *Chaucer* (if rightly interpreted) useth the word for blame. (sig. Tt4v) [Many citations in Tatlock & Kennedy.]

[With-sæggan] . . . to deny, to gainsay. *Chaucero*, with say. (sig. Vv1v) [Several citations in Tatlock & Kennedy.]

[Wlætan] . . . to nauseate, to loath . . . my stomacke turneth, loatheth or abhorreth. Hence *Chaucers* wlate, for loath, hate. (sig. Vv2r) [Chaucer uses *wlatsom* in *The Monk's Tale* and *The Nun's Priest's Tale*.]

[Wræc] . . . banishment. Hence *Chaucers* wrake, wrech, wreken, wrekery, for revenge. (sig. Vv3r) [Many citations in Tatlock & Kennedy.]

[Wreon] . . . to cover. Hence *Chaucers* wrene, wrine, for cover. (sig. Vv3v) [Chaucer uses *wryne* and *wrine* in *Romaunt of the Rose*.]

[Wununge] . . . a dwelling . . . *Chaucers* Wones, for dwellings. (sig. Vv4v) [Many citations for *wone* (and variations) in Tatlock & Kennedy.]

[Wyrde] . . . the fates, the destinies. *Chaucer* hath *Wyerds* in the same sence. (sig. Vv4v) [Chaucer uses *wyerds* (and variants) in *Boethius, Troilus and Criseyde,* and *The Legend of Good Women.*]

[Wyrnan] . . . to stop, to let, to hinder. Hence *Chaucers* werne, for deny, forbid: also his warned, for denied. (sig. Xx1r) [Many citations of *werne* (and variants) and *warned* in Tatlock & Kennedy.]

In an "Addenda," Somner cites Chaucer for the last time:

> Merke etiam *Chaucero* nostro pro darke. (sig. Sss2r) [*Merke* is not found in Tatlock & Kennedy.]

230. **WALKER, OBADIAH.** Περιαμμα 'επιδήμιον [Periamma 'epidemion]: *or, Vulgar Errours in Practice Censured.* W408. UMI 881: 19.

As MacKerness notes (*Notes and Queries*), Walker (1616–1699) cites Chaucer twice.

In chapter 2, "A Censure of the generall Scandall of some Professions, especially that of Physick," Walker paraphrases a quotation from *The General Prologue* (lines 437–38):

> I shall confine my Discouse to the *Profession* of *Physick*, the most common centre of reproachfull lines. This is evident from *Chaucer*'s verses,
>
> > Physicians know what is digestible,
> > But their study is but little in the Bible. (23)

In chapter 3, "A Censure of that common evill practice of Reproaching the Feminine Sex," Walker returns to Chaucer with a modernized couplet from *The Wife of Bath's Prologue* (lines 227–28):

> And *Catullus* . . . averreth that Wind and Water are of sufficient stability to receive the speeches of a *Woman* to him who is amorous, and would captivate her affection, and sues to her for matrimoniall entertainment. . . . One of our own Poets [in a shoulder note: "Chaucer"] agrees with these, and with his hobling feet thus tramples upon Female Credit:
>
> > Half so boldly there can none
> > Swear and lie as Woman can. (39–40)

231.   WITH, ELIZABETH. *Elizabeth Fools Warning.* W3139. UMI Thomason Tracts 242: E.2122 (1).

As the title page goes on to explain, Elizabeth With of Woodbridge regales readers with "a true and most perfect relation of all that has happened to her since her marriage. Being a Caveat for all young women to marry with old men." As Spurgeon notes (1: 237–38), With appears to allude to *The Clerk's Tale* when she writes of her miserable marriage:

> I had not been married one moneth unto him
> But in the Seas of sorrow I daily did swim;
> . . . .
> Instead of smiles he gave me a frown
> In his locking up my best silk gown,
> Which with my petty coats so neatly wrought
> Into his Sisters Chest after he brought;
> Which She lockt up upon that score
> That I should never have them more.
> How? patient Grisill what dost thou now say?
> Art thou contented with thy Gown of gray?
> . . . .
> When first these wasps at me did flie
> Then I would sit me down and cry:
> And many dayes I spent my tears in vain,
> At length I left this crying strain:
> And when old Naboth plaid his part,
> I did get patient Grisills heart. (4–5)

1660

232.   BAKER, RICHARD. *A Chronicle of the Kings of England.* B504. UMI 833: 14.

For references to Chaucer as John of Gaunt's brother-in-law, "the Homer of our nation," his association with Woodstock, his translation of *The Romaunt of the Rose*, his burial place in Westminster, and his association with Gower, see BAKER (1643) and (1653); in this edition, the passages are found on 144, 145–46, 168, 180, and sig. Mmm2r.

233.   CARTER, MATTHEW. *Honor rediviuus* [*sic*]: *or, An Analysis of Honor and Armory.* C659. UMI Thomason Tracts 239: E.1922 (1).

For a reference to Chaucer's escutcheon, see CARTER, C658 (1655); in this edition, the passage is found on 134.

    Another edition in 1660: C659A.

234.   *The Censure of the Rota upon Mr. Milton's Book.* H808. UMI 101: 10; UMI Thomason Tracts 151: E.1019 (5*).

In reprimanding Milton for his arguments in *A Ready and Easy Way to Establish a Free Commonwealth*, a clever satirist with Royalist sympathies alludes to *The Summoner's Tale* (lines 2249–50):

> [A] Common-wealth is like a great Top, that must be kept up by being whipt round, and held in perpetuall circulation, for if you discontinue the *Rotation*, and suffer the Senate to settle, and stand still, down it falls immediatly [*sic*]. And if you had studied this poynt as carefully as I have done, you could not but know, there is no such way under Heaven of disposing the Vicissitudes of Command and Obedience, and of distributing equall Right and Liberty among all men, as this of Wheeling, by which (as *Chauser* writes) a single Fart hath been equally divided among a whole Covent of Friers, and every one hath had his just share of the savour. (15)

235.   *Character of the Rump.* C2027. UMI Thomason Tracts 151: E.1017 (20).

As Spurgeon notes (1: 238), there is a reference to Chaucer in this short satire. In a passage about the parliamentary session that followed Colonel Thomas Pride's purging the "Long Parliament" of its controlling Presbyterian faction on 6 December 1648, the writer paraphrases a couplet from *The Prologue of The Summoner's Tale* (lines 1687–88). He writes:

> A Rump is the hinder part of the many-headed Beast, the Back-door of the *Devils Arse* . . . Tyranny and Rebellion ending in a Stink, the States *Incubus*, a Crab Commonwealth with the But-end formost. . . . [Y]ou may call it the tail of the Great Dragon, and 'tis a Thumper, for the devil's tail in Chaucer, being stuck in this, would look but like a maggot in a Tub of Tallow, and yet he saith
>
>> *That certainly Sathanas hath such a tail*
>> *Broader than of a Pinnace is the Sail.*

If you would reach me the Æquator, or rather one of the Tropiques, I would give a shrewd guesse at its abominable bignesse. . . . (1)

236.   FORDE, THOMAS. *Virtus rediviva: or, A Panegyrick for our Late King Charls [sic] the I.* F1550. UMI 2515: 36.

As Graves notes (*SP*), this work includes a collection of familiar letters with a separate title page, *Fænestra in Pectore: or, Familiar Letters.* In a letter addressed to "Mr. C. F.," Forde refers to Chaucer and alludes to *The Miller's Tale*:

Sir, . . . Truly I was informed, you were like to ruine your fortune, and that by one whom I know you esteem your friend. Therefore was I bold to advise you to provide an *Ark* against the *Deluge*: Not like the merry Scholar in *Chaucer*, that he might lie with the *Carpenters* wife. But I talk idle. Really, I had not said any thing, had I not been confident, you would take it with the *right hand*, as I gave it. . . . (43; sig. M7r)

Another edition: *Virtus rediviva*: *or, A Panegyricke*, F1550A (1661), same pagination.

Also found in: *Theatre of Wits*, F1548A (1661), fourth pamphlet, same pagination.

237.   GUILLIM, JOHN. *A Display of Heraldry*. G2219. UMI 1358: 27.

For quotations from *The Romaunt of the Rose*, a reference to Sir Payne Roet who is identified as Chaucer's father-in-law, a description of Chaucer's escutcheon, and a quotation from *The Knight's Tale*, see GUILLIM (1610) in Boswell & Holton No. 816; in this edition, the passages are found on 24, 286, 366, 398. Chaucer's name is also found in the index.

Another edition in 1660: G2219A (UMI 2656: 6), 24, 286, 366, 398, and index.

Other editions: G2220 (1664), 24, 286, 366, 398, and index; G2221 (1666), 24, 286, 366, 398, and index; G2222 (1679), 16, 215, 274, 310 and index.

238.   HOLLAND, SAMUEL. *Romancio-Mastrix*: *or, A Romance on Romances*. H2443. UMI 497: 18.

For a reference to "Sir Topaz," probably an allusion to Sir Thopas, and another reference to Chaucer, see HOLLAND (1656); in this edition, the passages are found on 2, 101–2.

239.   HOWELL, JAMES. *Lexicon tetraglotton, An English-French-Italian-Spanish Dictionary*. H3087. UMI 1594: 7.

For a reference to salty proverbs in Chaucer's works, see HOWELL (1659); in this edition, the passage is found in part 2, Παροιμιογραφια. *Proverbs: or, Old Sayed Sawes & Adages*, sig. ¶1r.

For an echo of a line from *The Reeve's Tale*, see 2 and 18; for an echo of a line from *The General Prologue*, see 17.

Other editions in 1660: H3088, sig. ¶r and 2, 17, 18; H3089, sig. ¶r and 2, 17, 18.

240.   PARKER, MARTIN. *The Famous History of That Most Renowned Christian Worthy Arthur King of the Britaines.* P437aA. UMI Thomason Tracts 151: E.1022 (2).

As Spurgeon notes (1: 238), in chapter 7, "How King Arthur instituted the order of the Round Table, and graced it with 150. Knights, with the reason of its institution to maintaine concord," Parker (d. 1656?) claims to have found the names of King Arthur's knights in "an old Chaucerian manuscript." Parker writes:

> 𝕶ing 𝕬rthur . . . instituted at the 𝕮ity of 𝖂inchester where he was then residing the ⽊rder of the 𝕽ound 𝕿able . . . and because 𝕵 find many of their names to be at this day great sirnames in the 𝕸onarchy of great 𝕭ritain, 𝕵 think it convenient . . . notwithstanding my promised brevity) to set down the names of the first 𝕶nights of the 𝕽ound 𝕿able in 𝕬lphabeticall order as 𝕵 found them long since in an old 𝕮haucerian manuscript. (13)

Another edition in 1660: P441E, same pagination.

241.   PHILLIPS, JOHN. *Montelion, 1660: or, The Prophetical Almanack.* A2109. UMI 1414: 29.

Phillips (1631–1706) identifies himself on the title page as "Montelion, knight of the oracle, a well-wisher to the mathematicks." He writes to would-be buyers of his almanac:

> *Gentlemen,* We do present you here with a new *Almanack*, whereby you may behold, how the three *fatal Sisters* do spin out the *Packthred* of your lives. It is as full of *Astrological predictions and Observations*, as an *Egg is full of meat.* . . . Now if you will buy it, the Book-seller saies he will either put ye in his next *Kalender* for Saints, or else name ye for his Benefactors . . . Therefore think upon't, and if you will forgoe Immortality, for a groat or sixpence, you may. (sig. A3v–4r)

Typical of the information he packs into his "Exact Chronologie of memorable things," Phillips notes that it has been eighty-one years "*Since Don Quixot wore Mambrino's Bason instead of an Head-piece*" and one hundred years "*Since the invention of Elder-guns*" and twenty years "*Since H. M. lay with the begger Wench*" (sig. A5r).

In his calendar, Phillips notes a few practical things such as times of sunrise and sunset and moon changes, but instead of noting saints's days and ecclesiastical feast days (as most almanac makers do), he substitutes literary and historical characters. For example in January, Country Tom is celebrated on the 3rd, Ovid on the 7th, and Fair Rosamond on the 28th. As Spurgeon notes (3: 4.73), Chaucer is celebrated on 13 January (sig. B1v). Shakespeare is celebrated on 4 May, "Ben. Johnson" on 4 July, and "Don Quixot" on 3 December.

242.   PRYNNE, WILLIAM, ed. Jan Hus's *A Seasonable Vindication of the Supream Authority and Jurisdiction of Christian Kings, Lords, Parliaments*. H3802. UMI Thomason Tracts 33: E. 190 (3).

Prynne (1600–1669) is identified on the title page as "William Prynne Esq; a Bencher of Lincolns Inne." As Dobbins notes (*MLQ*), Prynne cites Chaucer's contribution to the Protestant cause through the spurious work known as Chaucer's *Ploughman's Tale*. In "A Supplemental Appendix to the premised Disputation of John Hus, irrefragibly evidencing the Supream Jurisdiction of our Kings, Lords, and Parliaments, not only over the Persons, Liberties, Lives of our . . . Churchmen, in cases of High Treason, Rebellion, Disobedience, Contumacy and Disloyalty; but likewise over their Temporal Lands and Estates, to seise [*sic*] and confiscate them without Sacriledge or Injustice," Prynne writes:

> [I]t can be no Sacriledge or Impiety, but wholsom physick, for the King . . . to take away this *poyson* [i.e., great land holdings and possessions] from Bishops, and Cathedral Churches, which hath so much poysoned, corrupted them; and to reduce them to the condition of the Primitive Bishops. (41)

> Pierce Plowman his complaint of the Abuses of the World; Sir Geofry Chaucer in his Ploughmans tale . . . justified the lawfullness and necessity of taking away the Bishops abused temporalities which were such poyson to them. (42–43)

Another edition: H3803 (1668), 41–43.

243.   TOOKE, GEORGE. *The Belides: or, Eulogie of That Honourable Souldier Captain William Fairefax*. T1893A. UMI 676: 22.

For a reference that criticizes Chaucer for using language "from abroad," see TOOKE (1647); in this edition, the passage is found on sig. A2v.

244.   *Wandring Whore Continued*. No. 2. UMI Thomason Tracts 156: E1053 (3). Nelson and Seccombe 668.2.

This work, the second of a short-lived series in the mode of Pietro Aretino, is cast in the form of "A Dialogue between *Magdalena* a Crafty Bawd, *Julietta* an Exquisite Whore, *Francion* a Lascivious Gallant, and *Gusman* a Pimping Hector. Discovering their diabolical Practises at the Half-crown Chuck-Office." It also claims to include a "perfect List of the names of the Crafty Bawds, Common Whores, Wanderers, Pick-pockets, Night-Walkers, Decoys, Hectors, Pimps and

Trappanners" in and about London and suburbs (title page). As Harris notes (*PQ*), the author alludes to *The Summoner's Tale* (lines 2249–50). In a passage in which the four principals discuss the flourishing state of vice in London, Guzman reads a "proclamation" describing the charms of one of his whores:

> O Yes! O Yes! O Yes! Any man or woman, in City or Country, that will see an Ugly she-monster of deformed shape, impudent and brazen-fac'd carriage, uncivil behaviour, filthy constitutions, and preternatural disposition in her body, grindes Ginger in her a—hole betwixt her buttocks, and by that means hath weakened the retentive faculty in her posteriors . . . Let all such as fear not the losing of their Eye-sight, come put in their nose, as *Chaucers* twelve Fryers did at the dividing of a fart amongst them, and they may have it of a sluttish wench at the sign of, *Have you any wood to cleave*, &c. (12)

245. WINSTANLEY, WILLIAM. *Englands Worthies.* W3058. UMI Thomason Tracts 216: E.1736 (1).

Winstanley (1628?–1698) is identified on the title page as "William Winstanley, Gent." As Spurgeon notes (1: 238), Winstanley refers to Chaucer several times in this work. Apparently, however, Spurgeon did not notice that there is a small picture of Chaucer on the engraved title page that depicts forty-seven historical personages. Along with the easily recognizable William the Conqueror (No. 6), Sir Thomas More (No. 19), Sir Philip Sidney (No. 21), Sir Walter Raleigh (No. 30), Sir Francis Bacon (No. 33), Charles I (No. 42), and Oliver Cromwell (No. 47), No. 12 depicts Chaucer who is helpfully identified with the initials "J. C."

Winstanley lists Chaucer in "The Names of the Authors cited in this Book" (sig. A7v) and in "The Names of those whose Lives are written in this Book (sig. A8v).

In "The Life of King Edward the Third," Winstanley notes that Chaucer wrote the epitaph found in Westminster Abbey:

> [Edward III's] body was solemnly interred at *Westminster* Church, where he hath his monument, with this Epitaph engraven thereon, made by *Geffery Chaucer* the Poet.

> > *Hic decus Anglorum, flos regum præteritorum,*
> > *Forma futurorum, Rex clemens, pax popularum;*
> > *Tertius Edwardus, regni complens Jubilæum,*
> > *Invictus Pardus, pollens bellis Machabæum.*
> > *Here* Englands *Grace, the flower of Princes past,*
> > *Pattern of future,* Edward *the third is plac't,*
> > *Milde Monarch, Subjects peace, Wars Machabee,*
> > *Victorious Pard, his reign a Jubilee.* (79)

In a section headed "The Life of Geoffrey Chaucer," Winstanley writes:

> This famous and learned Poet *Geoffery Chaucer* Esquire, was supposed
> by *Leland*, to have been born in *Oxfordshire* or *Barkshire*; but as it is evi-
> dent by his own words he was born in the City of *London*, as we have it
> from him in his Testament of Love. 𝕬𝖑𝖘𝖔 𝖎𝖓 𝖙𝖍𝖊 𝕮𝖎𝖙𝖞 𝖔𝖋 𝕷𝖔𝖓𝖉𝖔𝖓, 𝖙𝖍𝖆𝖙
> 𝖎𝖘 𝖙𝖔 𝖒𝖊 𝖘𝖔 𝖉𝖊𝖆𝖗 𝖆𝖓𝖉 𝖘𝖜𝖊𝖊𝖙, 𝖎𝖓 𝖜𝖍𝖎𝖈𝖍 𝕴 𝖜𝖆𝖘 𝖋𝖔𝖗𝖙𝖍 𝖌𝖗𝖔𝖜𝖓; 𝖆𝖓𝖉 𝖒𝖔𝖗𝖊 𝖐𝖎𝖓-
> 𝖉𝖊𝖑𝖞 𝖑𝖔𝖛𝖊 𝖍𝖆𝖛𝖊 𝕴 𝖙𝖔 𝖙𝖍𝖆𝖙 𝖕𝖑𝖆𝖈𝖊 𝖙𝖍𝖊𝖓 𝖆𝖓𝖞 𝖔𝖙𝖍𝖊𝖗 𝖎𝖓 𝖍𝖞𝖊𝖗𝖙𝖍, 𝖆𝖘 𝖊𝖛𝖊𝖗𝖞 𝖐𝖎𝖓𝖉𝖊𝖑𝖞
> 𝖈𝖗𝖊𝖆𝖙𝖚𝖗𝖊 𝖍𝖆𝖙𝖍 𝖋𝖚𝖑𝖑 𝖆𝖕𝖕𝖊𝖙𝖎𝖙𝖊 𝖙𝖔 𝖙𝖍𝖆𝖙 𝖕𝖑𝖆𝖈𝖊 𝖔𝖋 𝖍𝖎𝖘 𝖐𝖎𝖓𝖉𝖊𝖑𝖞 𝖎𝖓𝖌𝖊𝖓𝖉𝖚𝖗𝖊, 𝖆𝖓𝖉 𝖙𝖔
> 𝖜𝖎𝖑𝖓𝖊 𝖗𝖊𝖘𝖙 𝖆𝖓𝖉 𝖕𝖊𝖆𝖈𝖊 𝖎𝖓 𝖙𝖍𝖆𝖙 𝖘𝖙𝖊𝖉𝖊 𝖙𝖔 𝖆𝖇𝖎𝖉𝖊) [*sic*] 𝖙𝖍𝖎𝖑𝖐𝖊 𝖕𝖊𝖆𝖈𝖊 𝖘𝖍𝖔𝖚𝖑𝖉 𝖙𝖍𝖚𝖘
> 𝖙𝖍𝖊𝖗𝖊 𝖍𝖆𝖛𝖊 𝖇𝖊𝖊𝖓 𝖇𝖗𝖔𝖐𝖊𝖓, 𝖜𝖍𝖎𝖈𝖍 𝖔𝖋 𝖆𝖑𝖑 𝖜𝖎𝖘𝖊 𝖒𝖊𝖓 𝖈𝖔𝖒𝖒𝖊𝖓𝖉𝖊𝖉 𝖆𝖓𝖉 𝖉𝖊𝖘𝖎𝖗𝖊𝖉.
> [black letter in text, *sic*]
>
> For his Parentage, although Bale, he termeth himself *Galfridus
> Chaucer nobili loco natus, & summa spei juvenis*, yet in the opinion of
> some Heralds (otherwise then his vertues and learning commended
> him) he descended not of any great House, which they gather by his
> Arms; and indeed both in respect of the name which is French, as also
> by other conjectures it may be gathered, that his Progenitours were
> Strangers; but whether they were Merchants, (for that in places where
> they have dwelled, the Arms of the Merchants of the Staple have been
> seen in the glass windows) or whether they were of other callings, it is
> not much necessary to search: but wealthy no doubt they were, and of
> good account in the Commonwealth, who brought up the son in such
> sort, that both he was thought fit for the Court at home, and to be
> employed for matters of State in Forreign Countreys.
>
> His Education, as *Leland* writes, was both the Universities of
> *Oxford* and *Cambridge*, as appeareth by his own words in his Book enti-
> tuled, The Court of Love; and in *Oxford* by all likelihood in *Canterbury*,
> or in *Merton Colledge*, with *John Wickliffe*, whose opinions in Religion
> he much affected: For who shall read his Works, will finde him not
> covertly, but with full mouth to cry out against the vices and enormities
> of the Priests of those times. Hear him in the Plough-mans tale.

> 𝕸𝖊𝖓𝖓𝖊𝖘 𝖂𝖎𝖛𝖊𝖘 𝖙𝖍𝖊𝖞 𝖜𝖔𝖑𝖑𝖊𝖓 𝖍𝖔𝖑𝖉,
> 𝕬𝖓𝖉 𝖙𝖍𝖔𝖚𝖌𝖍 𝖙𝖍𝖆𝖙 𝖙𝖍𝖊𝖞 𝖇𝖊𝖊𝖓 𝖗𝖎𝖌𝖍𝖙 𝖘𝖔𝖗𝖗𝖞;
> 𝕿𝖔 𝖘𝖕𝖊𝖆𝖐 𝖙𝖍𝖊𝖞 𝖘𝖍𝖆𝖑𝖑 𝖓𝖔𝖙 𝖇𝖊 𝖘𝖔 𝖇𝖔𝖑𝖉
> 𝕱𝖔𝖗 𝖘𝖔𝖒𝖕𝖓𝖎𝖓𝖌 𝖙𝖔 𝖙𝖍𝖊 𝕮𝖔𝖓𝖘𝖎𝖘𝖙𝖔𝖗𝖊𝖞,
> 𝕬𝖓𝖉 𝖒𝖆𝖐𝖊 𝖍𝖊𝖒 𝖘𝖆𝖞 𝖒𝖔𝖚𝖙𝖍 𝕴 𝖑𝖎𝖊,
> 𝕿𝖍𝖔𝖚𝖌𝖍 𝖙𝖍𝖊𝖞 𝖎𝖙 𝖘𝖆𝖜 𝖜𝖎𝖙𝖍 𝖍𝖊𝖗 𝖊𝖞𝖊.
> 𝕳𝖎𝖘 𝖑𝖊𝖒𝖒𝖆𝖓 𝖍𝖔𝖑𝖉𝖊𝖓 𝖔𝖕𝖕𝖊𝖓𝖑𝖞
> 𝕹𝖔 𝖒𝖆𝖓 𝖘𝖔 𝖍𝖆𝖗𝖉𝖑𝖞 𝖙𝖔 𝖆𝖘𝖐 𝖜𝖍𝖞.

Improving this time in the University, he became a witty Logician, a sweet Rhetorician, a grave Philosopher, a Holy Divine, a skilful Mathematician, and a pleasant Poet; of whom for the sweetness of his Poetry may be said, that which is reported of *Stefichorus*; and as *Cethegus* was tearmed *Suadæ Medulla*, so may *Chaucer* be rightly called the pith and sinews of Eloquence, and the very life itself of all mirth and pleasant writing: besides, one gift he had above other Authours; and that is, by the excellencies of his descriptions to possesse his Readers with a stronger imagination of seeing that done before their eyes which they read, then any other that ever writ in any tongue.

By his travel also in *France* and *Flanders*, where he spent much time in his young years, but more in the latter end of the Reign of King *Richard* the second, he attained to a great perfection in all kind of learning, as *Bale* and *Leland* report of him[25]. . . . About the Latter end of King *Richard* the Seconds dayes, he flourished in *France*, and got himself into high esteem there by his diligent exercise in learning. After his return home, he frequented the Court at *London*, and the Colledges of the Lawyers, which there interpretted [*sic*] the Laws of the Land; and among them he had a familiar Friend called *John Gower*, a *Yorkshire* man born, a Knight, as *Bale* writeth of him. This *Gower* in a Book of his entituled *Confessio Amantis*, tearmeth *Chaucer* a worthy Poet, and maketh him as it were the judge of his works.

He married a Knights Daughter of *Henault*, called *Paon de Ruet*, King of Arms, by whom he had issue his Son *Thomas*, to whom King *Edward* the Third (in recompense of his Fathers services in *France*) gave him in marriage the Daughter and Heire of Sir *John Burgersoe* Knight. This *Thomas Chaucer* had onely one Daughter named *Alice*, married thrice. . . .

But to return to our ancient Poet *Geffery Chaucer*, he had alwayes an earnest desire to inrich and beautifie our English Tongue, which in those dayes was very rude and barren; and this he did, following the example of *Dantes* and *Petrarch*, who had done the same for the Italian Tongue; *Alanus* for the French, and *Johannes Mena* for the Spanish: neither was *Chaucer* inferiour to any of them in the performance hereof; and *England* in this respect is much beholding to him, as *Leland* well noteth. . . .

Our England honoureth Chaucer Poet, as principal,
To whom her Countrey tongue both owe her beauties all.

---

[25] See **BALE** and **LELAND** in Boswell & Holton Nos. 161, 470.

He departed out of this world the 25. day of October, 1400. after he had lived about 72. years. Thus writeth *Bale* out of *Leland*: . . . *Chaucer* lived till he was an old man, and found old age to be grievous; and whilest he followed his causes at *London*, he died, and was buried at *Westminster*.

These old Verses which were written on his Grave at the first, were these.

> *Galfridus Chaucer vates & fama poesis,*
> *Maternæ hæc sacra sum tumulatus humo.*

But since, Mr. Nicholas Brigham did at his own cost and charges erect a Monument to him, with these Verses.

> *Qui fuit Anglorum vates ter maximus olim.* . . . [26]

It will not be amiss to these Epitaphs to adde the judgements and reports of some learned men of this worthy and famous Poet. And first of all *Thomas Occleve*, who lived in his dayes, writeth thus of him in his Book, *De regimine Principis* [*sic*].

> But welaway is mine hart woe,
> That the honour of English Tongue is dead,
> Of which I wont was consaile habe and reed,
> O maister dere, and fadre reberent:
> My maister Chaucer floure of Eloquence,
> Mirror of fructuous entendement.
> O unibersal fadre of science:
> Alas that thou thine excellent prudence
> In thy bed mortal mightest not bequeath.
> What eyld death, alas why would she thee sle:
> O death thou didst not harm singler in slaughter of him;
> But all the Land it smerteth.
> But natheless yet hast thou no power his name sle,
> His hie bertue asserteth
> Unslain fro thee, which ay us lifely herteth,
> With Books of his ornat enditing
> That is to all this land enlumining.

John Lidgate likewise in his Prologue of *Bocchas*, of the fall of Princes, by him translated, saith thus in his commendation.

---

[26] See FOXE in Boswell & Holton No. 285.

𝕸𝖞 𝕸𝖆𝖘𝖙𝖊𝖗 Chaucer 𝖜𝖎𝖙𝖍 𝖍𝖎𝖘 𝖋𝖗𝖊𝖘𝖍 𝖈𝖔𝖒𝖊𝖉𝖎𝖊𝖘
𝕴𝖘 𝖉𝖊𝖆𝖉, 𝖆𝖑𝖆𝖘! . . . [27]

Also in his Book which he writeth of the Birth of the Virgin *Mary*, he hath these verses.

𝕬𝖓𝖉 𝖊𝖐𝖊 𝖒𝖞 𝕸𝖆𝖎𝖘𝖙𝖊𝖗 Chaucer 𝖓𝖔𝖜 𝖎𝖘 𝖎𝖓 𝕲𝖗𝖆𝖛𝖊. . . . [28]

And as for men of latter time, Mr. *Ascham* and Mr. *Spenser* have delivered most worthy testimonies of their approving of him. Mr. *Ascham* in one place calleth him English *Homer*, and makes no doubt to say, that he valueth his Authority of as high estimation, as ever he did either *Sophocles* or *Euripides* in Greek. And in another place, where he declareth his opinion of English versifying, he useth these words: *Chaucer and Petrark, those two worthy wits, deserve just praise.* And last of all, in his discourse of Germany, he putteth him nothing behinde either *Thucidides* or *Homer*, for his lively descriptions of site of places, and nature of persons, both in outward shape of body and inward disposition of minde; adding this withall, that not the proudest that hath written in any Tongue whatsoever, for his time, have outstript him.

Mr. *Spenser* in his first Eglogue of his Shepards Kallender, calleth him *Tityrus*, the god of Shepards, comparing him to the worthiness of the Roman *Tityrus Virgil*: in his Faerie Queene, in his Discourse of Friendship, as thinking himself most worthy to be *Chaucers* friend, for his like natural disposition that *Chaucer* had; he writes, that none that lived with him, nor none that came after him durst presume to revive *Chaucers* lost Labours in that unperfect tale of the Squire, but onely himself: which he had not done, had he not felt (as he saith) the infusion of *Chaucers* own sweet spirit, surviving within him. And a little before he calls him the most renowned and Heroicall Poet; and his writings, the works of heavenly wit; concluding his commendation in this manner.

> *Dan* Chaucer, *well of English undefiled,*
> *On fames eternal Bead-roll worth to be filed;*
> *I follow here the scoring of thy feet;*
> *That with thy meaning so I may the rather meet.*

---

[27] See BOCCACCIO in Boswell & Holton No. 27.
[28] See LYDGATE in Boswell & Holton No. 19.

Mr. *Cambden* reaching one hand to Mr. *Ascham*, and the other to Mr. *Spenser*, and so drawing them together, uttereth of him these words. *De Homero nostro Anglico. . . .* [29]

The deservingly honoured Sir *Philip Sidney* in his defence of Poesy, thus writeth of him. *Chaucer* undoubtedly did excellently in his *Troylus* and *Crescid*, of whom truly I know not, whether to marvail more; either that he in that misty time could see so clearly, or that we in this clear age walk so stumblingly after him. And Doctor *Heylin* his his elabourate [sic] Description of the World, ranketh him in the first place of our chiefest Poets. Seeing therefore that both old and new Writers have carried this reverewd conceit of him, and openly declared the same by writing, let us conclude with *Horace* in the eighth Ode of his fourth Book.

Dignum Laude causa vetat mori.

Gower and *Chaucer* were both of the Inner Temple. Mr. *Buckley* a learned Gentleman of those times gives us an account of a Record he read in the same Inner Temple, wherein *Geofery Chaucer*, no friend to the convetous and leacherous Cleargy men of those times, was fined two shillings for beating of a Franciscan Frier in *Fleet-street*: a considerable sum, money was so scarce in those dayes. (91–98)

Other editions: W3059 (1684), title page, sig. a6v and sig. a7v, 102–3, 116–23 (and others).

Also found (revised and augmented) in *The Lives of the Most Famous English Poets: or, The Honour of Parnassus*, W3065 (1687), 23–32 (and others).

1661

246.   BLOUNT, THOMAS. *Glossographia, or a Dictionary.* B3335. UMI 1276: 8.

For a reference to "old Chaucer" and a quotation from *Troilus and Cryssede* and to Chaucer as an authority on language and word usage, see BLOUNT (1656); in this revised and augmented edition, the passages are found in the epistle (A4v), and in the definitions of *agroted* (B8r), *algebra* (C1r), *alnath* (C2v), *amortize* (C5r), *barbicane* (F5v), *benison* (F8r), *bordel* (G3v), *burlybrand* (G6r), *callot* (G8r), *covent* (L7v), *creance* (L8v), *disheviled* (N8r), *dulcarnon* (O5r–v), *frythe* (S2v), *gossymeare* (T1v), *lodemanage* (Aa3v), *losender* (Aa5r), *meriot* (Bb8v), *moiles* (Cc4v), *mortress* (Cc7v), *ouch* (Ee8v), *paraments* (FF5v), *pilgrim* (Hh1v), *rebeck* (Kk6v), *romance* (L17v), *superstition* (Pp5v), *taberd* (Qq2v), *tailage* (Qq3r).

[29] See CAMDEN in Boswell & Holton No. 439.

Note that *Agrise* and *cheve* are omitted altogether, and the definitions of *orfraies*, *romant*, and *strand* are altered so there is no mention of Chaucer. Among other revisions, new words were added, including two with references to Chaucer:

𝕭𝖔𝖔𝖓 (Sax. 𝕭𝖊𝖓𝖊, *Chaucer*, 𝕭𝖔𝖓𝖊) a petition or request. (sig. G3v) [Chaucer uses the term more than a dozen times: *The Knight's Tale*, lines 2269, 2669; *The Merchant's Tale*, line 1618; *The Second Nun's Tale*, lines 234, 356; *The Book of the Duchess*, lines 129, 834; *Parliament of Fowls*, line 643; *Troilus and Criseyde*, 1: 1027, 4: 68, 5: 594; *The House of Fame*, 3: 447, 3: 684; *The Legend of Good Women*, lines 1596, 2340.]

𝕷𝖊𝖈𝖙𝖊𝖗𝖓 or 𝕷𝖊𝖈𝖙𝖔𝖗𝖓, with *Chaucers* Interpreter, is a Desk; I suppose he means a Reading-Desk in a Church, which in old Latin is called *Lectrinum*. (sig. Z7r) [Neither spelling is found in Tatlock & Kennedy]

Another edition in 1661: B3335a, same pagination.

247. BRAMHALL, JOHN. *A Just Vindication of the Church of England from the Unjust Aspersion of Criminal Schisme.* B4227. UMI 1456: 5.

For a reference to Chaucer's portrayal of "the greediness and extortion of the Court of Rome" in the "Plowmans tale and elsewhere" (allusions to *The Canterbury Tales* and the spurious work known as Chaucer's *Ploughman's Tale*), see BRAMHALL (1654); in this edition, the passage is found on 134.

248. BRAMHALL, JOHN. *The Right Way to Safety after Ship-Wrack.* B4231. UMI 1144: 11.

Bramhall (1594–1663) is identified on the title page as "the most Reverend Father in God, John, Lord Archbishop of Armagh, primate and metropolitan of all Ireland." In this sermon preached before the House of Commons in St. Patrick's Church, Dublin, on 16 June 1661, Archbishop Bramhall cites Chaucer in a passage about confession of sins:

No man can doubt but the *Romanists* have grosly abused Confession, by tricking it up in the Robes of a Sacrament, by obtruding a particular and plenary enumeration of all sins, to man, as absolutely necessary to Salvation by Divine Institution, by making it with the commutations, a remedy rather for the Confessors purse, than the Confitents soul, by imposing ludibrious penances: as *Chaucer* observed, He knew how to impose an easie penance, where he looked for a good pittance, by making it a pick-lock to know the secrets of States and Families. . . . (18)

The passage is an allusion to the Frere in *The General Prologue*: "He was an esy man to yeve penaunce" (line 223).

Also found in Bramhall's *Works*: B4210 (1676), 974.

249.   CLEVELAND, JOHN. *Poems.* **C4695. UMI 658: 8.**

For an echo of a line from *The Manciple's Prologue*, see CLEVELAND (1644); in this edition, the passage is found on 182.

250.   FELL, JOHN. *The Life of the Most Learned, Reverend and Pious D'H. Hammond.* **F617. UMI 353: 19.**

Fell (1625–1686) is identified on the title page as "Dean of Christ-Church in Oxford." In his biography of Henry Hammond, Fell appears to echo a line from *The Reeve's Tale*: "The gretteste clerkes been noght wisest men" (line 4054). In a passage about Hammond's superlative judgement, he writes:

> His [i.e., Hammond's] *Judgement*, as in itself the highest Faculty, so was it the most eminent among his natural endowments: for though the finding out the similitudes of different things, wherein the Phansie is conversant, is usually a bar to the discerning the disparities of similar appearances, which is the business of Discretion, and that store of notions which is laid up in Memory assists rather Confusion then Choice, upon which grounds the greatest Clerks are frequently not the wisest men. (96–97)

Another edition: F618 (1662), 97–98.

251.   FORDE, THOMAS. *Virtus rediviva: or, A Panegyricke*, **F1550A. UMI 1947: 9.**

For a reference to Chaucer and an allusion to the *Miller's Tale*, see FORDE (1660); in this edition, the passage is found on 43 (sig. M7r).

Also collected in *Theatre of Wits*, F1548A (1661), fourth pamphlet, same pagination.

252.   G., E. Commendatory Poem in Martin Llewellyn's *The Marrow of the Muses: Express'd in That Excellent Facetious Poem Stiled Men-Miracles. The Second Edition.* **L2624. UMI 1425: 24.**

For a commendatory poem that links Chaucer with Spenser and Jonson and claims the soul of Chaucer lives on in Llewellyn, see G., E. (1646); in this edition, the poem is found on sig. A4r.

253.   LEIGH, EDWARD. *Choice Observations of All the Kings of England.* L987. UMI 944: 21.

Leigh (1602–1671) is identified on the title page as "Edward Leigh Esquire, and Master of Arts of Magdalen Hall in Oxford." In chapter 18, in a section about Henry IV, Leigh mentions Chaucer:

> In his time were two famous Poets *Chaucer* and *Gower*. (127) . . . *Gower* being very gracious with him, carried the name of the only Poet in his time. He and *Chaucer* were Knights. (129)

254.   MORGAN, SYLVANUS. *The Sphere of Gentry.* M2743. UMI 610: 15.

Morgan (1620–1693)—or perhaps Edward Waterhouse (1619–1670) to whom the work is also sometimes attributed—refers to Chaucer's escutcheon in book 2, chapter 3, "Of the third Honourable Ordinary, viz. The Pale":

> The Worthies that beare the Pale and Chief together, are . . . Parted per pale Argent and Sable, a bend counterchanged, by the name of *Geffery Chaucer* the famous English Poet. (234–35)

255.   MORLEY, GEORGE. *A Sermon Preached at the Magnificent Coronation of Charles II.* M2794. UMI Thomason Collection 257: E.184 (5).

Morley (1597–1684) is identified on the title page as "Lord Bishop of Worcester." His sermon at the coronation was preached at the Collegiate Church of St. Peter Westminster on 23 April 1661. Morley echoes a line from *The Reeve's Tale*: "The gretteste clerkes been noght wisest men" (line 4054). In a passage about the importance of a man's understanding and judgement, he writes:

> [T]hough a man have Read never so many Books . . . yet if he be not *naturally a man of judgement* and *understanding*, he may be a *Fool* for *all this*; nay he may be a much more *incurable Fool*, then he would be otherwise . . . which makes good our *English* Proverb, that *the greatest Clerks, are not always the wisest men*; or as it is more sharply express'd in the *Scotch* Dialect, *an ounce of Mother wit is worth a pound of Clergy.* (40)

256.   OWEN, JOHN. Θεολογουμενα παντοδαπα [Theologoumena pantodapa]: *sive, De natura, ortu, progressu, et studio veræ theologæ libri sex.* O810. UMI 1153: 29.

Owen (1616–1683) is identified on the title page as "Johanne Oweno." As Spurgeon notes (3: 4.73–74), Owen cites Chaucer and quotes conflated lines from *The Wife of Bath's Tale* (lines 17–18, 23–24). In book 1, chapter 8, under the running heads "De theologiæ naturalis" and "Corruptione et Amissione," in a passage about ubiquitous friars, Owen writes:

Ita *Chaucerus* nostras de fratrum conventu quodam suo temporere notissimo;

> 𝔉or there as wont to walken was an 𝔈lfe,
> 𝔗here walketh now the 𝔏imitor himselfe.
> 𝔍n every bush, and under every 𝔗ree
> 𝔗here nis none other incubus but he. (96)

257.   PHILLIPS, JOHN. *Wit and Drollery. Joviall Poems.* W3122. UMI 1112: 1.

For a reference to "ould Chaucer," see *Wit and Drollery* (1656); in this edition, the passage is found on 2.

258.   ROGERS, GEORGE. *The Horn Exalted: or, Roome for Cuckolds.* R1802. UMI Thomason Tracts 225: E.1808 (3).

The title page goes on to advise would-be readers that this work is "A Treatise concerning the Reason and Original of the word *Cuckold*, and why such are said to wear *Horns*. Very proper for these Times, when Men are Butting, and Pushing, and Goring, and Horning one another." As Spurgeon notes (3: 4.74), but does not transcribe, Rogers (1618–1697) cites Chaucer twice and quotes him without attribution several times.

There are, however, far more references and citations than Spurgeon records. In "A Treatise. Concerning the Reason and Original of the word Cuckold, and why such are said to wear Horns," Rogers attributes authorship of *The Remedy of Love* to Chaucer:

> And first, for that loth name cuckold. as *Chaucer* speaks, in in [*sic*] Remedy of love 'tis ransackt thus, C. for cold, O for old, K for knave, C for calot, a lewd woman whereof we have O or Wo,[30] L. for lewd, D for demeanure, so that 'tis a cold old knave,
>
> > *Cuckold himself weaning,*
> > *And eak a calot of lewd demeaning.* (1)

In a passage about delicate language for vulgar subjects, Rogers refers to Chaucer's use of *nicety*, possibly an allusion to *The Reeve's Tale*, "This millere smyled of hir nycetee" (line 4046), or *The Romaunt of the Rose*, "A jape, or elles nycete" (line 12):

---

[30] *Wo,* i.e., woe.

For coy and squeamish appetites disrelish many times the solid'st flesh and flood that is good and honest, when a quelq-chose, an andouille, codlins, or a nicety in *Chaucers* sence shall down with them. (2)

In a passage about the cuckoo, Rogers cites the Wife of Bath and attributes a quotation to her, alludes to *The Wife of Bath's Prologue*, "Whan that he wode han my *bele chose*" (line 510):

'Tis a mischievous timorous bird and of a low spirit. Hereby the Poets shewing us, that lofty dames must be sought, and addresst unto, by the artifice of submission, dejection, and all insinuing humiliations. So the wife of *Bath*

> *I loved him for his obeysance. . . .*

Chaucer sure hence brings in jealousie with a garland of gold-yellow, and a cuckow sitting on her fist. (3–4)

'Tis true the Greeks ascribe somewhat of horn to the Generative parts of both our sexes. . . . (7) [T]he Greeks call *Chaucers* Bellchose, Κύων, but whether they mean a shock, or a lap-dog, or a bull-dog judg [*sic*] ye. Though by a bull in Greek is meant a mans τῐῶω, which some call tool. (8)

[F]rom the first of *Genesis*, where of the Man 'tis said *Male and female created he them*. Yet in probability there is a great *pelleity* and propensity in both sexes, the man seeking to find his *rib*, and the Woman to be joyned to *his side* again.

> *Beast unto beast. the earth to water wan,*
> *Birds unto birds, and woman unto man.* (25)

The passage is marked with a shoulder note: "*Chaucer.*" The couplet is found in *The Court of Love* that was included in Stow's edition of Chaucer's *Works* (1561).

In a passage about adultery, Rogers alludes to a phrase in *Boethius*, "kerve asondir with his hook the bussches" (3: ml. 1. 610–15):

Indeed adultery is both murder and Theft, and therefore tis placed in the Ten Commandements twixt both: for as that steals the pleasures of another mans propriety, so (as *Chaucer speaks*) it *Kerves* in two and breaks asunder those that were of one flesh. (30)

In "An Appendix, Concerning Women and Jealousie," several more references and allusions may be found. In a passage about those who are reluctant to marry, Rogers quotes a somewhat modernized couplet from *The Miller's Prologue* (lines 3151–52) and follows it with a paraphrase of a line from *The Merchant's Tale*, "That is in marriage hony-sweete" (line 1396):

> Onely let me say this, that many and the most discreet, having past their prime, and made now their Passions cringe and stoup to their reasons, either venture upon the married condition for interest and conveniency, or else wholly avoid it for fear of the weighty cares, or the womans levity, that may accompany it.

> — *My leife brother* Oswold,
> *Who hath no wife, he is no Cuckold.*

[In a shoulder note: "*Chauc.*"] . . . But why this aversness and abhorrency (to speak *Chaucer*) of *hony-sweet-marriage*? (42)

> [I]f it be true what *Pliny* saies, the pith of a mans backbone in the sepulcher turnes to a serpent, and he was more subtile than any beast of the field.

> *Where is the trough of man? so God me save,*
> *For what they cannot get that would they have.*
> [In a shoulder note: "*Chauc.*"] (45)

The final quotation appears to be spurious.

In a passage about the temptations to betray marriage vows, Rogers mentions Pandarus, an allusion to *Troilus and Criseyde*, and paraphrases a couplet from *The Wife of Bath's Prologue* (lines 333–34):

> Avoid then their vitious temptations, and run from them. . . . [Y]our wit and virtue hath a nick of time, and criticall minute when to be surpriz'd. You being flesh and bloud, they know there's a *Pandarus* within to open the gates and betray you. (47) . . . [Wives] may be said with *Plinies Paphlagonian* partridges, to have two hearts, since they count that mouse but a silly rogue that hath but one hole to start to, and that *one life* so short requires more *loves than one*. All good Schollars to the wife of *Bath*, they think that Husband a *Monophagus*, and unkind man, that eats his morsell alone, and enjoyes his *bits* by himself, and as *Chaucer* speaks.

> *To great a niggard if that he yern*
> *A man to light his candle at his Lantern.* . . . . (52)

They are better skill'd in *Chaucers* sixteenth statute of love, and its canonicall hours, where duty was to be done the first, second, and third watch, and the Mantins bell to be rung one and twenty times a night, or the good mans head was to ake for't. (54)

In a passage about the nature of women, Rogers conflates modernized lines from *The Merchant's Tale* (lines 2271–72) and from *The Wife of Bath's Prologue* (lines 231–32):

By nature their veins are more hidden than mens, and by subtilty, their vices and vanities are more cover'd, what with the Sophistry of tears, still ready in their station for a watch-word, and what with other elusions, these false *Fidessa's* shall make men believe the Moon's made of green Cheese. Hear but the wife of *Bath's* confession.

> *For lack of answer none of them shall dien*
> *All had he see, a thing with both his eyen.*
> *A wise wife shall if that she can him good,*
> *Bere him in hond that the cow is wood.* . . . . (56)

Rogers goes on to cite Chaucer's usage of *chideress*, an allusion to *The Romaunt of the Rose* (lines 150, 4266), and quotes a somewhat modernized couplet from *The Merchant's Tale* (lines 1345–46):

A good wife as 'tis a *pillow* of ease, which *refreshes* the wearyed *with new work*, and *cooles with warm* embraces. As *Chaucer* speaks, she is no *Chideress*, nor understands any thing of *Xantippisme*, linked in hold bond, the conquers the hardship of commands, and freely submits to the enslavement of *Capricio's*. [In a shoulder note: "*Chaucer.*"]

> *She saith not once nay, when he saith ye,*
> *Do this saith he, a ready Sir saith she.* (58)

In a passage about the effects of neglecting marital duties, Rogers cites Chaucer's usage of the term *blanch-fever*, an allusion to *Troilus and Criseyde* (1: 916):

The discontinuance and neglect of which *Hippocrates* tell you, causes, head-ach, convulsions, dimnes of sight, giddiness, the blanch-fever, as *Chaucer* speaks, and Melancholy the forge of the Devill, fits also, &c. (65)

In a passage about the dangers of tyranny in love, Rogers quotes a modernized couplet from *The Franklin's Tale* (lines 765–66):

> Love will not endure to hear of maistry, as *Chaucer* speaks.
> > *When Maistry comes, the God of love anon,*
> > *Beateth his wings, and farewell he is gone.* (69)

In a passage about wandering wives and complacent husbands, Rogers attributes a quotation to Chaucer (actually from *The Court of Love* that was published in Stow's edition of Chaucer's *Works* [1561]) and follows it with a modernized couplet from *The Merchant's Tale* (lines 1671–72):

> Nay *Solon* gave leave for women to make use of some friends in case of husbands frigidity. [In a shoulder note: "*Chaucer.*"]
> > *And when thou maist the game no more assay*
> > *The statute bid thee pray for them that may.* . . . (71)

> If thy wife *spring a leck*, or be disloyall, drink thy wormwood sweetly, and swallow the pill without chawing. . . . This vitiousness [*sic*] of theirs may be our fiery tryall, to refine, and fit us that place celestiall, where no *Wives* shall be, though some *Women* may come, as *Dan Geffrey* speaks.
> > *She may be Gods mean, and Gods whip,*
> > *Then shall your soul up to Heaven skip.* (74–75)

Rogers warns against excessive sex in marriage, and to reinforce his point, he quotes modernized couplets from *Troilus and Criseyde* (5: 553–54) and *The Manciple's Tale* (lines 311–12):

> The taking too much of the smock off under the sheet, enervates and weakens us, and produces languors, and shortness of dayes. . . . Men . . . marry beauties which we so gaze on so long as they are coming, whence once prostrated, they loose their admiration, themselves being like the radish which helps our digestion, when itself remains most an end *undigested* and effensive [*sic*] to the stomach. [In a shoulder note: "*Chaucer.*"]
> > *Then fairwell Shrine of which the Saint is out*
> > *And ring of which the ruby is out fall.* . . . (79–80)

> However I think it unfit for any one to upbraid another for his misfortune, 'tis *Chaucers* advice.
> > *Tell no man never in your life*
> > *How that another man hath dight his wife.* (81–82)

259.   SMITH, JAMES. "The Preface to That Most Elaborate Piece of Poetry Entituled Penelope and Ulysses," in *Wit and Drollery*. W3132. UMI 1112: 2.

For a reference to a sharp disagreement about a poet's commendation of "ould" Chaucer, see SMITH (1656); in this edition, the passage is found on 2.

260.   STEVENSON, MATTHEW. *The Twelve Moneths: or, A Pleasant and Profitable Discourse of Every Action*. S5510. UMI 1241: 15.

As Harris notes (*PQ*), Stevenson (*fl.* 1654–1684) echoes a line from *The General Prologue* ["Whan Zepherus eek with his sweete breeth" (line 5)]. In "August," Stevenson writes:

> Now do the Reapers try their Backs and their Arms, and the lusty Youths pitch the sheafs into the Cart . . . *Zephyrus* now with his sweet breath cools and perfumes the parching beams of Titan. . . . (37)

261.   T., J. "Commendatory Poem" in George Rogers's *The Horn Exalted*. R1802. UMI Thomason Tracts 225: E.1808 (3).

As Spurgeon notes (3: 4.74), Chaucer is cited in a shoulder note in J. T.'s commendatory poem addressed "To His Most ingenuous Friend, The Authour of the Exaltation of Hornes":

> Read, and beware how that ye firk,
> Least the repentance stool o'th'Kirk
> Prove the reward of your queint wirk. (sig. *8v)

Queint is marked for a shoulder note: "*Chaucer.*" J. T. is probably alluding to *The Miller's Tale* (lines 3275–76).

262.   WALKER, CLEMENT. *Anarchia Anglicana: or, The History of Independency. The Second Part*. W318A. UMI 1900: 1.

Walker (1595–1651), identified on the title page as Theodorus Verax, was a prominent Presbyterian leader and a vigorous opponent of independency. Because of his *History of Independency*, he was committed to the Tower of London in 1649, and there he remained until his death in 1651. As Harris notes (*PQ*), Walker refers to Chaucer in an epistle addressed "To the Reader." Walker echoes a line from *The General Prologue*: "The wordes moote be cosyn to the dede" (line 742) as he writes:

> *It is a virtue to hate and prosecute vice. The Scripture tells us*, there is a perfect hatred, a holy Anger. *And our* Chaucer tells us, The words must be of kynn unto the deeds *otherwise, how can they be expressive enough?* (sig. A3r)

Also found in *The Compleat History of Independency* (1661): W324 (1661), sig. ²A3r; W324A (1661), sig. ²A3r; W324B (1661), sig. ²A3r; W324C (1661), sig. ²A3r.

263.   WOOLNOUGH, HENRY. *Fideles aquæ: or, Some Pious Tears Dropped upon the Hearse of the Incomparable Gentlewoman Mrs. Sarah Gilly.* W3529. UMI 2163: 15.

Sarah Gilly (d. ca. 1661?) is identified on the title page as "the only daughter of the loyal and worthy gentleman Matthew Gilly Esq." In addition to his own poems and elegies celebrating the life of Miss Gilly, Woolnough included some by "Mrs. Deval." These he introduces with "The Authour to the Incomparable Mrs. Deval; upon his inserting Her Verses into His Poems," in which Woolnough refers to "Learned Jeffry" and places him in company with Spenser, Jonson, Davenant. In a passage about the poor state of contemporary poetry and the superiority of Mrs. Deval's, Woolnough writes:

> Of all Poets thou art best;
> And *Apollo* for thy Layes
> Might bestow on the Bayes.
> Many Poets of great fame
> Have (I swear) been much to blame:
> Some ye most of 'em I ween
> Are scurilous, or obscene;
> Others very dull, the times
> Yield us store of Hymnes and Rhimes:
> Some do bite, and others claw;
> And the rest not worth a straw;
> Some are pious and yet plain;
> Others witty yet prophane;
> Some do prostitute their Muses
> Put up on 'em great abuses;
> Others two [*sic*] as bad I deem
> Do make Monks and Nuns of them:
> Few I think observe a right
> Just decorum as they might.
> But I dare say Madam you
> Are both Godly, witty too;
> Thicksculd [*sic*] wisdome, and the other
> *Thomas Sternhold* his sworn brother;
> Learned *Jeffry*, merry *Ben*
> *Spencer, Davenant,* such as them
> (Had they been alive to see
> Pretty one thy Poesie)
> Would I think have loved thee. (77–78)

1662

264.   ATWELL, GEORGE. *The Faithfull Surveyor.* A4164. UMI 1139: 22.

For an echo of *Troilus and Criseyde* 5: 1786, see ATWELL (1658); in this edition, the passage is found in "The Author to his Book" (no pagination, no signature).

265.   BAKER, RICHARD. *Theatrum redivivivum: or, The Theatre Vindicated.* B513. UMI Thomason Tracts 245: E.2269 (1).

Baker (1568–1645) is identified on the title page as "Sir Richard Baker." As Bowyer notes (*SP* 28), Baker seems to allude to *The Wife of Bath's Prologue.* Writing in response to Prynne's *Histrio-mastix,* Baker seeks to confute Prynn's "groundless Assertions against *Stage-Plays*" (title page). In passing, he mentions the "scurrility" of the Wife of Bath. Baker writes:

> [Prynne] would make us believe; *That all the attractive power in Plays, to draw Beholders, is meerly from scurrility*: as if it were no Play; at least no pleasing Play, without it. Wherein, besides his prejudice, he may be made to confess his ignorance: for let him try it when he will, and come himself upon the *Stage*, with all the scurrility of the Wife of *Bath*, with all the ribaldry of *Poggius*, or *Boccace*, yet I dare affirm, he shall never give that contentment o Beholders, as honest *Tarlton* did, though he said never a word. (34)

In a passage about Prynn's tendency to prolixity, Baker appears to echo a line from *The Reeve's Tale*: "The gretteste clerkes been noght wisest men" (line 4054). He writes:

> Others there are, of whom we may be bold to say, seeing the *Proverb* saith it, that *The greatest Clerks are not always the wisest men.* Bring them to a *Matter,* that is not meerly *Logical,* and you shall finde them oftentimes to be meerly *Irrational.* (98)

Another edition with a different title: *Theatrum Triumphans,* B514 (1670), 34, 98.

266.   CHARLES I, KING OF ENGLAND. Βασιλικα [Basilika]. *The Works of King Charles the Martyr.* C2075. UMI 2383: 6.

For an aphorism that the king attributes to Chaucer (but may allude to *The Squire's Tale*), see CHARLES I (1649); in this edition, the passage is found on ²166. *Another edition*: C2076 (1687), 80.

267.   CLEVELAND, JOHN. *Poems.* C4696. UMI 1305: 36.

For an echo of a line from *The Manciple's Prologue*, see CLEVELAND (1644); in this edition, the passage is found on 183.

268.   DAVENPORT, ROBERT. *King John and Matilda.* D371. UMI 2480: 3.

For an echo of a line in *The Wife of Bath's Tale*, see DAVENPORT (1655); in this edition, the passage is found on sig. G1v.

269.   *A Discourse of Artificial Beauty.*[31] *With Some Satyrical Censures on the Vulgar Errors of These Times.* G353. UMI 277: 18 (film is incomplete).

Harris notes (*PQ*) two allusions to Chaucer. In a section headed "Some Satyrical Censures on the Vulgar Errors of These Times," the author paraphrases Chaucer's description of the Physician in *The General Prologue* (lines 437–38) and later turns to *The Wife of Bath's Prologue* (lines 27–28):

> I shall confine my Discourse to the Profession of Physick, the most common centre of reproachfull lines. This is evident from Chaucer's verses,
>
> > 𝔓𝔥𝔶𝔰𝔦𝔠𝔦𝔞𝔫𝔰 𝔨𝔫𝔬𝔴 𝔴𝔥𝔞𝔱 𝔦𝔰 𝔡𝔦𝔤𝔢𝔰𝔱𝔦𝔟𝔩𝔢,
> > 𝔅𝔲𝔱 𝔱𝔥𝔢𝔦𝔯 𝔰𝔱𝔲𝔡𝔶 𝔦𝔰 𝔟𝔲𝔱 𝔩𝔦𝔱𝔱𝔩𝔢 𝔦𝔫 𝔱𝔥𝔢 𝔅𝔦𝔟𝔩𝔢. (223)
>
> The repute of *Women* hath been perplexed with Volumes of Invectives. . . . One of our own Poets agrees with these, and with his hobling [*sic*] feet thus tramples upon Female Credit:
>
> > 𝔋𝔞𝔩𝔣 𝔰𝔬 𝔟𝔬𝔩𝔡𝔩𝔶 𝔱𝔥𝔢𝔯𝔢 𝔠𝔞𝔫 𝔫𝔬𝔫𝔢
> > 𝔖𝔴𝔢𝔞𝔯 𝔞𝔫𝔡 𝔩𝔦𝔢 𝔞𝔰 𝔚𝔬𝔪𝔢𝔫 𝔠𝔞𝔫. (239–40)

270.   FELL, JOHN. *The Life of the Most Learned, Reverend and Pious Dr. H. Hammond.* F618. UMI 1149: 9.

For an echo of a line from *The Reeve's Tale*, see FELL (1661); in this edition, the passage is found on 97–98.

---

[31] *A Discourse of Auxiliary Beauty* (variously attributed to John Gauden, Jeremy Taylor, and Obadiah Walker) was also published in 1656 and 1692, but *Satyrical Censures* is not mentioned on either title page, nor is it found in the text.

271.   FOULIS, HENRY. *The History of the Wicked Plots and Conspiracies of Our Pretended Saints.* F1642. UMI 277: 5.

Foulis (ca. 1635–1669) is identified on the title page as a "Fellow of Lincoln-Colledge in Oxford." As Harris notes (*PQ*), he cites Chaucer and quotes from *The House of Fame* (lines 1579–82). In book 2, chapter 1, in a section about the "mischievous and impudent Contrivances and Innovations of the wicked long-Parliament," Foulis writes:

> [L]et us now think of his Majesties return from *Scotland*, in whose absence some of the Parliament had rais'd large reports of strange and terrible plots and designs against *John an Oaks*, and *John a Stiles*, by which means many people were endeavour'd to be whisper'd into dissatisfaction of the King; . . . and this was cunningly aimed at the King and his Favourites, by those who had their *Coy-ducks* in such obedience, that their Commands was not unlike that of Madam *Fame* to Æolus, in our ingenious *Chaucer* [in a shoulder note: "House of *Fame*, *lib*.3 *fol.* 320.*b*."].

> 𝔅ring eke his other claþioẃn
> 𝕿hat hight Sclaunder in eþery 𝕿oẃne,
> 𝖀ith ẃhich he ẃont is to disfame
> *𝕳em that me lyst and do *hem shame. (76–77)

[*Hem* is marked with an asterisk and furnished with a shoulder note: "Them."]

Shortly afterwards, Foulis alludes to *The Sommoner's Tale* and *The Parson's Tale* and then goes on to quote a quatrain from *The House of Fame* (lines 1389–92):

> And to make their Cause more favourable to the People, and to blast the Reputation of their Enemies, the promoted abundance of bawling Lecturers, most of them of no great Learning or Conscience . . . and for their dexterity and quickness they out-did a Mountebank; being alwayes as ready for the Pulpit, as a Knight-Errant for combate, never out of his way, let the Text be what it will; like the *Sompners Fryer* in *Chaucer*, (but nothing like the honest Parson in the same Poet) that is beyond admiration. . . . (80)

> And in this trade of vilifying, our Noncomformists were so expert and sedulous, that in a short while they had innumerable lying pamphlets and reports spread about the Nation, that in the first year or two of this Long Parliament, the hearers and believers, with the relatours of these slaunders, were so many, and all performed with that care and celerity, that Dame *Report* in *England* out-vapour'd Queen *Fame* in *Chaucer*, who

𝕳𝖆𝖉 𝖆𝖑𝖘𝖔 𝖋𝖊𝖑𝖊 𝖚𝖕 𝖘𝖙𝖆𝖓𝖉𝖎𝖓𝖌 𝖊𝖆𝖗𝖊𝖘
𝕬𝖓𝖉 𝖙𝖔𝖓𝖌𝖊𝖘, 𝖆𝖘 𝖔𝖓 𝖇𝖊𝖊𝖘𝖙 𝖇𝖊𝖓 𝖍𝖊𝖆𝖗𝖊𝖘,
𝕬𝖓𝖉 𝖔𝖓 𝖍𝖊𝖗 𝖋𝖊𝖙𝖊 𝖜𝖔𝖝𝖊𝖓 𝖘𝖆𝖜𝖊 𝕴
𝕻𝖆𝖗𝖙𝖗𝖎𝖈𝖍𝖊 𝖜𝖞𝖓𝖌𝖊𝖘 𝖗𝖊𝖉𝖎𝖑𝖞. (82–83)

[In a shoulder note: "House of Fame *Fol.* B. 329."]

In a passage about the reaction to debate in the House of Lords regarding bishops being seated there, Foulis alludes to *The Nun's Priest's Tale*:

And when the Lords by these unlawful and extravagant courses had been forced to agree with the Commons against the Bishops, good God! How did the Sectaries triumph! What bonefires? What bells ringing? What yelling and roaring in the streets? That the noise made by the neighbours, when *Don Russel* took Madam *Chaunteclere* away towards the Wood, was but a silence in respect of this Thundering Triumph . . . [In a shoulder note: "*Chaucer* fol. 104."] (92)

In a passage about Parliament's decision to take control of the militia, Foulis alludes to *The Summoner's Tale*:

Thus *Alexander* would but command the whole World. Thus . . . the crafty Fryer in the *Sumpners* tale, desired to his dinner only the liver of a Capon, and a roasted Pigs-head, knowing full well, that if he got those, he should not want his part of the Pigg and Capon too. And thus the Parliament only desired the Militia, that they might only command the King and all England. [In a shoulder note: "*Chaucer.* fol. 50"] (99)

In book 2, chapter 1, in a passage about Parliament's ill usage of the king, Foulis quotes lightly modernized lines of *The Clerk's Tale* (lines 529–32):

Thus are the best men violently opposed by the wicked, though the vertue and patience of the former might in reason mollifie the latter to obedience. How wishedly will some pitty . . . the patience of *Gryseld* in *Chaucer.* . . . (103)

If we perceive our selves grieved, resist we cannot but by Prayers and Obedience: To which purpose the ancient *Chaucer* instructs us, who certainly in this, sung according to the rule of his time, and therein, neither false Law, nor Gospel.

　　—𝕷𝖔𝖗𝖉𝖊𝖘 𝖍𝖊𝖘𝖙𝖊𝖘 𝖒𝖆𝖞 𝖓𝖔𝖙 𝖇𝖊 𝖋𝖆𝖞𝖓𝖊𝖉
　　𝕿𝖍𝖊𝖞 𝖒𝖆𝖞 𝖜𝖊𝖑 𝖇𝖊𝖜𝖆𝖞𝖑𝖊𝖉 𝖆𝖓𝖉 𝖈𝖔𝖒𝖕𝖑𝖆𝖎𝖓𝖊𝖉.

𝔅ut men must nedes unto *her lustre obey,
And so (wol 𝔍, there nis no more to sey. (104–5)

[*Her* is marked with a shoulder note: "their."]

In chapter 3, "The Inconstancy, villany, and monstrous Tyranny of the wicked Army! till the Restauration of his Majesty," in a section about the series of seventeen governments in England from the time of Charles I to the time of Charles II, Foulis again cites Chaucer and quotes *The Clerk's Tale* (lines 995–1001):

And what miseries the Nation underwent in these chopping, and changing of Models, is not yet forgot. This thing was today High-treason, which to morrow was good law; and the seduced people swore to maintain that, the contrary to which the next week they were constrain'd to defend: So that old *Chaucer's* complaint, may well be here revived [in a shoulder note: "Clerk of *Oxford's* tale *par* 6. *f.* 59.*a.*"]

𝔒 sterne people! 𝔘nsad, and untrewe,
Aye undiscrete, and chaungying as a fane,
Delyting ever in rumum that is new,
𝔉or like the 𝔐oon ever waxe ye, and wane,
𝔈ver full of clappying, dere enough a iane
𝔜our dome is false, your constaunce evel preveth,
A full great fool is he that on you leveth. (126)

In book 2, chapter 6, in a passage about the duplicity of Parliamentarians, Foulis alludes to *The Nun's Priest's Tale*:

And after this manner hath our former Rebels blanch'd over their designs: *Wat Tyler*, and his Companions, pretended onely to act against King *Richards* [*sic*] the seconds evil Counsel. . . . And the subtile Fox in *Chaucer*, profest he onely came to hear the Cock sing; but when by that craft he had once got hold of him, the case, and story was alter'd. [In a shoulder note: "The Tale of the *Nonne preest.* fol. 103."] (144–45)

Another edition: F1643 (1674), 77, 80, 83, 92, 99, 103, 104–5, 126, 144–45.

272.   FULLER, THOMAS. *History of the Worthies of England*. F2440. UMI 1092: 19.
Fuller (1608–1661) is identified on the title page as "Thomas Fuller, D. D." As Spurgeon notes and transcribes (1: 239–40 and 4: 74), there are references to generic Canterbury tales and Chaucer's *Canterbury Tales*; to Spenser's Chaucerian language; to Chaucer, the Homer of his age, who was probably born at

Woodstock; to Chaucer, "our English Ennius," and the expression Jack of Dover; and to Chaucer in contrast to Lydgate.

In chapter 10, "Writers," in a section headed "Writers on History," there is a reference missed by Spurgeon:

> Nor hath our Land been altogether barren of Historians since the Reformation. . . . Amongst these [who have been eminent in Poetry], some are additioned with the Title of *Laureat*, though I must confess, I could never find the root whence their Bays did grow in *England*, as to any solemn institution thereof in our Nation. Indeed I read of *Petrarch*, (the pre-coetanean of our *Chaucer*) that he was crowned with a Laurel, in the Capitol, by the Senate of *Rome, Anno* 1341. . . . Yet want there not those, who do confidently averr that there is always a Laureat Poet in *England*, and but one at a time, the Laurel importing Conquest and Sovereignty, and so by consequence soleness in that faculty; and that there hath been a constant succession of them at Court, who beside their salary from the King, were yearly to have a tun of win [*sic*], as very essential to the heightning of fancy. This last I conceive founded, on what we find given to *Geffery Chaucer*,

> > *Vigesimo secundo anno* Richardi *secundi concessum* Galfrido Chaucer *unum dolium vini per annum durante vitâ, in portu Civitatis* London, *per manus capitalis pincerna nostri.*

> But *Chaucer*, besides his poetical accomplishments, did the King service both in war and peace, as Souldier and Embassadour, in reward whereof, this and many other boons were bestow'd upon him. (27)

In the chapter on "Bark-Shire," in a passage about England's admiration of French things, there is another reference not recorded by Spurgeon. Fuller writes:

> We ape the French chiefly in two particulars. First in their language, (*which if* Jack *could speak, he would be a Gentleman*) which some get by travell, others gain at home with Dame *Eglentine* in *Chaucer.* [In a shoulder note: "In his Prologue of the Prioresse."]

> > *Entewned in her voice full seemly,*
> > *And* French *she spake full feteously*
> > *After the scole of* Stratford *at Bowe,*
> > *For* French *of* Paris *was to her unknow.* (86)

Spurgeon notes (but does not transcribe) a reference in the same chapter headed "Bark-Shire," in a section of "Memorable Persons" in the time of Henry IV:

THOMAS CHAUCER . . . was the sole son of *Geffery Chaucer*, that famous Poet, from whom he inerited fair lands, at *Dunnington-Castle* in this County, and at *Ewelme* in *Oxfordshire*. (106)

In the chapter on Kent, in a section on proverbs, Fuller quotes modernized lines 4347–48 from *The Cook's Prologue*:

A Jack of Dover. I find the first mention of this *Proverb* in our English *Ennius, Chaucer*, in his Proeme to the *Cook*:

And many a *Jack of Dover* he had sold
Which had been two times hot and two times cold.

This is no *Fallacy* but good *Policy* in an houshould, to lengthen out the Provision thereof, and though lesse toothsome may be wholsome enough: But what is no *false Logick* in a Family is *false Ethicks* in an *Inn*, or *Cook-shop*, to make the abused *Guest* to pay after the rate of *New* and *Fresh* for meat at the *second* and *third* hand. (²65)

In a section on Canterbury, in a subsection on proverbs, Fuller writes:

Canterbury-Tales. So *Chaucer* calleth his Book, being a collection of several *Tales*, pretended to be told by Pilgrims in their passage to the Shrine of Saint *Thomas* in *Canterbury*. But since that time *Canterbury-Tales* are parallel to *Fabula Milesia*, which are Charactered, *Nec vera, nec verisimilies*, meerly made to marre precious time, and please fanciful people. (²97)

In the chapter on Lancashire, in a section headed "The Manufactures," under the subhead "Fustians," Fuller cites Chaucer and quotes the *The General Prologue*, lines 75–76:

These anciently were creditable wearing in *England*, for persons of the primest quality, finding the *Knight* in *Chaucer* [in a shoulder note: "*Chaucer* in his Prologue."] thus habited.

𝔒f 𝔍ustian ꜧe ꞵeared a 𝔊ippon
Aꞁꞁ besmottreð ꞵitꜧ ꜧis Haubergion. (²106)

In the chapter on London, in a section on writers since the Reformation, Fuller notes Spenser's use of Chaucerian language:

EDMOND SPENSER . . . [was] especially most happy in English Poetry, as his works do declare. In which the many Chaucerisms used (for I will not say affected by him) are thought by the ignorant to be blemishes, known by the learned to be beauties to his book; which notwithstanding had been more falable, if more conformed to our modern language. . . . [D]ying for grief in great want, *Anno* 1598. was honorably buried nigh *Chaucer* in *Westminster*. . . . (²219–20)

In the chapter on Oxfordshire, Fuller writes of the conflicting accounts of Chaucer's birthplace:

JEFFREY CHAUCER was by most probability born at *Woodstock* in this County, though other places lay stiff claim to his Nativity.

Berk-shire title. Leland confesseth it likely that he was born in *Barechensi provincia*, and Mr. *Cambden* avoweth that *Dunnington-castle* nigh unto *Newwburie* was anciently his Inheritance. There was lately an old Oake standing in the Park called *Chaucers Oake.*

Londons title. The Author of his life, set forth 1602. proveth him born in *London*, out of these his own words in the *Testament of love*: Also in the Citie of London, that is to me too deare and sweete . . . Besides, Mr. *Cambden* praiseth Mr. *Edmund Spencer* the *Londoner* for the best Poet . . . Chaucer himself his fellow-citizen not being excepted.

Oxford shires title. Leland addeth a probability of his birth in *Oxford-shire*, and *Cambden* saith of *Woodstock, Cum nihil habeat quod ostintet, Homerum nostrum Anglicum, Galfredum Chaucerum alumnum suum fuisse gloriatur.* Besides, *I. Pits* is positive that his father was a Knight, and that he was born at *Woodstock*. And Queen *Elizabeth* passed a fair stone-house next to her Palace in that Town, unto the Tenant by the name of *Chaucers house*, whereby it is also known as this day.

Now what is to be done to decide the difference herein? Indeed *Appion* the Grammarian would have *Homer* (concerning whose Birth-place there was so much controversie) raised *ab Inferis*, that he might give a true account of the place of his Nativity. However our *Chaucer* is placed here, (having just grounds for the same) untill stronger reasons are brought to remove him.

He was a terse and elegant Poet, (the *Homer* of his Age) and so refined our *English* Tongue. . . . His skill in *Mathematicks* was great, (being instructed therein by *Joannes Sombus* and *Nicholas* of *Linn*) which he evidenceth in his book *De Sphara* [*sic*]. He being Contemporary with *Gower*, was living *Anno Dom.* 1402. (²337–38)

In the chapter on Suffolk, Fuller compares the language of Lydgate and Chaucer:

[B]oth in Prose and Poetry [Lydgate] was the best Authour of his Age. If *Chaucers Coin* were of a *greater weight* for *deeper learning*, *Lydgates* were of a more *refined Standard* for *purer language*, so that one might mistake him for a modern Writer. . . . [Yet he wrote] *For* Chaucer *that my Master was*. . . . (p. 168–69)

Spurgeon also notes (but does not transcribe) a reference in the chapter on Yorkshire, under the heading "Writers":

John Gower . . . was before *Chaucer*, as born and flourishing before him (yea by some accounted his Master,) yet was he after *Chaucer*, as surviving him two years, living to be stark blind, and so more properly termed our English *Homer*. (207)

"Jeffrey Chaucer" is also listed in "An Alphabetical Index to Fuller's Worthies of England" (45).
Another edition in 1662: F2441, same pagination.

273.   HACON, JOSEPH. *A Vindication of the Review: or, The Exceptions Formerly Made against Mr. Horn's Catechisme.* H178. UMI 740: 6.

Hacon (1603–1662) is identified on the title page as "J. H., Parson of Massinghamp. Norf." In an epistle addressed "To the Reader," he quotes a line from *Troilus and Criseyde*, "I am, til God me bettre mynde send, | At dulcarnoun, right at my wittes ende" (3: 930–31). Hacon writes:

I am quite put to silence in the respective partyiculars, and can finde out nothing to say in behalf of my self, but am at Dulcarnon, right at my wits end. (sig. A5r)

274.   *Iö Carole: or, An Extract of a Letter Sent from Parnassus.* I293. UMI 1485: 37.

This work is a collection of epigrams and odes written to commemorate the coronation of Charles II. The conceit is that Apollo presides over a jocular May Day feast; he calls on Homer, Virgil, Ovid, and others to read poems written in their style (or, perhaps more accurately, their language). In a prose bridge between the ancients and moderns, there is a reference to Chaucer:

The Latine Poëts having pretty well playd their parts, his Majesty and the whole company lookt all stedfastly now upon Du Bartas, *now upon* T. Tasso, *which was a sufficient signe what was expected from those two, hereupon they both stood forth, but instead of alling to the businesse in hand enterr'd into a dispute concerning their precedency one before the other, and appeal'd to* Apollo *which side of the Mountaine was the more fertile soile for witts, and whither had more righ to begin first the* French-man *or the* Italian; *his Majesty bade them both sit downe again for the present, and come again for judgement an* 100 *years hence; then turning towards the English Poëtts [sic], he thought to have brought old* Jeffery *upon the stage, but considering how littele difference there is both as to matter and stile between him and* Spencer, *he pitch't upon the last, who entertain'd us.* . . . (13–14)

275.   LOVEDAY, ROBERT. *Loveday's Letters Domestick and Forrein.* L3226. UMI 845: 20 (1662).

For a reference to Chaucer as a prophet and poet, perhaps an allusion to the spurious work known as "Chaucer's Prophecy," see LOVEDAY (1659); in this edition, the passage is found on 98–99.

276.   NEWCASTLE, MARGARET CAVENDISH. *Playes Written by the Thrice Noble, Illustrious and Excellent Princess, the Lady Marchioness of Newcastle.* N868. UMI 502: 11.

Although Lady Newcastle (1624?–1674) is described on the title page as the Marchioness of Newcastle, she was later created the Duchess of Newcastle.

In scene 37 of *The First Part of the Play Called Wits Cabal*, she writes of a group of ladies and gentlemen who discuss the merits of prose and poetry. Monsieur Vain-glorious says, "Rhime is a Veil to cover the face of Nonsense." Monsieur Censure remarks that no poem is esteemed that is not in gay, new-fashioned garb. Whereupon Mademoiselle Ambition defends Chaucer's poems and asserts their lasting value:

Then *Chaucers* Poems, which are in plain and old-fashion'd garments, which is Language, is to be despised, and his Wit condemned; but certainly *Chaucers* Witty Poems, and Lively Descriptions, in despight of their Old Language, as they have lasted in great Esteem and Admiration these three hundred years, so they may do Eternally amongst the Wise in every Age. (285–86)

In *The Second Part of the Play Called Wits Cabal*, Lady Newcastle appears to allude to *The House of Fame*. In the third act, scene 17 features Bon' Esprit, Ambition, Temperance, Faction, Portrait, Pleasure, and Superbe. Faction inquires of Bon' Esprit, "[W]here will your Tongue carry us?" And she responds: "As high as it can, even to the House of Fame, which stands on the highest pinacle of Heaven" (313).

In *The Unnatural Tragedy*, Lady Newcastle again appears to allude to *The House of Fame*. Scene 12 of the first act features a Matron and several Virgins. The First Virgin says, "I have observ'd that one pen may blur a Reputation; but one pen will hardly glorifie a Reputation." The Second Virgin replies, "No; for to glorifie, requires many pens and witnesses, and all little enough." The Fourth Virgin responds:

> It is neither here nor there for that: for merit will get truth to speak for her in Fames Palace; and those that have none, can never get in, or at least remain there: For have not some Writers spoke well of *Nero* . . . [a]nd have not some Writers done the like for *Claudius*, who was the foolishest of all the Emperours? yet they were never the more esteem'd in the House of Fame. And have not some Writers writ ill, and have indeavour'd to blot and blur the Renowns of *Julius Cæsar*, and *Augustus Cæsar*, and of *Alexander*, and yet they are never the worse esteem'd in the House of Fame. . . . (338)

In *The First Part of Bell in Campo*, Lady Newcastle appears to echo the description of the shipman in *The General Prologue*: "Of nyce conscience took he no keep" (line 398). In scene 25 Nell Careless asks Doll Pacify if she thinks it is a sin for a young woman to live as a widow. Doll replies that "it would be a case of Conscience to me if I were a Widow." Nell Careless responds: "By thy nice Conscience thou seem'st to be a Puritan" (605).

277.   PHILLIPS, EDWARD. *The New World of English Words: or, A General Dictionary.* P2069. UMI 574: 14.

For a pictorial representation of Chaucer on an engraved title page, see PHILLIPS, P2068 (1658); for references to Chaucer in the dedicatory epistle and the preface of this edition, see sigs. (a)3v and (b)4v. Chaucer is also mentioned in definitions of *Advenale* (sig. A4r), *Agiler* (sig. B1r), *Amalgaminge* (sig. B3r), *Amortize* (sig. B4r), *Appeteth* (sig. C3r), *Apprentice* (sig. C3r), *Arblaster* (sig. C3v), *Arretteth* (sig. C4r), *Arten* (sig. C4v), *Assise* (sig. D1r), *Assoyle* (sig. D1r), *Asterlagour* (sig. D1r), *Barm-cloth* (sig. D4v), *Baudon* (sig. E1r), *Bay* (sig. E1r), *Beau Sir* (sig. E1v), *Bend* (sig. E2r), *Burnet* (sig. F1v), *Caitisned* (sig. F2v), *Canceline* (sig. F3v), *Chastelyn* (sig. G4v), *Chekelaton* (sig. H1r), *Chelandri* (sig. H1r), *Chertes* (sig. H1r), *Chevesal* (sig. H1r), *Chimbe* (sig. H1v), *Chincherie* (sig. H1v), *Cierges* (sig. H2r), *Citriale* (sig. H3r), *Clergion* (sig. H3r), *Clicket,* (sig. H3r), *Curebulli* (sig. K4v), *Dennington* (sig. L4r), *Desidery* (sig. M1r), *Deslavy* (sig. M1r), *Digne* (sig. M2v), *Discure* (sig. M3r), *Divine* (sig. M4r), *Dowtremere* (sig. N1v), *Ebrack* (sig. N2v), *Gibsere* (sig. Q4r), *Giglet* (sig. Q4r), *Gourd* (sig. R1r), *Haketon* (sig. R3r), *Hanselines* (sig. R3v), *Magonel* (sig. Aa3v), *Rebeck* (sig. Kk2r), *Woodstock* (sig. Rr4r).

There are also at least two new references in this lightly revised and expanded edition:

Clinke, (old word) a key-hole; whose Diminutive is *Clicket*, a key: used by old *Chaucer*. (sig. H3r) [Chaucer uses *clicket* in *The Merchant's Tale*, lines 2046, 2117, 2121, 2123, 2151]

Jewise, rewarded by revenge: also a Gibbet; so *Chaucer's* Expositor. (sig. T2v) [*Jewise* is not found in Tatlock & Kennedy's *Concordance*.]

278.   PHILLIPS, JOHN. *Montelion, 1662: or, The Prophetical Almanack.* A2111. UMI 1414: 30.

As Spurgeon notes (3: 4.73), Phillips suggests that Chaucer's Miller be remembered and celebrated on 23 November 1662.

279.   SHAKESPEARE, WILLIAM. *The Bouncing Knight* in *The Wits: or, Sport upon Sport.* W3218. UMI 1112: 6.

In an epistle addressed to the readers, the stationer (Henry Marsh) writes that he has "undertaken to collect a Miscellany of all Humours which our Fam'd Comedies have exquisitely and aptly represented in the becoming dress of the Stage" (sig. A3r). The first droll in this collection is taken (without attribution) from Shakespeare's *Henry IV, Part I* and here is called *The Bouncing Knight: or, The Robers Rob'd.* Falstaff addresses the hostess as "dame partlet the Hen," an allusion to *The Nun's Priest's Tale.* See Shakespeare (1598), Boswell & Holton No. 613; in this collection, the passage is found on 9.

Another edition: W3219 (1672), 9.

280.   W., M. *The Comedy Called the Marriage Broaker: or, The Pander.* W84. UMI 337: 24.

In 2.1, Derrick the marriage broker refers the Wife of Bath as he speaks to Shift about widows. He says most widows solace themselves with memories of the past and with toothless gums chew over the pleasures of their youth. Only a few of them are so fortunate as to have had five husbands, an allusion to *The General Prologue*: "Housbondes at chirche dore she hadde fyve" (line 460).

> [B]ut few
> Can grace 5. fingers with five wedding-rings.
> And the example of the wife of *Bath*
> Is in my reading singular. (20–21)

Another edition in 1662 with a different title, *Gratiæ theatrales: or, A Choice Ternary of English Plays*: G1580, same pagination.

281.   WATKYNS [OR WATKINS], ROWLAND. *Flamma sine fumo: or, Poems With-out Fictions.* W1076. UMI 338: 5.

Watkyns is identified on the title page as "R. W." As Harris notes (*PQ*), there is a reference to "Wise Chaucer" in company with Jonson, Randolph, and Cleveland, all poets of modest means. In a poem headed "The Poets Condition," Watkyns may allude to Chaucer's "Complaint to His Purse"; he writes:

> A Poet, and rich? that seems to be
> A paradox most strange to me.
> A Poet, and poor? that Maxim's true,
> If we observe the Canting crue.
> What lands had *Randolph*, or great *Ben*,
> That plow'd much paper with his pen?
> Wise *Chaucer*, as old Records say,
> Had never but his length of clay:
> And by some men I have been told,
> That *Cleveland* had more brains than gold. [Etc.] (110)

1663

282.   A., J. Verses in John Batchiler's *Christian Queries to Quaking-Christians.* B1073aA. UMI 1029: 15 (as B97); UMI 2561: 11.

In a verse epistle addressed to the reader, J. A. echoes Chaucer's line, "Go, litel bok, go litel myn tragedye" (*Troilus and Criseyde* 5: 1786).

> Go little Book, *improve thy Scripture-skill,*
> *Advance the Truth, and throw down all self-will.* . . . (sig. A2r)

283.   BLOUNT, THOMAS. *The Academy of Eloquence.* B3323. UMI 2452: 11.

For an echo of the title of *The House of Fame*, see BLOUNT (1654); in this edition, the passage is found on 29.

284.   GAYTON, EDMUND. *The Religion of a Physician: or, Divine Meditations upon the Grand and Lesser Festivals.* G416. UMI 145: 7.

Gayton (1608–1666) is identified on the title page as "Edmund Gayton, Batch-elor of physick, and captain lieutenant of food to His Illustrious Highness James Duke of York." As Spurgeon notes (1: 240–41), Gayton quotes from *The General Prologue* (lines 437–38). In an "Epistle to the Favourable Reader," Gayton writes of his motivation for writing this collection of religious meditations:

'Tis true, that Sir Jeffrey Chaucer *had but an ill opinion of my Faculty, when he saith of a Doctor of Physick,*

> His meat was good and digestible,
> But not a word he had o'th'Bible.

To wipe off that stain and aspersion from our Botanick Tribe, *I wrote these* Meditations, *to shew the World, that it is possible for a Physician of the Lower Form to be* Theologue, *at leastwise to seem to be one.* (sigs. (*a*)4v–(*b*)1r)

285.   HILTON, JOHN. *Catch That Catch Can: or, A Choice Collection of Catches, Rounds & Canons.* H2038. No UMI.

For a reference to Chaucer's jape in a song, see HILTON (1652).

286.   JORDAN, THOMAS. *Tricks of Youth: or, The Walks of Islington and Hogsdon.* J1067. UMI 694: 6.

For a reference to "the wanton memory of Chaucer" and his "heathen" and "bawdy" English, see JORDAN (1657); in this edition, the passage is found on sig. E4v.

287.   *The Ladies Losse at the Adventures of Five Hours: or, The Shifting of the Vaile.* L156. UMI 1062: 16.

In an aside (as it were), following a passage about a lady whose "*Cunny* is not well *accoutred*," the anonymous rhymster alludes to *The Miller's Tale*:

> So fared it with *Absolon*,
> Who found a *Beard*, expecting *none*.
> When *Gossip* (to his great amazement)
> Turn'd *Tayle* for *Smeller*, out of *Cazement*,
> *Womanaging* so *cleaverly*,
> That *Nab* kist *Tout* full *savorly*,
> And started back, like *Horse* cryes *Wy-hee*
> At Female-Beard, to hear her *Ty-hee*. (5)

288.   LEIGH, EDWARD. *Fœlix Consortium; or, A Fit Conjuncture of Religion and Learning:* L995. UMI 387: 28.

For references to Chaucer grouped with other English poets, including Gower and Spenser, see LEIGH (1656); in this edition, the passages are found on sig. A5v–6r, 91, 160, 211, 328, and sig. Ccc3r.

289.   LEIGH, EDWARD. *Select and Choice Observations.* L1004. UMI 1362: 11.

For an echo of a line from *The Merchant's Tale*, see LEIGH (1647); in this edition, the passage is found on 424.

290.   LENTON, FRANCIS. *Characters: or, Wit and the World in Their Proper Colors.* L1095. UMI 153: 4

For an echo of a line in *The Manciple's Prologue*, see LENTON (1631) in the Appendix; in this edition, the passage is found on sig. H1v.

291.   LOVEDAY, ROBERT. *Loveday's Letters Domestick and Forrein.* L3227. UMI 1797: 28.

For a reference to Chaucer as a prophet and poet, perhaps an allusion to the spurious work known as "Chaucer's Prophecy," see LOVEDAY (1659); in this edition, the passage is found on 98–99.

292.   MENNES, JOHN. *Recreation for Ingenious Head-peeces: or, A Pleasant Grove for Their Wits to Walk In.* M1715. UMI 1346: 22 (identified as W3222).

For an epitaph "On our prime English Poet, *Geffrey Chaucer*," see MENNES (1641). The epitaph is originally from Lydgate's prologue to his translation of Boccaccio's *The Falle of Princes*; see BOCCACCIO (1494) in Boswell & Holton No. 27. In this edition, the passage is found on sig. O4r.

For a reference to Chaucer in an epitaph "On William Shake-speare," see *Wits Recreations* (1640) in Boswell & Holton No. 1377; in this edition, the passage is found on sig. O5r.

293.   PHILIPPS, FABIAN. *The Antiquity, Legality, Reason, Duty and Necessity of Prae-emption and Prourveyance, for the King: or, Compositions for His Pourveyance as They Were Used and Taken for the Provisions of the Kings Household.* P2004. UMI 472: 2.

In chapter 5, "Necessity that the King should have and enjoy his Ancient Right of Pourveyance," Philipps (1601–1690) cites Chaucer and quotes a quatrain from *The General Prologue* (lines 221–24):

> A freedom from the chargeable giving of great quantities of Lands for Chantries, and the *weaning* of that Clergy by the reformation of the Church of *England*, from their *over-sucking* or making sore the Breasts or Nipples of the common people, which the murmuring men of these times, would if they had as their forefathers tried it more then seven times, and over and over be of the opinion of *Piers* the *Plowman* in *Chaucer* (who being of the *Romish* Church, wrote in the unfortunate Reign of King *Richard* the second, when the *Hydra* of our late Rebellious devices

spawned by the not long before ill grounded Doctrines, and treasonable positions . . . complaining,

> 𝕿𝖍𝖆𝖙 𝖙𝖍𝖊 𝕱𝖗𝖎𝖆𝖗𝖘 𝖋𝖔𝖑𝖑𝖔𝖜𝖊𝖉 𝖋𝖔𝖑𝖐𝖊 𝖙𝖍𝖆𝖙 𝖜𝖊𝖗𝖊 𝖗𝖎𝖈𝖍,
> 𝕬𝖓𝖉 𝖋𝖔𝖑𝖐 𝖙𝖍𝖆𝖙 𝖜𝖊𝖗𝖊 𝖕𝖔𝖔𝖗, 𝖆𝖙 𝖑𝖎𝖙𝖙𝖑𝖊 𝖕𝖗𝖎𝖈𝖊 𝖙𝖍𝖊𝖞 𝖘𝖊𝖙;
> 𝕬𝖓𝖉 𝖓𝖔 𝕮𝖔𝖗𝖘 𝖎𝖓 𝖙𝖍𝖊 𝕶𝖞𝖗𝖐𝖊𝖞𝖆𝖗𝖉, 𝖓𝖔𝖗 𝖐𝖞𝖗𝖐𝖊 𝖜𝖆𝖘 𝖇𝖚𝖗𝖎𝖊𝖉,
> 𝕭𝖚𝖙 𝖖𝖚𝖎𝖈𝖐 𝖍𝖊 𝖇𝖊𝖖𝖚𝖊𝖙𝖍 𝖙𝖍𝖊𝖒 𝖔𝖚𝖌𝖍𝖙 𝖔𝖗 𝖖𝖚𝖎𝖙 𝖕𝖆𝖗𝖙 𝖔𝖋 𝖍𝖎𝖘 𝖉𝖊𝖙.
> [. . . a dozen more lines of *Piers Plowman*.]

And in his Prologue to his *Canterbury Tales* thus Characters such a *Frier*,

> 𝕱𝖚𝖑𝖑 𝖘𝖜𝖊𝖊𝖙𝖑𝖞 𝖍𝖊𝖆𝖗𝖉 𝖍𝖊 𝖈𝖔𝖓𝖋𝖊𝖘𝖘𝖎𝖔𝖓,
> 𝕬𝖓𝖉 𝖕𝖑𝖊𝖆𝖘𝖆𝖓𝖙 𝖜𝖆𝖘 𝖍𝖎𝖘 𝖆𝖇𝖘𝖔𝖑𝖚𝖙𝖎𝖔𝖓;
> 𝕳𝖊 𝖜𝖆𝖘 𝖆𝖓 𝖊𝖆𝖘𝖎𝖊 𝖒𝖆𝖓 𝖙𝖔 𝖌𝖎𝖇𝖊 𝖕𝖊𝖓𝖓𝖆𝖓𝖈𝖊,
> 𝕿𝖍𝖊𝖗𝖊 𝖆𝖘 𝖍𝖊 𝖜𝖎𝖘𝖍𝖙 𝖙𝖔 𝖍𝖆𝖇𝖊 𝖆 𝖌𝖔𝖔𝖉 𝖕𝖎𝖙𝖆𝖓𝖈𝖊. (315–17)

Another edition in 1663 with a different title, *Monenda: or, The Antiquity, Legality, Reason, Duty and Necessity of Præemption, or Pourveyance*: P2011A.

294.   PHILLIPS, EDWARD. *The New World of English Words: or, A General Dictionary.* P2070. UMI 1659: 24.

For a pictorial representation of Chaucer and for references to him in the dedicatory epistle and the preface, see PHILLIPS, P2068 (1658), and P2069 (1662); in this edition, these are found on sigs. (a)3v and (b)4v. Chaucer is also mentioned in definitions of *Advenale* (sig. A4r), *Agiler* (sig. B1r), *Amalgaminge* (sig. B3r), *Amortize* (sig. B4r), *Appeteth* (sig. C3r), *Apprentice* (sig. C3r), *Arblaster* (sig. C3v), *Argoil* (sig. C3v), *Arretteth* (sig. C4r), *Arten* (sig. C4v), *Assise* (sig. D1r), *Assoyle* (sig. D1r), *Asterlagour* (sig. D1r), *Autremite* (sig. D3r), *Barm-cloth* (sig. D4v), *Baudon* (sig. E1r), *Bay* (sig. E1r), *Beau Sir* (sig. E1v), *Bend* (sig. E2r), *Burnet* (sig. F1v), *Caitisned* (sig. F2v), *Canceline* (sig. F3v), *Chasteleyn* (sig. G4v), *Chekelaton* (sig. H1r), *Chelandri* (sig. H1r), *Chertes* (sig. H1r), *Chevesal* (sig. H1r), *Chimbe* (sig. H1v), *Chincherie* (sig. H1v), *Cierges* (sig. H2r), *Citriale* (sig. H3r), *Clergion* (sig. H3r), *Clicket,* (sig. H3r), *Clinke* (sig. H3v), *Curebulli* (sig. K4v), *Dennington* (sig. L4r), *Desidery* (sig. M1r), *Deslavy* (sig. M1r), *Digne* (sig. M2v), *Discure* (sig. M3r), *Divine* (sig. M4r), *Dowtremere* (sig. N1v), *Ebrack* (sig. N2v), *Gibsere* (sig. Q4r), *Giglet* (sig. Q4r), *Gourd* (sig. R1r), *Haketon* (sig. R3r), *Hanselines* (sig. R3v), *Jewise* (sig. T2v), *Losenger* (sig. Aa1r), *Magonel* (sig. Aa3v), *Rebeck* (sig. Kk2r), *Woodstock* (sig. Rr4r).

295.   S., W., in John Bullokar's *An English Expositor: Teaching the Interpretation of the Hardest Words Used in Our Language.* **B5430A. UMI 2718: 1.**

For a reference to Chaucer and *The Prologue to the Squire's Tale* in the definition of Chivancy, see S., W. (1654); in this edition, the passage is found on sig. D7r.

In this "Revised, Corrected, and very much augmented" edition by "a Lover of the Arts," a new reference to Chaucer and an allusion to *The Nun's Priest's Tale* is introduced for the first time into Bullokar's perennially popular work:

> *Chanticleer.* A word used by *Chaucer* for a Cock. (sig. D6r)

Other editions: B5431 (1667), sig. B11r; B5431A (1671), sig. B11r; B5432 (1676), sig. B11r; B5433 (1680), sig. B11r; B5434 (1684), sig. B11r; B5435 (1688), sig. B11r; B5435A (1695), sig. B11r; B5436 (1698), sig. B11r.

296.   Selden, John. *Mare clausum; The Right and Dominion of the Sea in Two Books. Formerly Translated into English, and Now Perfected and Restored by J. H. Gent.* **S2431. UMI 333: 8.**

For references to Chaucer in a Latin edition, STC 22175 (1635), see Selden (1635) in Boswell & Holton No. 1278; for references in a translation by Marchmont Needham, see Selden, S2432 (1652); in this edition, the passages are found on 191, 280–81.

297.   Shakespeare, William. *Mr. William Shakespeares Comedies, Histories and Tragedies.* **S2913. UMI 1858: 6.**

For multiple references and allusions to Chaucer and his works, see Shakespeare (1623), Boswell & Holton No. 1050.

For an echo of a line from *The Manciple's Prologue* in *Romeo and Juliet*, see Shakespeare (1597) in the Appendix; in this edition the passage is found on 646.

298.   *The True and Admirable History of Patient Grisel, a Poor Mans Daughter in France, and the Noble Marquis Salus. Written First in French, but Now Translated into English.* T2411. UMI 1644: 13

Although Chaucer writes of patient Griselde, this work appears to have no Chaucerian connection.

299.   Waterhouse, Edward. *Fortescutus illustratus: or, A Commentary on That Nervous Treatise, De labudibus legum Angliae, Written by Sir John Fortescue, Knight.* **W1046. UMI 161: 1.**

Waterhouse (1619–1670) is identified on the title page as "Edward Waterhous Esquire." He cites Chaucer and quotes slightly modernized lines from *The*

General Prologue (lines 309–10). In chapter 8, in a passage regarding the king's delegation of authority to judges to enforce the laws of the kingdom, Waterhouse writes:

> [S]ince the *King's* of *England* are furnished with learned Judges, Serjeants, Apprentices, and other men of learning in the Law . . . so that now, all the *King* is in this case to do, is, to give his mind to love and comprobate the Law, and in that delightful humour to please himself, such minutes as he can spare from action and pleasure. For though a Serjeant at Law, whose glory and grace it is, *Ut serviendo discat, & discendo alios perdiscat*, as men of that degree did at their *Parvise*, of which *Chaucer* speaks,
>
> > *A Serjeant at Law, wary and wise,*
> > *That often had ben at the* Pervise. (141)

In chapter 12, in free translation of verses from Juvenal's Satire 13, Waterhouse echoes a line from *The Manciple's Prologue*: "Sires, what! Dun is in the myre!" (line 5). He writes:

> *What day so sacred is, which cannot discover*
> *Theft, Perfidie, with Fraud, 'bout* Rome *to hover,*
> *In thee Gold is the Goddess men admire;*
> *They it by hook or crook reesolve t' acquire,*
> *Thus is the* Roman *virtue dun'd i'th' myre.* (188)

300.   WHARTON, GEORGE. "To my Very Honoured Friend," in Gaultier de Coste, Seigneur de La Calprenède's *Hymen's Præludia: or, Love's Master-Piece. Now Rendred into English, by Robert Loveday.* L112B. UMI 1723: 11.

For a reference to Chaucer and Gower as a pair who refined the English language, see WHARTON (1652); in this edition, the passage is found on sig. A4v.

1664

301.   BLOUNT, THOMAS. *The Academy of Eloquence.* B3324. UMI 1119: 14.

For an echo of the title of *The House of Fame*, see BLOUNT (1654); in this edition, the passage is found on 29.

302.   BOLD, HENRY. *Poems Lyrique Macaronique Heroique, &c.* B3473. UMI 127: 10. F.

Bold (1627–1683) is identified on the title page as "Henry Bold olim è N. C. Oxon." As Graves notes (*SP*), Bold mentions Chaucer in a poem headed "Marston Ale-House; April 13th 1648." Of the terrible service he and his friends received there, Bold writes:

> I and two *friends* of mine; who ne're had been there
> Did take a *walk* to *Marston*, after dinner
> ·
> We found a *shady place, where*, like *two* fine fooles,
> One on the *Grass* sate down, and two, on *Joynt-stooles*.
> And for a *Table*, where to set the *Water*;
> She brings the *Washingblock*—the *legs* came after.
> Then like to *Mother Gubbins mode* in *Chaucer*
> Sends out the *Flagon* coverd [*sic*] with a *Saucer*. (146)

303.   EVELYN, JOHN. *Sylva: or, A Discourse of Forest-Trees.* E3516. UMI 561: 15; UMI 593: 15.

Evelyn (1620–1706) is identified on the title page as "J. E. Esq"; As Spurgeon notes (1: 239), Evelyn refers to Chaucer in an essay delivered to the Royal Society in 1662. In chapter 29, in a passage about trees of remarkable size and quality of timber, Evelyn writes of the tradition that Chaucer planted trees:

> Nor are we to over-pass those memorable Trees which so lately flourished in *Dennington Park* neer *Newberry*; amongst which, *three* were most remarkable from the ingenious *Planter*, and *dedication* (if *Tradition* hold) of the famous English *Bard, Jeofry Chaucer*; of which one was call'd the *Kings*, another the *Queens*, and a third *Chaucers-Oak*. . . . *Chaucers Oak*, though it were not of these dimensions [i.e., not as large as the King's Oak or the Queen's], yet was it a very goodly Tree: And this account I receiv'd from my most honour'd friend *Phil. Packer* Esq. whose *Father* (as now the *Gentleman* his *Brother*) was proprietor of this *Park*: But that which I would farther remark, upon this occasion is, the *bulk*, and the *stature* to which an *Oak* may possibly arrive within less then three *hundred* years; since it is not so long that our *Poet* flourish'd (being in the *Reign* of King *Edward* the *fourth*) if at least he were indeed the *Planter* of those *Trees*, as 'tis confidently affirmed. I will not labour much in this enquiry; because an *implicit* faith is here of great encouragement. . . . (83)

Other editions: E3517 (1670), 153–54 (and in index sig. f1r); E3518 (1679), 166 (and index, sig. f1v).

304.   *A General Collection of Discourses of the Virtuosi of France, Render'd into English by G. Havers, Gent.* R1034. UMI 412: 11.

The work at hand is a translation of the first hundred conferences of the *Recueil général des questions traitéesés conférences du Bureau d'adresse.* In translating the debate of whether flesh or fish is the better food, George Havers inverts a phrase from Chaucer that had become proverbial:

> The fifth [speaker] said, That the Flesh of Animals is the rule of the goodness of Fish, which is the better the nearer it comes to Flesh; whence arose the Proverb, *Young Flesh, and old Fish*; because in time it acquires the consistince of Flesh. (179)

In *The Merchant's Tale*, Chaucer writes: "But one thing warn I you, my friendis dere, | I wol no old wife have in no manere. | She shall not passin sixtene yere certeine | Old fish, and young flesh woll I haue full faine" (lines 1415–18)

In considering the proposition that "all men naturally desire knowledge," Havers appears to echo a line from *The Reeve's Tale*: "The gretteste clerkes been noght wisest men" (line 4054). He writes:

> Moreover, there are some men who have not much less of the beast then of the man. And as the greatest Clerks (according to the Proverb) are not always the wisest men, so neither are they the most happy. (233)

305.   GUILLIM, JOHN. *A Display of Heraldry. The Fifth Edition.* G2220. UMI 1358: 28 (incomplete: 110–33 only).

For quotations from *The Romaunt of the Rose*, a reference to Sir Payne Roet who is identified as Chaucer's father-in-law, a description of Chaucer's escutcheon, and a quotation from *The Knight's Tale*, see GUILLIM (1610) in Boswell & Holton No. 816.

306.   HEATH, ROBERT. *Paradoxical Assertions and Philosophical Problems.* H1341A. UMI 2007: 2.

For a reference to Chaucer's mill, perhaps an allusion to *The Reeve's Tale*, see HEATH (1659); in this edition, the passage is found on ²12.

307.   LEIGH, EDWARD. *Analecta Caesarum Romanorum: or, Select Observations. Also Certain Choice French Proverbs.* L984. UMI 1062: 29.

For an echo of a line from *The Merchant's Tale*, see LEIGH (1647); in this edition, the passage is found on 424.

308. NEWCASTLE, MARGARET CAVENDISH. *CCXI Sociable Letters Written by the Thrice Noble, Illustrious, and Excellent Princess.* **N872. UMI 1553: 10.**

In the fifteenth letter in this collection of informal letters written to her neighbor, Lady Newcastle appears to allude to *The House of Fame.*

> Madam, Yesterday was the Lord *N. W.* To visit me, where amongst other Discourses we talk'd of the Lady *T. M.* not sooner was her name mentioned, but he seem'd to be rapt up into the third Heaven, and from thence to descend to declare her Praises. . . . [He said she] was had not a Temporal and Imperial Guard, yet she was guarded with virtue; and though she was not attended, waited and served with and by Temporal and Imperial Courtiers, yet she was attended, waited on, and served by and with the sweet Graces, and her Maids of Honour were the Muses, and Fame's house was her Magnificent Palace. (23–25)

309. NEWCASTLE, WILLIAM CAVENDISH. "On Her Book of Poems," in Margaret Cavendish's *Poems and Phancies.* **N870. UMI 721: 24.**

As Spurgeon notes (3: 4.74), the Marquis of Newcastle places his lady wife's poetry above that of Chaucer and Shakespeare in a commendatory poem headed "To the Lady Marchioness of Newcastle, On Her Book of Poems." In this second impression of her poems, he writes:

> I saw your *Poems*, and then Wish'd them mine,
> Reading the *Richer Dressings* of each Line;
> . . . .
> And Gentle *Shakespear* weeping, since he must
> At best, be Buried, now, *in Chaucers Dust*:
> Thus dark *Oblivion* covers their each *Name*,
> Since you have Robb'd them of their *Glorious Fame*. (sig. A2r)

The poem is not found in the first edition.
Another edition: N871 (1668), sig. A2r–v.

310. *Poor Robin. 1664. An Almanack After a New Fashion.* A2183. UMI 1517: 25.

Under the heading "Observations on April," we find "Patient Gryssell" is celebrated on the 24th (sig. A8r); this is perhaps a faint allusion to the protagonist of *The Clerk's Tale.*

311.   PRIDEAUX, MATHIAS. *An Easy and Compendious Introduction for Reading All Sorts of Histories.* P3442A. UMI 1938: 1.

For a reference to "diverse passages" in Chaucer's works that are "useful" for students of history, see PRIDEAUX (1648); in this edition, the passage is found on 349.

Another edition in 1664: P3443, 349.

312.   SANDYS, GEORGE, trans. *Ovid's Metamorphosis Englished.* O686. UMI 1768: 3.

For an echo of the title of *The House of Fame*, see SANDYS (1628) in Appendix; in this edition, the passage is found on 232.

313.   SHAKESPEARE, WILLIAM. *Mr. William Shakespeares Comedies, Histories and Tragedies.* S2914. UMI 1469: 15.

For multiple references and allusions to Chaucer and his works, see SHAKE-SPEARE (1623), Boswell & Holton No. 1050.

For an echo of a line from *The Manciple's Prologue* in *Romeo and Juliet*, see SHAKESPEARE (1597) in the Appendix; in this edition the passage is found on 646.

314.   SPELMAN, HENRY. *Glossarium archaiologicum.* S4925. UMI 194: 6.

Spelman (1564?–1641) is identified on the title page as "Henrico Spelmanno equite, Anglo-Britanno." Alderson & Henderson cite seven references to Spelman's citations of Chaucer's usage in the 1626 edition (see "A Collection," 195–96) in definitions of *bombarda, cololbium, defendere, drungus, leudis,* and *lushborow.* Spelman alludes to *The Prologue of The Wife of Bath's Tale, The Knight's Tale,* and *The Monk's Tale.* In this edition, the passages are found on 84, 137, 166, 185, 356–57, 371.

Boswell & Holton (No. 1097) add three others from the 1626 edition: *byrthinsak* (listed under *Bi*), *francling,* and *leta.* In this edition, the passages are found on 82, 246, 355.

In this augmented edition, Spelman (or more likely his editor or publisher) expands his definition of *bombarda,* quotes from *The House of Fame* (lines 1642–48):

Paulò post nostratibus cognitæ meminit Chaucerus, 3. book of *fame,* fol. 282. p. a. col. 2. speaking of *Eolus* Trumpet of evil Fame.

> Through out every Regien
> Went this foule trumpets soun,
> As swyfte as a Pellet out of a gonne
> When fier is in the pouder ronne.

And such a smoke gan out wend
Out of the foule Trompets end,
Black, blo, grenish, suartish, rede,
As doth, where that men melt lede. (84)

Spelman also expands his definition of *mona*, *monath*, cites Chaucer:

Et in *Chauceri* archæismo, fortie Winters old. (416)

Apparently Spelman was quoting from memory; Chaucer writes of forty days, forty nights, forty years, and forty fathoms, and also of twenty winters, thirty winters, a thousand winters, and ten thousand winters, but "fortie Winters old" does not show up in Tatlock & Kennedy's *Concordance*.

In the definition of *runcilus*, Spelman quotes a modernized line from Chaucer's description of the Shipman in *The General Prologue* (line 390):

[In] Anglicè a load horse. *Chaucer*. in Charactere *nautæ*.
He rode upon a Rowncy as he could. (493)

In the definition of *scrippum*, Spelman again cites Chaucer and attributes a line to *The Canterbury Tales* but is actually from the spurious *Ploughman's Prologue*:

In hisce autem sportulis, peris, *scrippis*, Cererem deferebant, & itineri necessaria, de quo *Chaucer* in apparatu coloni sui ad *S. Thomam* Cantuariensem peregrinantis,
In scrippe he bare both bread and leeks.
    Id est,
Thomipeta: in perâ porros cum pane ferebat. (507)

In the definition of *tassa*, there is another citation of Chaucer and a quotation from *The Knight's Tale* (line 1005):

[A] hay-cock, or stack.
Chaucer, in fabula Equites aurati f01.1.c01.4.
To ransake in the taas of bodies dead. (532)

Another edition: S4926 (1686), 82, 84, 137, 166, 185, 246, 355, 356–57, 371, 416, 493, 507, 532.

315.   WALDEN, RICHARD. *Parnassus aboriens: or, Some Sparkes of Poesie.* W290. UMI 1878: 15.

Walden is identified on the title page as "R. W. Philomus." In "To Erycina, Upon Her Retirement to Norwich," he quotes from *Parliament of Fowles* and "The Ten Commandments of Love" (the latter is no longer part of the canon, but was included by Stow in the 1561 edition and subsequent blackletter editions) and refers to Chaucer in two glosses:

> *Madam,*
> Sith 'tis your pleasure to deprive
> Us of that influence by which we live,
> Permit your poor *Devoto* to recount
> To what his infœlicities amount. (15)
> . . . .
> Yet all in vain, my heart doth still resent
> Those fires your absence will, I fear, augment.
> Though I had kept them secret they might then
> Have had the honour to have greater been.
> But cursed *Anteloquia*, whose tongue
> First did your matchless innocence that wrong,
> Was made a third, and cheated by her tears
> My hopes of their increase are turn'd to fears. (16–17)
> . . . .
> And when you enter *Hymen*'s bonds, and so
> Shall have a *Joynture* of a double woe,
> Should he be blind again, I dare assure
> *Pheron* might here obtain a second cure.
> Nor should you fear the *Stork*, nor to try all
> Your issue by the *Psylline Ordeal*. (20)

The poem is highly allusive, and Walden provides copious glosses which show off his learning; two of the glosses feature quotations from the 1603 edition of Chaucer's *Works*. For the passage about Anteloquia, *a third* is glossed: "Make privy to your dealing as few as you may, | For three may keep a counsel if twain be away. *Chauc: fo*: 323" (17) and is found in "The x. Commaundements of Love" in the stanza headed "Secretnesse." In the penultimate line, *Stork* is glossed: "The Storke wreker of Advoutrie *Chauc: fol*: 235" (20) and comes from *The Parliament of Fowles*, line 361.

316.   WALLIS, JOHN. *Grammatica linguæ anglicanæ.* W585. UMI 1878: 29.

For a reference to Chaucer's vocabulary, see WALLIS (1653); in this edition, this passage is found on 34.

317.   WILSON, JOHN. *The Cheats. A Comedy.* W2916. UMI 970: 9.

As Spurgeon notes (1: 240) and Graves repeats (*SP*), Wilson (1626–1696) cites *The Canon's Yeoman's Tale* as the source and inspiration for Erasmus's *Alcumistica* and Jonson's *Alchemist*. In an epistle headed "The Author to the Reader," Wilson defends himself from charges that his plot is not original. He writes:

> [T]*here is nothing which has not been before* . . . [Therefore] *there is hardly any thing left to write upon, but what either the Antients or Moderns have some way or other touch'd on; Did not* Apuleius *take the rise of his* Golden Asse *from* Lucian's Lucius? *and* Erasmus, *his* Alcumistica, *from* Chaucer's Canons Yeomans Tale? *and* Ben. Johnson, *his more happy* Alchymist, *from both*? (sig. A3r)

Other editions: W2917 (1671), sig. A3r; W2918 (1684), sig. A3r; W2919 (1693), sig. A3r; W2920 (1693), sig. A3r.

1665

318.   ATWELL, GEORGE. *The Faithfull Surveyor.* A4165. UMI 2452: 2.

For an echo of *Troilus and Criseyde* 5: 1786, see ATWELL (1658); in this edition, the passage is found in "The Author to his Book" (no pagination, no signature).

319.   BAKER, RICHARD. *A Chronicle of the Kings of England.* B505. UMI 756: 23.

For references to Chaucer as John of Gaunt's brother-in-law, "the Homer of our nation," his association with Woodstock, his translation of *The Romaunt of the Rose*, his burial place in Westminster, and his association with Gower, see BAKER (1643) and Baker (1653); in this edition, the passages are found on 144, 145–46, 168, 180, and sig. Bbbb2r.

Another edition in 1665: B505A, same pagination.

320.   BRATHWAITE, RICHARD. *A Comment upon the Two Tales of Our Ancient, Renpowned, and Ever-Living Poet S*[i]*r Jeffray Chaucer, Knight. Who, for His Rich Fancy, Pregnant Invention, and Present Composure, Deserved the Countenance of a Prince, and His Laureat Honour.* B4260. UMI 16: 1.

As Spurgeon notes (1: 242), this entire work is a running commentary on *The Miller's Tale* and *The Wife of Bath's Tale*. Under the heading "A Commentary upon Chaucer's Prologue to his Millers Tale," Brathwait (1588?–1673) writes:

> Our Famous and ever-living *Chaucer* . . . in his *Knight's Tale* expressed the sweet Comical passages of constant Love. . . . (1)

In commenting on the lines "What should I more say, but this Miller | He nolde his word for no man forbere," Brathwait writes:

> Here our ingenious *Chaucer* displays the Frontless boldness of a Rustick. On he will go with his Tale in spite of all opposition. In the end, our Poet, out of native and free-bred Modesty, as one doubtful, lest some passages might offend the chast of a modest hearer, he directs him to other historical Tales, plenteously stored with singular Precepts of Morality; which, together with his own Apology, he expresseth in these Lines, and so weaves up his Prologue. (6)

In his commentary on the lines "For trusteth well, it is an impossible | That any clerke would speake good of wives | But if it been of holy sainctes lives," Brathwait writes:

> It is not now as it was in *Chaucer*'s daies; Present times have Clarks, who can approve and love this Sex. . . . Now in the very last Verse mentioned by our Poet, this good wife of *Bath* shadows out such jealous Clarks; who, when they suspect their Wives affected to Company, or any way addicted to Liberty, they will pull out some antient Story or other, discoursing of the Lives of Saintly or Holy Women, to reclaim them from their Gadding, and restrain them in their Freedom of living. (131–32)

Following his commentary on the two tales, Brathwait adds "An Appendix" to justify his work. He writes:

> *After such time as the* Autor, *upon the instancy of sundry Persons of Quality, had finish'd his* Comments *upon these* Two Tales; *the Perusal of them begot that Influence over the clear and weighty Judgments of the Strictest and Rigidest Censors; as their high Approvement of them induced their Importunity to the* Author *to go on with the rest, as he had successfully done with these Two first: Ingenuously protesting, that they had not read any Subject discoursing by way of* Illustration, *and running Descant on such* Light, *but* Harmless *Fancies, more handsomly couched, nor modestly shadowed. All which, though urgently press'd, could make no Impression on the* Author: *For his Definite Answer was this:* "That his Age, without any Appellant, might render his Apology; and priviledge him from Commenting on Conceptions (were they never so pregnant) being interveined with Levity, saying;

> > Of such light Toyes Hee'd ta'n a long Adew,
> > Nor did He mean his Knowledge to renew.

Neither could he entertain any such thought of Perfection in these, being begun and finish'd in his Blooming Years; wherein the Heat of Conceipt, more than the Depth of Intellect dictated to his Pen. The Remainder of his Hours henceforth was to number his Daies: *But if Æson's Herb should revive him, and store him with a new Plumage, he was persuaded that his Youthful Genius could not bestow his Endeavour on any* Author *with more Pleasure nor Complacency to Fancy, than the Illustrations of* Chaucer.*"*

Amidst this Discourse, a Critick *stepping in, objected out of the Quickness of his Censure, much like that Phantastical Madam, who drew* Rapsodies *from her* Carpet, *that he could allow well of* Chaucer, *if his* Language *were* Better. *Whereto the* Author *of these Commentaries return'd him this Answer:* "Sir, It appears, you prefer Speech *before the* Head-piece; Language *before* Invention; *whereas Weight of Judgment has ever given* Invention *Priority before* Language. *And not to leave you dissatisfied, As the Time wherein these* Tales *were writ, rendered him incapable of the one; So his Pregnancy of Fancy approv'd him incomparable for the other." Which Answer still'd this Censor, and justified the Author; leaving* New-holme *to attest his Deserts; his* Works *to perpetuate his Honour.* (197–99)

Other editions in 1665: B4260A, 197–99; B4260B, 197–99.

321.   CLEVELAND, JOHN. *Poems.* C4697. UMI 958: 11

For an echo of a line from *The Manciple's Prologue*, see CLEVELAND (1644); in this edition, the passage is found on 183.

322.   LINDSAY, DAVID. *The Works of the Famous and Worthy Knight, Sir David Lindesay of the Mount.* L2315. UMI 1913: 18.

For a reference to Chaucer's skill as a poet in the prologue of *The Testament of Papingo,* see LINDSAY (1538) in Boswell & Holton No. 146; in this edition, the passage is found on sig. H9r.

For a passage that mentions the fable of *Troilus and Criseyde* in an epistle to the king that is set before the prologue to "The Dreme of Sir David Lindsay," see LINDSAY (1558) in Boswell & Holton No. 209; in this edition, the passage is found and appears on sig. K3r.

323.   LLOYD, DAVID. *The States-men and Favourites of England.* L2648. UMI 1781: 16.

Lloyd (1635–1692) is not named on the title page, but he signs an epistle addressed to the reader. In "Observations on the Life of Sir John Jeffrey," Lloyd seems to echo from *The Parliament of Fowls* (lines 22–25). He writes:

It's my Lord *Cook*'s Rule, "That . . . out of the old fields must spring and grow the new Corn." (193)

Also found in *State-worthies: or, The States-men and Favourites of England* (1670), L2646, 225.

324.   MENNES, JOHN. *Recreation for Ingenious Head-peeces; or, A Pleasant Grove for Their Wits to Walk In.* **M1715A. UMI 2356: 6.**

For an epitaph "On our prime English Poet, *Geffrey Chaucer*," see MENNES (1641). The epitaph is originally from Lydgate's prologue to his translation of Boccaccio's *The Falle of Princes*; see BOCCACCIO (1494) in Boswell & Holton No. 27. In this edition, the passage is found on sig. O4r.

For a reference to Chaucer in an epitaph "On William Shake-speare," see *Wits Recreations* (1640) in Boswell & Holton No. 1377; in this edition, the passage is found on sig. O5r.

325.   OGILBY, JOHN, trans. *The Fables of Æsop.* **A693. UMI 754: 23.**

For three references to Chanticleer the cock and one to "Partlet the Hen," perhaps allusions to *The Nun's Priest's Tale*, see OGILBY (1651); in this edition, the passages are found on 1, 103–4, 120.

326.   *Poor Robin. 1665. An Almanack After a New Fashion.* A2186. UMI 1517: 27.

Under the heading "Observations on April," Poor Robin notes that "Patient Gryssell" is to be celebrated on the 24th (sig. A8r); this is perhaps an allusion to the protagonist of *The Clerk's Tale*.

327.   SCARRON, PAUL. *Scarron's Novels.* **S833. No UMI.**

The work at hand is a translation by John Davies of Kidwelly (1625–1693) of a collection of Scarron's novels. In *The Fruitless Precaution*, Don Pedro sends a letter to Elvira. Davies translation appears to echo the description of the shipman in *The General Prologue*: "Of nyce conscience took he no keep" (line 398). He writes:

> *I am naturally a person of a very nice conscience, and therefore cannot without some remorse answer your proposal of marriage, you being a Widow but since yesterday.* (20)

Other editions: S834 (1667), 19; S834A (1682), 19; S834B (1683), 19; S835 (1694), 19; S836 (1700), 24.

Not found in *The Whole Comical Works of Monsr. Scarron* (1700), S829, a different translation.

328. SCOTT, REGINALD. *The Discovery of Witchcraft.* S945A. UMI 578: 3.

For references to Chaucer in a bibliography and for quotations from *The Cannon's Yeoman's Prologue and Tale* and *The Wife of Bath's Tale* and an echo of a line from *The Reeve's Tale*, see SCOTT (1651); in this edition, the passages are found on sig. (b4)v and 49, 202, 203–4, 205.

Another edition in 1665: S945, same pagination.

329. SMITH, JOHN. *The Mysterie of Rhetorique Unveil'd.* S4116B. UMI 876: 12 (identified as S2581).

For a reference to Spenser's imitation of Chaucer, see SMITH (1656); in this edition, the passage is found on 64.

330. *The Wanton Wife of Bath.* M3151. UMI: Tract supplement A5: 2 (C.20.f.8 [487]).

For a reference to Chaucer's writing of a wanton wife of Bath, see *The Wanton Wife of Bath* (1641). This version was printed on the verso of "The Lamentation of John Musgrave."

331. WHARTON, GEORGE. "To my Very Honoured Friend," in Gaultier de Coste, Seigneur de La Calprenède's *Hymen's Præludia: or, Love's Master-Piece. Now Rendred into English, by Robert Loveday.* L122. UMI 2008: 11.

For a reference to Chaucer and Gower as a pair who refined the English language, see WHARTON (1652); in this edition, the passage is found on sig. A4v.

332. WILSON, JOHN. *The Projectors. A Comedy.* W2923. UMI 1110: 19.

Wilson (1626–1696) mentions Chaucer's Friar, alludes to *The Pardoner's Prologue*, lines 350–51. In act 3, Driver says to Sir Gugeon Credulous:

> You know, Sir, we *English* men chiefly buzzle our heads about two things, That is to say, Religion, and Trade; — And truly you have luckily hit upon both, — The one, is a Project for a Divinitie-Mill, that shall go by any winde, and never stand still.
>   *Sir Gu.* But of what use?
>   *Dr.* Marry—To grind Controversie, and that so fine, and subtile, it shall hardly be perceptible, — and I'll undertake, make more Profelites, than ever did *Chaucers Frier* with his shoulder blade of the lost sheep. (37)

1666

333.   DRING, PETER. "Catalogue" in George Alsop's *A Character of the Province of Mary-land*. A2901. UMI 5: 7.

Under the heading "These Books, with others, are Printed for *Peter Dring*, and are to be sold at his Shop, at the sign of the *Sun* in the *Poultrey*, next door to the *Rose Tavern*," Dring lists a book with a Chaucerian connection: "A Comment upon the Two Tales of our Renowned Poet Sir *Jeffray Chaucer*, Knight" (sig. I8r). The reference is to Richard Brathwait's work published in 1665.

334.   DUGDALE, WILLIAM. *Origines juridiciales: or, Historical Memorials of the English Laws*. D2488. UMI 182: 4.

Dugdale (1605–1686) is identified on the title page as "William Dugdale Esq: Norroy King of Arms." As Spurgeon notes (1: 242–43), Dugdale cites *The Parson's Tale* in chapter 50 in a passage about robes worn by Serjeants at Law:

> I am of the opinion, that the form of the Robe, and the colour thereof, which they use at their Creation, is very antient: for in *Chaucer*'s time (which is 3. hundred years since) it is evident, that parti-coloured Garments were much in fashion; and that the people of that age were grown to a great exorbitancy therein; so that, in his *Parson's Tale* he sharply inveighs against the vanity thereof: and amongst other particulars, which he there instanceth, takes notice, that one half of their Hose was *White*, and the other *Red*. (136b, 137a)

In addition to the reference noted by Spurgeon, there is another in a chapter 57, "The Inner Temple." In a passage about the spoilage done by Wat Tyler's rebels, Dugdale cites Chaucer as an authority and quotes (somewhat modernized) from *The General Prologue* (lines 567–86):

> Howbeit, that they [the Knights Hospitalers of St. John of Jerusalem] were here seated in King *Edward* the third's time, is out of all doubt, from what our famous old Poet *Geffrey Chaucer* expresseth in his Prologue to the Manciple, concerning them (he having also been a Student of this House, as the History of his life, printed in the front of his works, sheweth) *viz*.
>
> A Manciple there was of the Temple,
> Of which all Catours might taken ensemple,
> For to been wise in buying of Uitaile:
> For whether he payd, or tooke by taile,
> Algate he wayted so in his ashate,

That he was aye before in good estate,
Now is not that of God a full faire grace,
That such a leude man's wit shall pace
The wisdome of an heape of learned men?
Of Masters had he mo than thrice ten,
That were of Law expert and curious;
Of which there was a dozen in that House,
Worthy to been Stewards of Rent and land
Of any Lord that is in England,
To maken him live by his proper good
In honour debtless, but if he were wood;
Or live as scarcely as him list desire,
And able to helpen all a Shire,
In any Case, that might fallen or hap;
And yet the Manciple sett all her Capp.

But notwithstanding this spoil by the Rebells, those Students so increased here, that, at length they divided themselves in two Bodies. . . . (145)

Other editions: D2489 (1671), 136b, 137a, 145; D2490 (1680), 136b, 137a, 145.

335.   GUILLIM, JOHN. *A Display of Heraldry*. G2221. UMI 1926: 1.

For quotations from *The Romaunt of the Rose*, a reference to Sir Payne Roet who is identified as Chaucer's father-in-law, a description of Chaucer's escutcheon, and a quotation from *The Knight's Tale*, see GUILLIM (1610) in Boswell & Holton No. 816; in this edition, the passages are found on 24, 286, 366, 398. Chaucer's name is also found in the index.

336.   MORGAN, SYLVANUS. *Armilogia: sive, Ars chromocritica. The Language of Arms by the Colours & Metals*. M2738. UMI 745: 25.

Morgan (1620–1693) is identified on the title page as "Sylvanus Morgan arms-painter." In chapter 3, "Of the Matter and Form of Coat Armour, conjunct in the Honourable Ordinaries," Morgan refers to Chaucer's coat of arms:

Many times Coats have more then one *Ordinary*, and are joyned with *Honourable Partitions*, and have very much significancy in them; for if we may believe the Author of the life of *Chaucer*, the Coat of *Jeffery Chaucer* our famous *English* Poet was taken from his skill in Geometry. . . . (82)

337. *Poor Robin. 1666. An Almanack after a New Fashion.* **A2185. UMI 1803: 18.**
Under the heading "Observations on April," we find "Patient Gryssell" cele-
brated on the 8th (sig. A8r); this is perhaps an allusion to the protagonist of *The
Clerk's Tale.*

1667

338. CAVENDISH, GEORGE. *The Life and Death of Thomas Woolsey, Cardinal.*
C1618. UMI 347: 10.
For a reference to Henry VIII's Queen Katherine of Aragon as a "patient Grissell," perhaps an allusion to *The Clerk's Tale,* see CAVENDISH (1641); in this edition, the passage is found on 34–35.

339. DENHAM, JOHN. *On Mr. Abraham Cowley His Death and Burial amongst
the Ancient Poets.* **D1003. UMI 180: 2.**
Denham (1615–1669) is identified on the title page as "the honourable Sir John
Denham." In a panegyric poem for Cowley, Denham places him in company
with Chaucer, Spenser, Shakespeare, Jonson, and Fletcher, and alludes to his
burial in Westminster Abbey:

> Old *Chaucer,* like the Morning Star,
> To us discovers Day from far;
> His light those Mists and Clouds dissolv'd,
> Which our dark Nation long involv'd;
> But he descending to the Shades,
> Darkness again the Age invades.
> Next (like *Aurora*) *Spencer* rose,
> Whose purple blush the day foreshews;
> The other three, with his own fires,
> *Phœbus,* the Poets God, inspires;
> By *Shakespeare, Johnson, Fletcher*'s lines,
> Our Stages lustre *Rome*'s outshines:
> These Poets neer our Princes sleep,
> And in one Grave their Mansion keep. (sig. A1r)

Also found in Denham's *Poems and Translaltions*: D1005 (1668), 89; D1006
(1671), 89–90; D1007 (1684), 89–90.

340.   EVELYN, JOHN. *Publick Employment and an Active Life Prefer'd to Solitude.* E3510. UMI 738: 4.

Evelyn (1620–1706) is identified on the title page as "J. E. Esq: S. R. S." In a passage about the solitary life of students and scholars, Evelyn echoes a line from *The Reeve's Tale*: "The gretteste clerkes been noght wisest men" (line 4054). He writes:

> Publick *Employment* is infinitely superior to it: If needs we will be *Learned* out of *Books* only, let it be in something more useful . . . for 'tis no *Paradox* to affirm, a man may be *learned* and know but *little*, and that the greatest *Clerks*, are not alwaies the wisest men. (89)

Other editions in 1667: E3511, 89; E3512, 89.

341.   FORD, SIMON. *The Conflagration of London Poetically Delineated.* F1479. UMI 493: 4; UMI 915: 5.

As Harris notes (*PQ*), in "The Author to the Graver, Upon occasion of a Draught of London in Flames, designed to have been prefixed as a Frontispiece to the Poem, but forborn upon second thoughts," in a passage about the value of a picture and the lamentable efforts of an engraver to depict properly the events described in his poem, Ford (1619?–1699) refers to Chaucer's "stale" language and alludes to *The Canterbury Tales*:

> If *all* these *miss'd* in thy *Picture* are,
> Not th' *hundreth part* of *Londons Woes* is there.
> *Hold* then: For *old Plays fashion* pleaseth not,
> Wherein, the *Prologue* onely told the *Plot*.
> Yet, (not I think on't) somewhat thou may'st do
> To stead the *Stationer*, and *Poem* too.
> The *Book* is sometimes turn'd for th' *Baby Letter*,
> And *sorry Cuts* help *Ballads* of the better.
> In *Chawcer*, since his *Language* grew so *stale*,
> Each *Picture* speaks more *English*, then its *Tale*.
> And in *Saints Legends* Romanists believe
> The *Cat's* [sic] do *best edification* give. (25)

Another edition: F1495 (1668), revised, no reference to Chaucer.

342. HALL, GEORGE. *The Triumphs of Rome over Despised Protestancie.* H338. UMI 629: 11.

For a reference to Chaucer, an allusion to *The Canterbury Tales*, and a quotation from *The Romaunt of the Rose*, see HALL (1655); in this edition, the passages are found on 30, 134–35.

343. HILTON, JOHN. *Catch That Catch Can: or, The Musical Companion.* H2039. No UMI.

Originally compiled by John Hilton (1599–1657), this edition of rounds and catches for three and four voices was continued by John Playford (1623–1686?). For a reference to Chaucer's jape, see HILTON (1652); in this edition, the passage is found on 65. Bond (*SP* 28) cites this edition.

344. MARVELL, ANDREW. *The Last Instructions to a Painter.* M871A. No UMI.

As Spurgeon notes (4: 75), Marvell (1621–1678) alludes to *The Nun's Priest's Tale* in a passage about the Speaker of Parliament:

> At Table jolly as a Country Host,
> And soaks his Sack with *Norfolk* like a Toast;
> At Night than *Chanticlere* more brisk and hot,
> And Serjeants Wife serves him for *Pertelot*.

Also found in *Poems on Affairs of State from the Time of Oliver Cromwell* (1697), P2719, 81.

345. MENNES, JOHN. *Recreation for Ingenious Head-peeces: or, A Pleasant Grove for Their Wits to Walk In.* M1716. UMI 2913: 5.

For an epitaph "On our prime English Poet, *Geffrey Chaucer*," see MENNES (1641). The epitaph is originally from Lydgate's prologue to his translation of Boccaccio's *The Falle of Princes*; see BOCCACCIO (1494) in Boswell & Holton No. 27. In this edition, the passage is found on sig. O4r.

For a reference to Chaucer in an epitaph "On William Shake-speare," see *Wits Recreations* (1640) in Boswell & Holton No. 1377; in this edition, the passage is found on sig. O5r.

Another edition in 1667: M1717, sigs. O4r, O5r.

346. PEERS, RICHARD. *Poems.* P1057. UMI 1974: 18.

Peers (1645–1690) is identified on the title page as "R. P. student of Ch. Ch. Oxon." In a poem addressed "To the Memory of the Incomparable Mr. Abraham

Cowley, lately Deceased," the poet or the printer notes Cowley's burial place between Chaucer and Spenser in Westminster Abbey. In stanza 13:

> For even they, who (while he liv'd) oppress'd
> His growing Merits and his worth defam'd,
> Confess him now of Modern Wits the best,
> And next Immortal *Spencer* to be nam'd.

"Next Immortal Spencer" is marked for a shoulder note: "Buried between *Chaucer* & *Spencer*" (14).
  Another edition in 1667: *Four Small Copies of Verses*, P1056, same pagination.

347.   *Poor Robin. 1667. An Almanack After a New Fashion.* A2186. UMI 1517: 27.
Under the heading "Observations on April," we find "Patient Gryssell" is celebrated on the 23rd (sig. A8r); this is perhaps an allusion to the protagonist of *The Clerk's Tale.*

348.   **Rookes, Thomas.** *The Late Conflagration.* R1917B. UMI 2317: 13.
The text begins:

> "*The late conflagration consumed my own, together with the Stock of Books (as it were) of the Company of Stationers,* London: *since that lamentable disaster, next my own loss; this doth trouble me, that when any of those few Ingenious Persons who desire books inquire after them, they are often answered by such as have them not, That they are all burnt, which discourageth any further enquiry, not only to the learned, but even of* Country Chapmen, *wherefore to let all men know notwithstanding the late dreadful Calamity, that there are Books yet to be had, And for the conveniencey of the Ingenious Buyers, I publish this ensuring Catalogue.*" (sig. A1r)

In the catalogue, under the heading "BOOKS in Large Folio," the bookseller advertises "Chaucers Works" (sig. A1r).

349.   **S., W.,** in John Bullokar's *An English Expositor: Teaching the Interpretation of the Hardest Words Used in Our Language.* B5431. UMI 1545: 13.
For a reference to Chaucer and *The Prologue to the Squire's Tale* in the definition of Chivancy, see S., W. (1654); in this edition, the passage is found on sig. B12r.
  For a reference to reference to Chaucer and allusion to *The Nun's Priest's Tale*, see S., W. (1663); in this edition, the passage is found on sig. B11r.

350.   SCARRON, PAUL. *Scarron's Novels.* S834. UMI 2058: 3.

For an echo of a line from *The General Prologue*, see SCARRON (1665); in this edition, the passage is found on 19.

351.   SPRAT, THOMAS. *History of the Royal Society of London.* S5032. UMI 477: 2.

Sprat (1635–1713) is identified on the title page as "Tho. Sprat." He mentions Chaucer twice. In a passage about modern writers, he writes of "admirable" Chaucer:

> But now it is time for me to dismiss this subtle generation of Writers: whom I would not have prosecuted so farr, but that they are still esteem'd by some men, the onely Masters of Reason. If they would be content, with any thing less then an Empire in Learning, we would grant them very much. We would permit them to be great, and profound Wits. . . . We would commend them, as we are wont to do *Chaucer*; we would confess, that they are admirable in comparison of the ignorance of their own Age; And, as Sir *Philip Sidney* of him, we would say of them; that it is to be wonder'd, how they could see so cleerly then, and we can see no cleerer now. . . . (21)

As Spurgeon notes (1: 244), Sprat refers to the growth of the English language since Chaucer's day:

> [I]f we observe well the *English Language*; we shall find, that it seems at this time more then others, to require some such aid to bring it to its last perfection. The Truth is, it has been hitherto a little too carelessly handled; and I think, has had less labor spent about its polishing, then it deserves. Till the time of *King Henry* the *Eighth*, there was scarce any man regarded it, but *Chaucer*; and nothing was written in it, which one would be willing to read twice, but some of his *Poetry*. (41–42)

In a passage about the glories of London, Sprat appears to allude to *The House of Fame*:

> [London] is the head of a *mighty Empire*, the greatest that ever commanded the *Ocean*: It is compos'd of *Gentlemen*, as well as *Traders*: It has a large intercourse with the *Earth*: It is, as the *Poets* describe their *House of Fame*, a City, where all the noises and business in the World do meet. . . . (87)

352.   Trench, David. *Catologus [sic] librorum venalium.* T2108B. UMI 2628: 11.

Trench is identified on the title page as "Davidem Trench, bibliopolam Edinbur-gensem." In his catalogue, under the heading "History Books, Poems, Romances, &c.," he lists "Chawcers Tales, 8" (26).

1668

353.   Charleton, Walter. *The Ephesian and Cimmerian Matrons, Two Notable Examples of the Power of Love & Wit.* C3670. UMI 87: 2.

In this edition *The Ephesian Matron* is augmented significantly with quotations from *The Book of the Duchess* and *The Legend of Good Women.* As was conventional in the seventeenth century, the quotations from Chaucer were set in a black let-ter font, so the Chaucerian passages stand out from the remaining text. In the story, an Ephesian woman, recently widowed, determines to join her husband in death, fasts for three days and nights and then conveys herself privily into the vault where her husband's remains were laid out. There she "sits down upon the damp earth, with her eyes fixt upon his Coffin" and contemplates the object of her love and devotion. Charleton (1619–1707) quotes *The Book of the Duchess,* lines 467–82:

> It was great wonder that Nature
> Might suffer any creature.
> To have such sorowe, and she not ded;
> Full piteous pale, and nothing red.
> She said a lay, a maner songe;
> Without note, withouten song;
> And was this, for full wel I can
> Reherse it, right thus it began.
>   I have of sorow so great wone,
> That joy get I never none;
> Nowe that I se my husband bright,
> Whiche I have loved with all my might,
> Is fro me deed, and is agone.
> And thus in sorowe left me alone,
> Alas Dethe, what yeleth the,
> That thou noldest have taken me?

This (you'l [sic] say) was a rare demonstration of a *Woman's constancy,* and ought not to be past over without admiration. (4–5)

As it happened, on that very same day, a notorious malefactor was executed, his corpse exhibited to the populace as an example, and a sentinel set to guard it. The sentry abandoned his post, went into the nearby tomb which was occupied by the grieving widow. Both were astounded to find another living creature there. Charleton again quotes from *The Book of the Duchess* (lines 509–18) slightly modified:

> For her sorowe, and holy thought
> Made her that, she herde him nought.
> For she had welnye lost her mind,
> Though Pan, that men clepeth god of kind,
> Were for her sorowes neuer so wrothe.
>   But at the last, so fain right sothe,
> She was ware of him, how he stood,
> Before her, and did of his hood,
> And had ygret her, ans best he coude,
> Debonairely, and nothing loude.
>   As Reverend Chaucer in his Dream. (sig. B2v)

The two young people looked at one another and almost instantly fell in love. The tale continues with a quotation from the "Legend of Dido" from *The Legend of Good Women* (lines 1232–39), again slightly modified to meet the situation:

> For the Souldier hath ikneled so
> And told her all his loue, and all his wo,
> And sworn so depe to her to be true,
> For well or wo, and change for so newe;
> And as a false Louer so well can plain,
> The selie Matron rewed on his pain;
> And toke him for husbond, and became his wife
> For euermore, while that him last life. (sig. D4r-v)

As the story continues, kinsmen of the slain malefactor steal the body, and the soldier, having been derelict in his duty, and facing certain death for his failure, blames womankind for his wretchedness, is about to fall upon his sword in utter despair when the pious matron flings herself into his arms to prevent his suicide. She rebuts his imprecations against women and concludes that they will substitute her dear husband's corpse for that of the criminal, and all will be well. In a section headed "Of Platonick Love," Charleton refers to Chaucer and quotes from "Praise of Women," a work no longer in the canon but was included in Thynne (1532) and subsequent blackletter editions:

> Here I cannot but cry out with Father, *Chaucer*, in his Ballad of the *praise of Women*.

𝔏o what gentillesse these women habe,
𝔍f we could knowe it for our rudeness.
𝔥ow busie thei be us to keepe and sabe
𝔅oth in heale, and also in sickness,
𝔄nd alwaie right sorie for our distress.
𝔍n ebery maner thus shewe thei routh,
𝔗hat in hem is all goodness and trouth.

    𝔉or all creatures that eber were get and born,
𝔗his wote ye well, a woman was the best.
𝔅y her was recobered the bliss that we had lorne:
𝔄nd through the woman we shall come to rest,
𝔄nd been isabed, if that our self lest.
𝔚herefore methinketh, if that we had grace,
𝔚e oughten honour women in ebery place. (78–79)

In an unsigned epistle addressed "To the Author of the Ephesian Matron,"
Charleton's friend refers twice to Chaucer and *The Wife of Bath's Prologue*, quotes
modernized lines 333–34, 321–22:

> My dearest Friend, . . . *When you were pleas'd last Summer, to send me your*
> Ephesian Matron, *with strict Command, that I should . . . mew her up in*
> *my Cabinet, from sight of the whole world . . . you would have had the Lady*
> *my Tenent at your will. . . . In a word, your Injunction to me, to retrain her*
> *from the conversation of all others, was not only tyrannical and inhumane in*
> *it self (for, as our great Moralist, and beloved Author,* Chaucer, *in the Wife*
> *of* Bath's *Prologue.*

>   𝔥e is to great a 𝔑iggarde, that will werne
>   𝔄 man, to light at candle at his 𝔏aterne;

> *But also inconsistent with both the goodness of her nature, and the freedome*
> *of my enjoying the pleasures thereof. . . . Besides, as the same Wife of* Bathe
> *speaks in the name of her whole sex,*

>   𝔚e lobe no man, that taketh keepe or charge
>   𝔚here that we go; we woll be at our large. (sig. F7r–8r)

He ends his epistle with an allusion to the Squire's *Prologue* and *Tale*:

>   𝔥ere endeth the 𝔖quiers 𝔓rologue,
>   and here after followeth his 𝔗ale. (sig. H2r)

In "The Cimmerian Matron," Charleton refers to Chaucer and January and May, quotes a baker's dozen lines from the *Merchant's Tale*, lines 2264–76.

> I cannot at any time reflect, without acknowledging the goodness of *Proserpine*, in keeping her promise made to the Lady *May* in *Chaucer*; which was that, in her answer to *Pluto*, who would fain restore to *January*, her Husband, his sight, that he might see his Esquire, *Damian*, making him *Cuckold* in a Pear-tree.

> You shall (quoth Proserpine) and well ye so?
> Now by my Mothers Soul, Sir, I swere,
> That I shall yeven her sufficient answere,
> And all women after for her sake;
> That though they ben in any gilte itake,
> With face bolde, they shullen hemselve excuse,
> And here hem doun, that wold hem accuse.
> For lack of answere, non of hem shull dien,
> All had he sey a thing with both his eyen:
> Yet should we women so bisage it hardely,
> And wepe, and swere, and chide subtelly;
> That men shall ben as leude as Gees.
> What recketh me of your auctoritees, &c. (30–31; sig. K1v–2r)

In "The Mysteries and Miracles of Love," Charleton refers to Chaucer and quotes from *Troilus and Criseyde* 1: 302–8:

> We will . . . conclude this Paragraph with a pertinent Stanza of that incomparable Critique in Love, old *Chaucer*: who in most lively and never-vading [*sic*] colours painting the surprize and astonishmen [*sic*] of *Troilus*, (till then a Woman-hater) at first sight of the fair *Creseide*, in her mourning habit, sparkling like a Diamond set in Jet; saith thus

> Lo, he that lete him selven so conning,
> And scorned hem that loves paines drien,
> Was full unware that love had his dwelling
> Within the subtel streams of her eyen;
> That sodainly him thought he felt dien,
> Right with her loke, the spirit in his herte.
> Blessed be love, that thus can folke converte. (68; sig. M4v)

Charleton concludes "The Mysteries and Miracles of Love" with another reference to Chaucer and a conflated quotation from *Troilus and Criseyde* (5: 1772–85), *The Legend of Good Women* (910–11, 920–21), and *The Shipman's Tale* (1623–24):

Let us, therefore, now . . . reserving what remains untouched of our Argument for another divertisement; and in the mean time, with our dearly beloved *Don Geffrey,*

> 𝔅eseeching every 𝔏ady bright of hewe,
> 𝔄nd every gentil woman, what she be,
> 𝔄lbeit that our 𝔐atrons were untrue,
> 𝔗hat for that gilte ye be not wroth with me.
> 𝔜e may in other 𝔅okes their gilte se.
> 𝔄nd gladder 𝔍 would write, if that ye leste,
> 𝔓enelopes truth, and faith of good 𝔄lceste.
>
> 𝔑e saie 𝔍 nat this all only for these men,
> 𝔅ut most for women that betraied be
> 𝔗hrough fals folke 𝔊od yeve hem sorowe,
> 𝔗hat with great witte and subtiltie (men)
> 𝔅etraien you; and this meveth me
> 𝔗o speke, and in effect you all 𝔍 praie,
> 𝔅ethe ware of men, and herkeneth what 𝔍 say.
>   𝔅ut 𝔊od forbid, but a woman
>   𝔅en as true and loving as a man.
>   𝔍for it is deintie to us men to finde.
>   𝔄 man, that can in love be trewe and kind.
> 𝔗hus endeth now my tale, and 𝔊od us sende
> 𝔊aling enough unto our lives ende. (76–77; sigs. M8v–N1r)

The passages quoted are not found in *The Ephesian Matron*, C3671 (1659), or *Matrona Ephesia*, C3683 (1665).

Other editions with different titles: *The Cimmerian Matron, to Which Is Added the Mysteries and Miracles of Love. By P. M. Gent.*, C3667 (1668), leaf 1v–2r [n.p.; n.s.], sigs. B2r (2nd signature B; pagination is garbled), D1v–2r, M4v, M8v–N1r; and *The Cimmerian Matron, a Pleasant Novel*, C3667a (1684), leaf 1v–2r [n.p.; n.s.], sig. B2r (2nd sig. B), D1v–2r, M4v, M8v–N1r.

354.   COWLEY, ABRAHAM. *The Works of Mr. Abraham Cowley.* **C6649. UMI 61: 7.**

For a reference to Chaucer's "rich rhymes," see COWLEY (1656), C6683; in this edition, the passage is found on 437 (sig. Aa1r).

For a reference to Cowley's burial place near Chaucer, see SPRAT (1668).

Other editions: C6650 (1669), 37 (sig. Aa2r); C6651 (1672), 37 (sig. Aa2r); C6652 (1674), 37 (sig. Aa2r); C6653 (1678), 37 (sig. Aa2r); C6654 (1680), 37 (sig. Aa2r); C6655 (1681), 37 (sig. Aa2r); C6656 (1681), 37 (sig. Aa2r); C6656A (1684), 37 (sig. Aa2r); C6656B (1684), no UMI; C6657 (1684), 37 (sig. Aa2r);

C6658 (1688), 37 (sig. Aa2r); C6659 (1693), 37 (sig. Aa2r); C6660 (1700), 96 (sig. Q4v).

355.   DENHAM, JOHN. *Poems and Translations.* **D1005. UMI 378: 12; UMI 1945: 6.**

For a reference to Chaucer in a cluster of other literary luminaries in a poem headed "On Mr Abraham Cowley, his Death and Burial amongst the Ancient Poets," see DENHAM (1667); in this edition, the passage is found on 89. Spurgeon (1: 244) cites this edition rather than the poem's first publication.

Other editions: D1006 (1671), 89–90; D1007 (1684), 89–90.

356.   FISHER, PAYNE. *The Catalogue of Most of the Memorable Tombes.* **F1014. UMI 1402: 17.**

Fisher (1616–1693) is described on the title page as "sometimes Serjant Major of Foot." In his catalogue of tombs, gravestones, plates, and escutcheons in London churches, extant and demolished, before the great fire, he notes a tomb with a Chaucerian connection. Fisher writes:

> *Richard Chaucer*, Vinter, father to Sir Geoffry Chaucer. (19)

357.   FORD, THOMAS. Αυτοκατακριτος [Autokatakritos]: *or, The Sinner Condemned of Himself.* **F1511. UMI 2208: 4**

Ford (1598–1674) is described on the title page as "One, that wisheth better to All, than most do to themselves." In this polemic against suicide, he appears to echo a line from *The Reeve's Tale*: "The gretteste clerkes been noght wisest men" (line 4054). Ford writes:

> Christ may be learn'd by the veriest Ideots, if they have but a willing mind, as soon, and as easily, as by the greatest Masters of Arts and Sciences. And in this case we may say, what hath been commonly said in a different sense, *That the greatest Clerks are not always the wisest men.* (230)

358.   LLOYD, DAVID. *Memoires of the Lives, Actions, Sufferings & Deaths of Those Noble, Reverend and Excellent Personages that Suffered by Death, Sequestration, Decimation, or Otherwise, for the Protestant Religion.* **L2642. UMI 190: 1.**

Lloyd (1635–1692) is described on the title page as "Da: Lloyd, A. M. sometime of Oriel-Colledge in Oxon." In his biography of Henry Hammond, Lloyd quotes Dr. John Fell who appears to echo a line from *The Reeve's Tale*: "The gretteste clerkes been noght wisest men" (line 4054). See Fell (1662); in the work at hand, the passage appears on 390.

Another edition: L2643 (1677), 390.

359. NEWCASTLE, WILLIAM CAVENDISH. "On Her Book of Poems," in Margaret Cavendish's *Poems and Phancies*. N871. UMI 612: 1.

For a reference to Chaucer in a commendatory poem, see NEWCASTLE (1664); in this edition, the passage is found on sig. A2r–v.

360. OGILBY, JOHN, trans. *The Fables of Æsop Paraphras'd in Verse*. A697. UMI 679: 12.

For three references to Chanticleer the cock and one to "Partlet the Hen," perhaps allusions to *The Nun's Priest's Tale*, see OGILBY (1651); in this edition, the passages are found on 1, 103–4, 120.

361. *Poor Robin. 1668. An Almanack after a New Fashion*. A2187. UMI 1803: 19.

Under the heading "Observations on March," "Chaucers miller" is celebrated on the 27th (sig. A7r).

Under the heading "Observations on April," "Patient Gryssell" is celebrated on the 24th (sig. A8r); this is perhaps an allusion to the protagonist of *The Clerk's Tale*.

362. PRYNNE, WILLIAM, ed. Jan Hus's *A Seasonable Vindication of the Supreme Authority and Jurisdiction of Christian Kings, Lords, Parliaments*. H3803. UMI 1642: 8 (identified as P4070a).

For a reference to Chaucer's contribution to the Protestant cause through the spurious *Ploughman's Tale*, see PRYNNE (1660); in this edition, the passage is found on 41–43.

363. SPARROW, ANTHONY. *A Rationale upon the Book of Common Prayer of the Church of England*. S4831. UMI 514: 14.

Sparrow (1612–1685), is identified on the title page as "Anth. Sparrow, D. D. Now Lord Bishop of Exon." At the conclusion of this expansion of an early work (first published in 1656), following the index, in a section headed "To your Liturgical Demands I make as good Return to you as I am able, on this wise," Sparrow comments on "Ember Weeks." He turns to Chaucer as an authority on language and cites him as a likely source of the word in English. The word *ember*, however, does not appear in the Tatlock & Kennedy's *Concordance*. Sparrow writes:

> The reason of the name is very uncertain. . . . As Lent, a Fast of weeks, so these, a Fast of daies. I believe it a Saxon word. Surely I have read it in *Gower* or *Chaucer*, our old Poets. Some think it betokens Fasting. . . . But look better into it. (sig. T10v)

Other editions: S4832 (1672), sig. R9r; S4833 (1676), sig. S3r; S4834A (1684), sig. S3r; S4834 (1684), sig. S3r.

364. SPRAT, THOMAS. "An Account" in *The Works of Mr. Abraham Cowley*. C6649. UMI 61: 7.

In "An Account of the Life of Mr. Abraham Cowley," Thomas Sprat notes that Cowley was buried near Chaucer:

> His Body was attended to *Westminster Abby*, by a great number of Persons of the most eminent quality, and follow'd with the praises of all good, and Learned Men. It lies near the Ashes of *Chaucer* and *Spencer*, the two most Famous *English* Poets, of former times. (sig. e2r–v)

Other editions: C6650 (1669), sig. c4r–v; C6651 (1672), sig. c4r–v; C6652 (1674), sig. c4r–v; C6653 (1678), sig. c4r–v; C6654 (1680), sig. c4r–v; C6655 (1681), sig. c4r–v; C6656 (1681), sig. B8r–v; C6656A (1684), sig. c4r–v; C6656B (1684); C6657 (1684), sig. c4r–v; C6658 (1688), sig. c4r–v; C6659 (1693), sig. d2r; C6660 (1700), sig. b5v.

365. WALLER, EDMUND. *Poems, &c. The Third Edition with Several Additions Never before Printed*. W515. UMI 882: 6.

Waller (1606–1687) is identified on the title page as "Edmond Waller, Esq:" As Spurgeon notes (1: 244), he comments on the difficulty of Chaucer's language for modern readers in a poem not found in earlier collections of Waller's works. In "Of English Verse," Waller writes:

> Poets may boast [as safely vain]
> Their work shall with the world remain
> Both bound together, live, or dye,
> The Verses and the Prophecy
> . . . .
>   Poets that lasting Marble seek
> Must carve in *Latine* or in *Greek*,
> We write in Sand, our Language grows,
> And like the Tide our work o're flows.
>   *Chaucer* his Sense can only boast,
> The glory of his numbers lost,
> Years have defac'd his matchless strain,
> And yet he did not sing in vain,
>   The Beauties which adorn'd that age
> The shining Subjects of his rage,
> Hoping they should immortal prove

> Rewarded with success his love,
>> This was the generous Poets scope
> And all an *English* Pen can hope
> To make the fair approve his Flame
> That can so far extend their Fame . . . (234–35)

Other editions: W516 (1682), 234–35; W517 (1686), 236–38; W518 (1693), 236–38; W519 (1694), 236–38; and W520 (1696), a bibliographical ghost.

366. WHARTON, GEORGE. "To my Very Honoured Friend," in Gaultier de Coste, Seigneur de La Calprenède's *Hymen's Præludia: or, Love's Master-Piece. Now Rendred into English, by Robert Loveday*. L122A. UMI 1529: 6.

For a reference to Chaucer and Gower as a pair who refined the English language, see WHARTON (1652); in this edition, the passage is found on sig. A4v.

367. WINSTANLEY, WILLIAM. *The New Help to Discourse: or, Wit, Mirth, and Jollity, Intermixt with More Serious Matters*. W3068. No UMI. Copy at BL (unique).

The transcription here is from the 1680 edition. In a discussion about the factors that make a city great, Winstanley (1628?–1698) cites Chaucer and quotes modified lines from *The General Prologue* (lines 16–17):

> The last, but not the least, is opinion of Sanctity, as was evidenced in former times by the City of *Canterbury*, to which Pilgrims from all places come to visit the Tomb of *Thomas Becket* Archbishop of *Canterbury*, who was there enshrined, as witnesseth *Chaucer*.

> 𝔉ro all England ꝺo they ꟃenꝺ
> 𝕿he 𝕳oly blissful 𝔐artyrs 𝕿omb to see. &c.

In a section about martyred Archbishop Thomas Becket, Winstanley (1628?–1698) mentions Chaucer and again quotes slightly garbled lines from *The General Prologue* (lines 15–18):

> Many miracles are said to be by him performed. . . . His Tomb was afterwards much enriched with costly gifts, and visited by Pilgrims from all places, according to what we find in *Chaucer*,

> *Fro every shires end*
> *Of England do they wend,*
> *The Holly blissful Martyrs Tomb to seek,*
> *Who hath them holpen wherein they be seke.*

Other editions: W3069 (1672), 19, 212; W3070 (1680), 15–16, 165; W3071 (1684), 19, 202; W3071A (1696), first reference deleted, 160.

1669

368.   CLEVELAND, JOHN. *Poems*. C4698. UMI 1353: 4.

For an echo of a line from *The Manciple's Prologue*, see CLEVELAND (1644); in this edition, the passage is found on 183.

369.   COWLEY, ABRAHAM. *The Works of Mr. Abraham Cowley*. C6650. UMI 684: 5.

For a reference to Cowley's burial place near Chaucer, see SPRAT (1668); in this edition, the passage is found on sig. c4r–v.

For a reference to Chaucer's "rich rhymes," see COWLEY (1656); in this edition, the passage is found on 37 (sig. Aa1r).

370.   FLAVEL, JOHN. *Husbandry Spiritualized: or, The Heavenly Use of Earthly Things*. F1165. UMI 492: 21.

Flavel (1630?–1691) is identified on the title page as "John Flavell minister of the gospel in Devon." In the second part, under the running head "Occasional Meditations," in a section headed "Meditations upon a Garden," the second meditation is titled "Upon the pulling up of a Leek." Here Flavel appears to echo lines from *The Reeve's Prologue*, "To have a hoor head and a green tayl, | As hath a leek" (lines 3878–79). He writes:

> A White head, and a green tail! how well doth this resemble an old wanton Lover! whose green youthful lusts are not extinguished, though his white head declares that nature is almost so. (259)

Other editions: F1165A (1671), 259; F1166 (1674), 259; F1167 (1678), 259; F1167A (1693), 317; F1168 (1700), 330–31.

371.   LOVEDAY, ROBERT. *Loveday's Letters Domestick and Forrein*. L3228. UMI 1915: 12.

For a reference to Chaucer as a prophet and poet, perhaps an allusion to the spurious work known as "Chaucer's Prophecy," see LOVEDAY (1659); in this edition, the passage is found on 98–99.

Another edition in 1669: L3228A, same pagination.

372.   PHILLIPS, EDWARD. *Tractatulus de carmine dramatico poëtrum veterum* in Johann Buchler's *Sacrarum prosanarumque phrasium poeticarum thesarurus.* B5303. UMI 2509: 5.

Spurgeon notes (1: 254), citing the 1679 edition, that Edward Phillips's work was printed with Buchler's and has its own title page. Phillips (1630–1696?), refers to Chaucer and places him in context (with Petrarch, Gower, Hoccleve, Churchyard, and Lydgate) under the heading "Poëtæ recentiores Angli & Scoti":

> Sub Henrico quarto, quinto & sexto floruit Galfridus Chaucerus Eques auratus, præclarissimus Anglorum Poetarum tam sui quam superiorum temporum, & quasi Petrarcha huius nationis, qui pene languentes scientias præcipue poeticam reflorere fecit: Non pauca sunt eius opera quæ extant, sed permulta desiderantur & eorum quæ extant quædam sunt manca & imperfecta, alia adhuc non typis commissa. Circiter idem tempus eminuerunt Gourius Eques Aratus, Oclevius, & Churchardus, ex quorum operibus præsertim Gourii, quædam superesse accepi, sed tanquam obsoleta una cum Chauceri operibus hac novorum studiosa ætate penitus neglecta. . . . Joannes Lydgatus Buryensis Monasterii Monachus Benedictinus proximus post Chaucerum æstimatus. . . . (395)

Other editions: B5304 (1670), 395; B5305 (1679), 395.

373.   *Poor Robin 1669. An Almanack after a New Fashion.* A2188. UMI 1494: 19.

Under the heading "Observations on April," we find "Patient Gryssell" is celebrated on the 26th of the month (sig. A8r); this is perhaps an allusion to the protagonist of *The Clerk's Tale.*

374.   SANDYS, GEORGE, trans. *Ovid's Metamorphosis Englished.* O687. UMI 1490: 12.

For an echo of the title of *The House of Fame*, see SANDYS (1628) in Appendix; in this edition, the passage is found on 232.

375.   SKINNER, STEPHEN. *An Etymologicon of the English Tongue: or, The Derivations of English Words.* S3946A. UMI 2856: 17.

Skinner (1623–1667) is identified on the title page as a "Steven Skinner of Lincoln, Doctor of Physic." In this prospectus for his dictionary, he advises would-be buyers that his work will include "the Derivations of all old Obsolete words, such as *Gower's, Chaucer's, Pierce Ploughman's,* and the like, that came up since the Conquest, and are now grown out of use" (title page).

376.   STONE, NICHOLAS. *Enchiridion of Fortification: or, A Handful of Knowledge in Martial Affaires.* S5733. UMI 2414: 2.

For a commendatory poem that faintly echoes Chaucer's line, "Go, litel bok, go litel myn tragedye" (*Troilus and Criseyde* 5: 1786), see STONE (1645); in this edition, the passage is found on sig. A3r.

377.   WEBB, JOHN. *An Historical Essay Endeavoring a Probability That the Language of the Empire of China Is the Primitive Language.* W1202. UMI 1243: 23.

Webb (1611–1672) observes the difficulty of Chaucer's language for contemporaries:

> [W]e our selves can scarcely now understand the Language that was used in the days of *Chaucer*. And yet nevertheless we know, that the *Latine* Tongue, hath from *Cæsars* time, maugre all conquests and intercourse whatsoever, received not the least alteration, but remaineth both in the Characters and reading the same. . . (39–40)

Reissued as *The Antiquity of China*, W1201 (1678), same pagination.

378.   WINSTANLEY, WILLIAM, compiler. *Poor Robin's Jests: or, The Compleat Jester. The Second Part.* W3075d. UMI 2142: 25.

After recounting an amusing anecdote about Ben Jonson, Winstanley (1628?–1698) comments on Jonson's memorial stone in Westminster Abbey, laments his placement far from Chaucer's tomb:

> I shall be here so serious as not to take any further notice of this Jest; but rather of a short inscription to Mr *Jonsons* memory, written on a little stone in one of the Long-walks of *Westminster* Abbey, the words are these
>
> O Rare Ben Jonson
>
> The Gentleman who was at this small cost (as he might be some poor Cavalier) is altogether unknown to me, perhaps his purse strings could not stretch further, or else he might do it out of an Ironie to the Court, that did not afford him a statelier Monument: I shall only make bold to affix these few lines
>
> > *What though our Nation could afford no room*
> > *Neer Chaucer, Spencer, Draiton for thy Tomb;*
> > *What's here ordain'd is for thy honour more*
> > *Than Pyres erect, or Marbles gilded ore;*
> > *Where when our Epitaphs cannot express*

> *Thy worth in writing more, we must write less*
> (63, really 65; sig. F1r)

Although the titles are quite similar, this work is not the same as *Poor Robin's Jests: or, The Compleat Jester*, W3075c (1668?), in which the passage is not to be found.

1670

379.   BAKER, RICHARD. *A Chronicle of the Kings of England*. B506. UMI 1323: 26.

For references to Chaucer as John of Gaunt's brother-in-law, "the Homer of our nation," his association with Woodstock, his translation of *The Romaunt of the Rose*, his burial place in Westminster, and his association with Gower, see BAKER (1643) and (1653); in this edition, the passages are found on 136, 138, 159, 171, and sig. Iiiii1r.

380.   BAKER, RICHARD. *Theatrum triumphans*. B514. UMI 198: 23.

Rather than the first edition, Spurgeon (1: 247) cites this one. For a reference to the "scurrility" of the Wife of Bath, see BAKER (1662); in this edition, the passage is found on 33–34. For an echo of a line from *The Reeve's Tale*, see BAKER (1662); in this edition, the passage is on 98.

381.   BLOUNT, THOMAS. *The Academy of Eloquence*. B3325. UMI 1544L 1.

For an echo of the title of *The House of Fame*, see BLOUNT (1654); in this edition, the passage is found on 29.

382.   BLOUNT, THOMAS. *Glossographia: or, A Dictionary*. B3336. UMI 784: 1.

For a reference to "old Chaucer," a quotation from *Troilus and Cryssede*, and references to Chaucer as an authority on the English language and word usage, see BLOUNT (1656) and (1661); in this revised and augmented edition, passages are found in the epistle (A4v), and in definitions of *agroted* (B8r), *algebra* (C1r), *alnath* (C2v), *barbicane* (F64), *benison* (F8v), *boon* (sig. G4v), *bordel* (G4v), *callot* (H1v), *covent* (M1r), *creance* (M2r), *dissheviled / disheviled* (O2r), *dulcarnon* (O8r), *frythe* (S6v), *gossymeare* (T5v), *lectern* (Aa4v), *lodemanage* (Bb1r), *losender* (Bb2v), *meriot* (Cc6v), *moiles* (Dd2v), *mortress* (Dd5v), *ouch* (Ff7r), *paraments* (Gg4r), *pilgrim* (Hh8v), *rebeck* (Ll6v), *romance* (Mm7v), *superstition* (Qq6v–7r), *tailage* (Rr5r).

In addition to the changes noted in the 1661 edition, there are other revisions in this edition: Blount alters the definition of *amortize* so there is no reference to Chaucer; he expands the definition of *taberd* to mention Chaucer by name and attributes a spurious quotation to him; and he adds two new words with definitions that include references to Chaucer:

𝔇𝔴𝔦𝔫𝔡𝔩𝔢 . . . to consume, to waste, to vanish, to moulder away by degrees. *Chaucer* used 𝔇𝔴𝔦𝔫𝔢𝔡, the Participle. (sig. O8r)
[*The Romaunt of the Rose*, line 360.]

𝔎𝔞𝔭 𝔞𝔫𝔡 𝔯𝔢𝔫, is a usual saying, even among the Vulgar, as to get all one can *rap* and *ren*: *Rap* comes from *rapio* to snatch: and *ren* from the Saxon *Ran*, i. rapine, or, *ren*, according to *Chaucer*, signified to *pull*. (sig. L15v)
[Chaucer uses the expression Arape and renne" in *The Canon's Yeoman's Tale*, line 1422.]

𝔗𝔞𝔟𝔢𝔯𝔡 or 𝔗𝔞𝔟𝔞𝔯𝔡 (Fr. *Taberre*) a Jacket, Jerkin, Mandilion, or sleeveless coat; a *chymere*. *Verstegan* says, it was antiently a short Gown that reach'd no further than the mid-leg; *Stow* in his Survey, 456. Says, 'twas a jacket or sleeveless Coat, whole before, open on both sides, with a square collar winged at the shoulders, of which thus *Chaucer*,
> He took his Tabard and his staff eke, &c.
It is now the name of an Heralds Coat, and is called their Coat of Arms in Service. It is also the sign of an Antient Inn in *Southwark*. (sig. Rr4r)
[Chaucer uses the term three times in *The General Prologue* (lines 20, 541, 719).]

383.   BLOUNT, THOMAS. Νομο-λεξικον [nomo-lexikon]: *A Law-Dictionary.*
B3340. UMI 168: 9.

Blount (1618–1679) is identified on the title page as "Thomas Blount of the Inner Temple, Esq." As Alderson & Henderson note, Blount cites Chaucer at least ten times as an authority on the English language and word usage.

𝔄𝔯𝔯𝔢𝔱𝔱𝔢𝔡 . . . That is convented before a Judge, and charged with a crime. . . . *Chaucer* useth the Verb 𝔄𝔯𝔯𝔢𝔱𝔱𝔢𝔱𝔥, *i*. Layeth blame, as it is interpreted. (sig. F1r)
[Blount alludes to *The Parson's Tale*, lines 580–85.]

𝔆𝔥𝔲𝔯𝔠𝔥-𝔎𝔢𝔟𝔢. A Church-Warden . . . of whom, thus *Chaucer*, speaking of the Jurisdiction of Archdeacons.
> 𝔒𝔣 𝔆𝔥𝔲𝔯𝔠𝔥-𝔎𝔢𝔟𝔢𝔰, 𝔞𝔫𝔡 𝔬𝔣 𝔗𝔢𝔰𝔱𝔞𝔪𝔢𝔫𝔱𝔰,
> 𝔒𝔣 𝔆𝔬𝔫𝔱𝔯𝔞𝔠𝔱𝔰, 𝔞𝔫𝔡 𝔩𝔞𝔠𝔨 𝔬𝔣 𝔖𝔞𝔠𝔯𝔞𝔪𝔢𝔫𝔱𝔰, &c. (sig. P2r)
[Chaucer uses *chirch-reeves* in *The Friar's Tale*, line 1305.]

𝔆𝔬𝔲𝔫𝔱𝔬𝔯𝔰 . . . Have been taken for such Serjeants at Law . . . of whom thus *Chaucer*,
> —𝔄 𝔖𝔥𝔢𝔯𝔦𝔣𝔣 𝔥𝔞𝔡 𝔥𝔢 𝔟𝔢𝔢𝔫, 𝔞𝔫𝔡 𝔞 𝔆𝔬𝔫𝔱𝔬𝔲𝔯,
> 𝔚𝔞𝔰 𝔫𝔬 𝔴𝔥𝔢𝔯𝔢 𝔰𝔲𝔠𝔥 𝔞 𝔴𝔬𝔯𝔱𝔥𝔶 𝔙𝔞𝔟𝔞𝔰𝔬𝔲𝔯. (sig. V2v)
[Blount cites *The General Prologue*, lines 359–60.]

𝕯𝖊𝖋𝖊𝖓𝖉 . . . Signifies, in our ancient Laws and Statutes, to prohibit or forbid. . . . Of which, thus *Chaucer.*

𝖂𝖍𝖊𝖗𝖊 𝖈𝖆𝖓 𝖞𝖔𝖚 𝖘𝖆𝖞 𝖎𝖓 𝖆𝖓𝖞 𝖒𝖆𝖓𝖓𝖊𝖗 𝖆𝖌𝖊,

𝕿𝖍𝖆𝖙 𝖊𝖛𝖊𝖗 𝕲𝖔𝖉 defended 𝕸𝖆𝖗𝖗𝖎𝖆𝖌𝖊. (sig. Y2v)

[Blount cites *The Wife of Bath's Prologue*, lines 59–60.]

𝕱𝖔𝖙𝖍𝖊𝖗 or 𝕱𝖔𝖉𝖉𝖊𝖗 (Sax.) Is a Weight (of Lead) containing Eight *Pigs*, and every *Pig* One and twenty Stone and a half, which is about a Tun, or a common Wain or Cart Load. *Speight in his Annotations upon Chaucer.* (sig. Hh1v)

[Chaucer uses *fother* twice: in *The General Prologue* (line 530) and *The Knight's Tale* (line 1908).]

𝕱𝖗𝖞𝖙𝖍. a Plain between two Woods, a Lawnd. *Chaucer* uses it for a Wood. (sig. Hh3v) [*Frith* is not found in Tatlock & Kennedy.]

𝕸𝖆𝖓𝖈𝖎𝖕𝖑𝖊 . . . An Officer anciently so called in the Inner-Temple . . . and still in Colledges, of whom *Jeoffrey Chaucer*, our ancient Poet, and a Student in this House, thus

𝕬 𝕸𝖆𝖓𝖈𝖎𝖕𝖑𝖊 𝖙𝖍𝖊𝖗𝖊 𝖜𝖆𝖘 𝖎𝖓 𝖙𝖍𝖊 𝕿𝖊𝖒𝖕𝖑𝖊,

𝕺𝖋 𝖜𝖍𝖎𝖈𝖍 𝖆𝖑𝖑 𝕮𝖆𝖙𝖔𝖚𝖗𝖘 𝖒𝖎𝖌𝖍𝖙 𝖙𝖆𝖐𝖊𝖓 𝖊𝖓𝖘𝖊𝖒𝖕𝖑𝖊. (sig. Tt2v)

[Blount cites *The General Prologue*, lines 567–68.]

𝕻𝖊𝖗𝖛𝖎𝖘𝖊, or 𝕻𝖆𝖗𝖛𝖎𝖘𝖊. . . . of which thus *Chaucer. Prolog. 9.*

𝕬 𝕾𝖊𝖗𝖏𝖊𝖆𝖓𝖙 𝖆𝖙 𝕷𝖆𝖜, 𝖜𝖆𝖗𝖊 𝖆𝖓𝖉 𝖜𝖎𝖘𝖊,

𝕿𝖍𝖆𝖙 𝖔𝖋𝖙𝖊𝖓 𝖍𝖆𝖉 𝖇𝖊𝖊𝖓 𝖆𝖙 𝖙𝖍𝖊 𝕻𝖆𝖗𝖛𝖎𝖘𝖊. (sig. Ccc2r)

[Blount cites *The General Prologue*, lines 309–10.]

𝕽𝖚𝖓𝖈𝖎𝖚𝖘 (from the Ital. *Runzio*) Is used in *Domesday* for a Load-horse, or Sumpter-horse; and sometimes a Cart-horse, which *Chaucer* calls a 𝕽𝖔𝖜𝖓𝖊𝖞. (sig. L112v)

[Chaucer uses *rouncy* in *The General Prologue*, line 390.]

𝖂𝖆𝖓𝖌 . . . the Cheek or Jaw, wherein the Teeth are set. Hence with *Chaucer* we call the Cheek-Teeth or Grinders Wang and Wang-teeth, which is also notified in that old way of sealing writings.

𝕬𝖓𝖉 𝖎𝖓 𝖜𝖎𝖙𝖓𝖊𝖘𝖘 𝖙𝖍𝖆𝖙 𝖙𝖍𝖎𝖘 𝖎𝖘 𝖙𝖍𝖆𝖙 𝖙𝖍𝖎𝖘 𝖎𝖘 𝖘𝖔𝖔𝖙𝖍,

𝕴 𝖇𝖎𝖙𝖊 𝖙𝖍𝖊 𝖂𝖆𝖝 𝖜𝖎𝖙𝖍 𝖒𝖞 𝖂𝖆𝖓𝖌 𝖙𝖔𝖔𝖙𝖍. (sig. Xxx1v)

[Chaucer uses *wang-tooth* in *The Monk's Tale*, line 3234; however, the quotation is not from Chaucer.]

Another edition: B3341A (1691), sigs. F2r, Q2r, X2v, Z2v, Kk1r, L11v, Zz1v, Hhh1r, Rrr1r, Eeee2r (and others).

384.   CLARKE, JOHN. *Phraseologia puerilis.The Fourth Edition.* C4474A.

For an echo of a line from *The Manciple's Prologue,* see CLARKE (1638) in the Appendix; in this radically revised and augmented edition, the passage is found on 100 under the heading "to Doubt."

385.   EVELYN, JOHN. *Sylva: or, A Discourse of Forest-trees. The Second Edition Much Inlarged and Improved.* E3517. UMI 665: 8.

For a reference to Chaucer's Oak, one of several trees said to have been planted by Chaucer, see EVELYN (1664); in this edition, the passage is found on 153–54. Chaucer is also cited in the index, sig. f1r.

386.   LE FÈRE, RAOUL. *The Destruction of Troy.* L930. UMI 604: 13; book 3 (as L939), UMI 1387: 29.

For two references to *Troilus and Criseyde,* see LE FÈVRE (1475) in Boswell & Holton No. 1; in this edition, the first reference to Chaucer's renaming Breseyda is omitted, but the second passage commending *Troilus and Criseyde* to readers is found in book 3, chapter 15, on 367.

387.   LEIGH, EDWARD. *Select and Choice Observations.* L1005. UMI 1126: 12.

For an echo of a line from *The Merchant's Tale,* see Leigh (1647); in this edition, the passage is found on 424.

388.   LINDSAY, DAVID. *The Works of the Famous and Worthy Knight, Sir David Lindesay of the Mount.* L2316. UMI 1574: 1.

For a reference to Chaucer's skill as a poet in the prologue of *The Testament of Papingo,* see Lindsay (1538) in Boswell & Holton No. 146; in this edition, the passage is found on sig. G10v.

For a passage that mentions the fable of *Troilus and Criseyde* in an epistle to the king that is set before the prologue to "The Dreme of Sir David Lindsay," see Lindsay (1558) in Boswell & Holton No. 209; in this edition, the passage is found and appears on sig. I3r.

389.   LLOYD, DAVID. *State-worthies: or, The States-men and Favourites of England.* L2646. UMI 964: 16.

For an echo of *The Parliament of Fowls* (lines 22–25), see Lloyd (1665); in this edition, the passage is found on 225.

390.   PATRICK, SIMON. *A Further Continuation and Defence: or, A Third Part of the Friendly Debate.* P805. UMI 726: 5.

Patrick (1626–1707), a prolific writer of devotional works, sermons, exegetical works, and polemics, rose through the ranks of the Church of England to become the Bishop of Chichester and Ely. The work at hand is an invective-filled screed against nonconformists. In a dialogue between "C." (a conformist) and "N. C." (a nonconformist or dissenter), the Conformist refers to Chaucer's Cook, but he actually alludes to Chaucer's description of the Serjeant of the Law in *The General Prologue*. Patrick writes:

> He may thank himself, who, like *Chaucer's* Cook, would needs be busie where ne needed not, taking much pains for which neither side will think themselves beholden to him. (51)

391.   PENN, WILLIAM. *The Great Case of Liberty of Conscience Once More Briefly Debated & Defended.* P1299. UMI 433: 7.

Penn (1644–1718) is identified on the title page as "W. P." As Dobbins notes (*MLN*), Penn cites Chaucer as a source for chapter six in the table of contents (8). And in the sixth chapter, "A Brief Collection of the Sence and Practice of the Greattest, Wisest, and Learnedst Common-Wealths, Kingdoms, and particular Persons of their Times, concerning Force upon Conscience," Penn writes:

> And here let me bring in honest *Chaucer*, whose Matter (and not his Poetry) heartely [*sic*] affects me: 'twas in a time when *Priests* were as rich, and lofty, as they are now, and Causes of Evil alike.

> *The time was once, and may return again,*
>   *(For oft may happen that hath been beforn)*
> *when Shepherds had none Inheritance,*
>   *ne of Land, nor Fee insufferance,*
> *But what might arise of the bare Sheep,*
>   *(were it more or less) which they did keep,*
> *Well ywis was it with Shepherds tho:*
>   *nought having, nought fear'd they to forgo,*
> *For P A N (God) himself was their Inheritance,*
>   *and little them serv'd for their Maintenance,*
> *The Shepherds God so well them guided,*
>   *that of nought were they unprovided;*
> *[. . . . . 15 lines . . . .]*
> *This was the first source of the Shepherds sorrow.*
>   *that nor will be quit, with bale, nor borrow.* (39–40)

The passage is marked with a shoulder note: "The primative State of things observed by a Poet, more then 300. year old; by which the Clergy may *read* their own Apostacy and Character" (39).

Another edition in 1670: P1298B (printed in Dublin), 26–27 (no shoulder note).

392.   PHILLIPS, EDWARD. *Tractatulus de carmine dramatico poëtrum veterum* in Johann Buchler's *Sacrarum prosanarumque phrasium poeticarum thesarurus.* B5304. No UMI.

For references to Chaucer who throve in the time of Petrarch, Gower, Hoccleve, Churchyard, and Lydgate, see Phillips (1669); in this edition, the passage is found on 395.

393.   *Poor Robin 1670. An Almanack After a New Fashion.* A2189. UMI 1434: 13.

Under the heading "Observations on April," we find "Patient Gryssell" is celebrated on the 28th of this month (sig. A8r); this is perhaps an allusion to the protagonist of *The Clerk's Tale.*

394.   PRESTON, RICHARD GRAHAM. *Angliae speculum morale.* P3310. UMI 507: 3.

Viscount Preston (1648–1695) is not named on the title page. As Harris notes (*PQ*), in a section headed "The Poet," Preston praises Chaucer and links him with Spenser:

> *England* hath produced those, who . . . have equall'd most of the Antients: and exceeded all the Moderns. *Chaucer* rose like the morning Starr of Wit, out of those black mists of ignorance; since him, *Spencer* may deservedly challenge the Crown. (67)

Another edition with different title, *The Moral State of England*: P3313 (1694), UMI 2213: 20, 67.

395.   RAY, JOHN. *A Collection of English Proverbs.* R386. UMI 398: 11.

Ray (1627–1705) is identified on the title page as "J. R., M. A. and Fellow of the Royal Society."

Under the heading "Proverbial Sentences," Ray includes a proverb that echoes a line from *The Wife of Bath's Prologue*: "A likerous mouth most han a likerous tayl" (line 466); he writes "A liquorish tongue a lecherous tail" (16).

In a section headed "Proverbs that are entire Sentences," Ray appears to echo a line from *The Reeve's Tale*: "The gretteste clerkes been noght wisest men" (line 4054). He writes:

> The greatest *clerks*, are not always the wisest men.
> For prudence is gained more by practise and conversation, then by study and contemplation. (71)

Under the heading "Proverbial Similies," in number 13 Ray appears to echo a line from *The Manciple's Prologue*: "Sires, what! Dun is in the myre!" (line 5). He writes: "As dull as dun in the mire" (202).

As Harris notes (*PQ*), Ray calls Chaucer "our English Ennius," and paraphrases a couplet from *The Prologue to The Cook's Tale* ("And many a Jakke of Dovere hastow soold | That hath been twies hoot and twies coold" [lines 4347–48]) in a section devoted to proverbs and sayings associated with Kent. For "A jack of Dover," Ray writes:

> I find the first mention of this Proverb in our *English Ennius, Chaucer* in his Poeme to the Cook.
>
> > *And many a* jack of Dover *he had sold,*
> > *Which had been two times hot, and two times cold.*
>
> This he makes parallel to *Crambe bis cocla*, and appliable to such as grate the eares of their Auditours with ungrateful tautologies, of what is worthless in it self, tolerable as once uttered in the notion of novelty, but abominable if repeated. (234)

Another edition: R387 (1678), 114, 169, 280, 315 (and another, 353).

396.   TALBOT, PETER. *A Treatise of Religion and Governmemt* [*sic*] *with Reflexions upon the Cause and Cure of Englands Late Distempers and Present Dangers.* **T118. UMI 1840: 1.**

Talbot (1620–1680) is not named on the title page. In a passage pleading for liberty of conscience in England for "Presbyterians and Fanaticks," the author appears to echo a line from *The Reeve's Tale*: "The gretteste clerkes been noght wisest men" (line 4054). In the preface he writes:

> I hope it will not be ill taken that I beg the same freedom and favor for Roman Catholicks, especially if I prove . . . that our principles are not only more sound in point of Christianity, but more safe in order to the government, then any others. And thoughn it be a common and true saying, that the greatest Clerks are not the wisest men, and by consequence, not so fit to prescribe rules for governing as as wordling that are not Divines. . . . (sig. &2r)

397. WOLVERIDGE, JAMES. *Speculum matricis Hybernicum; or, The Irish Mid-wives Handmaid.* W3319. UMI 161: 4.

Wolveridge (d. 1671) is identified on the title page as "James Wolveridge, M.D." In a valedictory poem, "The Author to His Book," Wolveridge echoes Chaucer's line, "Go, litel bok, go litel myn tragedye" (*Troilus and Criseyde* 5: 1786):

> Go little Book, I envy not thy hap,
> Mayst thou be dandled in the Ladies lap;
> I hope the Ladies will not thee disdain,
> Th'art clean, though in a home-spun dress, and plain:. . . . (sig. a4r)

Another edition with different title, *Speculum matricis; or, The Expert Midwives* (1671), 3319A, sig. a4r.

1671

398. CULPEPER, THOMAS. *Essayes or Moral Discourses and Essayes on Several Subjects.* E3301B. UMI 1001: 17 (identified as C7556).

Sir Thomas Culpeper (1626–1697) is not named on the title page. As Spurgeon notes (1: 247–48), he mentions Chaucer in an essay headed "Of Wit and Language." Culpeper writes:

> Every age hath generally a certain mode and manner of expression and wrighting, different, as we see tis now with us. . . . Nor do I believe it otherwise then a vulgar error to judge that the language we now speak and write, is more refined, then what they used, because we conceive it to be polished and enlarged by introducing some few French words, not considering, how many of the old, (perhaps of better signification as to our speech) are forgotten or wanted in their stead: I would willingly be resolved, if *caress, trepan, harange,* and the like had been written by *Chaucer,* whether they had not appeared as harsh and barbarous to us now, as any of the most obsolet used by him; so that it is an affectation of the present times, which gives a valew to words, rather then their apt-ness or weight. (109–10)

In another essay headed "Of Writing," Culpeper notes disapprovingly Spenser's use of Chaucerisms:

> Next to the writing of good matter, a gratious and eloquent Stile is to be endeavoured, it being the Glass, in which is to be discerned the Writ-ers thoughts; he that Pens obscurely, is hardly worth the study of his

Reader, who perhaps may want a Dictionary for his words: some have thought to honour Antiquity by using such as were obsolete, as hath been done by our famous *Spencer*, and others, though the times past are no more respected by an unnecessary continuing of their words then if wee wore constantly the same trimming to our Cloaths as they did, for it is not Speech, but things which render antiquity venerable, besides the danger of expressing no Language, if as *Spencer* made use of *Chaucers*, we should likewise introduce his. . . . (117–18)

399.   DENHAM, JOHN. *Poems and Translations*. D1006. UMI 1809: 22.

For praise of Chaucer in a poem headed "On Mr Abraham Cowley, his Death and Burial amongst the Ancient Poets," see Denham (1668); in this edition, the passage is found 89–90.

400.   DU BOSC, JACQUES. *The Accomplish'd Woman*. D2407AB. UMI 2482: 12.

For a reference to Chaucer's language being outdated, see Du Bosc (1655); in this edition, the passage is found on 117.

401.   DUGDALE, WILLIAM. *Origines juridiciales: or, Historical Memorials of the English Laws*. D2489. UMI 688: 21.

For a reference to *The Parson's Tale* and a quotation about the Manciple from *The General Prologue of The Canterbury Tales*, see Dugdale (1666); in this edition, the passage is found on 136b, 137a, 145.

402.   FLAVEL, JOHN. *Husbandry Spiritualized: or, The Heavenly Use of Earthly Things*. F1165A. UMI 2687: 35

For an echo of a line from *The Reeve's Prologue*, see Flavel (1669); in this edition, the passage is found on 259.

403.   HEAD, RICHARD, and FRANCIS KIRKMAN. *The English Rogue. The Third Part*. H1249A. UMI 102: 9.

The preface of this continuation of the life of Meriton Latroon and other extravagants is signed by "Fra. Kirkman" (1632–ca. 1680). As Atkinson notes (*MLN* 1944) Head (1637?–1686?) and/or Kirkman refer to generic "Canterbury Tales." In chapter 10, Mrs. Dorothy, the hostess of a country inn, tells of two old country men who came to her inn on a chilly morning and called for wine. The drawer brought it, and they then directed him to "rost it, that is put it to the fire and burn it." The serving man placed the wine pot before the fire to warm and went about his duties:

[T]he old men being busie in discourse forgot to look to it, when on a sudden they look'd, and the pot was melted almost half way down. . . . [T]he maid seeing it call'd out to them, what honest men do you melt your pot? Not we, said they . . . but you are like to pay for it, replyed the wench . . . at this mine Host came up, the maid tells how that these two old men had been telling their *Canterbury* tales so long that the pot was melted. . . . (134–35)

Other editions: H1250 (1674), 119; H1252 (1688), same title, different text.

404.   LLOYD, DAVID. *The Legend of Captain Jones*. L2633. UMI 1096: 12.

For a reference to Chaucer and *The Tale of Sir Thopas*, see Lloyd L2635 (1648); in this edition, the passage is found on 27.
    Another edition in 1671: L2634, 27.

405.   NEWCASTLE, MARGARET CAVENDISH. *Natures Pictures Drawn by Fancies Pencil to the Life*. N856. UMI 611: 10.

For an allusion to *The House of Fame*, see Newcastle (1656); in this edition the passage is found on 275, 278–79.

406.   PARKER, SAMUEL. *A Defence and Continuation of the Ecclesiastical Politie by Way of a Letter to a Friend in London*. P457. UMI 923: 14.

Parker (1640–1688) is not named on the title page. In his "Preface to the Reader," he appears to echo a line from *The Reeve's Tale*: "The gretteste clerkes been noght wisest men" (line 4054). Parker writes:

[M]*y Friends can never thank me enough for putting them to the penance of reading five or six hundred Pages, to no other purpose then to inform themselves that one* J. O. *is none of the greatest clerks, or the wisest men.* (sig. A3r)

407.   PHILLIPS, EDWARD. *The New World of Words: or, A General English Dictionary*. P2071. UMI 472: 10.

For a pictorial representation of Chaucer and for references to him in the dedicatory epistle and the preface, see Phillips (1658), (1662), (1663); in this edition, these are found on sigs. (a)3v and (b)4v. Chaucer is also mentioned in definitions of *Advenale* (sig. A4v), *Amalgaminge* (sig. C1r), *Amortize* (sig. C1v), *Appeteth* (sig. D1v), *Apprentice* (Chaucer reference not present in this edition), *Arblaster* (sig. D2r), *Argoil* (sig. D2v), *Arretteth* (sig. D3r), *Arten* (sig. D3v), *Assise* (sig. D4v), *Assoyle* (sig. D4v), *Asterlagour* (sig. D4v), *Autremite* (sig. E2v), *Barm-cloth* (sig. E4r), *Baudon* (sig. F1r), *Bay* (sig. F1r), *Beau Sir* (sig. F1v), *Bend* (sig. F2r), *Burnet* (sig. G3r), *Caitisned* (sig. G4r), *Canceline* (sig. H1v), Chasteleyn (sig. I3r), *Chekelaton* (sig. I3v), *Chelandri* (sig. I3v), *Chertes* (sig. I3v), *Chevesal* (sig. I3v), *Chimbe* (sig. I4r), *Chincherie* (sig. I4r), *Cierges* (sig. K1r), Citriale (sig. K1v), *Clergion* (sig. K2r), *Clicket*, (sig. K2r), *Clinke* (sig. K2v), *Curebulli* (sig. N1r), *Dennington* (sig. O1r), *Desidery* (sig. O1r), *Deslavy* (sig. O1r), *Digne* (sig. O3r), *Discure* (sig. O4r), *Divine* (sig. P2r), *Dowtremere* (sig. P3r), *Ebrack* (sig. Q1r), *Gibsere* (sig. V1v), *Giglet* (sig. V1v), *Gourd* (sig. V3r), *Haketon* (sig. X1v), *Hanselines* (sig. X2r), *Jewise* (sig. Z2v), *Losenger* (sig. Ee3r), *Magonel* (sig. Ff1v), *Rebeck* (sig. Pp2v), *Woodstock* (sig. Aaa1r).

408.   *Poor Robin 1671. An Almanack after a New Fashion.* A2190. UMI 1494: 20.

Under the heading "Observations on April," we find "Patient Gryssell" is celebrated on 25th of this month (sig. A8r); this is perhaps an allusion to the protagonist of *The Clerk's Tale*.

409.   S., W., in John Bullokar's *An English Expositor: Teaching the Interpretation of the Hardest Words Used in Our Language.* B5431A. UMI 2145: 2.

For a reference to Chaucer and *The Prologue to the Squire's Tale* in the definition of Chivancy, see S., W. (1654); in this edition, the passage is found on sig. B12r.

For a reference to reference to Chaucer and allusion to *The Nun's Priest's Tale*, see S., W. (1663); in this edition, the passage is found on sig. B11r.

410.   Skinner, Stephen. *Etymologicon linguæ anglicanæ.* S3947. UMI 779: 11.

Skinner (1623–1667) is identified on the title page as "Stephano Skinner, M.D." As Spurgeon notes (1: 243), Skinner refers to Chaucer throughout his work, but she transcribes one reference only from his "Præfatio" (sig. B3r). Of more than passing interest is a reference under the heading "Etymologicon Onomasticon" in which Skinner traces the etymology of Chaucer's name and calls him our English Homer:

> Chaucer, nostræ linguæ *Homerus* Poeseos Anglicanæ vel Parens, vel Instaurator, credo à Fr. G. *Chausseur*, olim *Chauceur*. . . . (sig. Mmmm2v)

411.   *Westminster-Drollery: or, A Choice Collection of the Newest Songs & Poems Both at Court and Theaters by a Person of Quality; With Additions.* W1457. UMI 371: 10.

In a song headed "The subtil and coy Girl," the author echoes a line from *The Manciple's Prologue*: "Sires, what! Dun is in the myre!" (line 5). In the second verse he writes:

> Is it because I have been so kind
> At all times to feed thy desire
> In Presents and Treatrs, thou hast chang'd thy mind
> And left me like Dun in the Mire? (34)

As Bond notes (*SP* 28, citing this, rather than the first edition), in "A Catch of
3 Parts" there is a reference to "a Jest as Chaucer meant" (48). See Hilton (1652).

Other editions in 1671: *Westminster-Drollery. With Additions*, W1458, 34,
"Catch" not included; *Westminster-Drollery: or, A Choice Collection*, W1459, 36,
"Catch," not included.

Other editions: *Westminster-Drollery: or, A Choice Collection*, W1460 (1672),
34, "Catch," nor included; *Westminster-Drollery: or, A Choice Collection*, W1462
(1672), "Catch," not included; *Westminster-Drollery, the Second Part*, W1463
(1672), "Catch," 48, "Subtil and Coy Girl" not included; *Westminster-Drollery: or,
A Choice Collection*, W1461 (1674), 27, "Catch," not included.

412.   WILSON, JOHN. *The Cheats. A Comedy.* **W2917. UMI 1452: 30.**

For a reference to *The Canon's Yeoman's Tale* as the source and inspiration for
Erasmus's *Alcumistica* and Jonson's *Alchemist*, see Wilson (1664); in this edition,
the passage is found on sig. A3r.

413.   WOLVERIDGE, JAMES. *Speculum matricis Hybernicum; or, The Irish Mid-
wives Handmaid.* **W3319A. UMI 2468: 23.**

For an echo of *Troilus and Criseyde* 5: 1786, see Wolveridge (1670); in this edition,
the passage is found on sig. a4r.

1672

414.   ASHMOLE, ELIAS. *The Institutions, Laws & Ceremonies of the Most Noble
Order of the Garter.* **A3983. UMI 341: 9.**

In chapter 1, section 5, "The Etymologie of Eques, Miles, Chevalier, Ritter and
Sir," Ashmole (1617–1692) links Lydgate and Chaucer:

> It is also noted, that the word used to denote the Degree of *Knighthood*
> . . . hath the same derivation, to wit, from a *Horse*; . . . concerning some
> of which hear also one of *Geoffry Chaucer*'s Scholars [in a shoulder note:
> "*Jo. Lydgate MS. of the Horse, Sheep, and Goos.*"]
>
>   Eques, *ab* Equo, is said of fiery rytht,
> And Chevalier, is said of Chebalrie,
> In which a Rider *called is a* Knight. . . . (17)

In chapter 26, "Of the Founder, the First Knights-Companions, and their Suc-
cessors," section 2, "A short view of the Founder's Wars," Ashmole mentions
Chaucer's role as a diplomat in the reign of Edward III:

[T]he Legate proposed a Marriage between *Richard* Prince of *Wales*, and the Lady *Mary* Daughter of the *French* King; which begot a private meeting shortly after at *Montrevile* by the Sea, and there Sir *Richard Dangle*, Sir *Richard Stan*, and Sir *Geoffry Chaucer*, Commissioners for King *Edward*. . . . (668)

Another edition: A3984 (1693), 17, 668.

415.　Chaucer's Ghoast, or, A Piece of Antiquity Containing Twelve Pleasant Fables of Ovid Penn'd after the Ancient Manner of Writing in England. O647. UMI 1509: 24.

The author of this work is identified on the title page as "a lover of antiquity." Spurgeon notes (1: 248) that there is no reference to Chaucer in this work other than the one in the title; indeed, she writes, "It is not the ghost of Chaucer, but of Gower, which is here revived." There is, however, a reference in a commendatory poem headed "The Authours Friend to the Readers upon his perusal of the Work":

> L*o here Antiquity, what think you Sirs,*
> *To see a Poem drest in Boots and Spur;*
> *A short Cloak, and long Breeches, in the fashion*
> *Of those that liv'd before us in this nation.*
> *'Tis pretty (faith) and pleasant for to see*
> *How we with Antiquity disagree.*
> *And to that purpose here my loving friend*
> *His Conjuring-glass into the World doth lend;*
> *Where both his worth appearing we may finde,*
> *And* Chaucer's *Ghoast, or else we all are blinde.* (123)

416.　CORBET, RCHARD. *Poems. Third edition*. C6271. UMI 377: 17.

For a reference to Chaucer's having written *The Romaunt of the Rose* near Bosworth Field, see Corbet (1647); in this edition, the passage is found on 18.

417.　COWELL, JOHN. Νομοθετης [Nomothet's]: *The Interpreter, Containing the Genuine Signification of Such Obscure Words and Terms Used Either in the Common or Statute Lawes of this Realm*. C6645. UMI 684: 18. [A&H]

This lexicon, originally compiled by John Cowell (1554–1611), this edition was revised and augmented by Thomas Manley (1628–1690) who is identified on the title page as "Tho. Manley of the Middle-Temple, Esq:" As the title page advertises this edition contains "many words omited by all former writers, and pertinent to this matter, with their etymologies as often as they occur."

As Alderson & Henderson note, Manley writes in the Preface that he "gleaned after" Blount's *Law Dictionary* of 1670, q.v. for Chaucerian references appearing under *Church-reve, Counters, Defend, Manciple, Pervise, Runcius, Wang,* see Blount (1670).

Another edition: C6646 (1684).

418.   Cowley, Abraham. *The Works of Mr. Abraham Cowley.* **C6651. UMI 812: 1.**

For a reference to Cowley's burial place near Chaucer, see Sprat (1668); in this edition, the passage is found on sig. c4r–v.

For a reference to Chaucer's "rich rhymes," see Cowley (1656), C6683; in this edition, the passage is found on 37 (sig. Aa1r).

419.   Garencieres, Theophilus de. Epistle in *The True Prophecies or Prognostications of Michael Nostradamus.* **N1399. UMI 468: 14.**

Garencieres (1610–1680) is identified on the title page as "Theophilus de Garencieres, doctor in Phisick Colleg. Lond." And the work at hand is his translation of *Prophéties* by Nostradamus. As Harris notes (*PQ*), in an epistle addressed "To the Courteous Reader," Garencieres compares the difficulty of the language of Nostradamus to that of Chaucer:

> *Reader,*
> Before thou goest on further in the perusing of this Work, thou art humbly intreated by the Authour, to forgive him his Anglicisme . . . . The very Antient *English* Language in this refined Age, is become both obsolete and unintelligible, as we may see in *Chaucer, Gower,* and others.
> no pagination, no signature

Another edition: N1400 (1685), same pagination.

420.   Lacy, John. *The Dumb Lady: or, The Farriar Made Physician.* **L143. UMI 280: 12.**

Lacy (d. 1681) is identified on the title page as "John Lacy, gent." He lifted various parts of this work from Molière's *Le médecin malagré lui* and *L'amour médecin.*

As Pierce notes (*N&Q*), near the end of the second act, a physician, having been asked to be the go-between for a pair of lovers and thinking he has been asked to play the pimp, paraphrases a couplet from *The Cook's Tale* (lines 4421–42):

> I begin to find that physick is but one part of a Doctors trade, and I shall gain the Character of *Chaucers* Semstriss; for says he,

> *She keeps a shop for countenance;*
> *But baudeth for her sustenance.* (28)

421. LINDSAY, DAVID. *The Works of the Famous and Worthy Knight, Sir David Lindsay of the Mount.* L2317. UMI 2173: 15.

For a reference to Chaucer's skill as a poet in the prologue of *The Testament of Papingo*, see Lindsay (1538) in Boswell & Holton No. 146; in this edition, the passage is found on sig. G3r.

For a passage that mentions the fable of *Troilus and Criseyde* in an epistle to the king that is set before the prologue to "The Dreme of Sir David Lindsay," see Lindsay (1558) in Boswell & Holton No. 209; in this edition, the passage is found and appears on sig. H6r.

422. MARVELL, ANDREW. *The Rehearsal Transposed.* M878. UMI 1036: 20. [A&H]

Marvell (1621–1678) is not named on the title page. As Alderson and Henderson note, in an Eighteenth Century edition of Marvell's collected works, there is a reference to "Chaucer's word" and "Limitour" which is an allusion to the description of the Friar in *The General Prologue*. There is, however, no such passage in the 1672 edition.

Another impression in 1672: M879, UMI 283: 6.

423. *Poor Robin 1672 An Almanack After a New Fashion.* A2191. UMI 1494: 21.

Under the heading "Observations on April," we find "Patient Grizel" is celebrated on the 28th of this month (sig. A8r); this is perhaps an allusion to the protagonist of *The Clerk's Tale*.

424. PRIDEAUX, MATHIAS. *An Easy and Compendious Introduction for Reading All Sorts of Histories.* P3444. UMI 1429: 1.

For a reference to "diverse passages" in Chaucer's works that are "useful" for students of history, see Prideaux, P3439 (1648); in this edition, the passage is found on 349.

425. RAMESEY (or RAMSAY), WILLIAM. *The Gentlemans Companion.* R206. UMI 367: 5.

Ramesey (1627–1675 / '76) is characterized on the title page as "a person of quality." As Spurgeon notes (1: 246 and 3: 4.76), Ramesey commends Chaucer's books as fit for a gentleman's study. In division 4, "Exercises within Doors," Ramesey writes:

A few good Books is better than a Library, and a main part of Learning. I shall here contract his [the Gentleman's] Study into these few Books Following; in which he may indeed reade all that is requisite, and of Substance. (127)

Homer, Horace, Virgil, Ovid, Buchanan the *Scot*, not inferiour to any Poet. And among our selves, old Sr. *Jeffery Chaucer, Ben. Johnson, Shakespear, Spencer, Beaumont* and *Fletcher, Dryden*, and what other Playes from time to time you find best Penn'd; And for a Diversion, you may read *Hudebras* [*sic*], and *Don Quixot*. . . . (129)

Another edition: R207 (1676), 132.

426.   S., R. *Ludus ludi literarii: or, School-boys Exercises and Divertisements.* **S134. UMI 2041: 3.**

The preface of the work at hand is signed "R. S." In this collection of recitations for schoolboys, "Some of them *Latine*, but most *English*; Spoken (and prepared to be spoken) in a *Private School* about *London*" (title page), in the thirty-ninth oration, "Upon a Glut of Doctors in Druina," the speaker attributes an "old Prophesie" to Chaucer:

[S]urely there are more *Doctors* than *Diseases* (there being some for every Disease, and some good for none) I know no better remedy than this, that there might be a *whisking Aniversary Pole*, set upon all unlearned persons, who go under that name. Thus we see an old Prophesie of *Chawcers* fulfilled, *The time is coming when Doctors and Knights will be a brief as Woodcocks and Snipes.* (110)

427.   SALMON, THOMAS. *A Vindication of an Essay to the Advancement of Musick from Mr. Matthew Lock's Observations.* **S419. UMI 226: 4.**

Salmon is identified on the title page as "Thomas Salmon, M. A. of Trin. Col. Oxon." In a passage about "translating a Greek Alstedius," he appears to echo lines from *The Reeve's Prologue*, "To have a hoor head and a green tayl, | As hath a leek" (lines 3878–79). Salmon writes:

I must confess not to understand, no more than our *Observer* . . . And then for that stinking story that savours of some old *Onion-like* Fornicator, with his *gray-head* and *green-tail*, I dismiss it as altogether unanswerable. (76)

428.   SAUL, ARTHUR. *The Famous Game of Chesse-Play.* S730. UMI 1468: 15.

For an echo of Chaucer's line, "Go, litel bok, go litel myn tragedye" (*Troilus and Criseyde* 5: 1786) in Saul's commendatory poem "To his Booke," see Saul (1614); in this edition, the passage is found on sig. A5v–6r.

429.   SELDEN, JOHN. *Titles of Honor. Third Edition Carefully Corrected. With Additions and Amendments by the Author.* S2240. UMI 579: 6.

For references to the Franklin, the Squire in *The General Prologue*, see Selden (1614), Boswell & Holton No. 890; in this edition, the passage is found on 519.

In this augmented edition, some references in the 1614 edition have been replaced with different ones and others have been added. In a section about the Order of Saint George, Selden quotes *The General Prologue* 52–53, 79–88 and *The Merchant's Tale* 1772–73:

For the Round Table was in special use in those ages for the drawing together of the braver Knights and Ladies. And in the Excellencies of his Knight, *Chaucer* thus mentions it.

Full oftentime he had the Bourd begon
Above all Nations—

And according to *Froissart* also . . . . (658)

The Saint of this Order was and is Saint *George* the great Martyr . . . . And the Order it self is stiled oftimes the Order of Saint *George*, as well as of the Garter. Whence *Chaucer* also thus writes to the Knights of the Order. [Here Selden attributes lines to Chaucer that are not found in Tatlock & Kennedy's *Concordance.*]

—for Gods pleasaunce
And his mother, and significaunce
Tyhat ye been of Saint Georges libere,
Doeth him serbice and Knightly obeisance
For Christes cause is his well known ye. (659)

In a section about the honorific *esquire*:

We may justly remember here amongst these occurring testimonies of the Title of Esquire, that of *Chaucer* in his Character of one. After the description of his Knight (whom as the rest he describes with such particulars as best design the nature of him) he says that

𝔚ith him there was his sonne a yong 𝔖quire
𝔄 lover and a lustie 𝔅achilere,
𝔚ith his locks crull as they were laid in presse
𝔒f twenty yeare of age he was as 𝔍 guesse.
𝔄nd he had be sometime in 𝔠hivauchie
𝔍n Flaunders, in Artois, in Picardie,
𝔄nd born him well, as of so little space,
𝔍n hope to stand in his 𝔏adies grace.
𝔠urteis he was, lowly, and serviceable;
𝔄nd kerft before his 𝔉ather at the table.

Here both his practice of Arms and his attendance on his Father being
a Knight are noted. His attendance being as that of those . . . *shield-
bearers*, or Esquires that waited on the old *Gaules* at their round Tables,
whereof *Possidonius* speaks in *Athenæus*. And for the necessary attendance of an Esquire upon every Knight in the elder ages long before
Chaucer; observe this . . . . *Chaucer* also in his Merchant's tale;

𝔄ll but a 𝔖quire that hight Damian
𝔚hich carft before the 𝔎night many a day.
𝔗he like is elsewhere also in him. (689–90)

Other editions in 1672: S2440A, same pagination; S2440B, same pagination.

430.   SHAKESPEARE, WILLIAM. *The Bouncing Knight* in *The Wits: or, Sport
upon Sport*. W3219. UMI 2539: 6.

For a reference to "Dame Partlet the hen," an allusion to *The Nun's Priest's Tale*,
see Shakespeare (1662) and Shakespeare (1598), Boswell & Holton No. 613; in
this edition, the passage is found on 9.

431.   SPARROW, ANTHONY. *A Rationale upon the Book of Common Prayer of the
Church of England*. S4832. UMI 476: 7.

For a reference to Chaucer as a likely source for the word *ember*, see Sparrow
1668); in this edition, the passage is found on sig. R9r.

432.   VEEL, ROBERT. *New Court-Songs, and Poems*. V169. UMI 479: 19.

The author is identified on the title page as "R. V. Gent." As Spurgeon notes (3:
4.76), in a commendatory poem addressed "To Mr. T. D. on his Ingenious Songs
and Poems," Veel (1648–1674?), or perhaps Robert Vine, notes Chaucer's changing place in the constellation of major poets:

How many Best *of* Poets *have we known?*
And yet how far those Best *have been out-done!*
When Chaucer *dy'd, Men of that Age decreed*
A Dismal Fate to all that shou'd succeed:
Yet when Great Ben, *and* Mighty Shakespear *wrote,*
We were convinc'd those Elder Times did dote.
After all These, our Juster Age allows
Laurels as Green, to as deserving Brows.
But no man's Muse *yet ever equall'd thine,*
Who seem'st to have One, *greater than the* Nine. (sig. A8r)

433. *Westminster-Drollery: or, A Choice Collection of the Newest Songs & Poems at Court and Theaters.* **W1460. UMI 1271: 9.**

For an echo of a line from *The Manciple's Prologue*, see *Westminster-Drollery* (1671); in this edition, the passage is found on 34.

434. *Westminster-Drollery, the Second Part.* **W1463. UMI 1271: 10.**

For a reference to "Chaucer's jape," see Hilton (1652); in this collection, the song is found on 48.

Also found in *The Last, and Now Only, Compleat Collection, of the Newest and Choisest Songs and Poems. Which Are Now Added to This Second Part of Westminster Drollery* (1672), L472, 48.

435. *Windsor-Drollery. Collected by a Person of Quality.* **W2980. UMI 1111: 4.**

The title page of this work promises "a more exact collection of the newest songs, poems, and catches, now in use, both in city and country. With additions." In "Song 142," there is a reference to Troylus and Cressed, perhaps an allusion to *Troilus and Criseyde*, but a spurious quotation:

> In a season all oppressed,
> With sad sorrows sore distressed
> *Troylus* said unto his *Cressed*,
> Yield, O yield thee, Sweet, and stay not. (79)

436. WINSTANLEY, WILLIAM. *The New Help to Discourse: or, Wit, Mirth, and Jollity, Intermixt with More Serious Matters.* **W3069. UMI 2320: 9.**

For two quotations from *The General Prologue*, see Winstanley (1668); in this edition, the passages are found on 19, 212.

437.   WOODHEAD, ABRAHAM. *The Roman-Church's Devotions Vindicated from Doctour Stillingfleet's Misrepresentation by O. N. a Catholick.* W3454. UMI 1516: 13.

"O. N." cloaks the identity of Abraham Woodhead (1609–1678) who writes here in response to Edward Stillingfleet's *Discourse Concerning the Idolatry Practised in the Church of Rome.* In a passage about "Mother Juliana's Revelations," he argues that Stillingfleet can hardly object to her works unless some of her words are "taken in a modern improper sence" and heresy imputed from her antique language. Woodhead continues:

> I hope this Author [Stillingfleet] will not put her in the List of his Fanaticks, unless he can make good the fame of them, or, that he can prove her old English to be Fanaticism, but then let Chaucer also look to himself. (112)

Also found in *A Collection of Several Treatises in Answer to Dr. Stillingfleet* by Serenus Cressy (1672), C689, same pagination, second treatise.

438.   WYVILL, CHRISTOPHER. *The Pretensions of the Triple Crown Examined in Thrice Three Familiar Letters.* W3782C. UMI 1055: 15 (identified as W3787).

In a passage about Roman Catholics' devotion to the Virgin Mary, Sir Christopher Wyvill (1614–1672?) writes that an old song in her praise can be understood only by studying's Chaucer's antique language:

> [T]he blessed Virgin did not only present to *Godric*, but sang to him, as well as taught him to sing, a short Song; which he by often repeating, committed to same memory, and thus it went: 𝕾𝖊𝖎𝖓𝖙 Marie, 𝖈𝖑𝖆𝖚𝖊 𝔙𝖎𝖗𝖌𝖎𝖓𝖊. . . . He that would master the Original must study *Chaucer* a long time. . . . (161–62)

1673

439.   CARTER, MATTHEW. *Honor redivius: or, The Analysis of Honor and Armory.* C661. UMI 911: 11.

For a reference to Chaucer's escutcheon, see Carter (1655); in this edition, the passage is found on 225 and indexed on 348.

440.   COOPER, WILLIAM. *The Philosophical Epitaph of W. C. Esquire.* C6072. UMI 784: 21.

At the end of this collection of chemical works by various hands and published by Cooper (*fl.* 1668–1688), we find "A Catalogue of Chymical Books which have been written Originally, or Translated into English." The first work listed is Elias Ashmole's "*Theatrum Chymicum Britanicum; Or, a Collection of our Famous English Hermetical and Poetical Philosophers*, (viz.) Th Norton, Geo. Ripley, Geofr. Chaucer . . . Lond. 1652" (sig. P1r), and later in the list: "Geof. Chaucer's *Channons Yeomans tale*" (sig. P3v).

441.   DARE, JOSIAH. *Counsellor Manners, His Last Legacy to His Son.* D247. UMI 1205: 4.

In a section related to birth, breeding, and behavior, Dare paraphrases a couplet from *The Wife of Bath's Tale*: "To do the gentil dedes that he kan; Taak hym for the grettest gentil man" (lines 1115–16). Dare writes:

Behave thy self as becomes one of thy *Birth*. . . . It was the saying of old *English Chaucer* that to do the gentle deeds, that makes the Gentleman. Have what thou wilt, without these thou art but a *three-half-penny fellow*: Gentry without Virtue is blood indeed. . . . (3–4)

In a section about foolish superstitions regarding dreams, Dare recounts an incident related by Chauntecleer in *The Nun's Priest's Tale*:

[T]wo Fellow Travellers riding together, came by night, to a certain Town, where they *parted*, the one to his *Friends* House, the other to a common *Inn*, he that lodged at his *Friends* House, *dreamt* that he saw his Companion that lodged at the *Inn* stand at his *Bed-side*, and desired him that he would arise and make haste to help him, or he should be *murthered* by his *Host*, but being very *drowsie* and *weary* with his *Journey* he arose not; wherefore in a short time after his Companion again appeared, and requested him more earnestly to *arise* and *succour* him; but he making no account of all this slept again; but he left him not so, but appeared unto him the *Third* time, all *bloody*, telling him that it was now too *late* to implore his *aid*, but yet he requested him to *avenge* his *Blood* upon the *Murtherer* his *Host*; who (as he told him) had *killed* and *buried* him in his *Dung-Mixon*, where he should find his *Corps*: at which the other *started* out of his *sleep*, and arose, and taking the *Officers* with him, *secured* mine *Host*, and upon further search found the Body of his Fellow Traveller, with his *Throat cut*: and so by this means *God disclosed* the *Murther*, and those that had an hand in it were brought to *condign* punishment.

My Son, if such foolish *Conceits* and *Phansies* as those which I have before mentioned, call at thy *Door*, use them as *vagrant* Passengers, with *slight* respect, let them not take up any *lodging* within thee. But though I would not have thee *superstitious*, yet I would have thee *devout*. (144–45)

Other editions: D247A (1676), 3–4, 144–45; D248 (1694), 3–4, 144–45; D248A (1698), 3–4, 144–45; D249 (1699), 3–4, 144–45.

442.   *Enchridion legum*: *A Discourse Concerning the Beginnings, Nature, Difference, Progress and Use, of Laws in General; and in Particular, of the Common & Municipal Laws of England*. E720. UMI 66: 6.

This work on the customary laws of England was published without an author's name attached. In chapter 4, "An answer to certain Objections usually made against the Laws of England," there is a reference to Chaucer's old-fashioned language

> [T]he most of our Law being in the ancient *French* (for so are the year Books until *Henry* the 7th his time inclusively) deserveth no more to be ill thought on for the language (although not spoken in our or in any Country) than *Plautus* his Comedies because they agree not with *Latine* Authors in their *Latine*, or *Chaucers* writings because in words & stile they differ so much from Sr. *Philip Sidneys* selected and exquisite phrase. (63–64)

443.   HEAD, RICHARD. *The Floating Island*: *or, A New Discovery*. H1253. UMI 72: 13.

This satire purports to relate the strange adventures of those aboard three ships, the *Pay-Naught*, the *Excuse*, and the *Least-in-Sight*, which traveled from Lambethana to Villa Franca (alias Ramallia, located eastward of Terra del Templo) under the command of Captain Robert Owe-much, and "Published by Franck Careless, one of the discoverers" (title page). In a section dealing with special cases in the law of Ramallia, in the last paragraph of the ninth case, Head (1637?–1686?) refers to patient Grizel, perhaps alludes to *The Clerk's Tale*:

> *Sarah* was much troubled that the patience of *Grizel* should exceed that of *Elenors* in suffering *Esther* to knock down *Cassandra* with a Churmstick into the dripping pan. (39)

444.   HICKERINGILL, EDMUND. *Gregory, Father-Graybeard, with His Vizard Off*: *or, News from the Cabal in Some Reflexions upon a Late Pamphlet*. H1808. UMI 983: 87.

Ostensibly writing to an old friend, Hickeringill (1631–1708) comments on *The Rehearsal Transpros'd*. In a passage about the possibility that Adam spoke Hebrew, he writes of the difficulty of Chaucer's English for contemporaries:

> I do not remember, it is a great while ago, but I think he did not . . . [W]ithout a miracle no one Tongue can be epidemical and universal

100 years together, different climates will make different pronuncia-
tions: *English* and *Dutch* was the same Tongue in our Forefathers the
Saxons, we scarce understand *Chaucer*'s English, nor do the *Dutch* born
in *England* readily understand the *Dutch* spoken in the Netherlands. . . .
(285–86)

445. HOWARD, EDWARD. *Poems, and Essays.* H2973. UMI 2405: 7.

The author is characterized on the title page as "a gentleman of quality." In
this collection of poems, Lord Howard (*fl.* 1669) includes "A Blank for Rhime"
which he deprecates Chaucer and Gower's use of rhyme as antiquated:

> Rhime is *Pernassus* Ballad-curse:
> . . . .
> A Cittern that most Quills can touch,
> An ancient Chime in Monkish Verse:
> *Chaucer*'s Grave-beard in it is seen,
> And *Gower* driv'ling his Prick-song.
> An old Plush Cloak the inside outward,
> Or high-crown'd Hat stuck with new Feathers,
> Fit for some Lawrel'd Gallants now,
> As well as Rhimers heretofore. (49; sig. E1r)

Another edition in 1674: H2973A, same pagination.

446. JACKSON, THOMAS. *The Works of the Reverend and Learned Divine,
Thomas Jackson.* J90. UMI 1232: 1.

For a reference to Chaucer, an allusion to *The Canterbury Tales*, and a comment
about Chaucer's increasing marginalization, see Jackson (1657); in this edition,
the passage is found in the third volume, 746.

447. LOCKE, MATTHEW. *The Present Practice of Musick Vindicated.* L2777.
UMI 154: 11.

Locke (1621/2–1677) is writing here in response to Thomas Salmon (1672), q.v.,
and he echoes lines from *The Reeve's Prologue*, "To have a hoor head and a green
tayl, | As hath a leek" (lines 3878–79). Locke writes:

> [W]hat has Green tail, and Onion-like Fornicatar to do with a differ-
> ence about the Gamut. But the Gentleman must be al a mode . . . [he]
> deserves to be convinc'd rather by Horse-Logick, than by replies of Pen
> and Ink. (64)

448.   LOVEDAY, ROBERT. *Loveday's Letters Domestick and Forrein.* **L3229. UMI 1797: 30 (1673).**

For a reference to Chaucer as a prophet and poet, perhaps an allusion to the spurious work known as "Chaucer's Prophecy," see Loveday (1659); in this edition, the passage is found on 98–99.

449.   MILTON, JOHN. *Poems of Mr John Milton.* **M2161A. UMI 643: 1; and UMI 1707: 8.**

For an echo of a line from *The Wife of Bath's Tale* and an allusion to *The Squire's Tale* in "Il Penseroso" and an allusion to Chaucer in "Mansus," see Milton (1645); in this edition, the passages are found on 41, 45–46; and ²75.

Another edition in 1673: M2161, same pagination.

450.   OGILBY, JOHN, trans. *The Fables of Æsop Paraphras'd in Verse.* **A700. UMI 1298: 6.**

For three references to Chanticleer the cock and one to "Partlet the Hen," perhaps allusions to *The Nun's Priest's Tale*, see Ogilby (1651); in this edition, the passages are found on 1, 123–24, 142.

451.   OSBORNE, FRANCIS. *The Works of Francis Osborn. The Seventh Edition.* **O505. UMI 1023: 8.**

For a reference to a bishop who boasted that he had never read a line of Calvin or Chaucer, see Osborne (1658); in this collection, the passage is found on 492.

452.   P., H. *A Looking-Glass for Children.* **P29. No UMI.**

In a commendatory poem, dated 12 December 1672, H. P., the editor of this collection, echoes Chaucer's line, "Go, litel bok, go litel myn tragedye" (*Troilus and Criseyde* 5: 1786):

> *Go little* Book, *and speak for them that be*
> *Lanch'd with great safety to Eternity.* (sig. unseen)

Other editions in 1673: P30, sig. A3v (UMI 2292: 24); P30A, sig. A4v.

453.   PENN, WILLIAM. *Wisdom Justified of Her Children from the Ignorance and Calumny of H. Hallywell.* **P1395. UMI 1236: 19.**

As Dobbins notes (*MLN*), Penn (1644–1718) commends the spurious work known as Chaucer's *Ploughman's Tale*. In response to Henry Hallywell's *Account of Familism as It is Revived and Propagated by the Quakers*, in a passage about tithes, Penn writes:

[I]t has been observed by the best Princes, Wisest Counsellors, and most moderate Clergy-Man, *that the Enrichment & Impovering* [*sic*] *of Church Officers, has been the* Kanker[32] *of the Church, and the* Moth *of the* State.

'Tis not my Business to write a History; but I recommend to the Inquisitive Reader, *Wickliff's Remonstrance, The Plow-man's Complaint, Chaucer's Plow-man's Tale* . . . Men that ought not to pass for, nor be reputed *Phanaticks*, especially by such who call themselves *Protestants.* (78)

Also collected in *Several Tracts Apologetical for the Principles and Practices of the People Called Quakers*, P1363 (1672–74), first tract, same pagination; *Five Tracts Apologetical*, P1291A (1672–74).

454.   PHILLIPS, JOHN. *Maronides: or, Virgil Travesty, Paraphrase upon the Sixth Book of Virgil's Æneids in Burlesque Verse.* **P2091. UMI 772: 7.**
The author is identified on the title page as "John Phillips Gent the author of the Satyr against hypocrites." As Spurgeon notes (1: 248), Phillips (1631–1706) places Chaucer in a glittering constellation of poets both ancient and modern. He writes of Elysium:

> There sits *Ben Johnson* like a Tetrarch,
> With *Chaucer, Carew, Shakespear, Petrarch,*
> *Fletcher* and *Beaumont,* and *Menander,*
> *Plautus* and *Terence,* (how I wander?)
> *Horace,* and *Cowley* with his Mistress;
> And *d'Amboise* now quite free from distress
> With *Chapman* spends his merry days. (108)

Other editions: P2090A (1672), fifth book only.
   Another edition in 1673: P2091 (1673), 108.
   Another edition: P2092 (1678), a reissue of P2090A and P2091, ²108.

455.   *Poor Robin. 1673 An Almanack After a New Fashion.* A2192. UMI 1084: 20.
Under the heading "April hath XXX.dayes": "Patient Grizel" is celebrated on the 9th (sig. A7v). Under the heading "May hath XXXI.dayes": "Chaucers millar" is celebrated on the 31st (sig. A8v). Under the heading "December hath XXXI days": "Chaucers Miller" is celebrated on the 25th (sig. B7v).

---

[32] *Kanker*: canker, an open lesion or ulcer that causes pervasive corruption.

456.   PRIDEAUX, MATHIAS. *An Easy and Compendious Introduction for Reading All Sorts of Histories.* P3444A. UMI 2254: 4.

For a reference to "diverse passages" in Chaucer's works that are "useful" for students of history, see PRIDEAUX (1648); in this edition, the passage is found on 349.

457.   RAMESEY (or RAMSAY), WILLIAM. *Conjugium conjurgium: or, Some Serious Considerations on Marriage. By William Seymar Esq.* R228. UMI 1429: 8.

On the title page, Ramsay (1627–1676?), a physician and astrologer, is identified with the anagram *Seymar.* As Harris notes (*PQ*), but cites the 1675 edition, Ramsay casts his treatise as a letter of advice to Philogynus, a friend who is thinking of marrying. Under the running head "Womens Piety considered," Ramsay attributes a quotation to "honest" Chaucer:

> Shew me, my *Pilogynus,* but two in thrice two Thousand that is not as I have described them [i.e., cross, sullen, perverse tormenters of men] . . . If *Women,* then, in general, be so bad *Philogynus, what an hazard is it then to Marry?* And if so, I admonish thee again, keep thy self as thou art, ['Tis best to be free, and at liberty.] [*Sic,* i.e., square brackets in Ramsay's text.] For as honest *Chauser* well observes,
>
> > 𝔐arriage is like a 𝔯ebel 𝔯out,
> > 𝔥e that is out would fain get in,
> > 𝔄nd he that's in would fain get out.
>
> And therefore, with the *Philosopher,* make answer to thy friends that importune thee to Marry, *Adhunc intempestivum,* 'Tis yet unseasonable, [and so let it always be.] [*sic*] (82–84)

In a section about how lust induces the unwary to marry, Ramsay quotes modernized lines from *The Knight's Tale* (lines 2077–79, 1361–66, and 2805–10), *The Romaunt of the Rose* (lines 4261–66), and *The Wife of Bath's Prologue* (lines 227–28, 615–16). He writes:

> AND now consider seriously, *Philogynus,* what I have said before, and thou wilt save mew a great deal of Labour touching this *Lust;* which in plain English is nothing but that which thou callest *Love.* . . . All that our *Poets,* both Ancient and Modern have wrote in this kind, tend only to explain unto us what the *Love burning Lust is,* The Lives and Deaths of these *Hair-brain'd Fools;* And so are most of our *Romances.* To what other end and purpose are, I pritheee, all those Love Letters and Bawdy Songs, but to discover what is in the brests of these *Dizards,* or to excite the same in their *Mistrisses* & Servants. Such as these, (a taste only, therefore, and proceed)

> He cast his Eye upon Emilia,
> And therewith he Blent and cryed Ah ha,
> As though he had been struck unto the Hearta. . . . (123–25)

And as *Chaucer* has it in the *Knights tale.*

> His Sleep, his Meat, his Drink is him bereft,
> That Lean he waxeth, and dry as a Shaft,
> His Eyes Hollow, and grisly to behold,
> His Hew Pale and Ashen to unfold;
> And solitary he was ever alone,
> And waking all the night making moan.

Nay, old Men as well as young can't resist, as the same *Chaucer* has it in the same *Tale.*

> —when he felt Death,
> Dusked been his eyes, and faded is his breath,
> But on his Lady yet casteth he his eye,
> His last word was, mercy Emely,
> His Spirit chang'd, and outwent there,
> Whither I cannot tell, ne where. . . . (127–28)

Art not thou a wise fellow to run made after *Toys*, *Shadows*, things of *no moment or substance*, a *bundle of Deceit and Villany*? Old honest *Chaucer* will tell you how they were in his time above three hundred years ago, in his *Romant of the Rose.*

> Ev'ry each of them hath some Vice,
> If one be full of Villanhy,
> Another hath a Liquerish Eye.
> If one be full of Wantonness,
> Another is a Childeress.

'Tis natural to them to be so. And as *Chaucer* notes elsewhere,

> For half so boldly there can non,
> Swear and Lye as Woman can.

Their Stars incline them, as the *wife of Bath* speaks from her own experience,

> I follow, aye mine Inclination,
> By virtue of my Constellation.

And now let us, *Philogynus*, proceed to consider *the second end of Marriage* [i.e., procreation], since they [women] are so still, and ever will be. (132–34)

Other editions: R228A (1674), 82–84, 123–25, 127–28, 132–34; R229 (1675), 49, 74–75, 77–78, 80; R230 (1684), 51 (*sic*, really 49), 74–75, 77–78, 80; R230A (1694), 51 (*sic*, really 49), 74–75, 77–78, 80.

458.   Saul, Arthur. *The Famous Game of Chesse-Play.* S730A. UMI 2774: 2.

For an echo of Chaucer's line, "Go, litel bok, go litel myn tragedye" (*Troilus and Criseyde* 5: 1786) in Saul's commendatory poem "To his Booke," see Saul (1614); in this edition, the passage is found on sig. A5v–6r.

459.   Smith, John. *The Mysterie of Rhetorique Unveil'd.* S4116C. UMI 876: 13 (identified as S2582).

For a reference to Spenser's imitation of Chaucer, see Smith (1656); in this edition, the passage is found on 64.

460.   S'too Him Bayes: or, Some Observations upon the Humour of Writing Rehearsals Transpros'd. S5740aA. M890. UMI 216: 21 (identified as M890).

As Harris notes (*PQ*), the author (sometimes thought to be Andrew Marvell) cites the spurious work known as Chaucer's *Ploughman's Tale* and quotes a somewhat modernized couplet from *The Reeve's Tale*: "Ay by his belt he baar a long panade | And of a swerd ful trenchant was the blade" (lines 3929–30). The author writes of Dryden:

> Well, this *Bayes* we are speaking of . . . *fam'd* the *Bishop* for *bravery*. . . .
> It is there describ'd however (that the *Bishop* might not *mistake* it seems)
> at large, in four *Wild-Irish* (I think) Verses. He might as well have took,
>> *Ay by His side he wore a long Pavade* [*sic*],
>> *And of his Sword full trenchant was the Blade.*
> Out of *Chaucer* (for they are better) but, I believe he durst not look in
> him for fear of meeting with *the Plow mans Tale.* (16–17)

461.   Verstegen (or Rowlands), Richard. *A Restitution of Decayed Intelligence in Antiquities.* V271. UMI 729: 17.

For references to Chaucer's translation of *The Romaunt of the Rose*, to his contributions to the English language, and to his diction, see Rowlands (1605) in Boswell & Holton No. 723; in this edition, the passages are found on 218, 222, 231, 274, sig. Bb5r.

1674

462.   BAKER, RICHARD. *A Chronicle of the Kings of England.* B507. UMI 706: 18.

For references to Chaucer as John of Gaunt's brother-in-law, "the Homer of our nation," his association with Woodstock, his translation of *The Romaunt of the Rose*, his burial place in Westminster, and his association with Gower, see BAKER (1643) and (1653); in this edition, the passages are found on 136, 138, 159, 171, and sig. Iiiii1r.

463.   BLOUNT, THOMAS. *Glossographia: or, A Dictionary. The Fourth Edition, with Many Additions.* B3337. UMI 809: 18.

Blount is identified on the title page as "T. B. of the Inner-Temple, Esq." For a reference to "old Chaucer" and a quotation from *Troilus and Cryssede* and to Chaucer as an authority on the English language and word usage, see BLOUNT (1656), (1661), and (1670); in this revised and augmented edition, the passages are found in the epistle (A4v), and in the definitions of *agroted* (B8r), *algebra* (C1r–v), *alnath* (C3r), *barbican* (F6v), *benison* (G1v), *boon* (G5v), *bordel* (G5v), *burlybrand* (G8v), *covent* (M3r), *creance* (M4r), *disheviled* (O5r), *dulcarnon* (P2v), *dwindle* (P3r), *fryth* (T1v), *lectern* (Aa8v), *lodemanage* (Bb5v), *losenger* (Bb7r), *meriot* (Dd3v), *moiles* (Dd7v), *mortress* (Ee3r), *ouch* (Gg4v), *paraments* (Hh1v), *pilgrim* (Ii6v), *rap and ren* (sig. Mm3v), *romance* (Nn6r), *superstition* (Rr6r), *taberd* (Ss3v), *tailage* (Ss4v).

In addition to omissions and additions noted in BLOUNT (1670), there is another reference in this edition:

𝕯iuinistre, so *Chaucer* calls an inferiour Divine: a smatterer in Divinity. (sig. O6r) [*The Knight's Tale*, line 2811.]

464.   BOLTON, EDMUND. *The Cities Great Concern.* B3505. UMI 1088: 14.

Bolton (1575?–1633?) is not named on the title page. In a section in which he examines "Whether Apprentiship extinguisheth Gentry," Bolton counts Chaucer as one London's greatest citizens:

[W]hosoever . . . were born in the City, they give to it the glory of *Arms*. And *Jeffery Chaucer*, Sir *Thomas Moore* Knight, with others born in *London*, communicate thereunto the Glory of Wits and Letters. (93)

465.   "CHAUCER JUNIOR." "A Character" in James Strong's *Joanereidos: or, Feminine Valour Eminently Discovered in Western Women. Reprinted (with Additions) for the Satisfaction of his Friends.* S5991. UMI 948: 14.

For a pastiche of lines from *The Prologue of The Canterbury Tales*, see "Chaucer Junior" (1645); in this edition, the passage is found on sig. D3r–v.

466.   COWLEY, ABRAHAM. *The Works of Mr. Abraham Cowley.* C6652. UMI 1438: 44.

For a reference to Cowley's burial place near Chaucer, see SPRAT (1668); in this edition, the passage is found on sig. c4r–v.

For a reference to Chaucer's "rich rhymes," see COWLEY (1656), C6683; in this edition, the passage is found on 37 (sig. Aa1r).

467.   FLAVEL, JOHN. *Husbandry Spiritualized: or, The Heavenly Use of Earthly Things.* F1166. UMI 1308: 39.

For an echo of a line from *The Reeve's Prologue*, see FLAVEL (1669); in this edition, the passage is found on 259.

468.   FOULIS, HENRY. *The History of the Wicked Plots and Conspiracies of Our Pretended Saints.* F1643. UMI 277: 6.

For quotations from and references and allusions to *The House of Fame*, *The Nun's Priest's Tale*, *The Summoner's Tale*, and *The Clerk's Tale*, see FOULIS (1662); in this edition, the passages are found on 77, 80, 83, 92, 99, 103, 104–5, 126, 144–45.

469.   GEARING, WILLIAM. *The History of the Church of Great Britain.* G435B. UMI 1670: 35; UMI 69: 15 (identified as G440).

In his account of the reign of Edward III, Gearing (or perhaps William Geaves or maybe George Geaves, to whom this work is sometimes attributed) mentions Chaucer:

> In his Reign also flourished . . . Sir *Geoffry Chaucer*, the *Homer* of our Nation. (113)

In the index, Chaucer is again mentioned: "Sir *Geoffry Chaucer*, when he flourished" (sig. L114r).

Another edition: G435D (1675), 113, sig. L114r.

470.   HEAD, RICHARD, and FRANCIS KIRKMAN. *The English Rogue: Continued in the Life of Meriton Latroon, and Other Extravagants. The Third Part.* H1250. UMI 1333: 5.

For a reference to old men telling "Canterbury tales," see HEAD and KIRKMAN (1671); in this edition, the passage is found on 119.

471.   HOWARD, EDWARD. *Poems, and Essays.* H2973a. UMI 2405: 8.

For a reference in which Lord Howard deprecates Chaucer's use of rhyme, see HOWARD (1673); in this edition, the passage is found on 49.

472.   HYDE, THOMAS. *Catalogus impressorum librorum bibliothecæ bodleianæ.* O864. UMI 967: 7.

The work at hand is identified on the title page as "Curâ & Operâ Thomæ Hyde è Coll. Reginæ Oxon. Protobibliothecarii." As Spurgeon notes (1: 240), Chaucer's *Works* (1561) and *The Plough-mans Tale* (1606) are listed under his name on 157. However, Hyde (1636–1703) lists others. Under the heading "Boëthius":

> De Consol. Philosophiæ, put into English Prose by Geffrey Chaucer.
> —G.2.16.*Th.*
> Same in English Verse. *Printed in the Monastery of Tavestock in Denshire*
> 1525. 40 L.71.
> *Art.* (95)

473.   PENN, WILLIAM. *Several Tracts Apologetical for the Principles and Practices of the People Called Quakers.* P1363. No UMI.

For Penn's commendation of the spurious work known as Chaucer's *Ploughman's Tale*, see PENN (1673); in this collection, the passage is found in the first tract.

The same collection with a different title: *Five Tracts Apologetical* (1674), P1291A, same pagination.

474.   *Poor Robin 1674. An Almanack after a New Fashion.* A2193. UMI 1603: 8.

Under the heading "Observations on April": "Patient Grizel" is celebrated on the 1st of this month (sig. A8r); this is perhaps an allusion to the protagonist of *The Clerk's Tale*.

475.   RAMSAY (or RAMESEY), WILLIAM. *Conjugium conjurgium: or, Some Serious Considerations on Marriage.* R228A. UMI 2357: 21.

For a spurious quotation attributed to Chaucer and genuine quotations from *The Knight's Tale*, *The Wife of Bath's Prologue*, and *The Romaunt of the Rose*, see RAMSAY (1673); in this edition the passages are found on 82–84, 123–25, 127–28, 132–34.

476.   RAY, JOHN. *A Collection of English Words Not Generally Used.* R388. UMI 435: 17.

Ray (1627–1705) is identified on the title page as "John Ray Fellow of the Royal Society." As Spurgeon notes (1: 249), but does not transcribe, Ray cites Chaucer's usage of several words. Under the running head "North Country Words," Ray writes:

> To *Rack* or *Reck*: . . . Chaucer hath *recketh*, for careth. (38)
>   [Tatlock & Kennedy cite more than twenty instances of Chaucer's use.]

A *Stot*: a young bullock or steer, a young horse in *Chaucer*. (45)
  [Chaucer uses *stot* twice, in *The General Prologue* and *The Friar's Tale*.]
To *Thole*; . . . *Chaucer* hath *Tholed*, for suffered. (48)
  [Chaucer uses tholed in *The Friar's Tale*, line 1546.]
To *Wite* . . . *Chaucer* useth the word for blame. (53)
  [Chaucer uses *wite* (and variants) more than a dozen times.]
Yare: Covetous, Desirous, . . . *Chaucero* etiam *Yare*, Paratus, promptus, &c. V. *Skinner*. (55)
  [Chaucer uses *yare* in *The Legend of Good Women*, line 2270.]
Yewd or *Yod*: *Chaucero* Yed, yeden, yode eodem sensu. *Spencer* also in his Fairie Queen, lib. 1.c.10. (55–56)
  [Chaucer uses *yede* (and variants) twice in *The Canon's Yeoman's Tale*, twice in *Troilus and Criseyde*, and four times in *The Romaunt of the Rose*.]

Under the running head "East and South Country Words," Ray adds:

Bucksome: Blithe, jolly, frolick, chearly, some write it *Buxome*; . . . quod eo confirmatur quod pud Chaucerum *Buxumness* exponitur *lowliness*, *Skinner*. (60).
  [Chaucer uses *buxumnesse* in *Truth*, line 15.]

Other editions: R389 (1691), 57, 70, 74, 82, 84–85, 85, 91.

477.   RYMER, THOMAS. "Preface of the Translator" in René Rapin's *Reflections on Aristotle's Treatise of Poesie*. R270. UMI 225: 1.

As Spurgeon notes (1: 249), Rymer (1641–1713) mentions Chaucer and the parlous state of the English language in his day in the unsigned "Preface of the Translator." In a section about unfortunate English poets who suffered because of their "ignorance or negligence of these fundamental Rules and Laws of Aristotle":

I shall leave the Author of the *Romance of the Rose* (whom Sir *Richard Baker* makes an *Englishman*) for the *French* to boast of, because he writ in their Language. Nor shall I speak of *Chaucer*, in whose time our Language, I presume, was not capable of any Heroick Character. Nor indeed was the most polite Wit of *Europe* in that Age sufficient for a great *design*. That was the Age of *Tales*, *Ballads*, and *Roundelays*. (sig. A6v)

Another edition: R271 (1694), sig. A5v.

478.   S., J. *The Case of the Quakers Relating to Oaths Stated.* S48. UMI 777: 13.

The author is identified on the title page as "J. S." In "Section III," he says he has "blown off the dust of false glosses from those sacred Texts, which the Quakers pervert to the condemnation of the universal practise of the Church of Christ . . . relating to Oaths and swearing. . . . It will be requisite therefore that I demonstrate the impertinency of those Examples which they alledge, and the want of either ingenjuity or honesty that they bewray in making of them" (37). He goes on to give over a dozen examples. In the fourth, he cites the spurious work known as Chaucer's *Tale of Jack Upland*, notes sardonically that he Chaucer is called "the dad of English Poets," and refers to "his Romance." J. S. writes:

> In the Plowmans Complaint is this, *viz. Lord, thou givest as a commandment of truth, ion bidding us say, yea yea, nay nay, and swear for nothing*; but Lord, &c.
>
> *Answer.* This I confesse comes home to the point, if the allegation be faithful, but if this Plowman be *Chaucers Jack-Upland*, (as by his stile he seems to be) I never read that he was Canonized a Martyr, or dub'd a Father of the Church, though he be the dad of English Poets; nor do I think his Romance will passe amongst rationall men for good authority. (39)

Another edition: S48A (1696), 39.

479.   SPEED, SAMUEL. *Fragmenta carceris: or, The Kings-Bench Scuffle; with the Humours of the Common-Side.* S4900. UMI 476: 9.

Speed (1631–1682) is identified on the title page as "Samuel Speed, a member of the Royal Society." As Spurgeon notes (1: 250), there is a reference to Chaucer in *The Legend of the Thrice-Honourable, Ancient, and Renowned Prince, His Grace Humphrey, Duke of St. Paul's Cathedral Walk.* Duke Humphrey "Perambulated to Ben Johnson's Tomb, | Where Shakespear, Spencer, Cambden, and the rest, | Once rising Suns, are now set in the West; | . . . [yet] some have fancied that they've heard them sing, | *Within this place is* Aganippe's *Spring.*" This sacred space is, however, tainted with doxies, pickpockets, and such like. Speed notes that Chaucer collected material for his tales from such bad company:

> Old *Chaucer*, who though sickly, full of ails,
> From hence collects a Book as full of Tales.
> His Neighbour *Drayton*, who was his *Amoris*,
> Studying to write *Encomium* on *Authoris*.
> The Learned *Cambden*'s Gravity appear'd,
> At which they starting, seem'd as if they fear'd. (sig. G1r)

Another edition: S4901 (1675), same pagination.

480.   STAVELEY, THOMAS. *The Romish Horseleech.* S5346. UMI 826: 4.

Staveley (1626–1684) is not named on the title page. In chapter 24, "Abbies, Monasteries, &c.," under the running head "Purgatory," in a passage about those who resisted the "ignorance" and "superstition" of the church of Rome, Staveley cites Chaucer as one whose work casts a light on a dark age:

> Yet in the darkest of these times, there wanted not some, that could dis-
> cern that all was not right, and that they were gotten into a very uncer-
> tain, and dangerous road; and in as much danger from their guides, as
> the enemy which they would avoid. Some of these, in a more serious
> way, protesting, and advising both against the Errour, and the danger
> of it, had their mouths stopp'd; when others more jocular, between jest,
> and earnest, as it were, made bold with the corruptions, and abuses of
> the time, witness the wits, and Satyrists of their respective times *Rob.* of
> *Glocester, John Harding, Jeffrey Chaucer, John Gower, Rob. Langland,* aliàs
> *Piers Plowman, Lydgate,* and many more, whose dull rimes carried a
> cutting sense with them. Indeed though the Lashes of a Satyrist seldom
> or never produce amendment of Epidemical vices, and Errors; yet in
> this they have their fruit, that thereby posterity is oftentimes more truly
> informed of the manners, and genius of times, than by the professed
> Historian, who rarely touches that string: And by these, the abuses,
> the cheats of Priests, Monks, and Fryers, in their Masses, Confessions,
> Shrifts, Penances, Pardons, Indulgences, Miracles, Reliques, &c. all
> serving to fill the people's brains with vain, and terrible apprehensions,
> and to empty their purses, were according to the wit of their respective
> Ages, to the warning of this, notably, and smartly detected, arraigned,
> and condemned. (202–3)

481.   WALLIS, JOHN. *Grammatica linguæ anglicanæ.* W586. UMI 1079: 10.

For a reference to Chaucer's vocabulary, see WALLIS (1653); in this edition, this passage is found on 24.

Another edition in 1674: W586A, same pagination.

482.   WHARTON, GEORGE. "To my Very Honoured Friend," in Gaultier de Coste, Seigneur de La Calprenède's *Hymen's Præludia: or, Love's Master-Piece. Now Rendred into English, by Robert Loveday.* L123. UMI 870: 1.

For a reference to Chaucer and Gower as a pair who refined the English language, see WHARTON (1652); in this edition, the passage is found on sig. A4v.

483. Whitehead, George. *The Case of the Quakers Concerning Oaths Defended as Evangelical.* **W1899. UMI 930: 10.**

Whitehead (1636?–1723) is not named on the title page. Writing in response to J. S.'s *The Case of the Quakers Relating to Oaths* (1674), q.v., Whitehead, a staunch Quaker, alludes to Chaucer's writing "against the usurping Clergy in his time" and cites the spurious works known as Chaucer's *Ploughman's Tale* and *The Tale of Jack Upland*. He writes:

> Our Example out of the Plow-man's Complaint against the Pope's Breaking Christ's Commandment, in making a Law to compel men to Swear; This *J. S. confesseth comes home to the Point, if the Allegation be faithful; but if this Plow-man be* Chaucer's Jack-upland, *as by his stile he seems to be, I never read,* saith he, *that he was canonized a Martyr, or dubbed a Father of the Church, though he be Dad* of English *Poets.* . . . And however he sleights or jeers *Chaucer,* hath he not been owned as . . . a Witness in his Method against the usurping Clergy in his time? (36–37)

Another edition: W1900 (1675), 36–37.

1675

484. Alsop, Vincent. *Anti-sozzo: sive, Sherlocismus enervatus.* **A2905. UMI 1084: 35.**

Alsop (1629/30–1703) is not named on the title page. Here he writes against some of the "great errors" espoused by William Sherlock in *Discourse Concerning the Knowledge of Jesus Chirst* (1674). In the third section of chapter three, "How unsafe it is to found Religion upon a Pretended Acquaintance with Christs Person," Alsop echoes a line from *The Manciple's Prologue*: "Sires, what! Dun is in the myre!" (line 5). He writes:

> I must needs observe to the Reader one piece of *cleanly conveyance* and *Legerdemain,* which our Author is forced frequently at a standing pull to serve himself of to *draw Dun* out o'th'Mire . . . (270)

Another edition: A2905A (1676), 270.

485. Cotton, Charles. *Burlesque upon Burlesque: or, The Scoffer Scoft. Being Some of Lucian's Dialogues, Newly Put into English Fustian.* **C6380a. UMI 89: 7.**

Cotton (1630–1687) is characterized on the title page as "one who never transgressed before, nor (if this may be pardoned) doe ever intend to offend again."

In the "Prologue," he refers to Patient Grizell, perhaps an allusion to *The Clerk's Tale*:

> *We in the Country do not scorn*
> *Our Walls with Ballads to adorn*
> *Of patient* Grizell, *and the Lord of* Lorne. (sig. A2r)

Other editions: C6380b (1686), sig. A2r; C6380c (1687), sig. A2r.

486.   G., R. *Ludus scacchia. A Satyr with Other Poems.* **L3471A. UMI 2212: 11.**

The author is identified on the title page as "R. G." In this poem about the game of chess, there is a reference to *Troilus and Criseyde* (3: 331, 333) and a note that explains the allusion:

> An Adverse Knight espi'd this, and leaping here
> And there about the Field, and every-where
> O're Neighbours Shoulders, at the last falls on
> The King and Bishop with his **Dulcarnon.*

Dulcarnon is marked for a note:

> * *The* Pythagorean Y, *and the* Logician's Dilemma, *are both of them* Horned; *Because they present two Objects of Choice, both dangerous, and one of them inevitable; rendring the mind anxious and perplex'd, being inforc'd to a Necessity of Election, yet not knowing which peril to choose. Chawcer, in his* Troilus *and* Cresseid, *when* Cresseid *was in a like Extremity, makes her say? [sic]*

> I am till God me better mind send
> At *Dulcarnon* right at my wits end.

> *Meaning, she was reduc'd to the same Condition as is affected by the Powers of the* Y, *or the* Dilemma, *for either of which Expressions,* Chawcer *substitutes, this new One of his Own, of the very same import, taking it from the Æra* Dhicarnain, *which was* Alexanders Æra: *Who, to establish that Opinion of his being the Son of* Jupiter Hammon *(who was* Corniger) *caus'd a coin to be stamp'd, having his Own Image on it with* Two Hornes *as well as his Father* Hammon; *whose Image also was on the* Reverse, *(a Coin of which I have by me) And the* Greeks, *in memory of* Him, *substituted* Another Æra *in place of their* Olimpiad *and calle'd it (*Æra Alexandrea) *Alexanders* Æra. *This* Æra, *the* Arabians calld' Æra Dhilcarnain, *viz.* Æra habentis duo

Cornua: *which our Excellent Poet, though in those dull times, saw as clearly as* Scaliger[33] *did after, and accordingly made use of.*

Whoever observes the Knight's *Cheque, That it equally threatens* Two Opposites, *and unavoidably destroyes* One, *will allow the Expression; and not take* Dulcarnon *for the name of the Knights Sword.* (13)

Another edition with title: *Ludus scacchiæ. A Satyr against Unjust Wars*: L3471B (1676), 13.

487. GADBURY, JOHN. *Obsequium rationabile: or, A Reasonable Service Performed for the Cælestial Sign Scorpio.* G95. UMI 1550: 37.

Gadbury (1627–1704) identifies himself on the title page as a "Student in Physick and Astrology." The work at hand is an attack on "that Grand (but Fortunate) Imposter Mr. William Lilly," (1602–1681), a well known astrologer and author of almanacks, who written unkind things about people born under the sign of Scorpio. Gadbury quotes from *The Wife of Bath's Prologue* (lines 615–16):

> It is a *sign* saith he *stigmatized by all Antient* and *modern Practicers in Astrology to be of evil signification.* . . . If it be an *impelling cause of evil, then Persons that are born under it are thereby necessitated to commit wickedness*, and need commute no otherwise for it, but lay the fault upon *their Horoscope*, with *Chaucer's Wife of Bath*.

> 𝔍 followed, aye, mine inclination,
> 𝔅y bertue of my Constellation. (13)

488. GEARING, WILLIAM. *The History of the Church of Great Britain.* G435D. UMI 1207: 3 (identified as G441) and 1670: 36.

For references to Chaucer, "the Homer of our nation," who flourished in the reign of Edward III, see GEARING (1674); in this edition, the passages are found on 113 and sig. L114r.

489. OGILBY, JOHN, trans. *The Fables of Æsop Paraphras'd in Verse.* A702. UMI 679: 14.

For three references to Chanticleer the cock and one to "Partlet the Hen," perhaps allusions to *The Nun's Priest's Tale*, see OGILBY (1651); in this edition, the passages are found on 1, 123–24, 142.

---

[33] Scaliger refers to Julius Caesar Scaliger (1484–1558), Italian humanist scholar.

490.   PENN, WILLIAM. *A Treatise of Oaths Containing Several Weighty Reasons Why the People Call'd Quakers Refuse to Swear.* P1388. UMI 1675: 14.

As Harris (*PQ*) and Langston (*N&Q*) note, in a section headed "Memorable Testimonies against Swearing, collected out of the Writings of Gentiles, Jews & Christians," Penn (1644–1718) quotes from the spurious work known as Chaucer's *Ploughman's Tale* and conflates lines from *The Parson's Tale* (lines 586–89). Penn writes:

> We will bring in here a Passage out of the *Plowman's Tale*, as it lyes in *GEFFRY CHAUCER*'s Works, not impertinent to our Purpose; whose Learning, Honour and Wit was great in the time he lived, which was about 1360. *John Wickliff*'s Contemporary.

> These Wollen make men to Swear
> *against Christ's Commaundment*;
> And Christ's Members all to tear,
> on rood as he were new yrent:
> Such Laws they maken by common Assent,
> each one it throweth as a Ball;
> Thus the Poor be fullshent;
> but ever Falshood foul it befal.

> He hath Expressions not less disliking Oaths in his *Parson's Tales*, where he makes the Parson to say,

> After those, then cometh Swearing, *expresly against the Commandment of God, and our Lord Jesus Christ, who saith by* St. Matthew's words, *Ne shall ye not Swear in all manner, or on no Account.* (122)

The passage is marked with a shoulder note: "*Geff. Chauc.* Works, fol. 86."
"Geff. Chaucer" is also listed in "A Catalogue of the Authors, Testimonies and Presidents cited in Favour of this Treatise" (5).

491.   PHILLIPS, EDWARD. *Theatrum poetarum: or, A Compleat Collection of the Poets Especially the Most Eminent, of All Ages.* P2075. UMI 191: 9.

As Spurgeon notes (1: 250–51), Phillips (1630–1696?) commends Chaucer in his "Preface":

> *Curteous* Readers, *let me plead a little for the well meaners only, as something Sympathising with those for whom I plead; Vertue will plead for it self, and needs no advocate; first let it considered that time* [*sic*; the passage is garbled] *some that had their Poetical excellencies if well examin'd, and chiefly*

among the rest Chaucer, *who through all the neglect of former-ag'd Poets still keeps a name, being by some few admir'd for his real worth, to other not unpleasing for his facetious way, which jyn'd with his old* English *intertains them with a kind of Drollery*. . . . (sig. ii2rv)

In a section headed "Eminent Poets Among the Moderns," alphabetized under the letter "G":

Sir *Geoffry Chaucer*, the Prince and *Coryphæus*, generally so reputed, till this Age, of our *English* Poets, and as much as we triumph over his old fashion'd phrase, and obsolete words, one of the first refiners of the *English* Language, of how great Esteem he was in the Age wherein he flourish'd, namely the Reigns of *Henry* the 4th, *Henry* the 5th, and part of *Henry* the 6th, appears, besides his being Knight and Poet Laureat, by the Honour he had to be allyed by Marriage to the great Earl of *Lancaster John* of *Gaunt*: How great a part we have lost of his Works above what we have Extant of him is manifest from an Author of good Credit, who reckons up many considerable Poems, which are not in his publisht Works; besides the Squires Tale, which is said to be compleat in *Arundel-house* Library. (50–51)

Sr *John Gowr*, a very Famous English Poet in his time, and counted little inferiour, if not equal to *Chaucer* himself; who was his Contemporary, and some say his Scholar and Successor in the Laurel: for *Gowr* was also both Poet Laureat and Knight. (109)

John Lane, a fine old Queen *Elizabeth* Gentleman, who was living within my remembrance, and whose several Poems, had they not had the ill fate to remain unpublisht, when much better meriting then many that are in print . . . [including] his Supplement to *Chaucers* Squires Tale. (112)

In "A Brief Supplement of some Persons and Things Omitted in the foregoing Treatises," there are three references to Chaucer (including one not mentioned by Spurgen):

Gaulfrid, one of the oldest of the Modern Poets . . . he is mentioned by *Chaucer* in his Description of *Chaunticleer* the Cock's being carried away by *Reynard* the Fox. . . . (223)

John de Mehunes, a French Poet, out of whom *Chaucer* is said to have borrowed his *Troilus and Cressida*, and some other of his Poems. (229)

Thomas Ocleave, a very famous English Poet in his time . . . and so much the more famous by being remember'd to have been the Disciple of the most fam'd *Chaucer*. (233)

492.   *Poor Robin. 1675. An Almanack after a New Fashion.* A2194. UMI 1347: 13.

Under the heading "Observations on April": "Patient Grizel" is celebrated on the 7th of this month (sig. A8r); this is perhaps an allusion to the protagonist of *The Clerk's Tale*.

493.   RAMSAY (or RAMESEY), WILLIAM. *Conjugium conjurgium: or, Some Serious Considerations on Marriage.* R229. UMI 774: 6.

For a spurious quotation attributed to Chaucer and genuine quotations from *The Knight's Tale*, *The Wife of Bath's Prologue*, and *The Romaunt of the Rose*, see RAMSAY (1673); in this edition the passages are found on 49, 75, 77–78, 80. Harris (*PQ*) cites this edition rather than the first.

494.   SHERBURNE, EDWARD. "A Catalogue" in *The Sphere of Marcus Manilius Made an English Poem.* M432. UMI 283: 3.

Sherburne (1618–1702) is identified on the title page as "Edward Sherburne, Esquire." In "A Catalogue of the most Eminent Astronomers, Ancient & Modern," he lists:

Galfridus Chaucer, a learned Knight, and Prince of *English* Poets, *Cui Veneres debet Patria lingua suas*, to use *Leland's* Encomium of him, merits a place in this Catalogue, for his Book of the *Astrolabe*, which he composed for the use and instruction of his Son. (38)

Leland's encomium to Chaucer is rendered by Kenneth Lloyd-Jones as "To whom our native tongue owes its graceful qualities." See LELAND (1589), Boswell & Holton No. 470.

In "The Table of Authors mentioned in the Catalogue," under the letter "C": "Chaucer Galfridus" (sig. Kkk1r).

495.   SPEED, SAMUEL. *Fragmenta carceris: or, The Kings-Bench Scuffle; with the Humours of the Common-Side.* S4901. UMI 851: 1.

For a reference to Chaucer's burial place in Westminster Abbey in very distinguished company and an allusion to *The Canterbury Tales*, see SPEED (1674); in this edition, the passage is found on sig. G1r.

496.   STILLINGFLEET, EDWARD. *An Answer to Mr. Cressy's Epistle.* S5556. UMI 826: 10.

Stillingfleet (1635–1699) is identified on the title page as "Edw. Stillingfleet D. D. Chaplain in Ordinary to His Majesty." In a section dealing with "perfection of poverty" found in Franciscan orders, Stillingfleet cites Chaucer's "plain Country-man" and quotes extensively from a spurious work; moreover, the shoulder note is bogus. Chaucer's "last edition" would have been Speght's second edition of 1602 (the next edition was published in 1687), but on 348 in that edition, no such passage is found.

> The plain *Country-man* in *Chaucer* asks the *Frier* a great many untoward *Questions* concerning their *Order*, which I doubt the *wisest* of their *Order* will not easily answer; as
>
> Freer, how many Orders be on erth, and which is the prefectest Order? Is there any perfecter Rule than Christ himself made? [in a shoulder note: "Chaucer. v. 348. last Edit."] If Christs Rule be most perfect, why rulest thou thee not thereafter? Why shall a Freer be more punished for breaking the Rule that his Patron made, than if he break the hests that God himself made? [The quotation goes on for eight pages.] . . . But if they woulden that their Freers saten above the Apostles in Heaven for the harder Religion that they keepen here, so would they sitten in Heaven above Christ himself for their more and strict observations, then so should they be better than Christ himself.
>
> In these *Questions*, (besides several others extant in *Chaucer*) we have the *hypocrisie* and *fraud* of these *Mendicant Friers* fully set forth by a Person who lived among them in the time of their greatest flourishing here in *England*. (221–32)
>
> [I]f we believe the concurrent testimony of these Historians, there were never greater Hypocrites known, since the Pharisees, and before the Jesuits, than these pretenders to *perfect Poverty*: who hated that in their hearts to which they made the greatest shew of Love. We may perceive by *Chaucer* what wayes they had of wheadling great persons into an opinion how much better it was to be buried among them, than any where else. . . . (234–35)

497.   TREVERS, JOSEPH. *An Essay to the Restoring of Our Decayed Trade.* T2129. UMI 1786: 9.

Following a commendatory poem by one R. B., Trevers also commends his book with an echo of Chaucer's line, "Go, litel bok, go litel myn tragedye" (*Troilus and Criseyde* 5: 1786):

Goe little Book into the world and see
  Who thou can'st find therein to welcome thee. . . . (sig. a2v)

Other editions: T2130 (1677), sig. a2v; T2130A (1678).

498. WHITEHEAD, GEORGE. *The Case of the Quakers Concerning Oaths Defended as Evangelical.* W1900. UMI 930: 11.

For references the spurious works known as Chaucer's *Ploughman's Tale* and *The Tale of Jack Upland*, see WHITEHEAD (1674); in this edition, the passages are found on 36–37.

1676

499. ALSOP, VINCENT. *Anti-sozzo: sive, Sherlocismus enervatus.* A2905A.

For an echo of a line from *The Manciple's Prologue*, see ALSOP (1675); in this edition, the passage is found on 270.

500. BRAMHALL, JOHN. *The Works of John Bramhall.* Dublin. B4210. UMI 204: 5.

For a reference to Chaucer's portrayal of "the greediness and extortion of the Court of Rome" in the "Plowmans tale and elsewhere" (allusions to *The Canterbury Tales* and the spurious work known as Chaucer's *Ploughman's Tale*), see BRAMHALL (1654); in this edition, the passage is found on 93.

For a reference to Chaucer and an allusion to the Frere in *The General Prologue*, see BRAMHALL (1661); in this edition, the passage is found on 974.

Another edition: B4211 (1677), same pagination.

501. BURNET, GILBERT. *A Relation of a Conference Held about Religion at London.* B5861. UMI 308: 3.

A conference about differences between the doctrines of the Roman Catholic Church and the Church of England was held in London on 3 April 1676. There Burnet (1643–1715) and Edward Stillingfleet (1635–1699) debated "some gentlemen of the Church of Rome" (title page). In a passage about changes in the English language since the days of William the Conqueror, Burnet writes:

Every one speaks the Language he heard his Parents, his Nurses, and others about him speak, when he was a Child. . . . Upon which, a man of wit and phancy might say a great many things, to shew it impossible any such change should ever have been made, as that we now should speak so as not to understand what was said five or six hundred years ago. Yet if I find *Chaucer*, or any other much ancienter Book, so written, that I can hardly make a shift to understand it, from thence, without any further reasoning how this could be brought about, I naturally must conclude our Language is altered. (117)

Other editions: B5862 (1679), no UMI; B5863 (1687), 45.

502.   COLES, ELISHA. *An English Dictionary.* C5070. UMI 1122: 3a.

Coles (1640?–1680) is identified on the title page as a "School-Master and Teacher of the Tongue to Foreigners." As Spurgeon notes (1: 252 and 3: 4.77), he cites Chaucer in his epistle addressed "To the Reader." Coles writes:

I have not only retain'd, but very much augmented the number of Old Words. . . . Those that I call Old Words are generally such as occurr in *Chaucer, Gower, Pierce Ploughman* and *Julian Barnes.* (sig. A3v)

Coles defines *Dennington* and notes the connection to Chaucer:

Dennington, a Castle in *Berks*, once the residence of Chaucer. (sig. K2r)

In his brief definition of *At Dulcarnon*, Coles also cites Chaucer and alludes to *Troilus and Criseyde*, 3. 931, 933:

At Dulcarnon, in a maze, at my wits end, *Chaucer, 1.3. fol. 161.* (sig. L3r)

And finally, in a section slightly garbled alphabetically:

Granson, a French Poet whom *Chaucer* translates. (sig. P4v)

Other editions: C5071 (1677), sigs. A3r, K2r, L3r, P4v; C5072 (1684), sigs. A3r, K2r, L3r, P4v; C5073 (1685), sigs. A3r, K2r, L3r, P4v; C5074 (1692), sigs. A3r, K2r, L3r, P4v; C5075 (1696), sigs. A3r, H4r, I4v, N1v.

503.   DARE, JOSIAH. *Counsellor Manners, His Last Legacy to His Son: Enriched and Embellished.* D247A. UMI 1809: 18.

For a paraphrase of a couplet from *The Wife of Bath's Tale* and a precis of an incident related by Chauntecleer in *The Nun's Priest's Tale*, see DARE (1673); in this edition, the passages are found on 3–4, 144–45.

504.   A FRIEND OF THE AUTHOR. "Commentary" in Walter Pope's *The Salsbury-Ballad.* P2915A. UMI 2037: 8.

This broadside ballad was written in praise of the River Avon and Salisbury (the city, cathedral, and bishop), and it is furnished with a learned commentary by "a friend to the authors memory." Spurgeon (1.329) cites a reprint of 1713 and attributes authorship to John Oldmixon, albeit with a query. The balladeer is taken to task for being unproductive in the fourteenth stanza of the first part; he takes issue and uses an expression which the commentator attributes to Chaucer:

> But when will this paltry Poet begin,
>> And shew us a touch of his Art?
> With a cup of old Sack, he'l wind up his Jack,
>> And twang it I' th' Second part.

Jack is marked for a shoulder note, and the commentator attributes a couplet to Chaucer: "His Engin wherewith he makes verses; so *Chaucer, As winding up makes a Jack go, so good wine makes good verses flow.*"

505.   G., R. *Ludus scacchiæ. A Satyr Against Unjust Wars.* L3471B. UMI 2212: 11

For a reference to *Troilus and Criseyde* and a note about the meaning of *dulcarnon*, see G., R. (1675); in this edition, the passage is found on 13.

506.   HARRIS, JOHN. *The Divine Physician.* H861A. UMI 534: 2.

Harris (1667?–1719) is identified on the title page as "J. H. M.A." In a commendatory poem headed "The Author to his Book," there is a faint echo of Chaucer's line, "Go, litel bok, go litel myn tragedye" (*Troilus and Criseyde* 5: 1786):

> Go little Book, and try thy fortune where
> More good thou may'st, for least thou can'st do here:
> Whil'st to a private shelf thou art confin'd,
> Thou as to publick good art still behind,
> Then venture forth, and freely shew thy kill,
> In curing such as shall thy Rules fulfil. (sig. A8v)

Another edition in 1676: H861B (UMI 2403: 16), sig. A8v.

507.   LE FÈVRE, RAOUL. *The Destruction of Troy.* L931. UMI 604: 14; UMI 1781: 8 (book 3 identified as L940).

For two references to *Troilus and Criseyde*, see LE FÈVRE (1475) in Boswell & Holton No. 1; in this edition, the first reference to Chaucer's renaming Breseyda is omitted, but the second passage commending *Troilus and Criseyde* to readers is found in book 3, chapter 15, on 367.

508. MASON, JOHN. *Mentis humanae metamorphosis: sive conversio, The History of the Young Converted Gallant.* M916. UMI 283: 9.

Mason (*fl.* 1676–1683) is identified on the title page as "J. Mason Gent. of Fordham in Cambridge-shire." Under the heading "Concerning Religious Pride and Gallantry," he appears to echo Chaucer's description of the Clerk in *The General Prologue*: "And gladly wolde he lerne and gladly teche" (line 308). In a passage giving advice to sectarians, he writes:

> And so 'twixt right and wrong the truth discern
> And gladly teach, and gladly also learn. (133)

509. *Poor Robin, 1676. An Almanack After a New Fashion.* A2195. UMI 1221: 12.

Under the heading "Observations on April": "Patient Grizel" is celebrated on the 6th of this month (sig. A8r); this is perhaps an allusion to the protagonist of *The Clerk's Tale*.

510. *Poor Robins Intelligence.* Nelson and Seccombe 548.212. Early English Newspapers 24: 1177.

In the issue covering events from 28 November through 5 December 1676, there is a reference to Chaucer and an allusion to the *Miller's Tale*:

> Whereas a Certain Astrologer, or Astrologers of the Western Climate (perhaps in imitation of the Fryer in *Chaucer*, who Predicted a Deluge, and wheadled a Silly Carpenter to build an Ark fro his Preservation, only with a design (in the meantime) to Cuckold him; have lately threatned the world with a Strange Monster. (sig. Mm1v)

511. RAMSAY (or RAMESEY), WILLIAM. *The Gentlemans Companion.* R207. UMI 1238: 3.

For a recommendation of Chaucer's books for a gentleman's diversion, see RAMSAY (1672); in this expanded edition, the passage is found on 132.

512. S., W., in John Bullokar's *An English Expositor: Teaching the Interpretation of the Hardest Words Used in Our Language.* B5432. UMI 1351: 8.

For a reference to Chaucer and *The Prologue to the Squire's Tale* in the definition of Chivancy, see S., W. (1654); in this edition, the passage is found on sig. B12r.

For a reference to Chaucer and allusion to *The Nun's Priest's Tale*, see S., W. (1663); in this edition, the passage is found on sig. B11r.

513.   SHAKESPEARE, WILLIAM. *The Tragedy of Hamlet Prince of Denmark.* S2950. UMI 297: 41.

For verbal parallels and contextual similarities that may indicate the influence of *The Legend of Good Women* and *The Monk's Tale*, see SHAKESPEARE (1604), Boswell & Holton No. 693.

Another edition in 1676: S2951.

Other editions: S2952 (1683); S2954 (1695); S2955 (1695).

514.   SPARROW, ANTHONY. *A Rationale upon the Book of Common Prayer of the Church of England.* S4833. UMI 514: 15.

For a reference to Chaucer as a likely source for the word *ember*, see SPARROW 1668); in this edition, the passage is found on sig. S3r.

1677

515.   BRAMHALL, JOHN. *The Works of John Bramhall.* Dublin. B4211. UMI 759: 28.

For a reference to Chaucer's portrayal of "the greediness and extortion of the Court of Rome" in the "Plowmans tale and elsewhere" (allusions to *The Canterbury Tales* and the spurious work known as Chaucer's *Ploughman's Tale*), see BRAMHALL (1654); in this edition, the passage is found on 93.

For a reference to Chaucer and an allusion to the Frere in *The General Prologue*, see BRAMHALL (1661); in this edition, the passage is found on 974.

516.   CLEVELAND, JOHN. *Clievelandi vindiciae: or, Cleveland's Genuine Poems, Orations, Epistles, &c.* C4669.

For an echo of a line in *The Manciple's Prologue*, see CLEVELAND (1644); in this collection, the passage is found on 67.

For a reference to Chaucer and an allusion to *The Pardoner's Prologue*, see CLEVELAND (1658); in this collection, the passage is found on 124.

Variant title pages: C4670 (1677), 67, 124; C4671 (1677), 67, 124.

517.   COLES, ELISHA. *An English Dictionary.* C5071. UMI 450: 27.

For references to Chaucer in Coles's epistle to the reader and in various definitions, see COLES (1676); in this edition, the passages are found on sigs. A3r, K2r, L3r, P4v.

518.   COOPER, WILLIAM. *Catalogus variorum & insignium librorum.* K422. UMI 944: 9.

Cooper began auctioning the library of Thomas Kidner, rector of Hitchin in Hertfordshire on 6 February 1677. In the catalogue, under the heading "English in Folio," lot 82 is listed as *"Chaucer's (Geffry)* Works. *London.* First Edition" (3).

519.   FLECKNOE, RICHARD. *Seventy Eight Characters.* F1234. UMI 184: 20.

Flecknoe (d. 1678?) is not named on the title page. He cites Chaucer and quotes (more or less) his description of the Sergeant of Law from *The General Prologue* (lines 321–22). In his characterization "Of a Busie Body," Flecknoe writes:

> He is too Busie a Body to have any head for business, yet he will have a hand in every thing. Chaucer seems to have Prophesied of him long since, when he said,
>
> > *A busier Man there nas,*
> > *And yet he seem'd more busie than he was.* (sig. G3v)

520.   LLOYD, DAVID. *Memoires of the Lives, Actions, Sufferings & Deaths of Those Noble, Reverend and Excellent Personages that Suffered by Death, Sequestration, Decimation, or Otherwise, for the Protestant Religion.* L2643. UMI 2127: 14.

For an echo a line from *The Reeve's Tale*, see LLOYD (1668); in this edition, the passage is found on 390.

521.   LOVEDAY, ROBERT. *Loveday's Letters Domestick and Forrein.* L3229B. UMI 1797: 31.

For a reference to Chaucer as a prophet and poet, perhaps an allusion to the spurious work known as "Chaucer's Prophecy," see LOVEDAY (1659); in this edition, the passage is found on 98–99.

522.   PLOT, ROBERT. *The Natural History of Oxford-Shire.* P2585. UMI 2625: 21

Plot (1640–1697) is identified on the title page as "Robert Plot, Doctor of Laws." As Spurgeon notes (1: 252), he discusses Chaucer's association with Woodstock. In a section about extraordinary echoes, Plot writes:

> As for *Polysyllabical articulate Echo's*, the strongest and best I have met with here, is in the Park at *Woodstock*, which in the day time, little wind being stirring, returns very distinctly seventeen syllables, and in the night twenty. . . . The object of which *Echo*, or the *Centrum phono-campticum*, I take to be the hill with the trees on the *summit* of it, about half a mile distant from *Woodstock* town . . . And the true place of the

Speaker, or *Centrum phonicum*, the opposite Hill just without the gate
at the Towns end, about thirty paces directly below the corner of a wall
inclosing some hay-ricks, near *Chaucers* house. . . . (7–8).

This work features an engraving that graphically illustrates the phenomenon of
echoes in general and in particular the one at Woodstock. The artist has rendered a vista that depicts the manor house of Woodstock in the distance, the
village church tower on the left, and Chaucer's house centered in the foreground.
The substantial two-storey house appears to be situated at the edge of town and
is surrounded by a garden wall. A guide identifies five of the geographical features in the illustration; item "C" is "Chaucers house" (following 16).
    Another edition in 1677: P2686, same pagination.

523.   POOLE, JOSUA. *The English Parnassus: or, A Help to English Poesie.* **P2815.
UMI 191: 11.**

For a reference to Chaucer in a bibliography of "Books principally made use of
in the compiling of this Work," see POOLE (1657); in this edition, the reference
is found on 33.

524.   *Poor Robin, 1677. An Almanack After a New Fashion.* A2196. UMI 1494: 22.

Under the heading "Observations on April": "Patient Grizel" is celebrated on
the 25th of this month (sig. A8r); this is perhaps an allusion to the protagonist
of *The Clerk's Tale.*

**525.   *Poor Robins Intelligence.* Nelson and Seccombe 248.411. Early English
Newspapers 24: 1177.**

In the issue covering events for 9–16 October 1677, a short prose narrative is
called a Canterbury tale, possibly an allusion to the *Canterbury Tales*. In a smug
little story from "Flint-shire," the writer fairly chortles over the "just desserts" of
one who dared to reach above his station in life. A "Worthy man of Art, vulgarly
dignified and distinguished by the Title of a Water-caster" is introduced by his
employer, a "merry gentleman," to a woman with a fortune of several thousand
pounds. Convinced of his own merit, the workman proposes marriage and is
quickly accepted. The lady, however, sees him as a crass adventurer and substitutes her serving woman as the bride.

[I]nstead of the *Weighty Heiress* he expected, 'twas quickly discovered
that he had tyed himself to a *Close-stool Caster*, whose Revenues . . .
reach'd no further than a Water-Mill, and a Wind-Mill, conveniently
supply'd with Sails of *Farrendine*; A Matrimonial Dose, 'tis confest
somewhat *bitter*, but very proper for cureing the Flatulent Tumours
of Ambitious Insolence, how it may agree with his Stomach we know

not, for we heard it onely as a *Canterbury* Tale, and so we leave it. (sig. L1111v)

A water-caster was a medical practitioner whose speciality was diagnosis through close examination of urine. Farrendine or farandine is cloth made from silk and wool.

526.   SANFORD, FRANCIS. *A Genealogical History of the Kings of England.* S651. UMI 510: 9.

Sanford (1630–1694) is identified on the title page as "Francis Sandford Esq; Lancaster herald of arms." As Harris notes (*PQ*), in book 5, chapter 4, section 13, in a passage about marriages of the Yorkist nobility, he mentions a Chaucerian connection. Sanford writes:

> *Elizabeth* of York . . . second daughter of *Richard* Duke of *York* and *Cecily Nevil*, was espoused to *John de la Pole* Duke of *Suffolke* (son of *William* Duke of *Suffolke*, by *Alice* his Wife, daughter and heir of Sir *Thomas Chaucer* Kt. son of Sir *Geoffry Chaucer* the famous *English* Poet, buried at *Westminster*). . . . (378–79)

Another edition: S651A (1683), 378–79.

527.   TREVERS, JOSEPH. *An Essay to the Restoring of Our Decayed Trade.* T2130. UMI 1216: 18.

For an echo of Chaucer's line, "Go, litel bok, go litel myn tragedye" (*Troilus and Criseyde* 5: 1786), see TREVERS (1675); in this edition, the passage is found on sig. a2v.

1678

528.   COOPER, WILLIAM. *Catalogus variorum & insignium librorum.* G942. UMI 916: 8.

Cooper began auctioning the libraries of John Godolphin (1617–1678, a civil lawer) and Owen Phillips on 11 November. In a group of philological works in folio, lot 44 is listed as "Geffry Chancers [*sic*] works, with his Progeny, Life, and the Explanat. Of the hard words — 1598" (sig. f2v); and lot 101 as "Geffry Chaucers Translation of Boetius de Consolatione Philosophiæ, in English, and Printed by William Caxton" (sig. g1r).

529.   COWLEY, ABRAHAM. *The Works of Mr. Abraham Cowley.* C6653. UMI 1421: 7.

For a reference to Cowley's burial place near Chaucer, see SPRAT (1668); in this edition, the passage is found on sig. c4r–v.

For a reference to Chaucer's "rich rhymes," see COWLEY (1656); in this edition, the passage is found on 37 (sig. Aa1r).

530.   DELONEY, THOMAS. *The Garland of Good-Will.* D946. UMI 350: 8.

For what may be a faint allusion to *The Clerk's Tale*, see DELONEY (1628) in Boswell & Holton No. 1116. In this edition, the passage is found in the second part, where number 2 is headed "Of Patient *Grissel* and a Noble *Marquess*" (sigs. E7r–F2v).

531.   DUNMORE, JOHN, and RICHARD CHISWELL. *Catalogus librorum in quavis lingua.* W3612. UMI 2122: 10.

The booksellers Dunmore and Chiswell began auctioning the books of Dr. Benjamin Worsley (1617/18–1677) "at the House over against the Hen and Chickens in Pater Noster Row" on 13 May 1678. Although the title page of the catalogue announces the sale of Dr. Worsley's books only, an epistle addressed to the reader notes that there are "three entire Libraries" up for sale, "which for the more ease and satisfaction of all Buyers, we have drawn up Alphabetically." The booksellers add an interesting note intended to inspire confidence in prospective buyers:

> [F]orasmuch as a Report has been spread, that we intend to use indirect means to advance the Prices, we do affirm that it is a groundless and malicious suggestion of some of our own Trade, not well pleased with our Undertaking: and that to avoid all manner of suspicion of such practice, we have absolutely refused all manner of Commissions that have been offered us for buying (some of them without limitation:) And do declare, that the Company shall have nothing but candid and ingenuous dealing from John Dunmore, Richard Chiswel. (sig. A2v)

In the second part of the catalogue, under the heading "English in Folio" lot 67 is listed as "*Chaucer's* (*Jeff.*) Works of Poetry. 1602" (sig. Aa1v).

532.   FLAVEL, JOHN. *Husbandry Spiritualized: or, The Heavenly Use of Earthly Things.* F1167.

For an echo of a line from *The Reeve's Prologue*, see FLAVEL (1669); in this edition, the passage is found on 259.

533. PHILLIPS, EDWARD. *The New World of Words: or, A General English Dictionary.* P2072. UMI 395: 24.

For a pictorial representation of Chaucer and for references to him in the preface, see PHILLIPS (1658), (1662), and (1671); in this revised edition, these are found on the engraved title page and sig. a2v. This edition has a different dedication that has no reference to Chaucer. Chaucer is mentioned in definitions of *Advenale* (sig. A4v), *Amalgaminge* (sig. C1v), *Amortize* (sig. C2r), *Arblaster* (sig. D3r), *Arretteth* (sig. E1r), *Arten* (sig. E1r), *Assoyle* (sig. E2r), *Asterlagour* (sig. E2v), *Autremite* (sig. E4v), *Barm-cloth* (sig. F2r), *Bay* (sig. F3r), *Bend* (sig. F4r), *Burnet* (sig. H1rBv), *Caitisned* (sig. H2v), *Chasteleyn* (sig. K2r), *Chekelaton* (sig. K2r), *Chelandri* (sig. K2r), *Chertes* (sig. K2r), *Chevesal* (sig. K2v), *Chimbe* (sig. K2v), *Chincery* (sig. K2v, spelled *Chincherie* in previous editions), *Cierges* (sig. K3v), *Citriale* (sig. K4v), *Clergion* (sig. L1r), *Clicket*, (sig. L1r), *Clinke* (sig. L1r), *Curebulli* (sig. N4r), *Desidery* (sig. P1r), *Deslavy* (sig. P1r), *Digne* (sig. P3r), *Discure* (sig. P4r), *Divine* (sig. Q1r), *Dowtremere* (sig. Q2v), *Ebrack* (sig. Q4r), *Gibsere* (sig. X1r), *Giglet* (sig. X1r), *Gourd* (sig. X2v), *Haketon* (sig. Y1r), *Hanselines* (sig. Y1v), *Jewise* (sig. Aa2r), *Losenger* (sig. Ff1r), *Magonel* (sig. Ff3v), see *Mangin* (really *Mangon*) (sig. Ff4v), *Rebeck* (sig. Qq2r), *Woodstock* (sig. Bbb1v).

In this revised edition, there are at least three new definitions with references to Chaucer:

To *Fonne*, (old word used by *Chaucer*) to be foolish. (sig. T4r)

Miswoman, (*old word* used by *Chaucer*) a Whore. (sig. Hh2v)

A *Pander*, one that procureth the hire of a Strumpet, a Bawd, or Pimp. The word signifies in *Dutch* taker of Pawns or Pledges, from whence we use it in a signification somewhat varied; unless *Skinners* conjecture please better, who is willing to deduce it from *Pandarus* the friend of *Troilus*, and by whose procurement he obtained the love of *Chryseis*. (sig. Mm1r)

Another edition in 1678: P2072A in which pagination differs from P2072. Chaucer references are found on the engraved title page, in the preface (sig. a2v), and in definitions of *Advenale* (sig. A4v), *Amalgaminge* (sig. C1v), *Amortize* (sig. C2r), *Arblaster* (sig. D3r), *Arret* (not spelled *Arretteth* in this edition) (sig. E1r), *Arten* (sig. E1r), *Assoyle* (sig. E2r), *Asterlagour* (sig. E2v), *Barm-cloth* (sig. F2r), *Bay* (sig. F3r), *Bend* (sig. F4r), *Burnet* (sig. H1r-v), *Caitisned* (sig. H2v), *Chasteleyn* (sig. K2r), *Chekelaton* (sig. K2r), *Chelandri* (sig. K2r), *Chertes* (sig. K2r), *Chevesal* (sig. K2v), *Chimbe* (sig. K2v), *Chincherie* (sig. K2v), *Cierges* (sig. K3v), *Citriale* (sig. K4v), *Clergion* (sig. L1r), *Clicket*, (sig. L1r), *Clinke* (sig. L1r), *Curebulli* (sig. N4r), *Dennington* (sig. O4r), *Desidery* (sig. P1r), *Deslavy* (sig. P1r), *Digne* (sig. P3r), *Dis-*

cure (sig. P4r), *Divine* (sig. Q1r), *Dowtremere* (sig. Q1v), *Ebrack* (sig. Q4r), *Fonne* (sig. T4r), *Gibsere* (sig. X1r), *Giglet* (sig. X1r), *Gourd* (sig. X2v), *Haketon* (sig. Y1r), *Hanselines* (sig. Y1v), *Jewise* (sig. Aa2r), *Losenger* (sig. Ff1r), *Mangon* or *Mangonel* (sig. Ff4v), *Miswoman* (sig. Hh3v), *Pander* (sig. Mm1r), *Rebeck* (sig. Qq2r), *Wood-stock* (sig. Bbb1v).

534.   PHILLIPS, JOHN. *Maronides: or, Virgil Travesty.* P2092. UMI 1675: 19.

For a reference to Chaucer placed in a glittering constellation of poets both ancient and modern in Elysium, see PHILLIPS (1673); in this edition, the passage is found on ²109.

535.   POOLE, JOSUA. *English Parnassus: or, A Help to English Poesie.* P2816. No UMI.

For a reference to Chaucer in a bibliography of "Books principally made use of in the compiling of this Work," see POOLE (1657).

536.   *Poor Robin, 1678. An Almanack After a New Fashion.* A2197. UMI 1414: 36.

Under "Observations on April": "Patient Grizel" is celebrated on the 28th of this month (sig. A8r), perhaps an allusion to *The Clerk's Tale.*

In the prognostications for the winter quarter, the writer quotes *The Romaunt of the Rose* (lines 71–72):

The days now be short, and the weather cold, the fields fruitless, trees leaveless, and Birds songless, as that great Astrologer *Don Chaucer* saith,

The Byrdes that had left her songe,
While they had suffred colde full stronge. (sig. C5v)

537.   RAY, JOHN. *A Collection of English Proverbs.* R387. UMI 774: 18.

For an echo of a line from *The Reeve's Tale,* see RAY (1670); in this edition, the pasage is found on 114.

For an echo of aline from *The Wife of Bath's Prologue,* see RAY (1670); in this edition, the pasage is found on 169.

For an echo of a line from *The Manciple's Prologue,* see RAY (1670); in this edition, the passage is found on 280.

For a reference to Chaucer as "our English Ennius" and a paraphrase of a couplet from *The Prologue to The Cook's Tale,* see RAY (1670); in this edition, the passage is found on 315.

In this augmented edition, there are other references.

In a section headed "Entire Sentences," Ray appears to echo lines from *The Reeve's Prologue,* "To have a hoor head and a green tayl, | As hath a leek" (lines 3878–79) when he comments on the proverb "Grey and green make the worst medley." He writes, "An old lecher is compared to an onyon, or leek, which hath a white head but a green tail" (149).

In a section headed "Proverbial Similies," Ray echoes a line from *The Manciple's Prologue*: "Sires, what! Dun is in the myre!" (line 5); he writes "As dull as dun in the mire" (280).

Smith (*SP* 28) cites this edition rather than the edition of 1670 as he notes another reference. In a section headed "Proverbs communicated by Mr. Andrew Paschall of Chedsey in Somersetshire,[34] which came not to hand till the copy of this Edition was delivered to the Bookseller, and so could not be referred to in their proper places," Ray attributes a proverb to Chaucer:

> *He that hath more smocks then shirts in a bucking,*[35] *had need be a man of good fore-looking.* Chaucer. (353)

538.   RYMER, THOMAS. *The Tragedies of the Last Age.* R2430. UMI 367: 18.

Rymer (1641–1713) is identified on the title page as "Thomas Rymer, of Grays-Inn, Esquire." In a discussion of *A King and No King*, he mentions "patient Grissel" and perhaps alludes faintly to *The Clerk's Tale*:

> We are let to know that the Queen-Mother was for removing the Usurper by poison, and for bringing all into the right channel agen. This we might expect to be a Woman *couragious*, and truly *Tragical*: yet we find her the veriest *patient Grissel* that ever was lain by a Monarch's side. (70)

Another edition: R2431 (1692), 70.

539.   SANDYS, GEORGE, trans. *Ovid's Metamorphosis Englished.* O688. UMI 1490: 13.

For an echo of the title of *The House of Fame*, see SANDYS (1628) in Appendix; in this edition, the passage is found on 232.

540.   TREVERS, JOSEPH. *An Essay to the Restoring of Our Decayed Trade.* T2130A.

For an echo of Chaucer's line, "Go, litel bok, go litel myn tragedye" (*Troilus and Criseyde* 5: 1786), see TREVERS (1675).

---

[34] Paschall: (1631?–1696), Church of England clergyman and advocate for a universal language. See A. J. Turner, *ODNB*.

[35] *Bucking*: washing.

541.   VOET, GISBERT. *Catalogus variorum librorum.* **V675. UMI 2537: 13.**

Among the works Voet offered for sale by auction of 25 November 1678, under the heading "English in Folio," lot 51 is listed as three works published in 1483 and bound together: "*Boethius de Consolatione* Englished [by Chaucer]. The Book of the Knight of the Tower. Æsop's Fables. *London.*" Lot 77 is listed as "Chaucer's (Geffrey) Works. 1602" (sig. Dd2v).

According to annotations in the catalogue, lot 51 went for 7*s* 10*d* and lot 77 for 19*s* 6*d*.

542.   WARD, NATHANIEL. "Commendatory verses" in Ann Bradstreet's *Several Poems.* **B4166. UMI 759: 15.**

For a reference to Chaucer (linked with Homer) in verses praising "the tenth muse" lately sprung up in New England, see WARD (1650); in this corrected and enlarged edition, the passage is found on sig. *a*4r.

543.   WEBB, JOHN. *The Antiquity of China: or, An Historical Essay Endeavoring a Probability That the Language of the Empire of China Is the Primitive Language.* **W1201. UMI 2377: 1.**

For a reference to the difficulty of Chaucer's language for contemporaries, see WEBB (1669); in this reissue, the passage is found on 39–40.

1679

544.   BAKER, RICHARD. *A Chronicle of the Kings of England.* **B507A. No UMI.**

For references to Chaucer as John of Gaunt's brother-in-law, "the Homer of our nation," his association with Woodstock, his translation of *The Romaunt of the Rose*, his burial place in Westminster, and his association with Gower, see BAKER (1653).

Other editions in 1679: B508, 132, 134, 155, 167, and sig. Hhhh4r; B508A, 132, 134, 155, 167, and sig. Hhhh4r.

545.   BAXTER, RICHARD. *Which Is the True Church?* **B1453. UMI 344: 7.**

In the third part, "A Defence of my Arguments to prove, That the Church of which the Protestants are members, hath been visible ever since the daies of Christ on Earth," Baxter (1615–1691) cites Chaucer in a group of writers critical of the Church of Rome. Baxter writes:

> My Eighth Proof of the Novelty of the Papal Sovereignty, was from Historical Testimony, that the Papal sovereignty was no part of the

Churches Faith, nor owned by the Ancients: This is done at large by . . .
Chaucer . . . and many other. (159)

546.   Brian, Thomas. *The Pisse-Prophet: or, Certaine Pisse-Pot Lectures.* B4438.
UMI 1725: 51.

For an echo of a line in *The Manciple's Prologue*, see Brian (1637) in the Appendix; in this edition, the passage is found on 46.

547.   Burnet, Gilbert. *A Conference Held at London.* B5862. No UMI.

For a reference to the difficulty of Chaucer's language for contemporary readers,
see Burnet (1676).

548.   C., H. *The Plain Englishman's Historian: or, A Compendious Chronicle of
England.* C45. UMI 1224: 16.

H. C. is characterized on the title page as a "Gent." In chapter 12, "King Edward
the Third," the author refers to Chaucer as "our English Homer":

> In his time lived Sir *Jeffery Chaucer,* our *English Homer,* who happily
> turn'd the Groves of *Woodstock* into the Banks of *Helicon.* (50)

549.   Cooper, William. *Catalogus librorum.* W1077. UMI 2558: 10.

Cooper began auctioning the libraries of the learned Stephen Watkins and
Thomas Sherley on 2 June 1679. In an appendix to the main catalogue, among
the works in folio, lot 104 is listed as "The Works of *Jeoffry Chaucer.* Wants the
end. [no date]" (sig. M1v).

550.   Croft, Herbert. *The Legacy of the Right Reverend Father in God, Herbert, Lord Bishop of Hereford, to His Diocess [sic]: or, A Short Determination of All
Controversies We Have with the Papists.* C6966. UMI 62: 2.

After a long flirtation with Roman Catholicism, Croft (1603–1691) returned
to the Church of England and rose steadily through the Church hierarchy for a
while, but he lost all his preferments during the Civil War and Commonwealth.
Afterwards, however, Charles II raised him to the bishopric of Hereford in 1661.

In the second sermon in this collection Croft uses as his text John 5:39:
"Search the Scriptures, for in them ye think ye have Eternal Life." In a paragraph
about the original languages of the Scriptures, he notes the difficulty of understanding the text and the evolution of English since Chaucer's time. Croft writes:

> Now many of the Primitive Fathers were either born, or much educated
> when those Languages [i.e., Hebrew, Syriac, and Greek] were naturally
> spoken; and thereby could much better judg [sic] of the propriety and

full signification of many words which we are much to seek in: and each Country Language hath several proverbial saying and antient forms of speech, which in process of time grow out of use and very hard to be understood: we see that very few now are able to understand old *Chaucers* Language, English being very much altered since. (34)

Another edition in 1679, *The Second Impression Corrected, with Additions by the Author*: C6967, 28–29.

551.   DRYDEN, JOHN. *Troilus and Cressida: or, Truth Found Too Late.* **D2388. UMI 208: 27; UMI 1382: 4; UMI 1440: 18.**

Dryden (1631–1700) is identified on the title page as "John Dryden servant to his Majesty." As Spurgeon notes (1: 254), he comments on the difficulty of Chaucer's language for Dryden's contemporaries. In the epistle dedicatory, Dryden writes:

It wou'd mortify an English man to consider, that from the time of *Boccace* and of *Petrarche*, the Italian has varied very little: And that the English of *Chaucer* their contemporary is not to be understood without the help of an Old *Dictionary*. (sig. A3v)

In "The Preface to the Play," Dryden mentions Chaucer again:

The Original story was Written by one Lollius *a* Lombard, *in Latin verse, and Translated by* Chaucer *into English: intended I suppose a Satyr on the Inconstancy of Women: I find nothing of it among the Ancients; not so much as the name once* Cressida *mention'd.* (sig. A4v)

Another edition in 1679: D2389 (UMI 688: 13), sig. A3v, A4v.
    Other editions: D2390 (1679 [*sic*], really 1692), sig. A3v, A4v; D2391 (1695), sig. A3v, A4v.
    Also collected in *The Works of Mr. John Dryden*: D2207 (1691), nineteenth work in volume; D2208 (1693), vol. 2; D2209 (1694), vol. 2; D2210 (1695), vol. 2.
    The Dramatick Works: D2211 (1695), vol. 2 (ninth work).

552.   DUNMORE, JOHN. *Bibliotheca Bissaeana: sive catalogus librorum.* **B6411. UMI 1351: 20.**

Dunmore offered the library of Sir Edward Bysshe for sale by auction on 15 November. In the sales catalogue, under the heading "English in Folio," lot 62 is listed as "Geff. Chaucer's Works of Ancient Poetry (best Edition). 1602" (sig. K1r).

553.   EVELYN, JOHN. *Sylva: or, A Discourse of Forest-trees. The Third Edition.* E3518. UMI 562: 1.

For a reference to Chaucer's Oak, one of several trees said to have been planted by Chaucer, see EVELYN (1664); in this edition, the passage is found on 166. Chaucer is also cited in the index, sig. f1v.

554.   G., E. "To the Author," in Martin Llewellyn's *Men Miracles.* L2627. UMI 1425: 25.

For a reference to Chaucer's "learned soul" and his influence on Spenser, see a commendatory poem by E. G., L2625 (1646); in this edition, the passage is found on sig. A4r.

555.   GUILLIM, JOHN. *A Display of Heraldry.* G2222. UMI 598: 19.

For quotations from *The Romaunt of the Rose*, a reference to Sir Payne Roet who is identified as Chaucer's father-in-law, a description of Chaucer's escutcheon, and a quotation from *The Knight's Tale*, see GUILLIM (1610) in Boswell & Holton No. 816; in this edition, the passages are found on 16, 215, 274, 310 and index.

In this expanded edition, there are others. In chapter 7, Guillim writes:

> What a Potent is, I have formerly shewed. . . . It may also be Blazoned a Cross crowche, for the resemblance that it hath of a Crutch, which *Chaucer* calleth a Potent, which is properly figetive. . . . (60)

Chaucer uses the term *potent* in *The Summoner's Tale* (line 1776), *Troilus and Criseyde* (5: 1222), and in *The Romaunt of the Rose* (lines 368 and 7415).

Moreover, Chaucer is listed in "An Alphabetical Table of the Names of the Nobility and Gentry Whose Coats are made Patterns of Bering in this Display of Heraldry" (sig. Aa2v).

556.   HALL, JOSEPH. *Contemplations upon the Remarkable Passages in the Life of the Holy Jesus.* H376. UMI 1463: 8.

Hall (1574–1656), identified on the title page as "late Lord Bishop of Excester," [*sic*] appears to echo a line from *The Reeve's Tale*: "The gretteste clerkes been noght wisest men" (line 4054). In a section headed "The Sages and the Star," he writes:

> Had these Sages met with the Shepherds in the villages near *Bethlehem*, they had received that intelligence of Christ which they did vainly seek from the learned Scribes of *Jerusalem*. The greatest Clerks are not alwaies the wisest in the affairs of God. (27)

557.   HOLLES, DENZIL. *A Letter to a Gentleman to His Friend, Shewing That the Bishops Are Not To Be Judges in Parliament in Cases Capital.* H2461A. UMI 1673: 3.

Baron Holles (1599–1680) alludes to *The Summoner's Tale* in a passage about an inconsistency in an argument about the role of bishops in criminal trials:

> How then can they say, we will have no part in condemning him? Is not this something like the Frier in *Chaucer*, that would have, *of a Capon the Liver, of a Pig the Head, yet would that nothing for him should be dead*: So they forsooth will take upon them to Judge his Pardon to be no Pardon, which brings on infallibly his condemnation, and yet say with that Frier, God forbid he should die for us, That we should have any hand in his bloud. . . . (66)

Other editions in 1679: H2461aA, 66; H2461.

558.   HOWELL, WILLIAM. *Medulla historiæ Anglicanæ. Being a Comprehensive History of the Lives and Reigns of the Monarchs of England.* H3139a. UMI 1690: 6

As Spurgeon notes (1: 254), under the running head "Richard II," Howell (1631 /32–1683) mentions Chaucer in the same breath as a knight who was famous for feats of arms:

> Now flourished Sir *John Hawkwood*, whose Chivalry had made him renowned through the Christian World. Sir *Geoffry Chaucer*, Poet-*Law-reat*, now also lived. (241)

Another edition in 1679: H3140, 241.
  Other editions: H3140a (1681), 249; H3141 (1683), 249; H3142 (1687), 176; H3142a (1694), 164.

559.   MASON, MARGERY, pseud. *The Tickler Tickled: or, The Observator Upon the Late Tryals of Sir George Wakeman, &c. Observed.* T1159. UMI 401: 10. [Harris]

As Harris notes (*PQ*), the narrator (described on the title page as "Spinster") attributes a quotation to Chaucer, really a paraphrase of *The Cook's Tale* (lines 4421–42). She says she began her life in service with a "Beautiful Lady of Great Quality about Court, as Superintendant of her Limbecks, Preserving-Pans, and Washes." For a while all goes well, but eventually she decides to leave service and go into business for herself:

> I thought fit to retire whilst I had some Money, and Beauty left; so accordingly did, into *Chancery*-Lane, turn'd Sempstress: where

> — *Shop I keep for Countenance*
> *But* — *is my Sustenance*. Chaucer.

And now having a little knack in Book-learning, I diverted myself this dead Vacation time with reading . . . . (1; sig. A2r)

Another edition in 1679: T1159aA.

560. PHILLIPS, EDWARD. *Tractatulus de carmine dramatico poëtrum veterum* in Johann Buchler's *Sacrarum prosanarumque phrasium poeticarum thesarurus.* B5305. UMI 1521: 21.

For references to Chaucer who thrived in the time of Petrarch, Gower, Hoccleve, Churchyard, and Lydgate, see PHILLIPS (1669); in this edition, the passage is found on 395.

561. *Poor Robin 1679. An Almanack of the Old and New Fashion.* A2198. UMI 1393: 5.

Under the heading "Observations on April": "Patient Grizel" is celebrated on the 28th of this month (sig. A8r); this is perhaps an allusion to the protagonist of *The Clerk's Tale.*

562. SPENSER, EDMUND. *The Works of That Famous English Poet.* S4965. UMI 77: 7.

For references and allusions to Chaucer, see Boswell & Holton No. 384. For a likely allusion to *The Squire's Tale* in *The Shepheardes Calender*, see SPENSER (1579) in the Appendix.

563. "A Summary of the Life" in *The Works of that Famous English Poet, Mr. Edmond Spenser.* S4965. UMI 77: 7.

In "A Summary of the Life of Mr. Edmond Spenser" (by an unknown hand, but sometimes attributed to Dryden) there is a reference to Spenser's burial near Chaucer:

> In this ill posture of his Affairs he return'd into *England*, where he his losses redoubled by the loss of his generous Friend Sir *Philip Sidney*; And thus, yielding to the impressions of a Fortune obstinately adverse to him, he died, without the help of any other Disease save a broken Heart; and was *Buried* in the Collegiate Church at *Westminster*, near the renowned *Chaucer* (as himself desired) at the Charge of the most Noble *Robert Earl of Essex*, in the year 1596. (sig. A1v)

564. *A Wife for a Husband, and a Husband for a Wife*: or, *A Popish Priest Turn'd Match-Maker Between a Knight and a Gentlewoman of Pretended Great Fortune, but Proved Otherwise*. W2094. UMI 950: 28.

The unknown writer of three short cautionary tales begins the first one (which gives its title to the whole tract) with a reference to Chaucer and *The Summoner's Tale*, from which he quotes somewhat garbled lines 1675–98:

> In the first place hear what Sir *Geffrey Chaucer* sayes in his Prologue
> before his *Sumpners Tale*, written about 300 years agone.

> Pardon ye have oft time heard tell
> How that a Frere ravished was to Hell;
> In Spirite once was by a Vision,
> And as an Angel led him up and doun
> To shew him the pains that there were,
> In all the place saw he not a Frere
> Of other Folke he sawe mow in two
> Unto the Angel spake the Frere tho
> Now Sir quoth he, have Freres soche a Grace
> That none of them shall come into this place?
> Yes quoth this Angel many a Millioun,
> And unto Sathanas ladde he him doun,
> And now hath Sathanas soche a Taile,
> Broder than of a Carike is the Saile
> Hold up thy taile thou Sathanas (quoth he)
> Shewe forth thine Erse, let the Frere se
> Where is the Nest of Freres in this place,
> And er that half a Forlong waie of space
> (Right as Bees swarmen out of an Hive)
> Out of the Devilles Erse they gan to drive
> Twentie thousande Freres on a rout
> And throughout Hell swarmed all about
> And come in again as fast as they were gone
> And into his Erse they crepten everie eak one. (3; sig. A2r)

565. WOODFORD, SAMUEL. *A Paraphrase upon the Canticles*. B2632A. UMI 783: 26; UMI 808: 13.

Woodford (1636–1700) is identified on the title page as "Samuel Woodford. D.D." As Alderson & Henderson note, Woodford notes the change in the English language since the days of Chaucer. In the preface, in a passage in praise of Milton's *Paradise Lost*, he writes:

[A]*s* Mr. Driden [*sic*] *has very well observed*, . . . "[*Paradise Lost* is] one of the greatest, most noble and most sublime Poems, take it altogether, which either this Age, or Nation has produced." *Nay, that it shall live as long as there are Men left in our* English *World to read, and understand it; and that many Ages hence translated into what-ever speech we shall be then changed (for changing we have been from* Chaucer's *time downward with a Witness, however it be call'd Refining) that shall survive the Language, wherein it stands written, and therein it self.* (sig. c3r)

Under the running head "Rimes," in an ode, "The Voyage," the protagonist is brought into the temple of his muse where "in Niches, on the Wall, | There did the lively Forms appear, | Of such who for their Verse the Laurel Sert did wear." There is a reference to Chaucer in company with "fair Orinda," i.e., Kathryn Philips:

> Thither I turn'd mine Eye, and in the Throng
> Of Crowned Heads, translated there,
> Whose very Names to could would be too long,
> From *Chaucer* downwards, (tho some Ancienter there)
> The fair *Orinda* did appear. . . . (171; sig. L16r)

1680

566. *Bibliotheca Digbeiana.* D1421. UMI 1307: 17.

The libraries of Kenelm Digby (1603–1665) and George Digby, Earl of Bristol (1612–1677), were offered for sale by auction on 19 April 1680. In the catalogue, under the heading "English in Folio," number 33 was: "*Chaucer's (Geffry)* Works. Lond. 1597" (81). And in "Pamphlets in Quarto," number 68, a gathering of twenty-four works, included "*Chaucer's* Plough mans Tale with expositions" (120).

567. *Catalogus variorum librorum in selectissimis bibliothecis doctissimorum viorum.* S6031. UMI 1515: 12.

The libraries of five eminent men, Mr. Henry Stubbe of London, Dr. Dillingham of Oundle in Northamptonshire, Mr. Thomas Vincent of London, Mr. Cawton of Westminster, and Mr. John Dunton, were offered for sale by auction on 29 November 1680. In the catalogue, under the heading "English Books in Folio, Large," number 53 is listed as "Chaucer's works—1602" (²2).

568.   COWLEY, ABRAHAM. *The Works of Mr. Abraham Cowley.* C6654. UMI 888: 1.

For a reference to Cowley's burial place near Chaucer, see SPRAT (1668); in this edition, the passage is found on sig. c4r–v.

For a reference to Chaucer's "rich rhymes," see COWLEY (1656), C6683; in this edition, the passage is found on 37 (sig. Aa1r).

569.   DUGDALE, WILLIAM. *Origines juridiciales: or, Historical Memorials of the English Laws.* D2490. UMI 688: 21.

For a reference to *The Parson's Tale* and a quotation about the Manciple from *The General Prologue of The Canterbury Tales,* see DUGDALE (1666); in this edition, the passage is found on 136b, 137a, 145.

570.   D'URFEY, THOMAS. *The Virtuous Wife: or, Good Luck at Last. A Comedy.* D2790. UMI 275: 18.

D'Urfey (1653–1723) was a prolific playwright whose plays were frequently panned by the critics but were very popular with audiences. In the prologue of this comedy (first acted by "His Royal Highness His Servants" at the Duke's Theater), one of the characters calls another "a Pimp, a Pandarus of Troy" (sig. A3v), possibly an allusion to *Troilus and Criseyde.*

571.   LE FÈVRE, RAOUL. *The Destruction of Troy.* L932. UMI 1953: 8 (book 3 as L941).

For two references to *Troilus and Criseyde,* see LE FÈVRE (1475) in Boswell & Holton No. 1; in this edition, the first reference to Chaucer's renaming Breseyda is omitted, but the second passage commending *Troilus and Criseyde* to readers is found in book 3, chapter 15, on 367.

572.   LITTLEBURY, ROBERT. *Catalogus bibliothecæ illustrissimi domini Gulielmi Ducie Vicecomitis Duni.* D2079. UMI 2847: 22.

Littlebury, a bookseller in London, published a catalogue of the library of William Ducie, first viscount Downe, and indicated that volumes might be purchased at his shop in Little Britain. In the catalogue, under the heading "English Books in Folio" he lists "Geffrey Chauce's Works. London 1602" (20).

573.   MILLINGTON, EDWARD. *Catalogus variorum librorum.* W1100D. UMI 2628: 27.

Millington began auctioning the library of Thomas Watson (M.A., "scholæ suttonianæ apud Charter-House, Londini nuperrime archididaschali") on 8 October 1680 at the Sign of the Lamb in Cornhill. In the catalogue, under the heading "Divinity, History, Philosophy, Poetry, &c. English In Folio," lot no. 28 is listed as "Chaucer's (Geffery [*sic*]) Works (*wanting the beginning, first Edit.*) [no date]" (18). Watson also owned copies of Katherine Phillips's poems, Spenser's *Shepherds Kalender* (1656), Milton's poems (1673), and Herbert's *Sacred Poems* (1674), along with countless theological works.

574. MILLINGTON, EDWARD. *Catalogus variorum librorum.* **S6031. UMI 1515: 12.**

Millington scheduled an auction beginning on 29 November 1680 at a house in Warwick Lane. He was selling off the libraries of "D. Hen. Stubb Nuperrime Londinensis" and "D. Dillinghami de Oundle Northamptoniensis" and "D. Thomæ Vincent Londinensis" and "D. Cautom Westmonsteriensis" and "Viri Johannis Duntoni" (title page). In the catalogue, under the heading "English Books in Folio, large," he lists lot 53 as "Chaucer's works — 1602" (32).

575. NABBES, THOMAS. *The Muse of New-market: or, Mirth and Drollery.* **M1869 and M3139. UMI 945: 20.**

In a farce "acted before the King and court at New-market," Nabbes (1605?–1645?) appears to echo the description of the Wife of Bath in *The General Prologue,* "For she koude of that art the olde daunce" (line 476). In *Love Lost in the Dark: or, The Drunken Couple,* he writes:

> My friend *Camillo* here's an Ass; what a Devil has he to do with Virgin Honour? when he should speak to the purpose, of the delight to meet in the old Dance between a pair of sheets, my Granam calls it the peopling of the World. (23)

Nabbes is closely following MASSINGER (1655), q.v.

576. *Poor Robin 1680. An Almanack after a New Fashion.* A2199. UMI 856: 5.

Under the heading "Observations on April": "Patient Grizel" is celebrated on the 25th of this month (sig. A8r); this is perhaps an allusion to the protagonist of *The Clerk's Tale.*

577. S., W., in John Bullokar's *An English Expositor: Teaching the Interpretation of the Hardest Words Used in Our Language.* **B5433. UMI 1844: 9.**

For a reference to Chaucer and *The Prologue to the Squire's Tale* in the definition of Chivancy, see S., W. (1654); in this edition, the passage is found on sig. B12r.

For a reference to Chaucer and allusion to *The Nun's Priest's Tale,* see S., W. (1663); in this edition, the passage is found on sig. B11r.

578.   SHADWELL, THOMAS. *The Woman-Captain. A Comedy.* S2887. UMI 400: 7.

Although he was sufficiently distinguished to be appointed poet laureate and historiographer royal, Shadwell (1642?–1692) is best remembered as the object of Dryden's satire in *Mac Fleknoe* and *Absalom and Achitophel.* As Graves notes (*SP*), at the end of the first act of *The Woman-Captain,* Gripe (a money lender) exults that he has attracted another prodigal who wishes to mortgage his property. Richard (his serving man) compliments his master as he refers to Gripe as "old Chaucer," i.e., a wise one:

> *Gripe.* See what becomes of foolish Sense-pleasers! Poor Puppies! Miserable Fools! I pity 'em: I'll not please one, not I
> *Richard*: Come, let's about this Business, and get my Lord to Seal.
> *Rich.* Well said, old *Chaucer,* say I.—
> 'Twould make one scratch where it does not itch,
> To see Fools live poor to dye rich. (12; sig. C2v)

Also found in Shadwell's *Works*: S2834 (1693), twelfth play, same pagination.

579.   STILLINGFLEET, EDWARD. *The Grand Question, Concerning the Bishops Right to Vote in Parlament* [sic] *in Cases Capital.* S5594. UMI 948: 15.

In the first chapter, "The Question stated; and general Prejudices removed," Bishop Stillingfleet (1635–1699) writing in response to a letter by an unnamed author (see HOLLES, 1679) cites Chaucer and alludes to *The Summoners Tale*:

> If the Bishops should give their Votes in the *Legislative* way to condemn a Person for Treason, and yet think they had not Voted in a *Case of Bloud*; they would then indeed be like *Chaucer's* Frier, mentioned by the *Authour* of the *Letter* [in a shoulder note: "Lett. *p.* 66"], that would have *of a Capon the Liver, and of a Pig the Head, yet would that nothing for him should be dead.* Doth a *Bill* of *Attainder* cut of [sic] a man's Head without making it a *Case* of *Bloud*? (4)

Another edition in 1680: S5594A .

580.   WINSTANLEY, WILLIAM. *The New Help to Discourse: or, Wit, Mirth, and Jollity, Intermixt with More Serious Matters.* W3070. UMI 2183: 5.

For references to and quotations from Chaucer, see WINSTANLEY (1668); in this edition the passages are found on 15–16, 165.

581.　WINSTANLEY, WILLIAM. *The Protestant Almanack.* A2224. UMI 1139: 12.

In "The Second Part," in a section headed "Brief Memorials of Popish Foppieries, believed by them as Sacred Oracles," in number 9, the almanac maker quotes from *The Summoners Tale* (lines 2099–106, 1839–42) and comments on Chaucer's fame:

> Now leave we the Bells and speak something of the *Fryers*; Our Ancient famous Poet *Geoffery Chaucer*, it seems was no great friend unto them, as appeareth in his *Canterbury-Tales*, where by the mouth of the *Sompner* he setteth them out in their proper colours, as where the *Fryer* perswading with the sick Farmer to make his Confession to him, rather than to his Parish Priest, having his hand upon his Half-peny, makes this request to the Bed-rid man lying upon his *Couch*.

> > Yeve me then of thy Gold to make our Cloister,
> > Quoth he, for many a Muskle and many an Oister,
> > When other men have been full well at ease
> > Hath been our Food: our Cloister for to rease,
> > And yet, God wot, unneath the Foundament
> > Performed is, ne of our Pavement
> > Is not a Tile; yet within our wones
> > By God we owen Fourty pound for stones.

And for their temperance in dyet, the same *Fryer* being asked of the Good-wife to stay and Dine, he tells her what a little would suffice him.

> > Have I of a Capon only the Liver,
> > And of your Whitebread but a shiver [*sic*],
> > And after that a roasted Pigshead,
> > For I would not for me no Beast were dead.

And in his Prologue to the *Sompners* Tale [lines 1675–98], he shews what becomes of Fryers at the last, which I shall give you in his own words.

> > Parde ye have often times heard tell,
> > How that a *Freere* ravished was to Hell,
> > In spirit once by a Vissyoun,
> > And as an Angel led him up and down,
> > To show him the pains that there were,
> > In all the place saw he not a *Freere*,
> > Of all other Folk he saw enough in wo;
> > Unto the Angel spake the *Freere* tho,

Now Sir quoth he, han *Freeres* such a grace,
That none of them shall come in this place,
Yes quoth the Angel, many a Millioun,
And unto *Sathanas* led he him down,
And now hath *Sathanas* such a Tail
Broader than of a Carkye is the Sail,
Hold up thy Tail thou *Sathanas* (quoth he)
Show forth thine erse, let the *Freere* see,
Where is the Nest of *Freeres* in this place,
And ere that half a Furlong way of space,
(Right as *Bees* Swarmen out of an hyve)
Our of the Devils erse they gan drive,
Twenty thousand *Freeres* on a Rout,
And throughout Hell swarmed all about,
And comen ayen as fast as they were gone,
And unto his erse they crepten every one. (sig. C4v–5r)

1681

582. BLOUNT, THOMAS. *Glossographia, or a Dictionary.* B3338. UMI 1416: 9.

For a reference to "old Chaucer" and a quotation from *Troilus and Cryssede* and to Chaucer as an authority on the English language and word usage, see BLOUNT (1656), (1661), (1670), and (1674); in this edition, the passages are found in the epistle (sig. A4v) and the definitions of *agroted* (sig. B8r), *algebra* (sig. C1v), *alnath* (sig. C3r), *barbican* (sig. F6v), *benison* (sig. G1v), *boon* (sig. G5v), *bordel* (sig. G5v), *burlybrand* (sig. G8v), *covent* (sig. M3v), *creance* (sig. M4v), *disheviled* (sig. O5r–O6r), *divinistre* (sig. O7r), *dulcarnon* (sig. P3r), *dwindle* (sig. P3v), *fryth* (sig. T2r), *lectern* (sig. Bb2r), *lodemanage* (sig. Bb7r), *losenger* (sig. Bb8r), *meriot* (sig. Dd5v), *moiles* (sig. Ee1v), *mortress* (sig. Ee4v), *ouch* (sig. Gg6v), *paraments* (sig. Hh3v), *pilgrim* (sig. Ii8v), *rap and ren* (sig. Mm5v), *romance* (sig. Nn8r), *superstition* (sig. Rr8r), *taberd* (sig. Ss5v), *tailage* (sig. Ss6v).

583. COLVILL, SAMUEL. *Mock Poem: or, Whiggs Supplication.* C5426. UMI 660: 11.

As Bond notes (*SP* 28), Colvill refers to Chaucer and Gower. Harris (*PQ*) cites the 1695 edition rather than this edition. In a section that satirizes the reading habits of the Scotch Presbyterians, Colvill writes:

[Many read, and like] drunken Asses flout
Not seeing the *Jewel* within the *Clout*:

Like Combs of Cocks, who take no heed
When they *Gower* or *Chaucer* read. (62)

Other editions with different title pages: *Whiggs Supplication, a Mock Poem*, C5428 (1687), 42; *The Scotch Hudibras: or, A Mock Poem*, C5427 (1692), 60–61; *Whiggs Supplication, a Mock Poem*, C5429 (1695), 42.

584.　Cooper, William. *Catalogus librorum.* **O600. UMI 431: 12.**

At Cooper's auction of books belonging to William Outram (1626–1679, late Canon of Westminster, and Thomas Gataker (1574–1654), under the heading "English in Folio," lot no. 46 is listed as *"Chaucer, (Jeff.) Works of Poetry, with his Life, best Edition. Lond.* 1602" (35; sig. G2r).

585.　Cowley, Abraham. *The Works of Mr. Abraham Cowley.* **C6655. UMI 685: 2.**

For a reference to Cowley's burial place near Chaucer, see Sprat (1668); in this edition, the passage is found on sig. c4r–v.

　　For a reference to Chaucer's "rich rhymes," see Cowley (1656), C6683; in this edition, the passage is found on 37 (sig. Aa1r).

　　Another edition in 1681: C6656, sig. B8r–v, 54 (sig. L6v).

586.　De Laune, Thomas. *The Present State of London: or, Memorials Comprehending a Full and Succinct Account of the Ancient and Modern State Thereof.* **D894. UMI 1945: 4.**

De Laune (d. 1685) is identified on the title page as "Tho. De-Laune, Gent." In a discussion of the distinguished people buried in Westminster Abbey, he notes that among them was *"Geoffrey Chaucer,* the Prince of *English* Poets in his time" (26).

　　Other editions: D894A (1683), 26; and with a different title: *Angliæ metropolis: or, The Present State of London* (1690), D889, 26.

587.　Dunmore, John. *Catalogus librorum.* **L2664. UMI 870: 8.**

Offered for sale by auction at Dunmore's auction house next door to the "Woollsack [*sic*]" in Ivy Lane near Pater Noster Row were works from the library of Rev. Nicholas Lloyd of Saint Marys, Newington. In the catalogue under the heading "English in Folio," lot no. 39 is listed as *"Geofferie Chaucer's* Works of Ancient Poetry. 1598" (25; sig. E1r)

588.   D'URFEY, THOMAS. *The Progress of Honesty: or, A View of a Court and City. A Pindarique Poem. By T. D.* D2764. UMI 490: 14.

In this satire on contemporary society, D'Urfey (1653–1723) describes an election for "Knights o' th' Shires." A nobleman ("in his intellect unknown," "a handsome publick Whore, | Infamous and contemn'd by th' wise and good, | And only useful to the lewd") appears at an assembly and presents the hand-picked candidate for Parliament ("a Peer") to the voters. D'Urfey refers to this paragon of a nobleman as "Sir Tophas," perhaps alludes to *The Tale of Sir Thopas.* In stanza 12, he writes:

> T' encourage all a Nobleman appears,
> For Wit and Valour famous many years,
> And choosing Knights o' th' Shires:
> . . . .
> In his right hand a Peer he led,
> Of whose worth more hereafter shall be said;
> With a young Baron fil'd, just fledg'd i' th' Laws,
> And newly then corrupted to the Cause,
> Usher'd by bold Sir *Tophas*: and in 'tother,
> A lean warpt canting Linsey-Wolsey Brother. (12–13)

Another edition in 1681: *The Second Edition*, 17–18.

589.   *Heraclitus Ridens: At a Diaglogue between Jest and Earnest, Concerning the Times.* Nelson and Seccombe 183.16. Early English Newspapers 24: 1173.

In issue No. 16, dated 17 May 1681, in a discussion of the recent innovation of printing the way Parliament voted on various issues, there is a reference to Chaucer and a modern paraphrase from *The Reeve's Tale* (line 4054). Jest inquires of Earnest:

> [P]ray Mr. *Earnest* what think you of Sir *F. W*'s Law, that the People constitute the House of Commons because they chuse them?
> *Earn.* I was reading to'ther day in Old *Chaucer* and there I met with an Old Saw, *That the greatest Clerks are not the wisest men*; but let that pass. (no pagination)

590.   HOWELL, WILLIAM. *Medulla historiæ anglicanæ.* H3140A. UMI 1690: 7.

For a reference to Chaucer as England's poet laureate in the reign of Richard II, see HOWELL (1679); in this edition, the passage is found on 249.

591.   MARVELL, ANDREW. *Miscellaneous Poems.* M872. UMI 216: 16.

Marvell (1621–1678) is described on the title page as "late Member of the Honourable House of Commons." As Spurgeon notes (3: 4.71–72), Marvell refers to Chaucer in "Tom May's Death":

> If that can be thy home where *Spencer* lyes
> And reverend *Chaucer*, but their dust does rise
> Against thee, and expels thee from their side,
> As th' Eagles Plumes from other birds divide. (37)

592.   MILLINGTON, EDWARD. *Catalogus librorum bibliothecis.* B6341. UMI 155: 2; 1379: 2.

An auction of books from the libraries of Ralph Button (sometime Canon of Christ's Church), Thankfull Owen (president of St. John's College in Oxford), and the Rev. William Howell of Sussex, was held on 7 November 1681 at Dunmore's auction house in Ivy Lane. In the catalogue for this sale, under "Miscellanies English, in Octavo and Duodecimo, &c.," lot number 9 is listed as "Comment on the two Tables of *Geffrey Chaucer, Miller's* Tale, &c.—1665" (212; sig. C2v). The work is by Richard Brathwait, and the full title reads *A Comment upon the Two Tales of our Ancient Renownd and Ever-Living Poet Sr Jeffray Chaucer, Knight Who for His Rich Fancy, Pregnant Invention and Present Composure Deserved the Countenance of a Prince and his Laureat Honor. The Miller's Tale and The Wife of Bath.* An annotation in the British Library copy of the catalogue indicates that Brathwait's book was sold to a Mr. Pullen for 9*d*.

593.   *A New Dialogue betwixt Heraclitus & Towzer Concerning the Times.* N619. UMI 1765: 29.

Heraclitus mentions the old ballad of Patient Grissel, perhaps a faint allusion to the *Clerk's Tale*:

> Now do you talk as dull as a Butterbox. 'Tis a sign what air you have suck'd in; dull phlegmatick Patience, we shall have you sing shortly the old ballad of Patient *Grissel.* (1)

594.   OLDHAM, JOHN. *Some New Pieces Never Before Publisht.* O248. UMI 614: 3b; UMI 946: 9.

As Spurgeon notes (1: 256), there is a reference to Chaucer in "Horace His Art of Poetry." Oldham (1653–1683) writes:

> 'Tis next to be observ'd that care is due,
> And sparingness in framing words anew:
> You shew your mast'ry, if you have the knack

So to make use of what known word you take,
To giv't a newer sense: if there be need
For some uncommon matters to be said;
Pow'r of inventing terms may be allow'd,
Which *Chaucer* and his Age n'eer understood. (5)

In the first of two pastorals bewailing the death of "Bion," i.e., John Willmot, second earl of Rochester, Oldham claims that Rochester will be mourned more than Chaucer, Milton, Cowley, Denham, and the matchless Orinda, Katharine Philips. Oldham implies that Chaucer is not as well appreciated as once he was. He writes:

Thou, sacred *Bion*, art lamented more
Than all our tuneful Bards, that dy'd before:
Old *Chaucer*, who first taught the use of Verse,
No longer has the tribute of our tears:
Milton, whose Muse with such a daring flight
Led out the warring *Seraphims* to fight:
Blest *Cowley* too, who on the banks of *Cham*
So sweetly sigh'd his wrongs, and told his fame:
and *He*, whose Song rais'd *Cooper*'s Hill so high,[36]
And made its glory with *Parnassus* vie:
And soft *Orinda*, whose bright shining name
Stands next great *Sappho*'s in the ranks of fame:
All now unwept, and unrelented pass,
And in our grief no longer share a place:
Bion alone does all our tears engross,
Our tears are all too few for *Bion*'s loss. (82–83)

Another edition: 0249 (1684), 5, 82–83.

Also collected in Oldham's *Works*: 0224 (1684), same pagination; 0225 (1684), same pagination; 0226 (1686), same pagination; 0227 (1686), same pagination; 0228 (1686), same pagination; 0229 (1692), same pagination; 0230 (1695), same pagination; 0231 (1698), same pagination.

Olden's tribute to Rochester is also found in some collections of Rochester's *Poems*: R1755 (1685), (not included); R1756 (1691), x–xi (sig. a2v–3r), cited by Spurgeon 1: 268; R1757 (1696), x–xi (sig. a2v–3r); R1758 (1683), (not included).

---

[36] "*He*" is Denham.

595. *Poor Robin 1681. An Almanack of the Old and New Fashion.* A2200. UMI 1084: 21.

Under the heading "Observations on April": "Patient Grizel" is celebrated on the 14th (sig. A6r); this is perhaps an allusion to the protagonist of *The Clerk's Tale*.

596. SCUDAMORE, JAMES, *Lord. Homer a la Mode. Second Part, in English Burlesque*: or, *A Mock-Poem upon the Ninth Books of Iliads.* S2133. UMI 616: 4.

In his burlesque of Homer's ninth book, "Invented for the median of Cambridge, where the pole of wit is elevated by several degrees," Lord Scudamore (1624–1668) attributes a bogus phrase to Chaucer:

> He heard no more, but left his place,
> And all with Soot besmear'd his face.
> Huge Horns he fasten'd on his head,
> And made his Cloaths all over red;
> Then to his Ar—a Tail he ties,
> But needs not to enlarge his eyes.
> (For they to use a Phrase of *Chaucers*,
> Were hugeous ones, and glar'd like Sawcers.) (67)

597. SELDEN, JOHN. *Jani Anglorum. Facies altera.* S2429 (1681). UMI 400: 1.

For references to *The General Prologue* and *The Summoner's Tale*, see SELDEN (1610) in Boswell & Holton No. 822. In this edition, the passage is found on 116.

598. SHAKESPEARE, WILLIAM. *Othello, the Moor of Venice.* S2940. UMI 297: 34.

For possible similarities to *Troilus and Criseyde*, see SHAKESPEARE (1622), Boswell & Holton No. 1035.

599. W., W. *Antidotum Britannicum*: or, *A Counter-Pest against the Destructive Principles of Plato Redivivus.* W140. UMI 854: 4.

In "The Preface to the Reader," the author criticizes the author of *Plato Redivivus*, alludes to *The Summoner's Tale*:

> The Bold Proposals of this Author, puts me in mind of the Crafty Friar in *Summer*'s Tale, who desired for his Dinner only the Liver of a *Capon* and a *Pig's* Head; well knowing, that if he got those we would not want his part of the *Pig* and *Capon* too. (sig. (a)2v–3r)

1682

600.   CHISWELL, RICHARD. *Bibliotheca Smithiana: sive catalogus librorum . . .*
Richardus Smith. S4161a (formerly S4151). UMI 1678: 10.

As Spurgeon notes (1: 256), Chiswell offered the library of Richard Smith
(1590–1675) for sale at the Auction House "known by the Name of the Swan" on
15 May 1682. In a note addressed "To the Reader," Chiswell writes that Smith
was "*a Person infinitely Curious and Inquisitive after Books, and who suffered nothing
considerable to escape him, that fell within the compass of his Learning. . . . He lived to
a very great Age, and spent a good part of it, almost intirely in the search of Books*" (no
pagination.; no signature).

In the catalogue, under the heading "English books in Folio," lot 77 is listed
as "*Chaucer's (Geoffery)* Works of Ancient Poettry; best Edition (with a MS. of a
Tale of *Gamelyn*, taken out of a MS. of *Chaucer's* Works in the University Library
of *Oxford* 1602" (274; sig. Aaaa1v, pagination is irregular).

601.   COOKE, EDWARD. *The History of the Successions of the Kings of England.*
C6000. UMI 60: 17.

Cooke is identified on the title page of the second edition of this work as "Edward
Cooke, of the Inner [*sic*] temple, Esquire." In a chapter headed "Edward the
Third, King of England and France, Lord of Ireland, and Duke of Aquitaine,
Surnamed of Windsor," in a section devoted to the children of Edward and
Philippa of Hainault, Cooke notes the connection between John of Gaunt and
Chaucer:

> *John* their fourth Son and sixth Child, was born at *Gaunt*. . . . His third
> Wife was *Katherine*, the widdow of Sir *Hugh Swinford*, a Knight in *Lin-*
> *colnshire*, eldest daughter and Co-heir of *Paen Roet* a *Gascoigne*, called
> *Guien*, King of Arms for that Country: His younger daughter being
> married to Sir *Jeoffry Chaucer*, the then Poet Laureat. (24)

Another edition with new title, *A Short Historical Account of the Kings of England*:
C6001A (1684), 24.

602.   COOPER, WILLIAM. *Catalogue Librorum Bibliothecæ Gualteri Rea Armi-*
geri. R423. UMI 1314: 11.

Cooper auctioned the library of Sir Walter Rea on 19 June 1682 at the Sign of the
Pelican in Little-Britain. In the catalogue, under the heading "English in Folio,"
number 50 is listed as "The works of Geffery Chaucer never before so compleated
—1542" (sig. D1v).

603.   Cooper, William. *Catalogus librorum bibliothecæ Joannis Humphry.* H3674. UMI 2007: 18.

Cooper scheduled an auction of the library of John Humpry of Rowell in Northamptonshire at Jonathan's Coffee House on 4 December 1682. In the catalogue, under the heading "English Miscellany Folio," lot 83 is listed as "*G. Chaucers* works with a Table, and *Chaucers* Life, —1598" (42).

604.   *Friendly Advice to the Correctour of the English Press at Oxford Concerning the English Orthographie.* F2215. UMI 960: 30.

As Harris notes (*PQ*), the author cites examples from *The Romant of the Rose* and *Testament in Love* (attributed to Chaucer) in his advice to the copy editor at the Oxford Press. He writes:

> [I]n our ancienter English Tongue, *tho* signifies quite another thing from what you intend it: as may appear from *Chauncer* [*sic*]; who uses it two wayes, But neither of them in your sense. For with him it signifies *Then*, and not *Though*; as in those verses quoted out of him, by his Publishers, (I should have said *Editors*) before his works, which are these.

> *I know that in fourm of speech is change*
> *Within an hundreth yeers; and words tho*
> *That hadden price, now wonder, nice and strange*
> *Think we them; and yet they speak them so;*
> *And sped as well in love as men now do*[.]

> These Verses are made in commendation of the English Language, even before *Chaucer*: and therefore his offence against our auncient Tongue, lesse excusable; that, contrary to his own judgment, he should endeavour to improve and imbellish it, by a number of Latine and French words brought into it, to the loss of as many, and as significant Teutonique words, and to the corruption of our Mother tongue, as *Verstegan* hath observed, and proved against *Chaucer*.[37] Yet is this brave Authour more excusable than many of this age, as using that liberty of innovating chiefly in Poetry, where it was evermore allowed, than in Prose, wherein he is much more sparing of forrein words. In *The Romant of the Rose*, being a translation of the French Authour *Clopinel* or *Meung*, he about the beginning, uses *tho* for *then*: and in his *Testament in* [*sic*] *Love*, fol: 301 of his *Workes*, sometimes he uses it for *then*, and sometimes for *those*: as *I have* (qd I tho) y nough: for quoth I then: And presently after, he thus uniteth [*sic*], *I would now* (qd I) *a little understand sithen all things*

---

[37]   See Boswell & Holton No. 723.

thus before en not [sic], whether thilking be of tho things. i.e. of *those things.*
Thus he: but you, for *tho,* or *those,* please to write *thos,* keeping neither to
old, nor modern Orthographie, but walking by your self, to the prejudice of the ususal pronunciation, which is thereby altered. (9)

605.   GIBBON, JOHN. *Introductio ad Latinam blasoniam. An Essay to a More
Correct Blason in Latine Than Formerly Hath Been Used.* **G650. UMI 531: 12.**
Gibbon (1629–1718) is identified on the title page as "Johanne Gibbono armorum
servulo, quem à Mantelio dicunt Cæruleo." As Atkinson notes (*MLN* 1936),
Gibbon uses Chaucer's coat of arms as an example to illustrate the term *counter-
changed*:

> Counterchanged, which is spoken of the Charge that is placed in Arms
> party of any sort. . . . And indeed in the Life of *Chaucer* (prefixt to
> his Works) I find his Arms (which are *party per pale Arg. Gules, a bend
> counterchanged*) thus blasoned in Latine, *Arma de argento & rubro colore
> partita per longitudinem Scuti cum benda ex transverso eisdem coloribus, sed
> transmutatis depicta.* (16)

606.   HEALE, WILLIAM. *The Great Advocate and Oratour for Women: or, The
Arraignment, Tryall and Conviction of All Such Wicked Husbands (or Monsters)
Who Held It Lawfull to Beate Their Wives.* **H1300B. UMI 1671: 16.**
This anonymously published work is attributed to Heale (1581 / '82–1627). In
chapter 4, in a discussion of civil and canon law, the author includes Chaucer
among those illustrious writers who defended women against calumnies:

> Are all women evil? then how came it to pass O grave *Plutarch* that thy
> wisdom so faild thee? O *Hesiod* who corrupted thy mature Judgment?
> Cælius, who beguiled thy witt? *Chauser,* [sic] how chance thy golden pen
> so miscarryed? . . . for deceived you all are if this position be received,
> who have severally written diverse Treatises in honour of honourable
> and deserving women. . . . (93–94)

Chauser is marked for a shoulder note: "Chancer."

607.   HOLLES, DENZIL. *Lord Hollis, His Remains: Being a Second Letter to a
Friend, Concerning the Judicature of the Bishops in Parliament.* **H2466. UMI 384: 3.**
Writing in response to Stillingfleet's *The Grand Question* (1680), q.v., Baron Hol-
les (1599–1680) alludes to *The Summoners Tale*:

[T]he Scribes and Pharisees . . . cryed out against our Saviour, Crucifie him, Crucifie him, but said it was not lawful for them to put any man to death. Is not this as good as *Chaucer's* Fryer that this Author quips me with p. 4.? (97)

608.   KEEPE, HENRY. *Monumenta Westmonasteriensia: or, An Historical Account of the Original Increase, and Present State of St. Peter's, or the Abby Church of Westminster.* K126. UMI 423: 10.

Keepe (1652–1688) is identified on the title page as "H. K. of the Inner-Temple, Gent." As Spurgeon notes (1: 255–56 and 3: 4.77), Keepe records Chaucer's burial spot near Spenser, Drayton, and Cowley:

And now come we to the first and last best Poets of the *English* Nation *Geffrey Chaucer,* and *Abraham Cowley,* the one being the Sun just rising, and shewing its self on the *English Horizon,* and so by degrees increasing and growing in strength till it came to its full *Glory* and *Meridian* in the incomparable *Cowley,* whose admirable *Genius,* hard to be imitated, but never equalled, hath set the bounds to succeeding times. *Chaucer* lies in an ancient Tomb, Canopied, of grey Marble, with his Picture painted thereon *in plano,* with some verses by; he died in the year 1400. [In a shoulder note: "*Geffrey Chaucer.* vid. Ep. 31."] (47)

Later Keepe adds a reference that was not picked up by Spurgeon:

Many more persons of note have been interred in this Church, whose Monuments are decayed and gone, or the inscriptions worn or torn off from their Grave-stones, as *Rachel Brigham,* Daughter of *Nicolas Brigham,* who had a marble stone laid over her, hard by *Chaucers* Tomb, *anno* 1557. (173)

Spurgeon also notes (3: 4.77) a reference to Chaucer's arms and his epitaph:

Arms. viz. 𝕮𝖍𝖆𝖚𝖈𝖊𝖗. Per pale Gules and Argent, a bend countercharged. [In a shoulder note: "*A. D.* 1400. *Galf. Chaucer.* vid. '37."]

31. *Epitaph.* viz.

M. S.
Qui fuit Anglorum Vates ter maximus olim,
Galfridus Chaucer, *conditur hoc tumulo,*
Annum si quæras domini, si tempora mortis,
Ecce notæ subsunt, quæ tibi cuncta notant.

25. *Octobris* 1400.
Ærumnarum requis Mors.
N. Brigham *hos fecit musarum nomine sumptus*, 1556. (210)

Another edition: K127 (1683), 47, 173, 210.

609. OSBORNE, FRANCIS. *The Works of Francis Osborn. The Eighth Edition.* O506. UMI 614: 6.

For a reference to a bishop who boasted that he had never read a line of Calvin or Chaucer, see OSBORNE (1658); in this collection, the passage is found on 441–42.

610. *Poor Robin, 1682. An Almanack after a New Fashion.* A2201. UMI 1494: 23.

Under the heading "Observations on August," we find "Chaucers Miller" is celebrated on the 26th of this month (sig. B4r).

In a section devoted to eclipses for the year, there is a faint allusion to *The House of Fame*:

> [T]he general Exchange for News is at the Coffee-house, where men are drinking their scalding hot *Ninny-broth*, a Coffee-house being like the Shop of *Fame*, that tatling Gossip, thus described by the Poet.
>> *She* [illegible] *enquireth into all the World,*
>> *And hath about her vaulted Palace burl'd*
>> *All rumours and reports, or true or vain,*
>> *What utmost Lands, or deepest Seas contain;*
>> *Her House is full of Echo made,*
>>> *Where never dies the sound,*
>> *And as her Brows the Clouds invade,*
>>> *Her feet do touch the Ground.* (sig. C2v–3r)

611. PRIDEAUX, MATHIAS. *An Easy and Compendious Introduction for Reading All Sorts of Histories.* P3445. UMI 1429: 2.

For a reference to "diverse passages" in Chaucer's works that are "useful" for students of history, see PRIDEAUX, P3439 (1648); in this edition, the passage is found on 379. Atkinson (*N&Q* 1936) cites this edition rather than the first.

612. SADLER, JOHN. *Rights of the Kingdom: or, Customs of our Ancestors Touching the Duty, Power, Election, or Succession of Our Kings and Parliaments.* S279. UMI 821: 27.

For a reference to Chaucer as an authority on the English language and British history, see SADLER (1649); in this edition, the passages are found on 45–46, 49, 177.

613. SCARRON, PAUL. *Scarron's Novels.* S834A. UMI 2676: 6.

For an echo of a line from *The General Prologue*, see SCARRON (1665); in this edition, the passage is found on 19.

614. SELDEN, JOHN. *The Reverse or Back-face of the English Janus. Concerning the Common and Statute-law of English Britanny.* Trans. Redman Westcot. S2436. UMI 294: 4.

For Latin editions of this work, see SELDEN (1610) in Boswell & Holton No. 822, and Selden (1681). As Alderson & Henderson note, Selden (1584–1654) cites and quotes inverted lines from Chaucer's description of the Parson in *The General Prologue* (lines 502, 501) and *The Summoner's Tale* (lines 2008–9). In book 2, chapter 13, in a passage about canon laws created by Thomas a Becket, regarding the word *leudemen*, Selden writes:

> As to what concerns our language, *John Gower* and *Jeoffry Chaucer*, who were the Reformers and Improvers of the same in Verse, do both make it good. Thus *Jeoffry* [in a shoulder note: "Chauc. in Prolog. of the Sumners tale"].
> No wonder is a leude man to rust
> If a Priest be foule on whom we trust.
> However, that is signifies an illiterate or unlearned person, as well as one not yet in orders; what he saith elsewhere, informs us.
> This every leud Vicar and Parson can say.
> And . . . others, use this expression; *as well Laymen as Scholars.* But let not *Chaucer* take it ill, that here he must give way to our *Gloucester* Muse. (77)

Also found in *Tracts Written by John Selden*, S2441 (1683), same pagination. Also found in *England's Epinomis*, S2442 (1683), 23–24.

615. SMITH, JAMES. "The Preface to That Most Elaborate Piece of Poetry Entituled Penelope and Ulysses," in *Wit and Drollery. Jovial Poems.* W3133. UMI 993: 12.

For a reference to a sharp disagreement about a poet's commendation of "ould" Chaucer, see SMITH (1656); in this edition, the passage is found on 212.

616. WALLER, EDMUND. *Poems, &c. Written upon Several Occasions.* W516. UMI 2102: 7; UMI 1452: 2.

For a reference to the difficulty of Chaucer's language for modern readers, see WALLER (1668); in this edition, the passage is found on 234–35.

617. *The Weekly Pacquet of Advice from Rome.* V. (24 Nov 1682) Nelson and Seccombe 477.514.

Under the heading "The Courant: or The Jesuits Memoirs," Henry Care (1646–1688) quotes lines from *The Summoner's Tale* and goes on to explicate:

> I Shall never forget *Chaucer*'s Frere:
> Have I of a Capon but the *Liver*
> And of your white brede but a Shiver [*sic*],
> And after that a rasted [*sic*] Pigges *hedde*,
> (But I nolde not for me no *Beest* were *dedde*)
> Thon had I inow for my suffisance
> For I am a man of *littel* sustenance.
>   — *Sompners Tale*, fo. 41.

> The good Father by no means would have any thing *Kill'd* for him; he only desired *Thomas's Wife* to provide him the *Liver* of the Capon and the *Head* of the Pigg—Much at this rate some folks talk; they are not offended with our writing against *Popery*, they object not against our *Historical part*,—but the *Courant*, the divelish *Courant*, alas! sticks in their Gizzard. . . .

618.   WHITLOCKE, BULSTRODE. *Memorials of the English Affairs.* W1986. UMI 556: 10.

Writing about events that transpired during the reign of Charles I and down to the Restoration of Charles II, Whitlocke (1605–1675/76) cites Chaucer on the subject of reverence:

> Our old English Poet *Chaucer* (whom I think not unproper to cite, being one of the greatest Clerks and Wits of his time) had a better Opinion of the state of a Sergeant, as he expresseth in his Prologue of the Sergeant.

> *A Sergeant at Law wary and wise,*
> *That oft had bin at the pervise,*
> *There was also, full of rich Excellence,*
> *Discreet he was, and of great Reverence.*

> And in his description of the *Franklyn*, he saith of him.

> *At Sessions there was he Lord, and Sire,*
> *Full oft had he bin Knight of the Shire;*
> *A Sheriff had he bin, and a Countor,*
> *Was no where such a worthy Vavasor.*

A *Countor* was a Sergeant, and a *Vavasour* was the next in degree to a *Baron*. (348)

In a passage about the role of a "Sergeant Countor" Chaucer is again cited as an authority on usage:

The were antiently called likewise *Countors* . . . and at this day every Sergeant at his creation, doth *count* in some real Action at the Common-Pleas Bar. . . . *Chaucer* calls them *Countors*. . . . (350)

1683

619. A., J. "Commedatory Poem" in *T. Lucretius Carus. The Epicurean Philosopher, His Six Books De natura rerum Done into English Verse, with Notes* [by **Thomas Creech]. L3448. UMI 606: 12.**

In a commendatory poem headed "To Mr. Creech on his Translation of Lucretius" and dated 1 January 1682 from King's College, Cambridge, J. A. writes that Chaucer drew inspiration from the local river.

Accept this Praise, & so much more your Due,
From one that envys and admires you too.
I thought indeed before I heard your Fame,
No Lawrels grew but on the banks of *Cham*;
Where *Chaucer* was by sacred fury fir'd,
And everlasting *Cowley* lay inspir'd.
Where *Milton* first his wondrous vision saw,
And *Marvel* taught the Painter how to Draw. (sig. c2v)

The poem is not found in the first edition.
    Other editions in 1683: L3449, sig. C4v; L3449B, sig. C4v.
    Other editions: L3449C (1699), sig. C4v; L3450 (1700), sig. C4v.

620. B. *The Arraignment of Co-Ordinate-Power; Wherein All Arbitrary Proceedings Are Laid Open to All Honest Abhorrers and Addressers: With a Touch at the London-Petition and Charter. B1. UMI 49: 27.*

As Harris notes (*PQ*), the author quotes *The Squire's Tale* (lines 147–52). Under the heading "Work for Another London-Petition, &c.," in a passage about corruption of government officials, he writes:

But for persons that are in Authority, wilfully to lie under Temptation, and to be satisfied in their Consciences and Duty to his Majesty, that to promote Petitions to his Majesty, and Presentments to His Majesties Justices in vindication of the unwarrantable Heats and Passions of the Commons, in opposition to His Majesties most Gracious Declaration, their kind of proceedings are matters of a more dangerous consequence, than the punishment by ordinary Fine and Imprisonment, and a Decree *tantum*, cannot satisfie the intention of these tarcelletts, which are to be discovered by wearing the Lady *Candaces* Ring in the Squires tale in *Chaucer*:

> Which that if it lust her farr to ware
> Upon her thumb or in her purse beare,
> There is noe fowle that flock under heaven
> That she we shall understond his stevyn,
> And know his meaneing openly and plain,
> And answer him in language againe.

These are not artiguous, but they are stupendious, comitial Distempers, they are to be cured by the touch of King *Edward* the Confessor's Ring at *Westminster*. . . . (5)

In a section headed "The Power of the Parliament of this Kingdom," in chapter 8, there are long modernized quotations from *The Squire's Tale* (lines 309–26, 156–67):

> If it so fall out, that the Priviledges of Parliament, and its Liberty in its use, exceed his bounds, doth mischief, and recoil upon the Electors of their own Representatives, then the People are likewise to understand, that their Rights are precedent to the Priviledges of such Representatives. . . . And so it was prophetically writ to the same purpose upon the front of the Abbey of *Leicester* before the dissolution.
>
> > *Has sacras Edes pietas quas stuxit avorum,*
> > *Tempore venturo ruinatur more Luporum.*

Sir *Jeffrey Chaucer*, in his Squire's Tale, by the Brazen-steed, the Ring and the Sword, presented to the King by the Knight from the King of *Araba*, shews the King how the distrubances during his Reign might be discovered and prevented.

> But finally, the King asked the Knight,
> The virtue of this Courser, and the might;
> And prayed to tell him of his governance.
> The Horse anon gan to trip and dance.

𝔚hen that this 𝕶night laid hand on his 𝕽ein,
𝕳e said, 𝕾id, there is no more to be sayne,
𝕭ut when you list to ride any where,
𝖄e must trill a pin that 'stout in 'his ear;
𝔚hich 𝕴 shall you tell betwixt us two;
𝖄ou must name him to what place also;
𝕺r to what 𝕮ountrey that ye list to ride;
𝕬nd when ye come there ye list abide,
𝕭id him descend, and trill another pyn;
𝕬nd therein lyeth the chiefest of all the gyn:
𝕬nd he will down descend, and do your will,
𝕬nd in that place he will abide still;
𝕿hough all the 𝕸orld hath contrary swore,
𝕳e shall not thence be draw ne bore;
𝕺r if you list, bid him thence gon,
𝕿rill this pin and he will banish anon,
𝕺ut of the sight of every manner of wight,
𝕬nd come again, be it by day or night:
𝔚hen that you clip him again,
𝕴n such a gyse as 𝕴 shall to you sayn,
𝕭etwixt you and me, and that right soon,
𝕽ide when you list, there no more to be done,
𝕴nformed when the 𝕶ing was, &c.

As to the naked Sword he saith.

𝕿his 𝕾word that hangeth by my side,
𝕾uch vertue hath that what man ye smite
𝕿hroughout his 𝕬rmour it will kein and bite,
𝕸ere as thick as branched 𝕺ake,
𝕬nd what man is wounded with the stroke,
𝕳e shall never be well till ye list of grace,
𝕿o strike him in the wound, and it will close,
𝕿his is very sooth, and it will glose.
𝕴t faileth not while it is in your hand.

Humane Laws are so made, that they oblige not in extream necessity, and so it is in conscience too. . . . (44–45)

In chapter 10, in a section about the rights and privileges of barristers, the writer quotes Chaucer's description of the Sergeant of the Law in *The General Prologue* (lines 323–26):

Concerning the priviledge of his profession . . . He casts off all his own
domestick affairs, that he may intend the good of others.

I find the best of Satyrists speak pleasantly of him; for when it hath
been enquired where a good man is to be found, they have forthwith
told you.

> —*Vir bonis est quis?*
> *Qui consulta patrum, qui Leges juraq; servat;*
> *Quo multæ magneq; secantur judice lites;*
> *Quo responsare, & quo causæ teste tenentur?*

> Where is the man you call good? Your fine
> And learned Barrister, that can outwine
> Statutes, quote Reports, Books of Entries, pare
> The Law, and split out Justice to a hair:
> He that can knowingly give Evidence.
> And smooth both parties to a Reference.

Which Sir *Jeffrey Chaucer* was so well pleased with, that he imitates him
to the same purpose.

> In tearms had he cause and doomes, all
> That fro the time of Kyng William were fall;
> Thereto he could indict, and make a thyng,
> There could no Wyght pinch at his Wryting. (53)

621.   BARNARD, JOHN. *Theologo-Historicus: or, The True Life of the Most Rever-end Divine, and Excellent Historian, Peter Heylyn.* B854. UMI 199: 7.

Barnard (d. 1683) is identified on the title page as "his [Peter Heylyn's] son in
law John Barnard D. D. rec. of Waddington near Lincoln." He cites the spurious
work known as Chaucer's *Ploughman's Tale* and advises the reader that he writes
"to correct the errors, supply the defects, and confute the calumnies of a late
writer" (title page). Barnard writes:

> I never met with such a Transcriber in all my days: For want of matter
> to fill up a *Vacuum*, of which his book was in much danger, he hath set
> down the Story of *Westminster*, as long as the Plowmans Tale in *Chaucer*,
> which to the Reader would have been more pertinent and pleasant. (14)

A reissue with different title page in 1683: B854A, same pagination.

622.   BLOUNT, THOMAS. *The Academy of Eloquence.* B3326. UMI 1223: 3.

For an echo of the title of *The House of Fame*, see BLOUNT (1654); in this edition, the passage is found on 29.

623.   C., D. Commendatory poem in *A Present for Youth.* P969C. UMI 2252: 20.

In a commendatory poem placed before the remaining works of Damaris Pearse, D. C. echoes Chaucer's line, "Go, litel bok, go, litel myn tragedye" (*Troilus and Criseyde* 5: 1786):

> Go, little *Book*, abroad, and tell mankind,
> What *graces* lodged in a *Virgins* mind.
> Declare the glorious wisdom, power and love
> Which did her *infant*-years to Vertue move;
> And fit for Heaven, when her childish days,
> Rather invited her to harmless plays. (sig. A2r)

624.   *The Case of Ministring at the Communion-Table When There Is No Eucharist.* A29. UMI 621: 2.

The Case is cast as an epistle addressed to "I. B." that was written on the occasion of the publication of a treatise by Richard Hart titled *Parish Churches Turn'd into Conventicles.* As Harris notes (*PQ*), the writer quotes modernized lines from *The Squire's* Tale (lines 221–24). In a passage about the dangers of clergymen pandering to the ignorant, the author writes:

> 'Tis an Argument the thing is very bad, which the Rout approves very much. Did you never hear of the Expert Master of Musick, who gave his Scholar a Box of the Ear when he took him playing to the Admiration of the Vulgar, Presuming he must needs be out, and play amiss, or the Common Sort would never have liked him so well? Which it were to be wished were not too often to be found in Popular Preachers, who the worse they Preach, the more they are applauded by such People whom *Chaucer* in his Squires Tale thus describes but too truely [*sic*].

> *As People deemeth commonly*
> *Of things that been more Subtilly*
> *Then they can in their leudness Comprehend,*
> *They deemen gladly to the badder end.* (31)

625.   COLERAINE, HENRY HARE. *The Situation of Paradise Found Out.* C5064. UMI 958: 15.

In "Section II," Baron Coleraine (1636–1708) refers to "the Tales of Chaucer." In a passage about the "Benefit and the Instructiveness of History," he points out that the historian is "tyed to the Laws of Truth" and must, therefore, reveal the faults as well as the virtues of his subject in order to set forth "a perfect and just Exemplar." In a passage about allegorical works, he writes:

> [N]or is this Allegorical *way of writing either improper, or new*. . . . Thus *was the* Theology, *and thus also was the* Philosophy *of the Ancients taught*; *whence some have writ large Volumes of the Heathen* Mythology. Thus *has* Xenophon *given the* pattern *of an excellent* Prince, *and* Plato *of a* Commonwealth; *and we have the latter ones of* New Atlantis, Utopia, Severambi, *&c. Not to instance in the* Tales *of* Chaucer, *the* Legends *of* Spencer, *and the jocular* Visions *of* Quevedo,[38] Pasquin, Heraclito-Democritus, *and others*. . . . (30–31)

626.   DE LAUNE, THOMAS. *The Present State of London*. D894A. No UMI.

For a reference to Chaucer's burial in Westminster Abbey, see DE LAUNE (1681); in this edition, the passage is found on 26.

627.   DUNTON, JOHN. *The Informer's Doom: or, An Amazing and Seasonable Letter from Utopia, Directed to the Man in the Moon*. D2629. UMI 1355: 17.

Dunton (1659–1733) is described on the title page as "a true son of the Church of England." He announces on the title page that this humorous work will be "Giving a full and pleasant Account of the Arraignment, Tryal, and Condemnation, of all those grand and bitter Enemies, that disturb and molest all Kingdoms and States, throughout the *Christian World*." Pope Innocent XI is the first enemy of Protestantism brought to the bar of justice, and he is followed by Mr. Implacable, a justice of the peace in Utopia, Mr. Hotspur (son of one Beastly), Mr. Envy-good, Mr. Violence, several witches, Mrs. Bad-wife (otherwise called Mrs. Tittle-tattle) and Sir John Fraud. The judge gives summary justice to most of these but begins to empanel a jury for Sir John; several prospective jurors are rejected and others called:

> [T]hree other men offered their Service to Sir *John*; the one said he was a Sumner, the other a Goaler, and third an Informer. Bless me (quoth the Judge) what a Gan is here gathered together! no doubt Hell is broke loose, and the Devil means to keep Holiday: I make Challenge against them all, as against worse men than those that gave evidence against Christ: for the Sumner, it boots me to say little more against him, that *Chaucer* did in his *Canterbury* Tales, who said he was a Knave, a Briber and Bawd: But leaving that Authority, although it be authentical, yet thus much I can say of my self, that these drunken, drowsie sons go a

---

[38] Francisco de Quevedo (1580–1645), Spanish writer and gadfly, author of *Los Sueños*.

tooting abroad (as they themselves term it) which is to hear if any man hath got his Maid with Child, or plays the Good-fellow with his Neighbors Wife. . . . Tush, what Bawdry is it he will not suffer, so he may have Money and good Chear? And if he like a Wench well, a Snatch himself; for they know all the Whores in a Country, and are as lecherous Champions as may be. To be brief, the Sumner lives upon Sins of People, and out of Harlotry gets he all his Gains. (102–3)

628.   HOWELL, WILLIAM. *Medulla historiæ anglicanæ.* H3141. No UMI.

For a reference to Chaucer as England's poet laureate in the reign of Richard II, see HOWELL (1679); in this edition, the passage is found on 249.

629.   KEEPE, HENRY. *Monumenta Westmonsteriensia: or, An Historical Account of the Original, Increase, and Present State of St. Peter's, or the Abby Church of Westminster.* K127. UMI 322: 1.

For a reference to Chaucer's burial spot near Spenser, Drayton, and Cowley, and to his coat of arms and his epitaph, see KEEPE (1682); in this edition, the passages are found on 47, 173, 210.

630.   LINDSAY, DAVID. *The Works of the Famous and Worthy Knight, Sir David Lindsay of the Mount.* L2318. UMI 1262: 22.

For a reference to Chaucer's skill as a poet in the prologue of *The Testament of Papingo,* see LINDSAY (1538) in Boswell & Holton No. 146; in this edition, the passage is found on sig. G4v.

For a passage that mentions the fable of *Troilus and Criseyde* in an epistle to the king that is set before the prologue to "The Dreme of Sir David Lindsay," see LINDSAY (1558) in Boswell & Holton No. 209; in this edition, the passage is found and appears on sig. H6v.

631.   MENNES, JOHN. *Recreation for Ingenious Head-peeces: or, A Pleasant Grove for Their Wits to Walk In.* M1718. UMI 1508: 10.

For an epitaph "On our prime English Poet, *Geffrey Chaucer,*" see MENNES (1641). The epitaph is originally from Lydgate's prologue to his translation of Boccaccio's *The Falle of Princes*; see BOCCACCIO (1494) in Boswell & Holton No. 27. In this edition, the passage is found on sig. O4r.

For a reference to Chaucer in an epitaph "On William Shake-speare," see *Wits Recreations* (1640) in Boswell & Holton No. 1377; in this edition, the passage is found on sig. O5r.

632.   MILLINGTON, EDWARD. *Bibliotheca Lloydiana.* **L2654. UMI 2050: 33.**

Millington began auctioning the libraries of the Rev. John Lloyd of North-Mimmes in Hertfordshire and Sir Thomas Raymond, sometime Justice of the Kings-Bench Court, on 3 December 1683. In the second part of the catalogue, under the heading "Miscellanies in Folio," lot 169 is listed as "Chaucer's Works —15-"; and lot 170 as "Another, with Explication of Words, (best Edit.) lettred —1602" (24; sig. Aa2v).

633.   OLDHAM, JOHN. *Poems, and Translations.* **O237. UMI 469: 4.**

Spurgeon (1: 256) notes that Oldham (1653–1683) refers to Chaucer in *Horace His Art of Poetry. Imitated in English*; however, it is *not* included in this edition.

634.   *Poor Robin 1683. An Almanack of the Old and New Fashion.* A2202. UMI 856: 6 (film imperfect: prognostication only)

Under the heading "Observations on August," we find that "Chaucers Miller" is celebrated on the 18th of this month (sig. B4r).

635.   S., J. *The Present State of England.* **C1844. UMI 206: 15.**

This continuation of Edward Chamberlain's *Angliæ notitia: or, The Present State of England* is by someone who signs an epistle addressed to the reader as "J. S." In the third part, in a section headed "Towns and Places of England eminent for some Remarkeable Accident, Person or Transaction," in a passage about famous folk who were born in London, the author writes:

> Other persons of eminent note and immortal memory were born at *London, viz* . . . Sir *Jeoffry Chaucer* the most famous of ancient *English Poets*, who flourisht in the Reigns of K. *Henry* the 4th, *Henry* the 5th, and part of K. *Henry* the 6th. . . . (149).

In a passage about Woodstock in Oxfordshire:

> [I]n the Town of *Woodstock* was brought up and educated that most renowned of *English* Poets Sir *Geoffry Chaucer.* (183)

636.   SANFORD, FRANCIS. *A Genealogical History of the Kings of England.* **S651A. UMI 1939: 1.**

For a reference to Chaucer's descendants marrying into the upper ranks of English nobility, see SANFORD (1677); in this edition, the passage is found on 378–79.

637.   SCARRON, PAUL. *Scarron's Novels.* S834B. UMI 2019: 11

For an echo of a line from *The General Prologue*, see SCARRON (1665); in this edition, the passage is found on 19.

638.   SELDEN, JOHN. *England's Epinomis.* S2442. UMI 702: 6.

Harris notes (*PQ*) this edition rather than earlier ones. For lines pertaining to lewd priests in *The General Prologue* and *The Summoner's Tale*, see SELDEN (1681); in this edition, the passage is found on 23–24.

Also found in *Tracts Written by John Selden*, S2441 (1683), 77.

639.   SHAKESPEARE, WILLIAM. *The Tragedy of Hamlet Prince of Denmark.* S2952. UMI 297: 42.

For verbal parallels and contextual similarities that may indicate the influence of *The Legend of Good Women* and *The Monk's Tale*, see SHAKESPEARE (1604), Boswell & Holton No. 693.

640.   SMITH, JOHN. *The Mystery of Rhetorique Unveil'd.* S4116E. UMI 2020: 11 (identified as S2582).

For a reference to Spenser's imitation of Chaucer, see SMITH (1656); in this edition, the passage is found on 64.

A variant imprint in 1683: S4116D, same pagination.

641.   SOAMES, WILLIAM, AND JOHN DRYDEN. An interpolation in Nicholas Boileau-Despréaux's *The Art of Poetry, Written in French by the Sieur de Boileau, Made English.* B3464. UMI 15: 2.

Spurgeon (1: 254) speculates that this translation of *L'art poétique* by Boileau-Desperéaux (1636–1711) was by Dryden; in point of fact, it is by Sir William Soames (but was revised by Dryden[39] who substituted English examples of literature for many of the French ones cited by Boileau). In an interpolation in a section headed "Satyr," there is a perceptive evaluation of Chaucer following comments on Juvenal and other Roman poets. Dryden writes:

> And *Juvenal*, Learn'd as those times could be,
> Too far did stretch his sharp Hyperbole;
> . . . .
> In all he Writes appears a noble Fire;
> To follow such a Master then desire,
> *Chaucer* alone fix'd on this solid Base;

---

[39] See O. B. Hardison, Jr., and Leon Golden, eds., *Horace for Students of Literature. The Ars Poetica and Its Tradition* (Gainesville: University Press of Florida, 1995), vii, 173.

In his old Stile, conserves a modern grace:
Too happy, if the freedom of his rhymes
Offended not the method of our Times. (24–25)

642.   TRYON, THOMAS. *A Way to Health, Long Life and Happiness: or, A Discourse of Temperance.* T3200.

Tryon (1634–1703) is identified on the title page as "Philotheos Physiologus." In chapter 19, "Of Marriage, and the Inconveniences of unequal Matches," he appears to echo lines from *The Reeve's Prologue*, "To have a hoor head and a green tayl, | As hath a leek" (lines 3878–79). Tryon writes:

> The Inconveniences that attend *Marriage* in *Age*, are many, the Benefits very few; how ill it looks to see the Spring of Wantonness arise in the *Autum* [sic] of Life, and a Man, (according to the Vulgar Proverb) appear like *an Onion with a Gray Head and a Green Tail.* (613)

Other editions: T3201 (1691), 457–58; T3201A (1691), 457–58; T3202 (1697), 416; T3202A (1697), 416; T3202B (1697), 416; T3203 (1698), no UMI.

1684

643.   BAKER, RICHARD. *An Abridgement of S*ʳ*. Richard Bakers Chronicle of the Kings of England.* B499. UMI 198: 22.

In the account of the reign of Edward III, Baker (1568–1645) refers to Chaucer in a passage about John of Gaunt:

> His third Wife was *Katherine*, the widdow of Sir *Hugh Swinford*, a Knight in *Lincolnshire*, eldest daughter and Co-heir of *Paen Roet* a *Gascoigne*, called *Guien*, King of Arms for that Country: His younger daughter being married to Sir *Jeoffry Chaucer*, then Poet Laureat. (24)

644.   BAKER, RICHARD. *A Chronicle of the Kings of England.* B509. UMI 783: 1.

For references to Chaucer as John of Gaunt's brother-in-law, "the Homer of our nation," his association with Woodstock, his translation of *The Romaunt of the Rose*, his burial place in Westminster, and his association with Gower, see BAKER (1643) and (1653); in this edition, the passages are found on 132, 134, 155, 167, and sig. Hhhh4r .

645.   BLOME, RICHARD. *An Essay to Heraldry.* B3211. UMI 809: 13; UMI 867: 16.

Under the heading "Examples of Counterchanges," Blome (d. 1705) cites Chaucer as his fourth example:

> *Per Pale* Argent and Gules, a *Bend Counterchanged* by the Name of *Chaucer.* [In a shoulder note: "Chaucer."] (67)

Other editions with title *The Art of Heraldry*: B3205 (1685), 67; B3206 (1693), 67.

646.   BUNYAN, JOHN. *The Pilgrim's Progress. The Second Part.* B5576. UMI 17: 14.

In "The Author's Way of Sending forth his Second Part of the Pilgrim," Bunyan (1628–1688) echoes Chaucer's line, "Go, litel bok, go litel myn tragedye" (*Troilus and Criseyde* 5: 1786):

> Go, *now my little Book, to every Place,*
> *Where my first* Pilgrim *has but shewn his Face,*
> *Call at their door: If any say* who's there?
> *Then Answer thou,* Christiana is here. (sig. A2r)

Other editions: B5578 (1686), sig. A2r; B5579 (1687), sig. A2r; B5580 (1690), sig. A2r; B5581 (1693), sig. A2r; B5582 (1696), sig. A2r.

647.   *Catalogus variorum librorum.* L3529. UMI 1710: 6.

The libraries of the late Rev. Thomas Lye and Thomas Jennings, both of London, were auctioned at Bridges Coffee-House on 17 November 1684. In the second part of the catalogue, under the heading "Large Folio, English Divinity," lot 77 is listed as "Chaucer (Jeffry) his works—1532" (2; sig. A1v).

647a.   CHARLETON, WALTER. *The Cimmerian Matron, a Pleasant Novel.* C3667a. UMI 2330: 4.

For references to *The Book of the Duchess, The Legend of Good Women, The Wife of Bath's Prologue, The Squire's Prologue and Tale, The Merchant's Tale, Troilus and Criseyde,* and *The Shipman's Tale,* see CHARLETON (1668); in this edition, the passages are found on leaves 1v–2r [n.p.; n.s.], sigs. B2r (2nd sig. B), D1v–2r, M4v, M8v–N1r.

648.   CHETWOOD, KNIGHTLY. "To the Earl of Roscommon" in Wentworth Dillon's *An Essay on Translated Verse*. R1930. UMI 437: 6.

As Spurgeon notes (1: 257), there is a reference to Chaucer (prominently placed in a constellation of other poets) in a commendatory poem by Knightly Chetwood headed "To the Earl of Roscomon on his Excellent Poem":

> As when by *labouring* Stars new Kingdoms rise
> The mighty *Mass* in *rude* confusion lies,
> A Court *unform'd*, *disorder* at the Bar,
> And even in *Peace* the *rugged Meen* of War,
> Till some wise States-man into *Method* draws
> The parts, and *Animates* the frame with *Laws*;
> Such was the case when *Chaucer's early* toyl
> *Founded* the *Muses* Empire in *our* Soyl.
> *Spencer* improv'd it with his painful hand
> But *lost* a *Noble* Muse in *Fairy-land*.
> *Shakspear* say'd all that *Nature* cou'd impart,
> And *Johnson* added *Industry* and *Art*.
> *Cowley*, and *Denham* gain'd immortal praise;
> And some who *merit* as they *wear*, the Bays. (sig. A3v)

Another edition: R1931 (1685), sig. A4v.

649.   COLES, ELISHA. *An English Dictionary*. C5072. UMI 1328: 2.

For references to Chaucer in Coles's epistle to the reader and in various definitions, see COLES (1676); in this edition, the passages are found on sigs. A3r, K2r, L3r, P4v.

650.   COOKE, EDWARD. *A Short Historical Account of the Kings of England*. C6001A. UMI 2462: 16.

For a reference to the connection between John of Gaunt and Chaucer, see COOKE (1682); in this edition, the passage is found on 24.

651.   COWLEY, ABRAHAM. *The Works of Mr. Abraham Cowley*. C6656A. UMI 2350: 16.

For a reference to Cowley's burial place near Chaucer, see SPRAT (1668); in this edition, the passage is found on sig. c4r–v.

For a reference to Chaucer's "rich rhymes," see COWLEY (1656) C6683; in this edition, the passage is found on 37 (sig. Aa1r).

Other editions in 1684: C6656B (1684); C6657, 37 (sig. Aa1r).

652. DENHAM, JOHN. *Poems and Translations. Third edition.* D1007. UMI 1439: 41.

For praise of Chaucer in a poem headed "On Mr Abraham Cowley, his Death and Burial amongst the Ancient Poets," see DENHAM (1668); in this edition, the passage is found on 89–90.

653. FISHER, PAYNE. *The Tombes, Monuments, and Sepulchral Inscriptions, Lately Visible in St. Pauls Cathedral.* F1041. UMI 1259: 39.

Fisher (1616–1693) is identified on the title page as "P. F. student in antiquities. Batchelor of Arts and heretofore one of His late Majesties majors of foot." In a description of the tomb of Sir Payne Roet, Fisher mentions Roet's relationship to Chaucer:

> His Second Daughter was *Anne Roet*, who was Married to Sir *Geof-fry Chaucer* our Famous Old *English* Poet, by whom He had that most Beautiful Daughter *Alice*, the lovely Countess of the then *THOMAS MONTECUTE* Earl of *Salisbury*, who as the Common Story goes, Dancing at *Windsor* Castle with King *Edward* the Third, Her Garter accidentally falling off, was catcht up and worn upon the Arm of that Couragious King; which the Common opinion is, was consequently the cause of the First Institution of that Illustrious Order. (64)

Another edition in 1684: F1042, 64.

654. LACY, JOHN. *Sir Hercules Buffoon: or, The Poetical Squire. A Comedy.* L147. UMI 461: 13.

As Graves notes (*SP*), in the first scene of act 3, Lacy (d. 1681) causes his characters to mention Chaucer. Hercules observes: "We can suffer as much abuse as any Family in England upon the score of Poetry" (20) and Overwise responds:

> Come kneel down, Sir: now fill every Gentleman a Bumper of Claret. You must know for six moneths [*sic*] together he must swallow daily two Verses, and by old custom he must begin with *Chaucer*, and so go through all the English Poets, till he come to Mr. *Bayes*. The ceremony is an ancient Copy of Verses, taken out of the Records of *Parnassus*. (21)

"Mr. Bayes" is Dryden's nickname.

In response to the question of whether people suffer agues in Parnassus, Overwise prescribes a pill wrapped up in two lines of Chaucer:

> *Here I produce a rare and precious Pill,*
> *Made by the Doctors of Parnassus hill:*

The virtue is, it will thy Brain inspire
With th' airy flames of brisk Poetick Fire:
Having in it the refin'd Quintescence
Of Wit, true Wisdom, and well-worded Sence:
It being wrapt up in two lines of Chaucer,
You must with reverence swallow it down your Maw, Sir. (21–22)

655.   LE FÈVRE, RAOUL. *The Destruction of Troy.* L933. UMI 605: 1; book 3 (as L941A), UMI 1761: 29.

For two references to *Troilus and Criseyde*, see LE FÈVRE (1475) in Boswell & Holton No. 1; in this edition, the first reference to Chaucer's renaming Breseyda is omitted, but the second passage commending *Troilus and Criseyde* to readers is found in book 3, chapter 15, 164.

656.   LIGHTFOOT, JOHN. *The Works of the Reverend and Learned John Light-foot.* L2051. UMI 463: 1.

Lightfoot (1602–1675) is identified on the title page as "late Master of Kather-ine Hall in Cambridge." In chapter 6, "Of Jewish Learning," he cites Chaucer and closely paraphrases a line from *The Reeve's Tale*, "The gretteste clerkes been nought wisest men" (line 4054):

How nimble Textualists and Grammarians for the [Hebrew] Tongue the Rabbins are, their Comments can witness. But as in *Chaucer the greatest Clarks are not the wisest men*, so among them, these that are so great Textualists, are not best at the Text. (997)

657.   LOVEDAY, ROBERT. *Loveday's Letters Domestick and Forrein.* L3230. UMI 1486: 51. (1684)

For a reference to Chaucer as a prophet and poet, perhaps an allusion to the spu-rious work known as "Chaucer's Prophecy," see LOVEDAY (1659); in this edition, the passage is found on 98–99.

658.   MAIMBOURG, LOUIS. *The History of the League Written in French by Monsieur Maimbourg; Translated into English by His Majesty's Command by Mr. Dryden.* M292. UMI 1290: 1.

In this translation by Dryden of *Histoire de la Ligue*, there appears to be an echo of a line from *The Reeve's Tale*: "The gretteste clerkes been noght wisest men" (line 4054). In book 3, in a passage about "President Brisson" who was alleged to have behaved in a self-serving manner, Dryden translates:

An action much unworthy of a man who had so high a reputation for his rare learning, who ought rather to have lost his life, than to have so

basely abandon'd his King, and to have made himself a Slave to the passions of his mortal Enemies, under pretence that all he did was onely
to shelter himself from the violence of the Faction, as he privately pro-
tested. But so it is, that the greatest Clerks are not always the wisest
Men. (450)

659.   MILLINGTON, EDWARD. *A Catalogue of the Libraries of Two Eminent Persons Deceased.* C1379. UMI 1710: 3.

Millington's auction was held on 16 June 1684 at Bridges Coffee-House. In the
catalogue, under the heading "Miscellanies, viz. History, Phisick, Law, Mathematicks, Romances, &c. In Folio," lot 34 is listed as *"Chaucer (Geofr.)* his whole
Works, with divers Additions—Guilt and Lett." (²1; sig. Aa1r). Under the heading "Miscellanies, viz. History, Physick, Law, Mathematicks, Romances, &c.
In Quarto," lot 38 is listed as *"Chaucer (Geofr.)* Loves of *Troylus* and *Cressida* in
Latine and *English* Verse.—1634" (²7; sig. Bb1r).

660.   OLDHAM, JOHN. *Some New Pieces Never Before Publisht.* O249. UMI
573: 1; UMI 1023: 1; UMI 1153: 24; UMI 1291: 3.

For references which imply that Chaucer is not so well appreciated as once he
was, see OLDHAM (1681); in this edition, a part of Oldham's *Works,* the passages
are found on 5, 82–83.

Also collected in *The Works of Mr. John Oldham* (1684) O224, same pagination; and O225, same pagination.

**661.   *The Politicks of Malecontents, Shewing the Grand Influence of the Jesuits
Have in All Their Desperate Undertakings.* P2769. UMI 847: 10.**

In a passage about the grasping nature of Jesuits, the writer alludes to *The Summoner's Tale*:

> But if you do give Money, let it be upon some grand Consideration. . . .
> It will be Prudence in you to imitate the crafty Fryer, who desired to his
> Dinner only the Liver of a Capon, and a Roasted Piggs Head, knowing
> full well, that if he got those, he would not want his part of the Pig and
> Capon too. (30)

662.   *Poor Robin, 1684. An Almanack after a New Fashion.* A2203. UMI 931: 64.

Under the heading "Observations on April": "Patient Griezel" is celebrated on
the 30th (sig. A6r); this is perhaps an allusion to the protagonist of *The Clerk's
Tale.*

663.   RAMSAY (or RAMESEY), WILLIAM. *Conjugium conjurgium: or, Some Serious Considerations on Marriage.* R230. UMI 2055: 16.

For a spurious quotation attributed to Chaucer and genuine quotations from *The Knight's Tale, The Wife of Bath's Prologue,* and *The Romaunt of the Rose,* see RAMSAY (1673); in this edition the passages are found on 51 (*sic,* really 49), 74–75, 77–78, 80.

664.   S., G. *Anglorum speculum: or, The Worthies of England, in Church and State.* S22A. UMI 438: 2 (identified as S672).

This work is a heavily edited and augmented version of Thomas Fuller's *The Worthies of England.* Although Spurgeon notes (1: 257) one reference to Chaucer's burial near Spenser, there are others.

In a chapter headed "Barkshire," in a section on noted sheriffs, G. S. (sometimes thought to be George Sandys, but he died in 1644) refers to Chaucer's son:

> *Th. Chaucer* sole Son to *Geffery Chaucer* the Famous Poet, from whom he inherited fair Lands at *Dunning-Castle* in this County, and at *Ewelme* in *Oxf.* He married *Maud* Daughter and Coheir of Sir *J. Burwash,* by whom he had *Alice* married to *Will. de la Pole* D. of *Suffolk.* (53)

In the chapter on Cambridgeshire, the author notes that Caxton printed Chaucer's works:

> *Will. Caxton* of *Caxton,* a diligent and learned Man . . . Collected and Printed all *Chaucer's* Works, and on many Accounts deserved well of Posterity, and dyed about 1488. (91)

In the chapter on Essex, under the heading "Noted Sheriffs," G. S. writes:

> *Brian Tuke,* Knight, was Treasurer of the *Chamber* to *H[enry]* 8 . . . *Lealand* says he was a very *Eloquent* Man and *Bale* affirms he wrote Observations on *Chaucer, &c.* (199)

In the chapter on Canterbury, under the heading "Proverbs," G. S. writes:

> *Canterbury Tales,* a Book of *Chaucer* so called; it is applied to all *Feigned* and *Pleasant* Stories, *&c.* such as the Miracles of Becket. (420–21)

In a section on writers of London since the reformation, in a passage about Edmund Spencer, the author notes Spenser's imitation of Chaucer and their burial near one another:

Edm. Spencer, bred in *Camb*. A great Poet who imitated *Chaucer* . . . was honourably buried nigh *Chancer* [*sic*] in *Westminster*. (497–98)

In the chapter on Norfolk, in a section headed "Seamen," we find an allusion to *A Treatise on the Astrolabe*:

Nich. of *Lynne*, bred in Oxford. . . . 'Tis said he wrote a Book of Discoveries. . . . *Chaucer* makes an Honourable mention of him. He died 1360. (523)

Another edition in 1684: S22B, same pagination.

665.   S., W., in John Bullokar's *An English Expositor: Teaching the Interpretation of the Hardest Words Used in Our Language*. B5434. UMI 1844: 11.

For a reference to Chaucer and *The Prologue to the Squire's Tale* in the definition of Chivancy, see S., W. (1654); in this edition, the passage is found on sig. B12r.

For a reference to Chaucer and allusion to *The Nun's Priest's Tale*, see S., W. (1663); in this edition, the passage is found on sig. B11r.

666.   SMALLWOOD, MATTHEW. *Catalogus librorum*. S4010. UMI 513: 12; UMI 1710: 1.

The library of the late Rev. Dr. Smallwood ("Decani de Lychfield") was offered for sale by auction on 2 May 1684 at Gresham College in Bishopsgate Street. In the catalogue, under the heading "English in Folio," number 84 is listed as "Chaucer the Ancient Poet (Geffray) his Works perfect and fair" (25). Under the heading "Bound Volumes of Tracts, &c. In Quarto," number 28 is "Amorum Troili & Creseide, Libr. 2. Anglico Latini" (35, really 37).

667.   SPARROW, ANTHONY. *A Rationale upon the Book of Common Prayer of the Church of England*. S4834A. UMI 2257: 2.

For a reference to Chaucer as a likely source for the word *ember*, see SPARROW 1668); in this edition, the passage is found on sig. S3r.

Another edition in 1684: S4834, sig. S3r.

668.   *The Wanton Wife of Bath*. W721A . No UMI. Pepys Ballad, vol. 2, 39.

For a reference to Chaucer's writing of a wanton wife of Bath, see *The Wanton Wife of Bath* (1641).

669.   WILSON, JOHN. *The Cheats. A Comedy.* W2918. UMI 1320: 32.

For a reference to *The Canon's Yeoman's Tale* as the source and inspiration for
Erasmus's *Alcumistica* and Jonson's *Alchemist*, see WILSON (1664); in this edition,
the passage is found on sig. A3r.

670.   WINSTANLEY, WILLIAM. *Englands Worthies.* W3059. UMI 1433: 12.

For a picture of Chaucer on the title page and references to Chaucer in Winstanley's bibliography and the table of contents, references to Chaucer's epitaph for
Edward III, and a life of Chaucer, see WINSTANLEY (1660) W3058; in this edition, the passages are found on sig. a6v and sig. a7v, 102–3, 116–23.

In this expanded edition that includes "The Life of Mr. Edmond Spenser,"
Winstanley writes:

> [H]e died *Anno* 1598. and was honourably buried nigh *Chaucer* in *West-*
> *minster*-Abbey, at the sole charge of *Robert*, first of that name Earl of
> *Essex.* . . . (226).

In "The Life of Mr. Michael Drayton," Winstanley notes his burial place near
Chaucer's:

> He changed his Lawrel for a Crown of glory, *Anno* 1631. and was buried
> in *Westminster-Abby*, near the South-door, by those two eminent Poets,
> *Jeffery Chaucer* and *Edmond Spenser.* . . . (341)

In "The Life of Mr. Wil. Shakespeare," Winstanley transcribes his epitaph that
mentions Chaucer:

> This our famous Comedian died, *Anno Domini* 16– – [*sic*] and was bur-
> ied at *Stratford* upon *Avon*, the Town of his Nativity, upon whom one
> hath bestowed this Epitaph.
> > *Renowned* Spenser, *lye a thought more nigh*
> > *To learned* Chaucer, *and rare* Beaumont *lye*,
> > *A little nearer* Spenser, *to make room for* Shakespear. . . . (346–47)

671.   WINSTANLEY, WILLIAM. *The New Help to Discourse: or, Wit, Mirth, and*
Jollity, Intermixt with More Serious Matters. W3071. UMI 1244: 22.

For two quotations from *The General Prologue*, see WINSTANLEY (1668); in this
edition, the passages are found on 19, 202.

1685

672.   BLOME, RICHARD. *The Art of Heraldry.* B3205. UMI 1031: 8.

For a description of Chaucer's coat of arms, see BLOME (1684); in this edition, the passage is found on 67.

Another edition: B3206 (1693), 67.

673.   BOLD, HENRY. *Latine Songs with Their English, and Poems.* B3471. UMI 127: 9.

Bold (1627–1683) is identified on the title page as "Henry Bold, formerly of N. Coll. in Oxon, afterwards of the Examiners Office in Chancery." In "Song XXXVII. Dear Friend," he echoes a line from *The Manciple's Prologue*: "Sires, what! Dun is in the myre!" (line 5). He writes:

> The King and the Prelates,
> Will Cudgel the Zealots,
> . . . .
> They'l [*sic*] serve to help Squire
> *Dun*, out of the mire. (117)

674.   CHETWOOD, KNIGHTLY. "To the Earl of Roscommon" in Wentworth Dillon's *An Essay on Translated Verse.* R1931. UMI 799: 29.

For a reference to Chaucer (prominently placed in a constellation of other poets) in a commendatory poem addressed to the Earl of Roscomon, see CHETWOOD (1684); in this edition, the passage is found on sig. A4v.

675.   COLES, ELISHA. *An English Dictionary.* C5073. UMI 1567: 6.

For references to Chaucer in Coles's epistle to the reader and in various definitions, see COLES (1676); in this edition, the passages are found on sigs. A3r, K2r, L3r, P4v.

676.   DELONEY, THOMAS. *The Garland of Good-Will.* D947. UMI 735: 11.

For what may be a faint allusion to *The Clerk's Tale*, see DELONEY (1628) in Boswell & Holton No. 1116. In this edition, the passage is found in the second part where number 2 is headed "Of Patient *Grissel* and a Noble *Marquess*" (sigs. E7r–F2v).

677.   EVELYN, JOHN. "The Immortality of Poesie" in *Poems by Several Hands, and on Several Occasions Collected by N. Tate.* T210. UMI 370: 6.

As Spurgeon notes (1: 258), there is a reference to Chaucer in a poem by John Evelyn, "The Immortality of Poesie. To Envy":

> Old *Chaucer* shall, for his facetious style,
> Be read, and prais'd by warlike *Britains*, while
> The Sea enriches, and defends their Isle. (91)

678.   GARENCIERES, THEOPHILUS DE. *The True Prophecies: or, Prognostications of Michael Nostradamus.* N1400. No UMI.

For a reference to the difficulty of Chaucer's language (comparable to the difficulty of Nostradamus's), see GARENCIERES (1672).

679.   A ghost.

680.   *Miscellany, Being a Collection of Poems by Several Hands.* Edited by Aphra Behn. M2230. UMI 190: 11.

As Harris notes (*PQ*), there is a reference to Chaucer in a poem headed "On the University of Cambridge. A Dialogue between Tutor and Pupil. By an Unknown Hand, Anno 84." In a passage extolling those who come from Cambridge, the author mentions Chaucer:

> They all of our great Learned Mother come,
> The Ingenious Offspring of her fruitful Womb;
> She *Chaucer* too, and *Cowly* first brought forth,
> Before in time, but not before in worth;
> In *Dryden's* Mighty self she claims a part,
> Tho he to *Oxford* has resign'd his heart. (249)

681.   *Miscellany Poems and Translations by Oxford Hands.* M2232. UMI 1235: 9.

As Spurgeon notes (1: 258) in a section headed "Some Elegies out of Ovid's Amours Imitated," in "Elegy the Fifteenth, Book the First Imitated. To detracting Censures, that the Fame of Poets is Eternal," an unidentified poet writes of Chaucer's lasting fame:

> Ill-natur'd Censurer desist for shame
> With thy malicious Tongue to stab my Fame
> How durst thou think I live dissolv'd in ease
> Or call brave Verse the effects of Idleness?
> . . . .

And to gain Gold, damnation, and renown,
Turn a meer Prostitute to all the Town;
With Mercenary breath cant out the Laws,
And take mens Money to betray their Cause?
But all these servile things must with us dye,
The Fame, I seek, shall know Eternity:
My Wit a lasting Monument shall raise,
And all the world shall loudly sing my Praise.
Chaucer shall live, whilst this our *Brittish* Land,
Or the vast *Cornwall-Mount* in it shall stand:
Or whilst (almost a Sea it self) the *Thames*
To th'Ocean rowls his tributary Streams. (155)

682.   MONTAIGNE, MICHEL DE. *Essays of Michael, Seigneur de Montaigne in Three Books.* **M2479. UMI 818: 1.**

In this translation by Charles Cotton of Montaigne's *Essais*, there appears to be an echo of a line from *The Reeve's Tale*: "The gretteste clerkes been noght wisest men" (line 4054). In book 1, chapter 24, "Of Pedantry," Cotton translates Rabelais's line *magis magnos Clericos, non sunt magis magnos sapientes* as "The greatest Clerks are not the wisest men" (211).

Other editions: M2480 (1693), 191; M2481 (1700), 191.

683.   PARKHURST, THOMAS. *Catalogus variorum librorum ex bibliothecis selectissimis.* **P491. UMI 157: 3; UMI 1710: 12.**

The bookseller Thomas Parkhurst offered the libraries of "two Learned Men deceased" (sig. A2r) for sale by auction at Bridges Coffee House in Popes Head Alley in Cornhill on 19 October 1685. In the sales catalogue for this vast collection, under the heading "English Books of Poetry and Playes, in large Folio," lot 115 is listed as "Chaucer (Jeffery) his works. — 1532" (31). Another work touches on Chaucer; under the heading "Poetry, in small Octavo and Twelves, English," lot 511 is listed as "Chaucers ghost, a piece of Antiquity, contain. [*sic*] 12 pleasant Fables" (76).

684.   PHILLIPS, EDWARD. *The Mysteries of Love and Eloquence.* **P2067. UMI 1202: 6.**

For a witty saying attributed to Chaucer, see PHILLIPS (1658); in this edition, the passage is found on 196.

685.   PLOT, ROBERT. *De origine fontium.* **P2583. UMI 1154: 23.**

Plot (1640–1696) is identified on the title page as "Rob. Plot. L. L. D. Custodiæ Musæi Ashmoleani Oxoniæ præpositum et Regiæ Societis Londoni Secretarium." In a Latin quotation of a passage from Josiah Sylvester's rendition of Du Bartas's *Divine Weeks*, Plot writes:

> *Unde sitim longas in luces millia sedant*
> *Præter quæ excurrunt; avido properantia cursu*
> Chauceri *alluere inde pedes prope* Donningtonam. (44–45)

Donningtonam is marked for a foot note: "Donnintonæ *castellum, quondam sedes* Galfridi Chauceri *Eq. Aur. nobillisimi* Anglorum *Poetæ, juxta hunc rivulum situm est*" (45).

For Du Bartas, see Boswell & Holton No. 838.

686.   *Poor Robin, 1685. An Almanack of the Old and New Fashion*. A2204. UMI 1084: 22.

Under the heading "Observations on August": "Chaucers Miller" is celebrated on the 16th of the month; this is no doubt an allusion to *The Canterbury Tales* (sig. B4r).

687.   RYVES, BRUNO. *Mercurius Rusticus: or, The Countries Complaint of the Barbarous Outrages Committed by the Sectaries of This Late Flourishing Kingdom.* R2449. UMI 1578: 6.

Ryves (1596–1677) echoes a line from *The Wife of Bath's Prologue*: "A likerous mouth most han a likerous tayl" (line 466) in describing an event in which soldiers had raided a gentleman's house and upon breaking in "the Ladies Closet," discovered provisions for hospitable entertainment. Ryves writes:

> [A] common Soldier, who seeing him [an officer] feed greedily on a Gally-pot, and presuming his judgment to be good in the choice, (for the Proverb is true which end soever you put formost [*sic*], *A liquorish tail hath a liquorish tooth*), rudely thrust his whole fist all begrimed and besmeared in blood and powder, into the pot with him. . . . (11)

688.   SHAKESPEARE, WILLIAM. *Mr. William Shakespeares Comedies, Histories and Tragedies*. S2915. UMI 1294: 21.

For multiple references and allusions to Chaucer and his works, see SHAKE-SPEARE (1623), Boswell & Holton No. 1050.

For an echo of a line from *The Manciple's Prologue* in *Romeo and Juliet*, see SHAKESPEARE (1597) in the Appendix; in this edition the passage is found on 2308.

Variant editions in 1685: S2916; S2917, same pagination.

689. TALLENTS, FRANCIS. *A View of Universal History.* T129A. UMI 2373: 13 and UMI 1558: 14 (identified as T130).

In his chart of historical events from the creation down to the year 1680, Tallents (1619–1708) includes a list of eminent writers for the modern periods. In the period 1300–1400, he includes "Dantes," "Fra: Petrarch," and "Boccace," and notes that the latter "reforms ye Italian." At the end of the century he lists "Geffr. Chaucer *p*[*oet*]" and "Joh. Gower *p*[*oet*] *&c.*" (no pagination; no signatures).

Other editions: T 130 (1695), same pagination; T131 (1700?), same as 1695 edition.

690. TYTON, FRANCIS. "A Catalogue" in John Flavel's *Pneumatologia, A Treatise of the Soul of Man.* F1176. UMI 960: 22.

In "A Catalogue of Books Printed for, and Sold by Francis Tyton Bookseller at the Three Dagges in Fleetstreet near the Temple-Gate," among "Books in small," i.e., 80, 120, and 240, we find: "*Chaucer*'s Ghost" (no pagination; no signatures).

691. WESLEY, SAMUEL. *Maggots: or, Poems on Several Subjects.* W1374. UMI 907: 1.

As Spurgeon notes (1: 258), Wesley (1662–1735) refers to Chaucer in an explanatory note for the line "E're my brisk feather'd Bell-man will tel me 'tis day":

> *Meaning* Chaunticleer, — *as Grandsire* Chaucer *has it*; *or in new* English, *no better nor worse than a* Cock, — *that* Baron Tell-Clock of the Night, — *as* Cleveland *christens him.* (97)

1686

692. *Bibliotheca Anglicana: or, A Collection of Choice English Books.* B2819. UMI 1790: 4.

An auction of books was held at Jonathan's Coffee-House on 5 May 1686. In the catalogue, lot 27 is listed as "*Chaucers* Works, best Edition, with his Life 1598" (no page; no signature). In the margin of the British Library copy, someone noted that the book sold for £1.

693. *Bibliotheca Baconia.* B273. UMI 12299: 33.

The library of "Mr. Francis Bacon, lately deceased," was offered for sale by auction on 19 May 1686 at Jonathan's Coffee House in Exchange Alley, Cornhill, London. Lot 29 is listed as "*Chaucers* Works, imperfect at the end" without date or place of publication. The marked catalogue in the British Library indicates that it sold for 7s 8d.

694.   BRITAINE, WILLIAM DE. *Humane Prudence: or, The Art by Which a Man May Raise Himself & Fortune to Grandeur. The Third Edition: Corrected and Very Much Enlarged.* B4805B. UMI 1808: 7.

Britaine attributes a quotation to Chaucer in this revised and augmented edition of his book of good counsel. Although this book went through thirteen printings between 1680 and 1730, Britaine has been neglected by *ODNB*. His witty epigrams (e.g., "A Woman is a Book, and often found | To prove, far better in the Sheets than Bound") suggest that he may be ripe for revival. In section headed "Of Riches, and the right use thereof," in a passage that urges folk to enjoy their estates while they are alive, Britaine writes:

> And when you are dead, you are no more concerned in that you shall leave behind you, than you were in that which was before you were born; therefore get well to live, and then study to live well.
> Many times, with *Chaucer*, I scratch my Head where it doth not itch, to see Men live poor to dye rich. (55)

Other editions: B4805C (1689), 167, in which the context changes and "Chaucer's" sentiments are presented in verse; B4806 (1693), 120; B4807 (1697), 99; B4807A (1700), 99.

695.   BUNYAN, JOHN. *The Pilgrim's Progress. The Second Part.* B5578. UMI 1663: 27.

For an echo of Chaucer's line, "Go, litel bok, go litel myn tragedye" (*Troilus and Criseyde* 5: 1786), see BUNYAN (1684); in this edition, the passage is found on sig. A2r.

696.   *A Catalogue Containing Variety of English Books.* C1257. UMI 1326: 29.

An auction of books was held on 20 December 1686 at Bridges Coffee-House in Popes Head Alley, Cornhill. In the sales catalogue, under the heading "Appendix, Folio, Quarto, Octavo," number 6 is listed as "*Chaucers* Works, wants a Title at the beginning—" (47).

697.   *Catalogus variorum librorum.* B4103. UMI 1303: 10.

The libraries of the Reverend Doctors John Bradford and William Cooper, both of London, were offered for sale at Bridges Coffee-House in Popes-Head Alley in Cornhill on 14 June 1686. Among the works was one by Chaucer. In the catalogue, under the heading "An Appendix, English Folio," lot 21 is listed as "Sir

Jeffery Chaucers Works, with his Life, the best Edition.—1662" (69); the date should probably be read as 1602.

698. COTTON, CHARLES. *Burlesque upon Burlesque: or, The Scoffer Scoft. Being Some of Lucian's Dialogues, Newly Put into English Fustian. Second edition.* **C6380b. UMI 684: 1.**

For a reference to Patient Grizell, perhaps an allusion to *The Clerk's Tale*, see COTTON (1675); in this edition, the passage is found on sig. A2r.

699. DAVIES, JOHN. *A Memorial for the Learned: or, Miscellany of Choice Collections from Most Eminent Authors.* **D395. UMI 63: 3 (identified as D38).**

In a chapter headed "Notable Events in the Reign of King Edward the III," Davies (1625–1693) mentions Chaucer. Davies writes:

> In this King's Time lived the so much famed Sir *Geoffry Chaucer*, the famous *English* Poet. [In a shoulder note: "*Chaucer.*"] (68)

Chaucer is also listed in "An Alphabetical Table to the Historical Part."

700. JEVON, THOMAS. *The Devil of a Wife: or, A Comical Transformation.* **J731. UMI 108: 10.**

As Graves notes (*SP*), in the second act of this farce "Acted by Their Majesties Servants at the Queens Theatre in Dorset Garden" (title page), Jevon (1652–1688) interpolates a popular ballad that refers to Chaucer's writing about the Wife of Bath. The ballad was first published as *The Wanton Wife of Bath* (1641), q.v.; in this play, the passage is found on 26.

Other editions: J731A (1693), 26; J732 (1695), 21–22.

701. JOHNSON, RICHARD. *The Famous History of the Seven Champions of Christendom. The Third Part.* **J806. UMI 2032: 7**

Richard Johnson (1573–1659?) was one the most successful English writers of chivalric romance. Based on medieval lore, the first part of his *Seven Champions* appeared in 1596 and proceeded to enjoy numerous editions as well as sequels and abridgments right on through the seventeenth century and for many years thereafter. As Spurgeon notes (3: 4.78), thirty or so years after his death, this "Third Part" appeared. In an epistle addressed "To the Curteous Reader," Johnson notes that the English language has changed since Chaucer's eloquent lines were in vogue. He writes:

> The general acceptance which the two first Parts of this Renowned History have received, hath invited my Pen to the prosecution thereof in a third Part which I have raked out of the must Records of old moth-

eaten Authors, almost worn out by length of time, and indeed the two first Parts do seem imperfect without a third. . . . If I have soared above the height of the Language of the two former parts, know that our speech is refined since they were writ, *Chaucer* whose lines did excel for Eloquence in his days, is now despised for plain and rustick, even by those who scarcely know what language is. . . . (sig. A3r–v)

Other editions: J804 (1696), sig. A3r–v.

702.   LINDSAY, DAVID. *The Works of the Famous and Worthy Knight, Sir David Lindsay of the Mount.* L2319. No UMI.

For a reference to Chaucer's skill as a poet in the prologue of *The Testament of Papingo,* see LINDSAY (1538) in Boswell & Holton No. 146.

For a passage that mentions the fable of *Troilus and Criseyde* in an epistle to the king that is set before the prologue to "The Dreme of Sir David Lindsay," see LINDSAY (1558) in Boswell & Holton No. 209.

703.   MILLINGTON, EDWARD. *Bibliotheca Castelliana.* C1223. UMI 1546: 20.

Millington began auctioning the library of Dr. Edmund Castell, Professor of Arabic at Cambridge, on 30 June 1686 at the Sign of the Eagle and Child in Cambridge. In the catalogue, under the heading "Divinity, History, &c. in Folio," lot 62 is listed as "The Works of Geffray Chaucer, with his Life, and an explanation of the obscure Words, and Difficulties, His Effigies, &c.—1598" (24). Someone marked the British Library copy of the catalogue to indicate that the volume sold for 19*s.*

704.   MILLINGTON, EDWARD. *A Collection of Choice Books . . . Curiously Bound.* C5119. UMI 1438: 12 and UMI 1710: 20.

Millington conducted an auction at Bridges Coffee House in Popes-Head Alley on Monday, 8 February 1685/86. In the catalogue, under the heading "Poetry, Plays, Romances, Novels, &c. Fol.," lot 6 is listed as "Chaucer (Geffrey) Works of Antient Poetry, with his Life and exposition of his Terms—1598" (20).

705.   OLDHAM, JOHN. *The Works of Mr. John Oldham.* O226. UMI 2010: 7.

For a reference to Chaucer's penchant for coining new words in "Horace His Art of Poetry" and a reference to the diminished appreciation of Chaucer's poetry in a tribute to the Earl of Rochester, see OLDHAM (1681); in this collection, the passages are found on 5, ²82–83.

Other editions in 1686: 0227, same pagination; 0228, same pagination.

706.   PHILIPPS, THOMAS. *Bibliotheca Angleseiana.* A3166. UMI 1472: 3.

The library of Arthur Annesley, Earl of Anglesey, was offered for sale by auction beginning 25 October 1686 at the Sign of the Black Swan. In the catalogue, under the running head "Miscellanies in Folio, viz. History, &c.," number 196 is listed as "*G. Chaucers* Works, with the Seige and Destruction of the City of *Theb.* by *Lidgate* 1561" (²28). Under the heading "Libri Manuscripti Diversis Voluminibus," number 5 is "*Geffery Chaucer* the Ancient *English* Poet, his Works most curiously written upon Vellum and the great Letters Guilded, with flourishes in Gold and Colours. *Folio*" (²77).

707.   PIERCE, THOMAS. *The Law and Equity of the Gospel: or, the Goodness of Our Lord as a Legislator.* P2185. UMI 1621:25.

Pierce (1622–1691) is identified on the title page as "Chaplain in Ordinary to his Majesty, and Dean of Sarum." In a sermon titled "Satan's Masterpiece as a Tempter to Worldly Greatness," Pierce appears to echo the description of the shipman in *The General Prologue*: "Of nyce conscience took he no keep" (line 398). He writes (Satan speaks to Jesus):

> *Thou seest it goes* best *with the* worst *of men; and that the men of nice* Conscience *are quite* undone *by their* Integrity. (548)

708.   *The Pleasant and Sweet History of Patient Grissel. Translated out of Italian.* P2532. UMI 2150: 28.

Other than the name, an allusion to *The Clerk's Tale*, this account "shewing how she from a poor mans Daughter came to be a great Lady in France, being a pattern for all Vertuous Women" has little or nothing to do with Chaucer.

709.   PLOT, ROBERT. *The Natural History of Stafford-shire.* P2588. UMI 819: 5.

Plot (1640–1696) is identified on the title page as "Robert Plot. LLD. Keeper of the Ashmolean musæum and professor of chymistry in the University of Oxford." As Harris notes (*PQ*), Plot mentions Chaucer's association with Oxfordshire. In a section on monstrous or imperfect births, he writes:

> Nor has it been usual only amongst the *Natural Historians* to transmit to posterity such *imperfect births* as these; but he most perfect ones too, when they have proved *extraordinary*: whence it is that the birth-places of *Princes*, and *Men* any way *famous*, either for *Arts*, or *Arms*; for *Piety*, or *Munificence*; have been constantly noted: and if by chance so neglected that they have become *dubious*; what contention has there been between *Citys* and *Countries* for the honour of the *birth* of a *famous Man*? Thus no less than *seven Cities* strove for the birth of *Homer*; and thus *Middlesex* and *Oxfordshire* contest the birth of *Chaucer* our famous English *Poet* [in

a footnote: "*See the Life of Chaucer by John Speght.*"]; and here in *Oxford-shire Ewelm* and *Wood-stock* both pretend to him. (272)

710. *Poor Robin. 1686. An Almanack of the Old and New Fashion.* A2205. UMI 1393: 6.

Under the heading "Observations on April": "Patient Grizell" is celebrated on the 25th of this month (sig. A8r); this is perhaps an allusion to the protagonist of *The Clerk's Tale*.

Under the heading "Observations on August": "Chaucers Miller" is celebrated on the 13th of this month (sig. B4r).

711. **WALLER, EDMUND.** *Poems, &c. Written upon Several Occasions.* W517. UMI 588: 4.

For a reference to the difficulty of Chaucer's language for modern readers, see WALLER (1668); in this edition, the passage is found on 236–38.

712. **WRIGHT, THOMAS.** *The Glory of God's Revenge against the Bloody and Detestable Sins of Murther and Adultery.* W3709. UMI 995: 19.

Wright is described on the title page as "M. A. of St. Peters Colledge in Cambridge." In this collection of "histories," Wright appears to plagiarize Scarron, q.v. In this work, the passage is found on 273. There Scarron's translator appears to echo the description of the shipman in *The General Prologue*: "Of nyce conscience took he no keep" (line 398).

1687

713. **BASSET, THOMAS.** "Catalogue" in Hugo Grotius, *Christ's Passion. The Second Edition.* G2093. UMI 598: 16.

At the end of this work is found "A Catalogue of some Books, Printed for, and to be Sold by Thomas Basset, at the George in Fleet-Street." In the catalogue, under the heading "Folio's" he lists "*Chaucer's* Works" (sig. H7r).

714. **BOWMAN, THOMAS.** *Catalogus librorum.* C1448. UMI 933: 24.

In an epistle addressed "to the readers," Bowman (*fl.* 1664–1687) writes that it would be presumptuous of him to explain the advantages of selling books by auction, for "they are already sufficiently known to all the Curious in Learning here, and beyond Sea." Encouraged by the success of two previous auctions, he gives the learned gentlemen of Oxford another at his place of business on High Street. The sale was scheduled to commence at 8 o'clock in the morning of 28 February

1686/87 and, with a two-hour break for dinner, finish at 5 o'clock, "continuing dayly till all the Books are Sold."

In the catalogue under the heading "English Books in Divinity, Law, Physick, Mathematicks, History Poetry, &c. Folio," Bowman lists "Chaucer's (Geoffrey) Works—Lond. 1561" (sig. A*1v).

Under the running head "English Books in Divinity, Law, &c. In Quarto," number 173: "Loves of *Troilus* and *Cresseid*, in Lat. And English Verse - - *Oxf.* 1635" (sig. E*1r). This work is, of course, Kynaston's translation of *Troilus and Criseyde*.

In the same sale, three volumes of Ben Jonson's works, several works by the Duchess of Newcastle, two copies of Spenser's works (1679), John Harington's translation of *Orlando Furioso* (1607), Shakespeare's plays, second folio edition (1632), the poems of Mrs. Katharine Philips, and *Don Quixot* (1675) were offered up for auction.

715.   BUNYAN, JOHN. *The Pilgrim's Progress. The Second Part.* B5579. UMI 2950: 9.

For an echo of *Troilus and Criseyde* 5: 1786, in "The Author's Way of Sending forth his Second Part of the Pilgrim," see BUNYAN (1684); in this edition, the passage is found on sig. A2r.

716.   BURNET, GILBERT. *Relation of a Conference Held about Religion at London.* B5863. UMI 839: 8.

For a reference to the difficulty of Chaucer's language for contemporaries, see BURNET (1676); in this edition, the passage is found 45.

717.   *A Catalogue of Books of the Several Libraries of the Honorable Sir William Coventry, and the Honorable Mr. Henry Coventry.* C6626. UMI 487: 11.

The Coventry libraries were auctioned at the residence of Henry Coventry, sometime Secretary of State to King Charles II, at the upper end of the Hay-Market on 9 May 1687. In the catalogue, under the heading "English Books in Folio," lot 75 is listed as "Jeff. Chaucer's Works - - [n.p., n.d.]" (15). Under the heading "English Folio," lot 31 is listed as "Gef. Chaucers Works - - Lond. 1602" (36).

718.   *A Catalogue of Choice Books.* C1298a. UMI 2587: 12.

An enterprising bookseller held an auction in the Flesh Market at New Castle upon Tyne on 1 August 1687. In the catalogue, under the heading "Books in Folio, of various Subjects. Eng. and Lat.," lot number 61 is listed as "The Works of *Jeffery Chaucer*; with a Clavis - - 1687" (11).

719. *A Catalogue of Choice English Books.* C1302. UMI 1304: 17.

A collection of books "Consisting of divinity, history, physick, and Variety of other subjects" was exposed for sale by auction on 10 January 1687 at Jonathan's Coffee-House in Exchange Alley in Cornhill. In the catalogue, under the heading "Divinity, History, Physick, Miscellanies, in Folio," lot number 57 is listed as "Geof. Chaucer's Works Lettered. (wants a little at the end) [no date of publication given]" (2). Among books in quarto, lot 116 is listed as "Sir *Fr. Kinaston*'s Translation of *Chaucer*'s *Troilus* and *Cresida*—1635" (8).

720. *A Catalogue of Choice English Books.* C1302A. UMI 2587: 14

An auction of books on various subjects was held at Wellington's Coffee-House in Threadneedle Street on 18 July 1687. In the catalogue, under the heading "Divinity, History, Physick, &c. in Folio," lot number 247 is listed as "Sir *Jeff. Chaucers* Works [n.p.; n.d.]" (6).

721. *A Catalogue of Latin, French, and English Books.* C1352. UMI 624: 3 and **Early English Books: Tract Supplement: D7: 3 (S.C.922.[2]).**

A book auction was held on 17 October 1687 at Wellington's Coffee-House on the back side of the Royal Exchange. In the catalogue, under the heading "Divinity, History, &c. in Octavo and Twelves," lot 535 is listed as "Chaucers Ghost, or a piece of Antiquity—1671" (35). And in "Appendix," lot 25 is listed as "Chaucer (Geof.) His works, with his Life and Progeny—1598" (sig. A1r, following 40).

722. *A Catalogue of the Libraries of Mr. Jer. Copping . . . and Anscel Beaumont.* C6107. UMI 60: 18.

An auction was held at Jonathan's Coffee-House in Exchange-Alley in Cornhill on 21 March 1686/87 to sell the libraries of Jeremiah Copping, late of Sion College, and Anscel Beaumont, late of the Middle Temple. In the first part of the catalogue, under the heading "Divinity, History, &c. in Folio," lot 281 is listed as "*Geof. Chaucer's* Works; wants end—[no place, no date]" (6). In quarto, lot 33 is listed as "*Chaucer*'s Loves of *Troilus* and *Cresida*, in Latine and English; by Sir *Fr. Kinaston* (no date)" (7). In octavo, lot 132 is listed as "Chaucer's Ghost or a Piece of Antiquity; with the History of Prince *Corniger*" (8).

723. CHARLES I, KING OF ENGLAND. Βασιλικα [Basiliká]. *The Works of King Charles the Martyr. The Second Edition.* C2076. UMI 652: 7.

For an aphorism that the king attributes to Chaucer (but may allude to *The Squire's Tale*, lines 220–24), see CHARLES I (1649); in this edition, the passage is found on 80.

724. CHAUCER, GEOFFREY. *The Works of Our Ancient, Learned, & Excellent English Poet, Jeffrey Chaucer: As They Have Lately Been Compar'd with the Best Manuscripts; and Several Things Added, Never Before in Print. To Which Is Adjoyn'd, The Story of the Siege of Thebes, by John Lidgate, Monk of Bury. Together with the Life of Chaucer, Shewing His Countrey, Parentage, Education, Marriage, Children, Revenues, Service, Reward, Friends, Books, Death. Also a Table, Wherein the Old and Obscure Words in Chaucer are Explained, and Such Words (Which Are Many) That Either Are, by Nature or Derivation, Arabick, Greek, Latine, Italian, French, Dutch, or Saxon, Mark'd with Particular Notes for the Better Understanding Their Original.* C3736. UMI 59: 1.

As Spurgeon notes (1: 259), this edition is basically a reprint of Speght's second edition of 1602. At the end is an "Advertisement to the Reader" signed J. H., presumably Joseph Hindmarsh, the printer.

For a likely allusion to *The Knight's Tale*, see LYDGATE (1497); in this edition, the passage is found on 650.

725. CHAUCER JUNIOR. *Canterbury Tales: Composed for the Entertainment of All Ingenious Young Men and Maids at Their Merry Meetings.* C455A. UMI 1419: 32.

As Spurgeon notes (3: 4.77), Chaucer's connection with this jest book is solely by the title.

726. CLEVELAND, JOHN. *The Works of Mr. John Cleveland.* C4654. UMI 1713: 20.

For an echo of a line from *The Manciple's Prologue*, see CLEVELAND (1644); in this edition, the passage is found on 67.

For a reference to Chaucer and an allusion to *The Pardoner's Prologue* in "A Letter sent from a Parliament Officer at Grantham," see CLEVELAND (1658); in this collection, the passage is found on 95–96.

For Cleveland's citation of Chaucer and his reference to Jack Straw's riot in *The Nun's Priest's Tale*, see CLEVELAND (1654); in this collection, the passage is found on 424.

Another edition: C4655 (1699), 67, 95–96, 424.

727. CLIFFORD, MARTIN. *Notes upon Mr. Dryden's Poems in Four Letters.* C4706. UMI 348: 5.

Clifford (d. 1677) is identified on the title page as "late Master of the Charter-House in London," In the second letter, he quotes Shakespeare's allusion to *Troilus and Criseyda*:

Pistol defies his Rival in these words:

> *Fetch from the Powdring-Tub of Infamy*
> *That Lazar-Kite of Cressids kind.* (6)

728.   COLVILL, SAMUEL. *Whiggs Supplication, a Mock Poem.* C5428. UMI 1665: 15.

For a reference to cockscombs who pay insufficient attention when they read Chaucer, see COVIL (1681); in this edition, the passage is found on 42.

729.   COOPER, WILLIAM. *Catalogus librorum bibliothecæ instructissimae Eduardi Wray de Barling in comitatu Lincolniensis armigeri.* W3666. UMI 2122: 12.

"At the usual hours of 9 in the Morning, & 2 in the Afternoon, & so to continue daily till all are sold," on 20 June 1687, at the sign of the Pelican in London's Little-Britain, Cooper began auctioning the library of Edward Wray of Barlings in Lincolnshire. In an epistle to the readers, Cooper informs us that Wray was "a Gent. Well known for his skill in Arts and Languages, and his singular judgment in the choice of his Library, as well as curiosity of their Binding."

In the catalogue, under the heading "Philology in Folio, English," lot 105 is listed as "Gef. Chaucers Works, with the Siege & Destr. of the City of Thebes, compiled by J. Lidgate"; and 106 as "Another of the same, the best edition – – – Lond. 1687" (34; sig. I1v).

730.   COOPER, WILLIAM. *Catalogus librorum bibliothecæ viri cujusdam literati.* C1434. UMI 1304: 20.

In an epistle to the reader, Cooper notes that "the Sail of these books will begin the 14th. Day of February next 1686/7. At the Pelican in Little-Britain London, at the usual Hours of Nine in the Morning and Two in the Afternoon (if but twenty Buyers be present)." In the catalogue under the heading "Philology in Quarto," lot 214 is listed as "*Geof. Chaucer* (the English *Homer*) of the Laws [*sic*] of *Troilus* and *Cresida* in Latin and English [no date]" (21).

731.   COTTON, CHARLES. *Burlesque upon Burlesque: or, The Scoffer Scoft. Being Some of Lucian's Dialogues, Newly Put into English Fustian. Second edition.* C6380c. UMI 978: 20.

For a reference to Patient Grizell, perhaps an allusion to *The Clerk's Tale*, see COTTON (1675); in this edition, the passage is found on sig. A2r.

732.   DRYDEN, JOHN. *The Hind and the Panther. A Poem in Three Parts.* D2281. UMI 489: 11; and UMI 914: 7 (identified as D2284).

Dryden (1631–1700) is not named on the title page. In the third part of this allegory/fable, he uses the names *Partlet* and *Chanticleer* to allude to nuns and monks and may thus allude to *The Nun's Priest's Tale.* Dryden writes:

The World was fall'n into an easier way,
This Age knew better, than to Fast and Pray.

Good Sence in Sacred Worship would appear
So to begin, as they might end the year.
Such feats in former times had wrought the falls
Of crowing Chanticleers in Cloyster'd Walls.
Expell'd for this, and for their Lands they fled,
And Sister Partlet with her hooded head
Was hooted hence, because she would not pray a Bed. (130)

A Law, the Source of many Future harms,
Had banish'd all the Poultry from the Farms;
With loss of Life, if any should be found
To crow or peck on this forbidden Ground.
For *Chanticleer* the white, of Clergy kind. . . . (132–33)

After a grave Consult what course were best,
One more mature in Folly than the rest,
Stood up, and told 'em, with his head aside,
That desp'rate Cures must be to desp'rate Ills apply'd:
And therefore since their main impending fear
Was from th' encreasing race of *Chanticleer*:
Some Potent Bird of Prey they ought to find,
A Foe profess'd to him, and all his kind. . . . (135)

In his "translation" of Chaucer (*Fables Ancient and Modern* [1700]), Dryden consistently called Pertelote "Dame Partlet."

Other editions in 1687: D2282, printed in Edinburgh, 81, 82, 83–84; D2283, printed in Dublin, 57, 58, 59; D2284, second edition, printed in London, 130, 132–33, 135; D2285, third edition, London, 130, 132–33, 135.

Also found in *The Works of Mr. John Dryden*: D2207 (1691), thirty-fourth work in volume; D2208 (1693), in vol. 4; D2209 (1694), vol. 4; D2210 (1695), vol. 4.

733.   HOWELL, WILLIAM. *Medulla historiæ anglicanæ.* H3142. UMI 764: 5.

For a reference to Chaucer as England's poet laureate in the reign of Richard II, see HOWELL (1679); in this edition, the passage is found on 176.

734.   LEIGH, RICHARD. *Poems, upon Several Occasions, and, to Several Persons.* L1019. UMI.

Leigh (1649/50–1728) is identified on the title page as "the author of The censure, of the Rota." In a poem headed "On the Oxford Theater," he alludes to *The House of Fame*:

Those glorious *Heights* which *Art* of old did raise,
Liv'd uncommended in their own first *Days*
. . . .
But had the beauteous *Frame* been rear'd of old,
What *Divine Tales* the *Wits* had of it told!
. . . .
Their *Fairy Seats* they had from this deriv'd,
And all their *Scenes* of *Bliss* like this contriv'd.
This then had been, though with another name,
The *Palace* of the *Sun* and *House* of *Fame*. (9–11)

735. MILLINGTON, EDWARD. *Bibliotheca Jacombiana.* **J113. UMI 1035: 9, 1710: 26.**

Millington began auctioning the library of Thomas Jancombe on 31 October 1687. In the catalogue, under the heading "Miscellanies, in Folio," lot 74 is listed as "*Geffry Chaucers* Works, with a Table —1570" (80).

In his will, Jacomb said he paid nearly £2000 for his books, but the auction realized only £1300 (*ODNB*).

736. MILLINGTON, EDWARD. *Bibliotheca Maynardiana.* **M1449. UMI 1710: 25.**

Millington auctioned the library of John Maynard of Mayfield (Sussex) on 13 June 1687. In the catalogue, under the heading "Miscellanies, History, &c. in Folio," number 45 is listed as "*Chaucer* (*Geoffry*) Works. Wants a Title—[no date]" (54).

737. MILLINGTON, EDWARD. *Catalogue of Choice Books.* **C1299. UMI 2587: 13.**

Millington's began auctioning some of his stock of "Choice Books in Divinity, History, Physick and Poetry, Romances, Travels, &c." at Richards Coffee-House in Fleetstreet on 9 May 1687. In the catalogue, under the heading "Divinity, History, &c. In Folio," lot 166 is listed as "*Chaucer* (Sir *Geoffrey*) Works with his Life—1687" (4).

738. MILLINGTON, EDWARD. *Catalogue of English Books.* **M1580. UMI 1312: 11.**

Millington began auctioning the stock of Charles Mearnes, "late Bookseller to His Majesty," at Richard's Coffee House in Fleetstreet on 17 February 1687. In the sales catalogue, under the heading "English Miscellanies in Folio," lot 162 is listed as "Chaucer's Works with his Life and an Explicat.of the old and obscure, and from what Tongue or Dialect derived, &c.—1602" (15).

739. *Poor Robin, 1687. An Almanack of the Old and New Fashion.* A2206. UMI 1084: 23.

Under the heading "Observations on April," "Patient Grizell" is celebrated on the 30th (sig. A8r); this is perhaps an allusion to the protagonist of *The Clerk's Tale.*

Under the heading "Observations on August," "Chaucers Miller" is celebrated on the 21st (sig. B4r), no doubt an allusion to *The Canterbury Tales.*

740. SHAKESPEARE, WILLIAM. *Othello, the Moor of Venice.* S2941. UMI 297: 35.

For possible similarities to *Troilus and Criseyde*, see SHAKESPEARE (1622), Boswell & Holton No. 1035.

741. SHAKESPEARE, WILLIAM. *Titus Andronicus: or, The Rape of Lavinia.* S2949. UMI 297: 40.

For a reference to *The House of Fame*, see SHAKESPEARE (1594), Boswell & Holton No. 547; in this edition "alter'd" by Edward Ravenscroft (1654?–1707), the passage appears on 18.

742. SPELMAN, HENRY. *Glossarium archaiologicum. Editio tertia auctior & correctior.* S4926. UMI 824: 38.

For quotations from Chaucer, see SPELMAN (1626), Boswell & Holton No. 1097. For more spurious attributions from *The Plowman's Prologue* and quotations from *The House of Fame*, *The General Prologue*, and *The Knight's Tale*, see SPELMAN (1664); in this edition, the passages are found on 82, 84, 137, 166, 185, 246, 355, 356, 357, 371, 416, 493, 507, 532.

743. *Spencer Redivivus Containing the First Book of the Fairy Queen.* S4969. UMI 825: 2.

As Millican notes (*SP* 28), the author (identified on the title page as "a person of quality") refers to Spenser's use of Chaucerian language. In "The Preface" he writes:

> [W]hy he should he should not conceive himself oblig'd to impart the Tongue of that season as curant as he found it, I cannot apprehend.
> Unless he was resolv'd, as is reported of him [Spenser], to imitate his ancient Predecessor Chaucer, or affected it out of design to restore our Saxon English. (sig. A7v)

744.   WHARTON, GEORGE. "To my Very Honoured Friend," in Gaultier de Coste, Seigneur de La Calprenède's *Hymen's Præludia*: *or, Love's Master-Piece. Now Rendred into English, by Robert Loveday.* L124. UMI 1126: 1.

For a reference to Chaucer and Gower as a pair who refined the English language, see WHARTON (1652); in this edition, the passage is found on sig. A4v. Spurgeon cites this edition rather than the first one.

745.   WINSTANLEY, WILLIAM. *The Lives of the Most Famous English Poets*: *or, The Honour of Parnassus.* W3065. UMI 197: 3.

As Spurgeon notes (1: 261) but does not transcribe, there are numerous references to Chaucer in this expanded edition of Winstanley's brief biographies published in 1660 and 1684. Moreover, this edition is embellished with a frontispiece engraved by F. H. Van Hove that features a laurel-crowned bust of a poet that looks quite similar to William Shakespeare. The bust sits on a pedestal that is flanked by a pair of obelisks with the names of Cowley and Chaucer inscribed on the bases. A winged figure hovers above Shakespeare and holds a laurel wreath above each obelisk. [40]

There is also a reference to Chaucer in the table of contents (sig. a4r).

For Winstanley's biographical sketch of Chaucer, see WINSTANLEY (1660); in this edition, the passage is found on 23–32 where the text has been lightly edited and expanded, notably at the end, where Winstanley writes:

> The Works of this famous Poet, were partly published in Print by *William Caxton*, Mercer, that first brought the incomparable Art of Printing into *England*, which was in the Reign of *Henry* the Sixth. Afterward encreased by *William Thinne*, Esq; in the time of King *Henry* the Eighth. Afterwards, in the year 1561. in the Reign of Queen *Elizabeth*, Corrected and Encreased by *John Stow*; And a fourth time, with many Amendments, and an Explanation of the old and obscure Words, by Mr. *Thomas Speight*, in *Anno* 1597. Yet is he said to have written many considerable Poems, which are not in his publish'd Works, besides the *Squires Tale*, which is said to compleat in *Arundell-house* Library. (32)

In the life of John Gower, Winstanley writes of his relationship with Chaucer:

> This our *Gower* was contemporary with the famous Poet *Geoffry Chaucer*, both excellently learned, both great friends together, and both alike endeavour'd themselves and employed their time for the benefit of their Country. And what an account *Chaucer* had of this our *Gower* and of his

---

[40] See Jackson C. Boswell, "Yet Another 'New' Shakespeare Image," *Shakespeare Quarterly* 60.3 (Fall 2009): 341–47.

Parts, that which he wrote in the end of his Work, entituled *Troilus* &
Cressida, do sufficiently testifie . . . (18–19)

> He was before *Chaucer*, as born and flourishing before him, (yea,
> by some accounted his Master) yet was he after *Chaucer*, as surviving
> him two years, living to be stark blind, and so more properly termed our
> *English Homer*. (20)

In the life of John Lydgate, Winstanley writes:

> [B]oth in Prose and Poetry [Lydgate] was the best Author of his Age, for
> if *Chaucer*'s Coin were of greater Weight for deeper Learning, *Lydgate*'s
> was of a more refined Stantard [*sic*] for purer Language; so that one
> might mistake him for a modern Writer. (33)
>
> Now if you would know further of him, hear him in his Prologue to
> the Story of *Thebes*. . . . This Story was first written in *Latine* by *Geoffry
> Chaucer*, and translated by *Lydgate* into *English* Verse. . . . (34–35)
>
> He writ (saith my Author) partly *English*, partly *Latine*; partly in
> Prose, and partly in Verse, many exquisite learned Books, saith *Pitseus*,
> which are mentioned by him and *Bale*, as also in the latter end of *Chau-
> cer*'s Works; [t]he last Edition. . . . (37)

Under the heading "Thomas Kid, Thomas Watson, &c.," Winstanley writes:

> There also flourish'd about the same time *Thomas Watson* . . . with some
> others, especially one *John Lane*, whose Works though much better
> meriting than many that are in print, yet notwithstanding, had the ill
> fate to be unpublish'd, but they are still reserved in Manuscript, namely
> . . . his Supplement to *Chaucer's Squires Tale*. (100)

For references to Chaucer in the lives of Spenser, Drayton, and Shakespeare, see
WINSTANLEY (1684); in this edition, the passages are found on 88–93 (the life of
Spenser), 105–108 (Drayton), 130–33 (Shakespeare).

1688

746. BARNES, JOSHUA. *The History of that Most Victorious Monarch Edward
III^d^*. B871. UMI 52: 6.

Barnes (1654–1712) is identified on the title page as "Bachelor of Divinity, and
one of the senior fellows of Emmanuel College in Cambridge." As Alderson &
Henderson note, he refers to Chaucer's service as a diplomat. Near the end of

this work, in book 4, chapter 14, section 12, Barnes writes of yet another failed negotiation for a peace treaty between France and England:

> [T]he Legates seeing all things like to break to pieces, in Pious sub-telty began to propose a Match between *Richard*, the Young Prince of *Wales*, and the Lady *Mary*, Daughter to the *French* King. Which Pro-posal coming to the Ears of both the Kings, begat another private meet-ing shortly after at *Montrevil* by the Sea, where Sr. *Guischard Dangle*, Sr. *Richard Sturry*, and Sr. *Geoffry Chaucer* (the Prince of our *English Poets*) met . . . Commissioners from the *French* King. And here they treated earnestly about the Marriage. . . . (906)

747.   BEHN, APHRA. Interpolation in Bernard Le Bovier de Fontenelle's *History of Oracles, and the Cheats of the Pagan Priests*. F1413. UMI 29: 11.

In this translation of *Histoire des oracles* by M. Bernard Le Bovier de Fontenelle (1657–1757), Aphra Behn (1640–1689), the translator, interpolates a reference to Chaucer in "The Second Discourse," chapter 5, "That if Heathenism had not been abolish'd, yet Oracles would have ceased." In a discussion of the role of poetry in ancient works of religion, morality, natural philosophy, and astrology, Behn writes:

> [T]he Muses have of late days mightily deviated from their original Gravity. Who would imagine that the *Old Statutes* should by right have been written in Metre, and *Chaucer*'s *Tales* in Prose? (209)

Another edition: F1413A (1699), 134.

748.   A ghost.

749.   *Bibliotheca selecta*. B2852. UMI 1564: 9.

Among the works auctioned on 21 May 1688 at the Sign of the White Hart, there was one by Chaucer. In the catalogue, under the heading "Divinity, His-tory, &c. in Folio," lot 91 is listed as "Sir *Gef. Chaucer*'s Works, best Edition — 1686" (²2; sig. A1v).

750.   *Catalogus variorum in pluriis facultatibus variisq[ue] linguis insignium librorum*. C1455. UMI 2587: 18.

An auction began on 23 January 1688 "at the Sign of the White Horse, over against the South Door of St. *Paul*'s Church, (amongst the Woollen-Drapers) in St. *Paul*'s Church-Yard, continuing Day by Day, the first five Days every Week, till all the Books are sold, from the Hours, of Nine in the Morning to Twelve, and from Two to Six in the Evening." In the sales catalogue, under the heading

"Divinity and Miscellanies, in Quarto," one of the items mentions Chaucer. Lot 35 is listed as "Vision of Pierce Plow-man, an Antient Piece of Poetry before *Chaucer*—[no date or place of publication]" (²23).

751.   COOPER, WILLIAM. *Catalogi variorum librorum Richardi Davis. Pars Tertia.* **D428. UMI 913: 22.**

In the midst of Davis's "Misfortunes," Cooper conducted an auction of a portion of his fellow bookseller's stock in Oxford beginning 25 June 1688. In the catalogue, under the heading "English Miscellanies in Quarto," lot 260 is listed as "*Chaucer*'s Loves of Triolus [*sic*] and Chersida [*sic*]—1635" (80).

752.   COWLEY, ABRAHAM. *The Works of Mr. Abraham Cowley.* **C6658. UMI 685: 3.**

For a reference to Cowley's burial place near Chaucer, see SPRAT (1668); in this edition, the passage is found on sig. c4r–v.

For a reference to Chaucer's "rich rhymes," see COWLEY (1656), C6683; in this edition, the passage is found on 37 (sig. Aa2r).

753.   DELONEY, THOMAS. *The Garland of Good-Will.* **D948. UMI 959: 15.**

For what may be a faint allusion to *The Clerk's Tale*, see DELONEY (1628) in Boswell & Holton No. 1116. In this edition, the passage is found in the second part, where number 2 is headed "Of Patient *Grissel* and a Noble *Marquess*" (sigs. E7r–F2v).

Another edition around 1688: D947A (UMI 2847: 14), sig. D5v–10r.

754.   *An Historical Relation of Several and Learned Romanists Who Did Imbrace the Protestant Religion.* H2108. UMI 497: 31.

In "A Catalogue of sundry great Persons of the Roman Catholick Religion, who have all along Oppos'd the Tenents of the Church of Rome," the unidentified author alleges that Chaucer was a proto-Protestant:

> In the next Century from 1300, to 1400 . . . may be deservedly added,
> *Dante, Petrarch,* and *Chaucer,* who all found fault with the *Roman* Faith,
> as well with her Manners. . . . And as for *Chaucer* there is no man more
> Satyrical against Shrifting, Relicks, Purgatory, Pardons, and Meritori-
> ous Works than he is, up and down in his Poems. (30–31)

755.   HOLME, RANDLE. *The Academy of Armory.* **H2513. UMI 634: 10.**

Holme (1627–1699) is described on the title page as being "of the city of Chester, gentleman sewer in extraordinary to his late Majesty King Charles 2. and sometimes deputy for the Kings of Armes."[41] In book I, chapter 5, in a section headed "Of the Cross Potent," he attributes a quotation to Chaucer:

> THESE kinde of Crosses resemble the heads of Crowches, which in Elder days were called 𝔓otents or 𝔓otans, as saith old *Chaucer.*
> *When lust of youth wasted be, and spent*
> *Then in his hand he takes a Potent.* (45)

Chaucer does indeed use the term *potent* in *The Summoner's Tale* (line 1776), *Troilus and Criseyde* (line 5: 1222), and in *The Romaunt of the Rose* (lines 368 and 7415).

In book I, chapter 7, in a section headed "Of Tinctures of Feilds [*sic*], Holme again cites Chaucer's use of the word *potent*:

> By Tinctures, I mean the colour or colours of Feilds. . . . [The term *potent counter potent* comes from] its resemblence to Crowches head which *Chaucer* call a potens; is reckoned by him to be a Furre. . . . (68)

In book III, chapter 2, in a section on arms displaying a crutch, Holme cites Chaucer as an authority yet once more:

> The Crutch is of some termed (and that vulgarly) a 𝔠rich, but more usually a 𝔠rutch 𝔖taff, which by Old Sir *Geffrey Chaucer*, was called a 𝔓otence. It is a 𝔖taff with a Cross piece on the head of it, which Lame Persons put under their Arm holes, thereby to support and stay them in their going, without which they were not able to stir. (224)

In book III, chapter 8, in a section about arms displaying the wheel:

---

[41] As Atkinson notes (*MLN* 1940) the 1688 edition of Holme's work is incomplete. In part 2, book 4, section 5, Holme quotes from *The Knight's Tale* in a passage about mantles. He writes:
  Of this kind of habite the famous Sir Geffrey Chaucer makes mention in the Knights tale: where describing the habits and Ornaments of two combatants entering the list, hath these verses
  Came riding like the God of Armes Mars
  His coate of Armour was of cloth of Thrace
  A Mantle of his shoulder hanging
  Beautifull of Rubies red as fire sparkling.
  From whence we may collect, that frome the hanging on his shoulders it did cast itselfe in so many plaits (as naturally all garments of large size doe) which form of plaiting in the art of painting is termed drapery or fouldage, but in the termes of Herauldry is blazoned, Doubling. (*The Academy of Armory*, ed. I. H. Jeayes [London: for the Roxburghe Club, 1905], 320.)

𝔚𝔥𝔢𝔢𝔩𝔰 are born in Arms whole, or by half, or by quarters as the examples following manifest.

    G. 3 Wheels O. This was the Coat of Sir *Payne Roet*, Knight, whose Daughter Married to the famous *English* Poet Sir *Geffrey Chaucer*. (²331)

In book III, chapter 13, Holme cites Chaucer in a passage about towers and battlements being featured in coats of arms:

    Some take it for a 𝔖𝔢𝔫𝔱𝔦𝔫𝔞𝔩 𝔥𝔬𝔲𝔰𝔢, or 𝔖𝔠𝔬𝔲𝔱 𝔥𝔬𝔲𝔰𝔢.Sir *Gefforey* [*sic*] *Chaucer* useth the word *Barbican*, for a Watch Tower . . . (²474)

Another edition: H2513A (1693), 45, 68; ²24, ²321, ²474.

756.   MILLINGTON, EDWARD. *Bibliotheca Massoviana*. M1029. UMI 1446: 15.

Millington auctioned Monsieur Massauve's library on 1 February 1688 at the Sign of the Black-Swan in St. Paul's Church-Yard. Massauve was, he says, "sometime Counsellor of Parliament at Montpellier" and a great collector of well printed books. In the catalogue, under the heading "English Books, Divinity History, &c. in Folio," lot 164 is listed as "Chaucers Works with the Explication of the hard and obscure words — 1602" (60).

757.   MILLINGTON, EDWARD. *A Catalogue of Choice and Valuable Books English and Latin*. C1295. UMI 624: 2.

Millington's auction was held at the Unicorn in Pater Noster Row on 30 April 1688. In the catalogue, under the heading "Books in Folio, on several Subjects," lot 27 is listed as "The Works of our ancient, learned and excellent Poet, Jeffrey Chaucer; with a Key for obscure Words — 1687" (50); and lot 139 as "the Works of our Learned English Poet Jeffery Chaucer, with a Key explaining the obscure Words. — 1687" (54).

758.   *A New Song of the Misfortunes of an Old Whore and Her Brats*. N767aA. UMI 1994: 20.

The unidentified author of this broadside satire on "the old hag of Rome" echoes a line from *The Manciple's Prologue*: "Sires, what! Dun is in the myre!" (line 5):

    And the young Welchman's Sire,
      Stuck like *Dun* in the Mire
  With revengeful Despair looks around him,
    And then Curses the Crowd,
      That with Suffrages loud
  Shouted (*Vive le Roy*) when they Crown'd him.

759.   PARSONS, ROBERT. *A Treatise of Three Conversions of England.* **P575. UMI 1154: 1.**

For a reference to "the Poem of *Chaucer*" as an obviously fictional work, see PARSONS (1603), Boswell & Holton No. 692; in this edition, the passage is found on 199.

760.   *Poor Robin, 1688. An Almanack of the Old and New Fashion.* A2208. UMI 1603: 9.

Under the heading "Observations on August": Hudibras is celebrated on the 22nd, "Chaucers Miller" on the 23rd (sig. B4r).

761.   S., W., in John Bullokar's *An English Expositor: Teaching the Interpretation of the Hardest Words Used in Our Language.* **B5435. UMI 1545: 15.**

For a reference to Chaucer and *The Prologue to the Squire's Tale* in the definition of Chivancy, see S., W. (1654); in this edition, the passage is found on sig. B12r.

For a reference to Chaucer and allusion to *The Nun's Priest's Tale*, see S., W. (1663); in this edition, the passage is found on sig. B11r.

762.   SCOT, WALTER. *A True History of the Several Honourable Families of the Right Honourable Name of Scot in the Shires of Roxburgh and Selkirk, and Others Adjacent.* **Edinburgh. S948. UMI 2043: 13.**

In the second part of this work is found a dedicatory poem addressed to Sir Francis Scot of Thirlston. There Captain Walter Scot (ca. 1614–1694), "an old souldier, and no scholler, and one that can write nane, but just the letters of his name," writes of several men named John Scot, one of whom was a poet in the same league with Chaucer and Sidney:

> John Scot the Squire of Newburgh-hall,
> *Alias* of Rennal-burn as men him call.
> To the first John Scot of Rennal-burn late,
> He was the Son, and Heir to his Estate,
> Who was the Son of that Sir John Scot of worth,
> The Prince of Poets, and Knight of New-burgh,
> Chancer Glovet [*sic*], and Sir Thomas Moir [*sic*],
> And Sir Philip Sidney, who the Lawral wear:
> They never had a more Poetical Vein,
> Than New-burgh's John, that was Mr. Arthurs Son.
> And Mr. Arthur was a learned Man. . . . (9–10)

763.   SMITH, JOHN. *The Mystery of Rhetorique Unveil'd.* S4116F. UMI 876: 14 (identified as S2584).

For a reference to Spenser's imitation of Chaucer, see SMITH (1656); in this edition, the passage is found on 64.

764.   WALFORD, BENJAMIN. *Catalogus librorum instructissimæ bibliothecæ.* L615. UMI 1425: 19.

Walford auctioned works from the library of Richard Maitland, Earl of Lauderdale, on 30 October 1688. In the catalogue, under the heading "English Miscellanies in Folio," lot 151 is listed as "*Geff. Chaucer's* Works—1687" (131). Under the heading "English Manuscripts," lot 1 is listed as "The Works of Sir *Geoffry Chaucer*, curiously written upon Vellum, and Gilded, very Antient—[no date]" (146).

1689

765.   B., T. "A Dedication" in Michael Drayton's *England's Heroical Epistles. Newly Corrected and Amended.* D2144B. No UMI.

As Spurgeon notes (1: 267), but cites the 1695 edition rather than this one, T. B.'s commendatory poem mentions Chaucer in conjunction with Spenser and Jonson. In a poem headed "A Dedication of These and the Foregoing Verses in Mr. Drayton's Heroick Epistles," T. B. writes:

Eternal Book, to which our *Muses* flye,
In hopes of gaining Immortality.
Time has devour'd the Younger Sons of Wit,
Who liv'd when *Chaucer, Spencer, Johnson* writ:
Those lofty Trees are of their Leaves bereft,
And to a reverend Nakedness are left.
But the chief Glory of *Apollo's* Grove,
Drayton, who taught his *Daphne* how to Love;
Drayton, that sacred Lawrel seems to be,
From which each *Sprig* that falls must grow a *Tree.* [Etc.] (sig. A4r)

Other editions: D2145 (1695), sig. A4r; D2146 (1697), sig. A4r.

766.   BRITAINE, WILLIAM DE. *Humane Prudence.* B4805C. UMI 732: 6.

For a spurious quotation attributed to Chaucer, see BRITAINE (1686); in this edition, the passage is found on 167, and here the context changes and "Chaucer's" sentiments are presented in verse.

767.   *A Catalogue of Very Good English and Latin Books.* UMI Early English Books: Tract Supplement: D1: 1 (S.C.1035[4]).

An auction was held on 9 September 1689 at the sign of Three Half-Moons. In the catalogue, under the heading "Miscellanies, in Folio," number 32 is listed as "Chaucer, imperfect—[no date]" (14).

768.   GADBURY, JOHN. Εφημερις [Ephemeris]: *or, A Diary Astrological, Astronomical, Meteorological for the Year of our Lord, 1689.* A1768. UMI 908: 32.

Gadbury (1627–1704) is identified on the title page as a "student in physick and astrology." In a section of chronological observations about outstanding events relating to Westminster Abbey, he refers to the death and burial of Chaucer, "our English Homer":

> [Event number] 27. Sir *Geoffery Chaucer* Kt., our English *Homer*, died, and was buried in *Westminster Abbey.* [Year happened] 1400 [Years elapsed] 288[.] (sig. C5v)

769.   HOGARTH, RICHARD. *Gazophylacium Anglicum: Containing the Derivation of English Words, Proper and Common.* G426. UMI 739: 24.

Hogarth (1663/64–1718) is not named on the title page. In a section headed "Etymologicon Onomasticon: or, An Etymological Explication of the Proper Names of Men and Women," there is a reference to Chaucer:

> Chaucer, the *Homer* or Parent of all English Poetry; possibly from the Fr. G. *Chausseur*, formerly *Chauceur*, Part. of the Verb *Chausser*, formerly *Chaucer*, to put on ones shoes, q. d. a Shoe-maker. So *Skinner.* (sig. Bb8v)

Another edition with a different title: *A New English Dictionary* (1691), N637a, same pagination.

770.   HOWARD, EDWARD. *Caroloiades: or, The Rebellion of Forty One. A Heroick Poem.* H2966. UMI 535: 4.

As Spurgeon notes (1: 261–62), in Book 5 Howard mentions Chaucer and Spenser in a passage about "Powerfull Sons of Phebus":

> And wit this islands Glory far display'd,
> Through Powerfull Sons of *Phebus* by whose sence
> The Mighty Nine best raptures did dispense.
> With these around their brows were Lawrells lac'd,
> Large next to those *Apollo's* Temples Grac'd:
> Of which, he *Chaucer*, *Spencer*, much beheld,
> And where their Learned Poems most excell'd. (137)

Another edition in 1689: H2967, 137.

Also found in *Caroloiades Redivivus: or, The War and Revolutions in the Time of King Charles the First. An Heroick Poem*, H2968 (1695), same pagination.

771. MILLINGTON, EDWARD. *Bibliotheca Carteriana.* C652. UMI 2616: 15.

Millington began auctioning the library of Edward Carter, late deacon of St. Albans, at his widow's house in St. Albans on 5 August 1689. In the catalogue, under the heading "Divinity, History, Philology, in Folio, &c." lot 93 is listed as "*Chaucer* (*Jeffery*) Works (*gilt back*)" (10).

772. MILLINGTON, EDWARD. *Bibliotheca Skinneriana, & Hampdeniana.* S3942. UMI 2153: 14.

Millington began auctioning the libraries of two men named Skinner and Hampden on 13 February 1698/99. In Skinner's catalogue, under the heading "English Books in Folio," number 78 is listed as "Jeffrey Chaucer's Works with his Life— 1687" (26).

773. MILLINGTON, EDWARD. *A Catalogue of Valuable Books.* C1416. UMI 1419: 2 and UMI 469: 2 (identified as O274).

Millington held an auction at Mrs. Elizabeth Oliver's house in Norwich on 16 December 1689 for the benefit and entertainment of the clergy, gentry, and citizens of the environs. In the catalogue, under the heading "Miscellanies in Folio," lot 77 is listed as "*Chaucer's* Works (*wants Title*) old Edit—[no date]" (19).

774. OSBORNE, FRANCIS. *The Works of Francis Osborn. The Ninth Edition.* O507. UMI 1364: 15.

For a reference to a bishop who boasted that he had never read a line of Calvin or Chaucer, see OSBORNE (1658); in this collection, the passage is found on 441–42.

775. *A Poem on the Coronation of King William and Queen Mary.* P2690. UMI 1511: 11.

The poet (not named on the title page) invokes Chaucer in his commendatory poem on the new king and queen:

> WHere are you all, you lewd ignoble Race,
> Who even *Tyrants* with your *Praise* disgrace?
> . . . .
> Since all the Scrib'ling *Herd* beside refuse,
> *Love* now, as *anger* once, shall make a Muse:
> I'de have a certain rugged bravery shine,
> In honest sense thro' each *true English* Line:

Plain truth, must, since 'tis *natural*, needs be *Wit*,
Such as Old *Chaucer*, or Young *Oldham* writ;
And since my Verse is truth and *Reason* too,
John Hopkins, or *John Bunyans Rhimes* will do. (sig. B1r–v)

776.   *Poor Robin, 1689. An Almanack of the Old and New Fashion*. A2208. UMI 1603: 9.

Under the heading "Observations on August": Hudibras is celebrated on the 22nd, "Chaucers Miller" on the 23rd. (sig. B4r)

777.   PRINCE, VINCENT. *The Protestant Almanack*. A2229A. UMI 2224: 5.

Prince is identified on the title page as "Philoprotest, a well-willer to the mathematicks." In an epistle addressed "To the Truly Christian Reader," he quotes from the spurious work known as Chaucer's *Ploughman's Tale*. Following a lengthy list of the means and methods used by the Church to acquire worldly wealth and power, Prince writes:

By these helps hath the Papal Crown attained to the Dignity it is now at; far different from the condition of St. *Peter*, whose Successor they brag themselves to be, who told the Criple that expected Almes of him, *Gold nor Silver have I none*; they swiming [*sic*] in all manner of wealth and luxuriousness, as the antient Poet *Geoffry Chaucer* thus expresseth in the *Plow-mans tale*.
    Popes, Bishops, and Cardinals,
    Cannons, Parsons, and Vicare,
    In Gods service I trow been fals,
    That Sacraments sellen heve,
    Band been as proud as Lucifer.
    Each man look whether that I lie,
    Who so speaketh ayenste her power
    It shall be holden Heresie. (sig. A3v–4r)

778.   SHANNON, FRANCIS BOYLE. *Several Discourses and Characters Address'd to the Ladies of the Age. Wherein the Vanities of the Modish Women are Discovered*. S2965B. UMI 297: 44.

In "The Sixth Discourse. Against Maids Marrying for meer Love, or only to please their Parents Inclinations, tho' quite contrary to their own," Lord Shannon (1623–1699) refers to the marriage of January and May, perhaps a faint allusion to *The Merchant's Tale*.

[M]ost Parents make it more their concern to match Fortunes than Children, or to suit inclinations or ages, when 'tis but a kind of Reversing

Nature it self, it being as feasible to unite two contraries, and make Fire and Water agree, and *May* and *January* meet, as by the Magick of Matrimony to make a very old Man, and a very young Woman to be but one flesh and temper. (93)

Another edition in 1689: S2965A (UMI 1130: 8), 93.

779.   *The Third Part of the Collection of Poems on Affairs of State.* T913. UMI 298: 32.

This collection of poems features "Rochester's Farewel," a satire of "the noysome Follies of the Age," ostensibly by John Wilmot, Earl of Rochester. The unnamed poet appears to allude to *The House of Fame* as he writes of "Lust and Devotion, Zeal and Letchery":

> Important use Religion's made,
> By those who wisely drive the Cheating Trade;
> As Wines Prohibited securely pass,
> Changing the Name of their own Native place.
> So Vice grows safe, drest in Devotions Name,
> Unquestion'd by the Custom-house of Fame. (29)

Also found in *Poems on Affairs of State*, P2719A (1697), 159.

1690

780.   A ghost.

781.   BLOUNT, THOMAS POPE. *Censura celebriorum authorem.* B3346. UMI 123: 3.

Blount (1649–1697) is identified on the title page as "Anglo-Britannus baronettus." As Spurgeon notes (1: 262), he collects a number of testimonials to Chaucer in a section headed "Galfredus Chaucerus." Blount writes:

> Apud *Woodstock* non longè ab *Oxonio* in *Angliâ* claris parentibus natus, patrem habuit Equestris Ordinis virum, & ipse tandem aratus factus est eques.
>   Vir belli pacisque artibus mirè florens. Antequam virilem ætatem attigisset, erat Poëta elegans, & qui *Poësim Anglicam* ita illustravit, ut *Anglicus Homerus* merito haberetur. Rhetor etiam disertus, Mathematicus peritus, Philosophus acutus, *Theologus* denique non contemnendus. Maximè conatus est, ut materna excolatur lingua, & in *Anglico* sermone

eloquentiæ *Romanæ* expressa appareant vestigia. Illi duo viri *Joannes Gouerus* & *Galfredus Chaucerus* attulerunt certè nostro Idiomati tantus splendoris & ornamenti, quantum ante illos prorsus nemo. Nam sibi mutuò calcar addiderunt, & uter patriæ plus afferret honoris, uterque vinci & vincere ambiens, amanter contenderunt. *Pitsæus* de Illustr. Angl. Script.

Fuere & in *Britannorum* idiomate & eorum vernaculo sermson e aliqui Poëtæ ab eis summo in pretio habiti, inter quos *Galfredus Chaucerus* vetustior, qui multa scripsit, Thomas Viatus, ambo insignes equites. *Lil. Gyrald.* de Poëtis.

Galfredus Chaucerus Anglus Poëta, linguam Patriam magnâ ingenii solertiâ ac culturâ plurimùm ornavit; interque alia, cùm *Joannis Mone* poëma de Arte amandi *Gallicè* tantùm legeretur, *Anglico* illud metro feliciter reddidit. *Vossius* de Hist. Lat.

Oppidum *Woodstock*, cùm nihil habeat quod ostentet, Homerum nostrum *Anglicum Galfredum Chaucerum* alumnum suum fuisse gloriatur. De quo, & nostris Poëtis Anglicis illud verè asseram, quod de *Homero* & *Græcis* ille *Italus* dixit:
　—*Hic ille est cuius de gurgite sacro*
　Combibit arcanos vatum omnis turba furores.
Ille enim extra omnem ingenii aleam positus, Poëtastros nostros longo post se intervallo relinquit. *Camden.* in *Britann.*

Galfridus Chaucerus, Poëtarum nostrorum princeps, acris judicii, non lepidi tantum ingenii, vir. Is Philosopnhicis, Theologicisque haud mediocriter imbutus fuit. *Henr. Savil* Præfat. ad *Bradwardin.* lib. contra *Pelag.*

De *Chaucero Lelandus* inter Epigrammata sua sic scribit:

Prædicat Algerum *meritò* Florentia Dantem,
　Italia *& numeros tota* Petrarcha *tuos.*
Anglia Chaucerum *veneratur nostra Poëtam,*
　Cui veneres debet patria lingua suas.

Till the Time of King Henry *the Eighth, there was scarce any Man regarded the English Language but* Chaucer; *and nothing was written in it, which one would be willing to read twice, but some of his* Poetry. *But then it began to raise it self a little, and to sound tolerably well.* Sprat's *History of the Royal Society,* 42.

Sir Geoffry Chaucer, *the* Homer *of our Nation*; *and who found as sweet a Muse in the Groves of* Woodstock, *as the Ancients did upon the banks of* Helicon. Baker *in the Reign of* Edward *the Third*.[42]

Verstegan *condemns* Chaucer *for spoiling the purity of the* English Tongue, *by the mixing of so many* French *and* Latin *Words*.[43]

Of some things I must advertise the Readers; *as first, That in* Chaucer *they shall find the* Proper Names *oftentimes much differing from the* Latin *and* Greek, *from whence they are drawn*; *Which they must not condemn in him as a Fault*: *For both he and other Poëts, in translating such Words from one Language into another, do use, as the* Latins *and* Greeks *do, the sundry species of* Metaplasmus: *As* Campaneus *for* Capeneus: Atheon *for* Acteon: Adriane *for* Adriadne. *Which* Chaucer *doth in other Words also*: *as* gon *for* begon: leve *for* beleve: peraunter *for* peradventure: loveden *for* did love: woneden *for* did won. *It is his manner likewise, imitating the* Greeks, *by two* Negatives *to cause a greater* Negation: *As*, I ne said none ill. *Also many times to understand his* Verb: *As*, I not what men him call, *for* I know not, *&c. And, for the Author, to name some part of his Work*: *as*, Argonauticon *for* Apollonius Rhodius. *And that sometime is the* Genetive Case *a former* Substantive *being understood*; *as, read* Æneidos: Metamorphoseos: *for the Authors of those Works. See the* Pref. *before* Chaucer's *Works, printed in Fol.* 1602.

Ex hoc male sano novitatis pruritu, *Belgæ Gallicas* voces passim civitate suâ domando, patrii sermonis puritatem nuper non leviter inquinaverunt, & *Chaucerus* Poëta, pessimo exemplo, integris vocum plaustris ex eadem Galliâ in nostram linguam invectis, eam, nimis anteà à *Normannorum* victoriâ adulteratam, omni ferè nativâ gratiâ & nitore spoliavit, pro genuinis coloribus fucum illinens, pro verâ facie larvam induens. Vide *Stephan. Skinner.* In Præfat. Præfix. Etymologico suo linguæ *Anglic.*

Londini senex obiit, & apud *Westmonasterium* honorificè sepultus est cum hac *Inscriptione*:

Qui fuit Anglorum *Vates ter maximus olim*
      Galfredus Chaucer, *conditur hoc tumulo.*
Annum si quaras Domini, si tempor a mortis,
      Ecce notæsubsunt, quæ tibi cunct a notent.
            25. *Octobris* 1400. (312–13)

The passage is marked with a shoulder note: "Clar. An. Dom. MCCCLXXX."

---

[42] Baker, i.e., Richard Baker, q.v.
[43] See Boswell & Holton No. 723.

782.   BROWN, THOMAS. *The Late Converts Exposed: or, The Reasons of Mr. Bays's Changing His Religion. Considered in a Dialogue. Part the Second.* B5061. UMI 345: 15.

Brown (1663–1704) is not named on the title page. He satirizes Dryden's conversion to Roman Catholicism in this work that is cast as a dialogue. In a conversation with Eugenius and Crites, Mr. Bays mentions "the Tragedy of Troilus and Cressid," a faint allusion to *Troilus and Criseyde*:

> [O]nce upon a time an Assignation being made between *Hector* and his Cousin *Ajax* to determine the war in a single Combat, just before the Trumpets sounded, *Hector* tells his Noble Kinsman, that if he certainly knew which part of his Body was *Trojan*, and which was *Grecian*, he'd spare the one out of a respect to his pious Aunt, but slash, cut and mortifie the other like Lightning. The whole passage you may find in the Tragedy of *Troilus* and *Cressid*. (2)

Another edition: *The Second Edition with Additions* (1591), B5070, the allusion is lost in the revision.

783.   BULLORD, JOHN. *Bibliotheca curiosa.* B2823. UMI 1564: 7.

Bullord auctioned the library ("most of them either large Paper, or Gilt-back") of the late Robert Bruce, Earl of Ailesbury, on 19 May 1690 at Roll's Coffee-House. In the catalogue, under the heading "English Miscellanies in Folio," number 91 is listed as "Chaucer's Works, the last Edition [no date]" (21, really 23; sig. G1r). In this same group one also finds works by Katharine Philips, Boccaccio, and Shakespeare.

784.   BULLORD, JOHN. *Bibliotheca realis & instructissima, sive catalogus variorum librorum.* S2077. UMI 1294: 7.

Bullord began auctioning the library of the Reverend Dr. Peter Scott on 28 April 1690. In the catalogue, under the heading "English Miscellanies in Folio," lot 39 is listed as *"Jeff Chaucers* Works — [Lond. 1591]" (25). In the British Library copy of the catalogue, an annotation indicates that the book fetched 6*s.*

785.   BUNYAN, JOHN. *The Pilgrim's Progress. The Second Part.* B5580. UMI 1248: 9.

For an echo of *Troilus and Criseyde* 5: 1786, in "The Author's Way of Sending forth his Second Part of the Pilgrim," see BUNYAN (1684); in this edition, the passage is found on sig. A2r.

786.   DE LAUNE, THOMAS. *Angliæ metropolis: or, The Present State of London.* D889. UMI 813: 13.

For a reference to Chaucer's burial in Westminster Abbey, see DE LAUNE (1681); in this edition, the passage is found on 26.

787.   DRYDEN, JOHN. *Amphitryon: or, The Two Socia's.* D2234. UMI 208: 33 and UMI 351: 2

Dryden's comedy, adapted from Plautus and Molière, was performed at the Theatre Royal with music composed by Henry Purcell. In 2.2, Dryden (1631–1700) alludes to *The Nun's Priest's Tale.* Mercury responds to Bromia's calling him a "Dunghill-Cock":

> Hold your peace, Dame *Partlet*, and leave your Cackling. (21)

In his "translation" of Chaucer (*Fables Ancient and Modern*), Dryden consistently called Pertelote "Dame Partlet."

> *Another edition*: D2235 (1691), 21.
> Also found in *The Works of Mr. John Dryden*: D2207 (1691), twenty-fourth work in volume; D2208 (1693), in vol. 3; D2209 (1694), vol. 3; D2210 (1695), vol. 3. Also included in *The Dramatick Works* (1695), D2211, vol. 3.

788.   *The Muses Farewel to Popery and Slavery. Second edition.* M3141. UMI 769: 25.

In this edition there are many new songs and poems that do not appear in the first edition, M3140 (1689). In part five of "Cæsar's Ghost" there is reference to January and May, likely an allusion to *The Merchant's Tale*:

> Here an old batter'd *Tangieren* he beheld,
> More mawl'd by Love than e're he was in Field;
> Yet wondrous Amorous still, and wondrous gay,
> Old *January* dizen'd up in *May*;
> His Zeals as Trophies of his Victory Graces,
> But all adorn'd with many Looking-glasses,
> In which he practises *Bon Mien* and Faces. (205)

789.   *Poor Robin, 1690. An Almanack of the Old and New Fashion.* A2209. UMI 2088: 1.

Under the heading "Observations on August," "Chaucers Miller" is celebrated on the 30th of this month.

790.   SANDYS, GEORGE, trans. *Ovid's Metamorphosis Englished.* O688A. UMI 1490: 14.

For an echo of the title of *The House of Fame*, see SANDYS (1628) in Appendix; in this edition, the passage is found on 232.

791.   *The Secret History of K. James I and K. Charles I.* S2339. UMI 1536: 10.

The Secret History is sometimes attributed to John Phillips (1631–1706) and sometimes to Nathaniel Crouch (1632?–1725?). Whoever the author, he paraphrases an unnamed bishop who bragged that he had never read a line of Chaucer because he was linked (in the bishop's mind) with Luther and Calvin:

> [T]o avoid the very Imputation of Puritanism (a greater rub in the way of Preferment than Vice) our Divines, for the generality . . . [were] more conversant with the F—[44] than the Fathers; scoffing in their ordinary Discourse at *Luther* and *Calvin*, but especially at the last; so as a certain Bishop thank'd *God* he never (though a good Poet himself) had read a Line in him or *Chaucer.* The same used this simile at Court, *That our Religion, like the Kings-Arms, stood between Two Beasts, the* Puritans *and* Papists. (13–14)

Other editions with a different title, *The Secret History of the Four Last Monarchs of Great-Britain*: C7346 (1691), 6; and C7347 (1693), 7.

792.   *The Wanton Wife of Bath.* W723. No UMI.

For a reference to Chaucer's writing about a wanton wife of Bath, see *The Wanton Wife of Bath* (1641).

1691

793.   *The Athenian Mercury.* Volume 2: 14. Nelson and Seccombe 21.0204.

As Spurgeon notes (1: 263), in the issue dated 11 July 1691, a correspondent inquires:

> *Which is the best* Poem *that ever was made and who in your Opinion, deserves the* Title *of the best* Poet *that ever was?*
>   *Answ.* . . . But since we can't go through all the World, let's look home a little. *Grandsire Chaucer*, in spite of the Age, was a Man of as

---

[44] "F—", i.e., friars.

much wit, sence and honesty as any that have writ after him. (no pagination)

794.   *The Athenian Mercury*. Volume 3: 16.

In the issue dated 19 September 1691, an anonymous correspondent wishes to
know:

> *Whether there's any such thing as the Perfection of a Language, and wherein
> it consists, and whether our Language is now in its heighth, or when it was
> so?*
>
> *Answ.* . . . [H]ere in *England*; the old *Saxon* is undoubtedly the
> proper *English* Tongue . . . and yet our present *English* is as absolutely a
> different Language from it as the old *Greek* is from the *Roman*. But still,
> which is more to our present purpose, old *Chaucer, Gower*, and their
> Contemporaries were call'd great Refiners of our *English* Language,
> and undoubtedly were thought to have brought it to as great a Perfection
> by their Contemporaries. . . . (no pagination)

**795.   BLAGUE, DANIEL. *A Catalogue of Latine Greek & English Books*. C1356.
UMI Early English Books: Tract Supplement D1: 2 (821.i.9[10]).**

Blague is identified on the title page as a bookseller. Blague's auction was held
on 15 June 1691 at "Mr. John Martins at Guild-Hall Coffee-House." In the
catalogue, under the heading "Latin and English Books, in Folio," number 44 is
listed as "Chaucers works 1687" (7).

**796.   BLOUNT, THOMAS. Νομο-λεξικον [Nomo-lexikon]: *A Law-Dictionary*.
The Second Edition. B3341a. UMI 836: 15.**

For references to Chaucer as an authority on the English language and word
usage, see BLOUNT (1670); in this augmented edition, the passages are found on
sigs. F2r, Q2r, X2v, Z2v, Kk1r, L11v, Zz1v, Hhh1r, Rrr1r, Eeee2r.

As Alderson and Henderson note, Blount (1618–1679) also refers to Chaucer
in definitions of *Lodemerege* and *Portuass*. Blount writes:

> Lodemerege. . . . *Chaucer* expounds it to be the Skill or Art of Naviga-
> tion. (sig. Yy1v) [Chaucer uses *lodemenage* in *The General Prologue*, line
> 403.]

> Portuass. . . . I suppose it the same which *Chaucer* calls a Porthose,
> and which I find elsewhere written Porteos & Portvos. It was that
> Book which is now called a *Breviary*, of which thus *Chaucer*, For on my
> Porthose I make an Oath. (sig. Iii1v)
> [Blount cites *The Shipman's Tale*, line 1321.]

797.   BULLORD, JOHN. *A Catalogue of Books of Two Eminent Mathematicians.*
C1287. UMI 2552: 1.

At a sale held on 21 May 1691 at Rolls's Coffee-House on the north side of St.
Paul's Church Yard, among the books John Bullord offered for sale by auction,
under the heading "Books in Folio, Latin, French, English, &c." lot 87 is listed
as "Chaucer's Works — [no date]" (3; sig. B2r).

798.   BULLORD, JOHN. *A Catalogue of Excellent Greek, Latine and English Books.*
C1330. UMI Early English Books: Tract Supplement: D1: 2 (821.i.9[24]).

Bullord's auction was held at the Sign of the Black Bear and Star, near the little
north door of St. Paul's on 13 October 1691. In the catalogue, under the heading
"English Miscellanies in Folio," number 246 is listed as "Chaucers works [n.p.;
n.d.]" (27, really 30).

799.   BULLORD, JOHN. *A Catalogue of Latin and English Books.* C1348. UMI
Early English Books: Tract Supplement: D1: 1 (S.C.1035[2]).

Bullord held an auction at Rolls's Coffee-House on 11 May 1691. In the catalogue, under the heading "English and Latin Books in Folio," lot 93 is listed as
"*Chaucers* Works, last edition — 1687" (2).

800.   *A Catalogue of Books in Folio.* C1283. UMI Early English Books: Tract
Supplement D1: 2 (821.i.9[13]).

An auction was held at Tom's Coffee-House on 31 July 1691. In the catalogue,
under the heading "English Books Omitted. In Folio," the first item is listed as
"Chaucers Works [n.p.; n.d.]" (22, really 20).

801.   DRYDEN, JOHN. *Amphitryon: or, The Two Socia's.* D2235. UMI 739: 9 and
UMI 1382: 4.

For a reference to "Dame Partlet," an allusion to *The Nun's Priest's Tale*, see
DRYDEN (1690); in this edition, the passage is found on 24.

802.   DRYDEN, JOHN. *The Works of Mr. John Dryden.* D2207. UMI 208: 8.

For references to the difficulty of Chaucer's language for Dryden's contemporaries and to Chaucer's having translated the story of Troilus and Criseyde from
the Latin of "one Lollius a Lombard," see DRYDEN (1679); in this collection, the
play is the nineteenth work.

    For an allusion to *The Nun's Priest's Tale* in *Amphitryon*, see DRYDEN (1690);
in this collection, the twenty-fourth work.

    For an allusion to *The Nun's Priest's Tale* in *The Hind and the Panther*, see
DRYDEN (1687); in this collection, the poem is the thirty-fourth work.

The volume consists of Dryden's previously published plays and poems; therefore, according to what editions were available at the time the sets were made up, the contents of the sets vary slightly.

Other editions and collections: D2208 (1693), D2209 (1694), D2210 (1695).

Also found in *The Dramatick Works*, D2211 (1695), but *The Hind and the Panther* is not included.

803. *The English Part of the Library of the Late Duke of Lauderdale.* L611. UMI 1724: 10.

This collection of books belonging to the late John Maitland, Duke of Lauderdale (1616–1682), "All Curiously Bound and Gilt on the Back, many in Turkey Leather and of the Large Papers" were to be auctioned as of May 27, 1690, at Sam's Coffee House in Ave-Mary-Lane near Ludgate-Street (title page). Under the heading "English in Folio," number 69 is listed as *"Chaucers (Jeffery) Works in Ancient Poetry—Lond.* 1561" (2)

804. **GIBSON, EDMUND.** "Notes" in William Drummond's *Polemo-middmia. Carmen macaronicum.* D2204. UMI 1256: 17.

As Spurgeon notes (3: 4.80–81), Edmund Gibson (1669–1748) cites Chaucer several times in his comments on this Latin version of *Christ's Kirk on the Green* by Drummond (1585–1649).

In a footnote, Gibson quotes part of a line from *The Clerk's Tale* (line 974): "She gan the house to dight, *Chaucer*" (4).

In another footnote, Gibson learnedly glosses with a line from *The Romaunt of the Rose* (line 4116): "For want of it I grone and grete. *Chaucer*" (9).

In yet another footnote, Gibson quotes a line from *The Parson's Tale* (line 630–35): "Guering, brawling. *Chaucer.* Better is a morsell or little gobbet of bread with joy, than an house filled full of delices, with chiding and guerring" (10).

In the Scots version of the poem (supposedly by King James V), Gibson continues to gloss various passages.

For the line "To dance these Damosels them dight," Gibson glosses *dight*: "prepare, provide . . . *Vox Chaucero usitatissima.* Dighteth his dinner.—To bed thou wold the dight.—His instruments would he dight.—He was aie the first in armes dight.—He doth his shippes dight.—*& sæpius alibi*" (11). [The first example is not Chaucerian. The others: *The Romaunt of the Rose* (line 2555), *The Romaunt of the Rose* (line 4240), *Troilus and Criseyde* (line 3: 1773), *The Legend of Good Women* (line 1288).]

For the line "Her lyre was like the Lilly," Gibson glosses *lyre*: "complexion, countenaunce . . . *Cui consonant illa Chauceri*—Saturne his lere was like the lede.—Thy lustie lere overspredde with spottes blacke. . . . *Huic concinit & istud*

Chauceri—ᚐnꝺ nere ꝉ ꞇꝏent anꝺ gan to lere.—" (12). [None of the examples is Chaucerian.]

For the lines "The Miller was of manly make | To meet with him it was no mowes," Gibson glosses *it was no mowes*: "it ꞇꝏas no jesting matter. Of the foule moꞇꝏes anꝺ of the reproꝏes that men saieꝺ to him. *Chaucer*" (17). [Not Chaucerian.]

For the lines "The bushment whole about him brake | And bickered him with Bowes," Gibson glosses *bickered*: "pelteꝺ, inꝏaꝺeꝺ. ꝏe tꞇꝏo shall haꝏe a biker. *Chaucer*" (17). [*The Legend of Good Women* (line 2661).]

805. HOGARTH, RICHARD. *A New English Dictionary.* N637a. UMI 1955: 8.

For a reference Chaucer and to the etymology of the name *Chaucer*, see HOG-ARTH (1689); in this edition, the passage is found on sig. Bb8v.

806. LANGBAINE, GERARD, THE YOUNGER. *An Account of the English Dramatick Poets.* L373. UMI 281: 1.

As Spurgeon notes (1: 262–63), Langbaine (1656–1692) refers to Chaucer three times. In a passage about Abraham Cowley, he writes:

> He was Buried in *Westminster* Abby, near Two of our most English Bards, *Chaucer* and *Spencer*. (86)

In a passage about Sir John Denham:

> [He] was Buried the Twenty-third Instant [March 1668] at *Westminster*, amongst those Noble Poets, *Chaucer*, *Spencer*, and *Cowley*. (127)

In his discussion of Dryden's *Troilus and Cressida: or, Truth Found Out Too Late*, Langbaine credits Chaucer's plot:

> The Plot of this Play was taken by Mr. *Shakespear* from *Chaucer's Troilus and Cressida*; which was translated (according to Mr. *Dryden*) from the Original Story, written in Latine Verse, by One *Lollius*, a *Lombard*. (173).

In his annotated list of Ben Jonson's works, Langbaine notes the connection of *The Masque of Queens* with *The House of Fame*: He writes:

> *Masque of Queens*, celebrated from the House of Fame, by the Queen of *Great Britain* with her Ladies, at Whitehall, *Febr.* 2.1609. This Masque is adorned with learned Notes, for the Explanation of the Author's Design. (293)

This connection is noted in Boswell & Holton No. 797.

Another edition with a new title: *The Lives and Characters of the English Dramatick Poets*, L375 (1699), with additions.

807. MIEGE, GUY. *The New State of England under Their Majesties K. William and Q. Mary.* **M2019. UMI 2108: 7.**

Miege (1644–1718?) is identified on the title page as "G. M." In the second part, "An Account of the Inhabitants, their Original, Genius, Customs, Religion and Government; [etc.]," the first chapter is titled "Of the Inhabitants of England . . . with an Account of the most famous Men of this Nation, either for Souldiery or Learning." Following a section on scholars of note, Miege includes one "For Men of other Studies." There Chaucer is enshrined along with other notable poets. Miege writes:

> For Poetry, *Gower*, and *Lydgate*, a Monk of Bury.
> The famous *Geofry Chaucer*, Brother in Law to John of Gaunt, the great Duke of Lancaster.
> Sir Philip *Sidney*, and the Renowned *Spencer*.
> *Sam. Daniel*, and *Michael Drayton*, That the Lucan, and This the Ovid of the English Nation.
> *Beaumont*, and *Fletcher*, not inferiour unto Terence and Plautus.
> And lastly, *Ben. Johnson*, equal to any of the Ancients for the exactness of his Pen, and the Decorum he kept in the Dramatick Poems, never before observed on the English Theater. (pt. 2, 20)

Other editions in 1691: M2019A, part 2, 20;
   Other editions: M2020 (1693), part 2, 17; M2021 (1694), part 2, 17.
   Also found in *The New State of England, Under Our Present Monarch K. William III*, M2022 (1699), part 2, 9–10.

808. N., J. *Catalogus variorum librorum.* **L610. UMI 1724: 9.**

Part of the Duke of Lauderdale's library was auctioned on 26 March 1691 at Tom's Coffee-House. In the catalogue, under the heading "English Divinity, History, Poetry, Travels and Miscellanies in Folio," lot 70 is listed as "*Chaucer's* Works (Imperfect)—[no date]" (30; sig. H1v); and number 134 as "*Jeffery Chaucee's* [*sic*] Works—*Lond.* 1687" (31; sig. H2r).

809.   OLDHAM, JOHN. "A Pastoral" in the Earl of Rochester's *Poems, &c. On Several Occasions*. R1756. UMI 777: 10.

For a reference that says Rochester will be mourned more than Chaucer, see OLDHAM, *Some New Pieces* (1681); in this edition, the passage is found on x–xi (sig. a2v–3r)

   Another edition: R1757 (1696), same pagination.

810.   "On John Burnyeat's Book" in Burnyeat's *The Truth Exalted*. B5968. UMI 272: 4.

The opening line of a commendatory poem headed faintly echoes Chaucer's line, "Go, litel bok, go, litel myn tragedye" (*Troilus and Criseyde* 5: 1786):

> Go, *Little Book*, speak out the Praise
> Of him, that did thy *Author* Raise
> An *Eminent Apostle* of our Days. (sig. A4v)

811.   PRINCE, VINCENT. *The Protestant Almanack for the Year 1691*. A2231. UMI 2828: 16.

The author is identified on the title page as "Philoprotest, a well-willer to the mathematicks." Following the almanac for July, in a section headed "Several Officers in the Popish Church," Prince[45] quotes from the spurious work known as Chaucer's *Ploughman's Tale*:

> *Deacons*, had charge to relieve Widows and Orphans, and other poor faithful people, and to distribute unto them the Alms which devout Christians had given to that intent. But of these, and their other higher Officers, see what Chaucer saith of them in the *Ploughman's Tale*.

> *Popes, Bishops, and Cardinals,*
> *Chanons, Parsons, and Vicare,*
> *In Goddes Service I trow bene fals,*
> *That Sacraments sellen here,*
> *And been as proud as* Lucifere,
> *Eche man look whether that I lie, Sir.* (sig. B3r)

---

[45] Attributed to Prince by Wing but to William Winstanley by Bernard Capp, *English Almanacs, 1500–1800: Astrology and the Popular Press* (Ithaca, NY: Cornell University Press, 1979), 339.

812.   RAY, JOHN. *A Collection of English Words Not Generally Used.* R389. UMI 774: 19.

For references to Chaucer's usage of quaint words, see RAY (1674); in this edition, the passages are found on 57, 70, 74, 82, 84–85, 85, 91.

813.   RAY, JOHN. *The Wisdom of God Manifested in the Works of the Creation.* R410. UMI 474: 1.

Ray (1627–1705) is identified on the title page as "John Ray, M. A. sometimes Fellow of [Trinity-College in Cambridge], and now of the Royal Society." In "some common places delivered in the chapp[el] of Trinity-College, in Cambridge," he appears to be an echo of a line from *The Reeve's Tale*: "The gretteste clerkes been noght wisest men" (line 4054). In a passage about "Scurrilous Words, Scoffing and Jeering, Flouting and Taunting," Ray writes:

> [T]here may be some Wit shewn in Scoffing and Jesting upon others, yet it is a Practice inconsistent with true Wisdom. The Scorner and the Wise man are frequently posed in Scripture . . . It is a Proverbial saying, *The greatest Clerks are not always the wisest men.* I think the saying might as often be verified of the greatest Wits. (238)

Another edition: R411 (1692), ²164.

814.   *The Secret History of the Four Last Monarchs of Great Britain.* C7346. UMI 90: 4.

This work is sometimes attributed to Nathaniel Crouch (1632?–1725?) and sometimes to John Phillips (1631–1706). For a reference to an unnamed bishop who bragged that he had never read a line of Chaucer because he was linked (in the bishop's mind) with Luther and Calvin, see *The Secret History* (1690). As Harris notes (*PQ*), in this edition, the passage is found 6.

Another edition: C7347 (1693), 7.

815.   *Some Modest Remarks on Dr. Sherlocks New Book about the Case of Allegiance Due to Sovereign Powers, &c.* S4525. UMI 2178: 1.

As Harris notes (*PQ*), the unidentified author casts this work as a letter written to a friend about William Sherlock's *Case of Allegiance Due to Sovereign Powers.* The author observes that Sherlock's chief authority is "his dearly beloved Darling, Bishop *Overall*'s Convocation Book" (17). In a passage about convocations held during the reign of James I, he writes:

'Tis a thousand to one, but that same Bishop might be a Member of
this Convocation, who thank'd God, he had never read a Line either in
Chaucer or *Calvin*. (17)

For a similar sentiment in a different context, see *The Secret History* (1690).
    Another edition in 1691, *The Second Edition Corrected and Enlarged*: S4526, 17.

816.   TRYON, THOMAS. *A Way to Health, Long Life and Happiness: or, A Discourse of Temperance.* T3201. UMI 1451: 15.

For an echo of a line from *The Reeve's Prologue*, see TRYON (1683); in this edition,
the passage is found on 457–58.
    Another edition in 1691: *The Second Edition, with Amendments. By Thomas
Tryon, Student in Physick,* T3201A, 457–58. UMI 2083: 35

817.   WALFORD, BENJAMIN. *Catalogus variorum & insignium.* C1453. UMI
2384: 3.

Walford held an auction of the stock of the bankrupt publisher and stationer
Adiel Mill of Amen Corner beginning on 9 February 1691 at the Sign of the
Bear in Ave-Mary-Lane. In the catalogue, under the heading "English Miscellanies in Folio," lot 63 is listed as "[Works] of Geoffry Chaucer—ib. [i.e., Lon-
don] 1598" (102).

818.   WALFORD, BENJAMIN. *Catalogus variorum & insignium librorum ex
diversis Europæ partibus advectorum.* C1453. UMI 2384: 3.

Walford held an auction at the Sign of the Bear in Ave-Mary-Lane on 19 October 1691. In the catalogue, under the heading "English Miscellanies, in Folio,"
number 112 is listed as *"Geffery Chaucer's* Works—(Wants the Title)—[n.p.;
n.d.]"; lot 113 as "—The same with Additions—*Ibid.* [i.e., London] 1602" (102).

819.   WOOD, ANTHONY À. *Athenæ Oxonienses. An Exact History of all the Writers and Bishops Who Have Had their Education in the University of Oxford. The
First Volume.* W3382. UMI 117: 5.

Spurgeon notes (1: 264) four references to Chaucer in Woods's first volume, but
there are others.
    In his biographical sketch of Stephen Hawes, Wood (1632–1695) notes his
study of Chaucer. Wood writes:

[H]e could repeat by heart most of our *English* Poets; especially *Jo.
Lydgate* a Monk of *Bury,* whom he made equal in some respects, with
Geff. Chaucer. (col. 6)

As Spurgeon notes (1: 263–64), Wood notes William Thynne's work on Chaucer:

This Person who was poetically given from his Youth, did make a search after all the works of *Jeffery Chaucer* the Prince of our English Poets, many of which were then in MS. At length having collected all the ancient Copies of that Author, he took great pains to correct and amend them. Which being so done, he put notes and explanations on, and printed them altogether in one Volume in Folio, (not in double columns as they have been since) and dedicated them to K. *Hen.* 8. an. 1542, having been partly and imperfectly done several Years before by *Will. Caxton.* Afterwards *Joh. Stow* the Chronologer did correct, increase and publish, them with divers ample notes collected out of several *records* and monuments. All which he delivering to his Friend *Tho. Speght* a *Cantabrigian*, he drew them into good form and method, mixed them with his own, and published them 1597. (sig. E1v–2r col. 52–53)

In his sketch of Ralph Radcliff, a schoolmaster in Hertfordshire, Wood notes that he wrote dramatic works for his students to perform. Two of his comedies that have Chaucerian connections: "Patient Greseld [*sic*]" and "Chaucers Melibie." (sig. F3r col. 73).

Wood records Nicholas Brigham's admiration for Chaucer:

When he [Brigham] continued in the University, and afterwards in one of the Inns of Court, he exercised his muse much in Poetry, and took great delight in the works of *Jeffry Chaucer*: For whose memory he had so great a respect, that he removed his bones into the South cross Isle or trancept of St. *Peters* Church in *Westminster*, in the Year 1556. Which being so done, he erected a comely Monument over them, with *Chaucers Effigies*, and an Epitaph in Prose and Verse; which to this day remains against the East Wall of the said Isle. . . . This ingenious and curious Person . . . yeilded [*sic*] up his last breath to the great regret of all those that knew his worth, within the City of *Westminster* in the month of *Dec.* in Fifteen hundred fifty and nine, (which was the second year of Queen *Elizabeth*) but where buried, unless near to the bones of *Chaucer*, I cannot tell. (sig. H1v col. 99)

In his biographical sketch of the musician and poet Richard Edwards (1525–1566), Wood notes that he wrote a comedy in two parts called "Palæmon and Arcyte . . . Acted before Qu. *Elizab.* in *Ch. Ch.* hall 1566. which gave her so much content, that sending for the Author thereof, she was pleased to give him many thanks, with promise of reward for his pains. . . . In the said play was acted a cry of hounds on the quadrant, upon the train of a fox in the hunting of *Theseus*" (sig. I1r col. 118). It appears likely that Edwards took at least part of his plot from *The Knight's Tale*.

Wood notes that he has seen several works written by Nicholas Grimald, including "*Troilus Chauceri*, com. — with several suchlike things" (col. 140).

Regarding Francis Thynne, Wood says:

> What other things our Author *Thynne* hath written I know not, nor any thing else of him, only that he died in sixteen hundred and eleven. But that which I have forgotten to let the Reader know farther of him, is, that he had several *Notes on, and corrections of, Chaucer's Works* lying by him; with the helps of which, he did intend to put out that author, with a comment in our English tongue, as the Italians have *Peteark* [*sic*] and others in their language. But he having been taken off from that good work, he did assist *Tho. Speght* of *Cambridge* with his notes and directions, as also with considerable materials for the writing *Chaucer's life*. Whereupon the said *Speght* published that author again in 1602. (having in the former edition 1597. had the notes and corrections of *Joh. Stow* the Chronologer for his assistance,) whereby most of *Chaucer*'s old Words were restored, and Proverbs and Sentences marked. See more in *Will. Thynne*, under the year 1542. from whom, if I mistake not, this *Francis* was descended. (sig. X2r col. 319–20)

1692

820.   *The Athenian Mercury*. Volume 5: 18.

In the issue dated 30 January 1691 [1692], a correspondent asks:

> *What is the meaning of the word Fame, and whether do you think a man famous or infamous for an ill Action?*
> *Answ.* . . . [T]he word *Famous* as well as *Fame*, is used by the *Latins* in a *middle Sence*, tho' we believe for the most part in a *bad one*, contrary to our English, as in *Horace*, where he brings in old *Lucilius* (the *Chaucer* of the *Romans*) attacking *Lupus*, whoever he was, with *Famosis versibus*, which we shou'd render Lampoons, or Defamatory Verses, in which Sence the middle Finger is also stiled *Famosus Digitus*. . . . (no pagination)

821.   BULLORD, JOHN. *A Catalogue of Extraordinary Greek and Latin Books.* C1331. UMI 1774: 15.

Bullord began auctioning the library of the lately murdered Andrew Clench, M.D., at Toms Coffee-House on 1 June 1692. In the catalogue, under the heading "English Books in Folio," number 100 is listed as "Chaucers Works, the best Edit. wants Title [no date]" (17; sig. E1r)

822.   CARTER, MATTHEW. *Honor redivius: or, The Analysis of Honor and Armory.* C661A. UMI 2526: 13.

For a reference to Chaucer's escutcheon, see CARTER (1655); in this edition, the passage is found on 225 and indexed on 348.

823.   *A Catalogue of Books to be Sold by Auction.* C1291. UMI 1791: 23.

An auction was held on 14 October 1692 at Wills (formerly Rolls's) Coffee House. In the catalogue, under the heading "Books in Folio," lot 61 is listed as "*Chaucers* Works. *Boccas* Fall of Princes together—[no date]" (2).

824.   COLES, ELISHA. *An English Dictionary.* C5074. UMI 450: 28.

For references to Chaucer in Coles's epistle to the reader and in various definitions, see COLES (1676); in this edition, the passages are found on sigs. A3r, K2r, L3r, P4v.

825.   COLVILL, SAMUEL. *The Scotch Hudibras: or, A Mock Poem.* C5427 (1692). UMI 310: 10.

For a reference to cockscombs who pay insufficient attention when they read Chaucer, see COVIL (1681); in this edition, the passage is found on 60–61.

826.   DRYDEN, JOHN. *Troilus and Cressida: or, Truth Found Too Late.* D2390. UMI 1549: 1; UMI 2353: 2.

For references to the difficulty of Chaucer's language for Dryden's contemporaries and to Chaucer's having translated *Troilus and Criseyde* from the Latin of Lollius, see DRYDEN (1679); in this edition, the passages are found on sig. A3v, A4v.

827.   DUNTON, JOHN. *The Young-Student's-Library.* D2635. UMI 1187: 6.

As Harris notes (*PQ*), Dunton was a bookseller at the Sign of the Raven in the Poultry. In "An Essay upon All Sorts of Learning Written by the Athenian Society," in a section about poetry, Dunton prints a list of poets that the Society recommends. Dunton introduces the lists with a caveat: "We shall only . . . here place the *Chief* of the Latin and English Poets, which are to be preus'd with great Care and Regard." The list of Latin poets begins with Virgil, Horace, Ovid, and Catullus and ends with Buchannan. The list of nineteen English poets begins with Chaucer:

> *Chaucer.* | *Spenser.* | *Shakespear.* | *Johnson.* | *Beaumont* and *Fletcher.* | *Drai-*
> *ton. Daniel.* | Sr. *John Suckling.* | Sr. *John Denham.* | *Crashaw.* | *Cowley.*
> | Sr. *William Davenant.* | Dr. *Donn.* | Mr. *Dryden.* | Mr. *Otway.* | Mr.
> *Lee.* | Mrs. *Behn.* | Mrs. *Phillips.* | Several Collections of Poems. (xiii)

828.   FINCH, CHARLES. "Bellositum" in *Musarum Anglicanarum analecta, sive, Poemata quædam melioris notæ.* M3135. UMI 468: 3 and 1490: 17 (as O898).

In this collection of miscellaneous poems is found a long poem headed "Bellositum: sve de regione Oxonium circumjacente." There "Caroli Finch Baronis de Daventriæ, ex Æde Christi" notes Chaucer's association with Oxford:

> Hic etiam ônullis obliviscenda poëtis
> *Chauceri* domus, antiquæ domus hospita Musæ
> Usque stat, immunis stati, viridisque juventâ:
> Sponte suâ erumpunt laurus, hederæque frequentes
> Intexunt vernâ tecti fastigia scenâ,
> Sic post Thebanas superest illæsa ruinas
> Una domus, fruiturque perenni Pindarus ævo.
> Quin age, Nam facilem spondet titi, Musa, loquelam
> *Chauceri* nomes; similem tibi spiritus æstum
> Inspirat, sacrosque in vate resuscitat ignes.
> Prisca refer, quotquot juxta hic monumenta supersunt;
> Gestaque, supremasque ducum testata favillas. (14)

Another edition: M3135A (1699), 14.

829.   GILDON, CHARLES. *The Post-Boy Rob'd of His Mail: or, The Pacquet Broke Open.* G735A. UMI 1461: 44.

This work is a collection of "five hundred letters to person of several qualities and conditions. With observations upon each letter" (title page). The conceit of the collection is that letters have been sent to the wrong address and have been forwarded to the editor for comment. "Letter XCVIII" is "From a Lover to his Mistriss, in absence." In the letter, the lover (who signs himself "Poor Charles") eloquently bewails his unhappiness because it has been almost four days since he saw the face of his mistress except in his dreams. Apparently the editor passes letters around to in-house readers, collects their comments, and passes them on to the public readers. One of them quotes from *The Knight's Tale* (lines 1361–66) to buttress his observation that "Love is the most violent of passions" and another (named Brook) comments on Chaucer's language:

> *Absence to him that truly loves must be the greatest of Torments, as Love is the most violent of Passions. As 'tis excellently describ'd by old* Chaucer (pursu'd I) *in his* Knights Tale:

> His Sleep, his Meat, his Drink is him bereft,
> That lean he waxeth, and dry, as a Shaft,
> His Eyes hollow, and grisly to behold;

His Hew pale, and Ashen to unfold.
And solitary he was ever alone,
And waking all the night, making moan.

Rare indeed (said Brook) *are all the effects of a desperate Passion, natural and beautiful, tho' drest in so antiquated a phrase.* [Another reader attributes five lines to Spenser.] . . . *These Poets* (said River) *drew their Picture from Nature; since 'tis evident Love triumphs over our other passions, Ambition it self being forc'd to submit, when once Love opposes it.* (267–68)

830.   HARINGTON, JAMES. "The Introduction," in Anthony à Wood's *Athenæ Oxonienses. An Exact History of all the Writers and Bishops Who Have Had their Education in the University of Oxford. The Second Volume.* W3383. UMI 301: 10.

As Spurgeon notes (1: 263–64), Harington mentions Chaucer's role in refining the English language. In "The Introduction" in a passage about ancient Britons and the changing nature of the English language, Harington writes:

As to the Poetry of the Age, the beauty of Speech, and the Graces of measure and numbers, which are the inseparable ornaments of a good Poem, are not to be expected in a rude and unsettled Language; And tho Chaucer, *the Father of our Poets, had not taken equal care of the force of expression, as of the greatness of thought; yet the refining of a Tongue is such a Work, as never was begun, and finished by the same hand. We had before only words of common use, coin'd by our need, or invented by our passions: Nature had generally furnish'd this Island with the supports of Necessity, not the instruments of Luxury; the elegance of our speech, as well as the finess of our garb, is owing to foreign Correspondence. And as in Clothes, so in Words, at first usually they broke in unalter'd upon us from abroad; and consequently, as in* Chaucer's *time, come not over like Captives, but Invaders: But then only they are made our own, when, after a short Naturalization, they fit themselves to our Dress, become incorporated with our Language, and take the air, turn, and fashion of the Country that adopted them.* (sig. A1v)

831.   *An Historical Dictionary of England and Wales.* H2103a. UMI 106: 5.

The entry for Chaucer portrays him as a polymath:

Chaucer, *Geofry,* b. at *London,* was an excellent Poet, the *Homer* of his age, and the Refiner of the English Tongue. A great *Mathematician,* witness his book *de Sphera.* He was also an acute Logician, a sweet Rhetorician, a grave Philosopher. He died in the year 1400. (sig. C2r–v)

832.   HUSSEY, CHRISTOPHER. *This Catalogue of Books, Bound and in Quires.*
T924. No UMI.

Hussey held an auction at Rolls's Coffee-House in St. Paul's Churchyard on 4
January 1691/92. In the catalogue, under the heading "English Miscellany, &c.
in Folio," number 153 is listed as "*Chaucer* (Sir *Ge.*) His Works, best Edit. [n.p.;
n.d.]" (10; sig. D1v).

833.   JONSON, BENJAMIN. *The Works of Ben Jonson.* J1006. UMI 359: 1.

For an echo of lines from *The General Prologue* and *The Wife of Bath's Prologue*, see
JONSON (1605) in this edition, the passage is found on 145–46.
      For an echo of a line describing the Cook in *The General Prologue*, see JON-
SON (1641); in this edition, the passage is found on 539.

834.   OLDHAM, JOHN. *The Works of Mr. John Oldham.* O229. UMI 724: 1.

For a reference to Chaucer's penchant for coining new words in "Horace His Art
of Poetry" and a reference to the diminished appreciation of Chaucer's poetry in
a tribute to the Earl of Rochester, see OLDHAM (1681); in this collection, the passages are found on 5, 82–83 (second pagination).

835.   RAY, JOHN. *The Wisdom of God Manifested. The Second Edition, Very
Much Enlarged.* R411. UMI 1044: 8.

Here Ray (1627–1705) is identified as "John Ray, Fellow of the Royal Society."
For an echo of a line from *The Reeve's Tale*, see RAY (1691); in this edition, the
passage is found on 2164.

836.   ROLLS, NATHANIEL. *Bibliotheca ornatissima: or, A Catalogue of Excellent
Books.* B2845. UMI 1710: 28.

Rolls held an auction of books and manuscripts at Will's (formerly Rolls's) Coffee-House on 18 April 1692. In the catalogue, under the heading "English Miscellanies, in Folio," lot 168 is listed as "Geffry Chaucers Works—[no date]"; and
number 169 as "The same with Additions and with his Life—Lond. 1687" (101,
really 57; sig. Q1r)

837.   RYMER, THOMAS. *The Tragedies of the Last Age.* R2431. UMI 475: 7.

For a possible allusion to *The Nun's Priest's Tale*, see RYMER (1678); in this edition, the passage is found on 70.

838.   SAUNDERS, FRANCIS. "Catalogue of Books" in Nahum Tate's *A Present
for the Ladies.* T212. UMI 1662: 9.

At the end of Tate's work is found "A Catalogue of Books Sold by F. Saunders in the New Exchange in the Strand." In addition to the works of Cowley,

Shakespeare, Beaumont and Fletcher, Jonson, Katharine Philips, and "*Spencer*'s Fairy Queen" in a section headed "Poetry and Plays. Folio's," number 10 is "*Chaucer*'s Works" (sig. I8r).

839. *The Wanton Wife of Bath*. W722. No UMI.

For a reference to Chaucer's writing of a wanton wife of Bath, see *The Wanton Wife of Bath* (1641).

840. WINSTANLEY, WILLIAM. *The Protestant Almanack. By Philoprotest.* A2232. UMI 1114: 13.

As Harris notes (*PQ*), under the heading "Of the Eclipses this Present Year, 1692," Philoprotest (a pseudonym for William Winstanley) refers to Chaucer and quotes from *The Summoners Tale* (lines 2099–2106). In a passage about the Catholic practice of fasting, he writes:

> [W]e may with much confidence predict from hence [an eclipse of the sun on 9 February], that the Popish Monks, Fryers and Nuns, will be as abstenious this Year as ever; and will Fast from Flesh on *Wednesdays* and *Frydays*, that they may with the better Appetite feed on Fish. Do not these men undergo sharp penance? Is not this terrible Fasting? As bad as the Fryer inflected on himself, who desired but
> *Round about the Crible Loaf an inch thick sliver,*
> *Of the Goose only the Liver:*
> *Of the Pig no more but the head;*
> *For him he wisht nothing should be dead.* (sig. A2r)

Shortly thereafter, he refers to Chaucer by name and quotes from *The Summoners Tale* (lines 2099–2106):

> Now as by the last Eclipse we predicted, that the uncleanness and lasciviousness of the Popish Clergy would be equivalent to the precedent Ages; so by this Eclipse it is plainly demonstrated, that their covetousness, avarice, and wayes of getting money to enrich themselves, their Abbeys, Nunneries, and other Religious Houses, as they call them, will be no less this year than heretofore, especially their working on the Consciences of dying men, that by their gifts and benevolence they might be prayed out of Purgatory. The Fryer in *Chaucer* perswading with the sick Farmer top make his confession to him rather than to his Parish Priest, having his hand upon his half-penny, makes this request to the Bed-rid man lying upon his Couch.

Yeve me then of thy Gold to make our Cloyster,
Quod he, for many a Muskle and many an Oyster,
When other men have been full well at ease
Hath been our food: our Cloister for to rease:
And yet God wot, unneath the foundament
Performed is, ne of our Pavement
Is not a Tile yet within our wones
By God we owen fourty pound for stones. (sig. A2v–3r)

841. WOOD, ANTHONY À. *Athenæ Oxonienses. An Exact History of all the Writ-ers and Bishops Who Have Had their Education in the University of Oxford. The Second Volume.* W3383A. UMI 301: 10.

For references to Chaucer's role in refining the English language in James Har-ington's introduction to Wood's second volume, see HARINGTON (1692).

In "The Introduction," in a passage about English poetry, Wood notes Chaucer's contributions. Wood writes:

As to the Poetry of the Age, the beauty of Speech, and the Graces of measure and numbers, which are the inseparable ornaments of a good Poem, are are not to be expected in a rude and unsettled Language; And tho *Chaucer,* the Father of our Poets, had not taken equal care of the force of expression, as of the greatness of thought; yet the refining of a Tongue is such a Work, as never was begun, and finished by the same hand. We had before only words of common use, coin'd by our need, or invented by our passions: Nature had generally furnish'd this Island with the supports of Necessity, not the instruments of Luxury; the elegance of our speech, as well as the fitness of our garb, is owing to foreign Correspondence. And as in Clothes, so in Words, at first usu-ally they broke in unalter'd upon us from abroad; and consequently, as in *Chaucer's* time, come not over like Captives, but Invaders: But then only they are made our own, when, after a short Naturalization, they fit themselves to our Dress, become incorporated with our Language, and take the air, turn, and fashion of the Country that adopted them. (2–3)

As Spurgeon notes (1: 264), Wood (1632–1695) mentioned Chaucer in his entry for Sir Francis Kinaston. Wood writes:

Our Author *Kinaston* did . . . [translate] from English into Lat. *Jeff. Chaucer* his *Troilus* and *Cresseid* which he entit. *Amorum Troili & Crese-idæ libri duo priores Anglico-Latini.* Oxon. 1635. qu. Which being beheld as an excellent translation, was usher'd into the world by 15 copies of Verses made by *Oxford* men. . . . (11)

For Kenneth Lloyd-Jones's splendid translations of the commendatory verses in Kinaston's translation, see KINASTON (1635), Boswell & Holton No. 1265.

There are at least two other references that Spurgeon overlooked. In his entry for John Denham, Wood notes his burial place near Chaucer:

> He died at his Office . . . and was buried on the 23 of the same month [March], in the s. cross isle or trancept of the Abby Church of S. *Peter* in *Westminster*, near to the graves of *Jeffry Chaucer* and *Abr. Cowley*. (303)

In his entry for Abraham Cowley, Wood writes:

> He died . . . [and was conveyed to Westminster Abbey] on the 3 of *Aug.* following, accompanied by divers persons of eminent quality, and there . . . was buried near to the place where the reliques of *Jeffr. Chaucer* had been lodged. (799)

1693

842.   ASHMOLE, ELIAS. *The Institutions, Laws & Ceremonies of the Most Noble Order of the Garter.* A3984. UMI 782: 29.

For references to Chaucer's relationship with Lydgate and to his role as a diplomat in the reign of Edward III, see ASHMOLE (1672); in this edition, the passages are found on 17, 668.

843.   *The Athenian Mercury.* Volume 12: 1.

As Spurgeon notes (1: 265–66), in the issue for 24 October 1693, in "Questions from the Poetical Lady," question 4 is:

> *What Books of Poetry wou'd you Advise one that's Young, and extreamly delights in it, to read, both Divine and other?*
>   *Answ.* . . . For others, Old Merry *Chaucer*, [etc.]. . . . (no pagination)

844.   BARNARD, JOHN AUGUSTINE, AND EDMUND BOHUN. *A Geographical Dictionary.* B3454. UMI 975: 12.

As the publisher notes on the title page, this work was "Begun by Edmund Bohun, Esquire [1645-1699]. Continued, corrected, and enlarged with great additions throughout . . . by Mr. Bernard [*sic*; b. 1660/61]."

In the entry for Sheffield, Barnard alludes to a line in *The Reeve's Tale*: "A Sheffeld thwitel baar he in his hose" (line 3933):

𝔖𝔥𝔢𝔣𝔣𝔦𝔢𝔩𝔡, a large well-built Market-town in the West riding of *York-shire* . . . of particular note for Iron Wares, even in *Chaucer*'s time, who describes a Person with a *Sheffield Whittle* by his side. . . . (376)

Another edition: B3455 (1695), 376.

845.   *Bibliotheca insignis*: *or, A Catalogue of Excellent . . . Books*. B2832. UMI Early English Books: Tract Supplement: D1: 1 (S.C.1035[9]).

A sale was held at Rolls's Auction House in St. Paul's Churchyard on 12 June 1693. In the catalogue, under the heading "English Miscellaneous Books . . . in Folio," lot 25 is listed as "*Geffery Chaucers* Works—*Lond*. 1602" (24).

846.   BLOME, RICHARD. *The Art of Heraldry*. B3206. UMI 1119: 10.

For a description of Chaucer's coat of arms, see BLOME (1684); in this edition, the passage is found on 67.

847.   BRITAINE, WILLIAM DE. *Humane Prudence*. B4806. UMI 2125: 5.

For a spurious quotation attributed to Chaucer, see BRITAINE (1686); in this edition, the passage is found on 120.

848.   BROME, JAMES. "The Life of Mr. Somner" in *A Treatise of the Roman Ports and Forts in Kent by William Somner*. S4669. UMI 194: 4.

In his biographical sketch of Somner, Brome lists his contributions to linguistic scholarship, including Somner's "*Glossography*" to the works of *Chaucer*" (62).

849.   BUNYAN, JOHN. *The Pilgrim's Progress. The Second Part*. B5582. UMI 1683: 2.

For Bunyan's echo of Chaucer's line, "Go, litel bok, go litel myn tragedye" (*Troilus and Criseyde* 5: 1786), see BUNYAN (1684); in this edition, the passage is found on sig. *A*2r.

850.   *A Collection of Excellent English Books*. C5145. UMI Early English Books: Tract Supplement: D1: 1 (S.C.1035 [7]).

An auction was held at Batson's Coffee House near the Royal Exchange in Cornhill on 23 May 1693. In the catalogue, under the heading "English, in Folio" number 16 is listed as "*Jeffery Chaucer's* Works, with his Life; the last Edition. —1687" (13; sig. D1r).

851.   *A Collection of Modern English Books*. C5147. UMI 1775: 3.

An auction of books was held at Batson's Coffee House in Cornhill on 31 October 1693. In the catalogue, under the heading "English History, Miscellanies,

&c. In Folio," number 32 is listed as *"Jeffery Chaucer's* Works, the last Edition, with his Life—1687" (9).

852. COWLEY, ABRAHAM. *The Works of Mr. Abraham Cowley.* C6659. UMI 685: 4.

For a reference to Cowley's burial place near Chaucer, see SPRAT (1668); in this edition, the passage is found on sig. e2r.

For a reference to Chaucer's "rich rhymes," see COWLEY (1656); in this edition, the passage is found on 37 (sig. ⁴Aa2r).

853. CROUCH, NATHANIEL. *Martyrs in Flames: or, Popery (in Its True Colours) Displayed.* C7344A. UMI 2665: 3.

After detailing the persecution of Protestants in Piedmont, Bohemia, Germany, Poland, Lithuania, France, Italy, Spain, Portugal, Holland, Scotland, and Ireland, Crouch (1632?–1725?) mentions Chaucer in a section headed "The Cruelties, Plots, and Treasons of the Papists against the Protestants in England." He says that "the Papists impertinently urge against us the Newness of our Religion," so he traces the English roots of Protestantism back to the days of King Alfred. Crouch writes:

> [I]n every Year it pleased God to raise up several learned and worthy men to testify against the Horrid Corruptions of *Rome*, both by Speaking, Writing and Disputing against them . . . [among them] Doctor *John Wickliff, Jeoffery Chaucer, William Wickam* Bishop of *Winchester*, and many other Learned men.
>
> All these gave ample Testimony by their publick Writings against the many Corruptions evil Doctrines and Superstitious Worship of the *Romish* Church, with the hazard of their Lives, Honours, Liberties, Estates and Fortunes. (123–24)

854. DRYDEN, JOHN. "Dedicatory Epistle" in *The Satires of Decimus Junius Juvenalis. Made English by Mr. Dryden* [and others]. J1288. UMI 212: 7.

As Spurgeon notes (1: 264–65), in Dryden's dedicatory epistle, dated 18 August 1692 and addressed to Charles Sackville (1638–1706), sixth earl of Dorset and first earl of Middlesex, there is a reference to Spenser's imitation of Chaucer's language in a couple of sections about Milton:

> As for Mr. *Milton* . . . His Antiquated words were his Choice, not his Necessity; for therein he imitated *Spencer*, as *Spencer* did *Chaucer.* And tho,' perhaps, the love of their Masters, may have transported both too far, in the frequent use of them; yet in my Opinion, Obsolete Words may then be laudably reviv'd. . . . (viii)

But as he endeavors every where to express *Homer,* whose Age had not arriv'd to that fineness, I found in him a true sublimity, lofty thoughts, which were cloath'd with admirable *Grecisms,* and ancient words, which he had been digging from the Mines of *Chaucer,* and of *Spencer,* and which, with all their rusticity, had somewhat of Venerable in them. (viii, 1)

Other editions: J1289 (1697), xiii–xiv; J1290 (1697), xiii–xiv.

855.   DRYDEN, JOHN. *The Works of Mr. John Dryden, in Four Volumes.* D2208. UMI 1382: 4.

For references to the difficulty of Chaucer's language for Dryden's contemporaries and to Chaucer's translation of *Troilus and Criseyde* from the Latin of "one Lollius a Lombard," see DRYDEN (1679); in this collection, the play is in vol. 2.

For an allusion to *The Nun's Priest's Tale* in *Amphitryon,* see DRYDEN (1690); in this collection, the play is in vol. 3.

For an allusion to *The Nun's Priest's Tale* in *The Hind and the Panther,* see DRYDEN (1687); in this collection the poem is in vol. 4.

856.   EDWARDS, JOHN. *A Discourse Concerning the Authority, Stile, and Perfection of the Books of the Old and New-Testament.* E202. UMI 1422: 26a.

Edwards (1637–1716) is identified on the title page as "Sometime Fellow of St. John's College in Cambridge." In the first volume, in a section headed "Of the Truth and Authority of the Holy Scriptures," in chapter 7, in a passage about the meaning of *dulcarnon* (an allusion to *Troilus and Criseyde* 3: 931, 933), Edwards writes:

Alexander is called *Dulcarnain,* in the Alcoran by *Mahomet.* . . . And 'till some others give a better Interpretation of *Chaucer*'s [at *Dulkernoon*] I presume to say it signifies as much as to be *in a maze,* to be at ones wits end, to be dilemma'd, to be push'd at one side and the other. . . . (247)

Another edition in 1693: E202aA, same pagination.
    Other editions: E202A (1694), 247; E203 (1696), 247.

857.   FLAVEL, JOHN. *Husbandry Spiritualized: or, The Heavenly Use of Earthly Things.* F1167A. UMI 1907: 23.

For an echo of a line from *The Reeve's Prologue,* see FLAVEL (1669); in this edition, the passage is found on 317.

858.   H., S. "To his Ingenious Friend," in Joseph Aicken's *The English Grammar: or, The English Tongue Reduced to Grammatical Rules.* A799. UMI 47: 22.

In a commendatory poem by S. H. headed "To his Ingenious Friend Mr. Jos. Aickin upon his Book Intitul'd the English Grammar," the poet characterizes Chaucer as the first to refine the English language. He begins by saying English no longer depends on Latin because of Aicken's efforts:

> *Others with painful toyl the work begun:*
> *But did not or else could not carry't on:*
> *You did on their foundation build and sought,*
> *And found what they neglected or forgot.*
> *To their defects you give a large supply,*
> *Which may be seen by the discerning Eye:*
> *Great* Chaucer *did at first the Tongue refine*
> *But you from all its dregs have clear'd the mine.* (sig. A2r)

Another edition in 1693: A799A, sig. A2r.

859.   HACKET, JOHN. *Scrinia reserata: A Memorial Offer'd to the Great Deservings of John Williams, D. D.* H171. UMI 533: 3.

Hacket (1592–1670) is identified on the title page as "Late Lord Bishop of Litchfield and Coventry." As Graves notes (*SP*), in the second part of this biography of John Williams, sometime Lord-Keeper of the Great Seal of England, Bishop of Lincoln, and Archbishop of York, Hacket turns to *Troilus and Criseyde* (5: 1857) for an apt word. Hacket writes:

> 'Tis custom to Toll a little before a Passing-bell ring out: and that shall
> be done in a Moral strode; as *Chaucer* calls it. (pt. 2, 18)

As Harris notes (*PQ*), Hacket quotes a modernized couplet from the second book of *The House of Fame* (lines 785–86). In a passage about the undeserved bad reputation of the Welsh, Hacket writes:

> [W]e that live in the *South* slander them, if their common men be not
> Filchers and Thieves.
>
> > *And though it were piped by a Mouse,*
> > *It must needs come to Fame's House;*
>
> says noble *Chaucer.* (pt. 2, 217)

As Graves notes (*SP*), Hacket quotes conflated lines from a modernized version of the third book of *The House of Fame* (lines 1628-30, 1788-89). In a passage about slander, he writes:

> Few consider how odious the voice of Slander is before the God of Truth. . . . If the Slanderer have recourse for his own Apology to common Report and Fame, his Judgment marcheth after the Devil's Drum. Our time honoured *Chaucer*, in his pretty Fiction of the House of Fame, condemns the Giddiness of common Talk, in a very pleasant Art: That Æolus brought two Trumpets to Fames House, one of Laud, another of Slander; That Fame would not suffer Æolus to wind out the Praise of some, though most deserving; bad him cry up others of no merit; authoriz'd him to disgrace divers, that had done things worthy of Renown.

> *Speak of them Harm and Shrewdness,*
> *Instead of Good and Worthiness:*
> *For thou shalt Trumpet all contrair,*
> *If that they have done well and fair:*
> *Some new thing, I wot not what,*
> *Tydings, either this or that.*

> When Æolus's foul Blasts are over, which will not continue long, the Glory of this Archbishopp, and his Innocency, will mount above the Envy and Credulity of his Foes. . . . (pt. 2, 221-22)

Ambrose Philips of St. John's College (Cambridge), published an abridged version of this work in 1700, but all the references to Chaucer were cut.

860.   HOLME, RANDLE. *The Academy of Armory.* H2513A. No UMI.

For references to Chaucer's use of words as authoritative and to Chaucer's marriage to the daughter of Sir Payne Roet, see HOLME (1688); in this edition, the passages are found on 45, 68, ²24, ²321, ²474.

861.   HOUGHTON, JOHN. *Collection for Improvement of Husbandry And Trade.* **Nelson and Seccombe 49.067.**

Houghton (1645-1705) is identified as a Fellow of the Royal Society in the issue for 10 November 1693. In a review of John Evelyn's book of trees (see No. 555), he notes that Evelyn writes of Chaucer's oak:

> The Ingenious *John Evelyn Esq*; in his Discourse of *Earth* and *For-est-Trees*, and Third Edition, gives several Accounts of *Clay*. . . . And

Chaucer's great Oak, mentioned *Page* 166, grew in a *gravelly Clay*, moistned with small and frequent Springs. . . .

862. JEVON, THOMAS. *The Devil of a Wife: or, A Comical Transformation.* **J731A. UMI 1465: 1.**

For a reference to Chaucer and the Wife of Bath, see JEVON (1686); in this edition, the passage is found on 26. See also *The Wanton Wife of Bath* (1641).

863. MIEGE, GUY. *The New State of England under Their Majesties K. William and Q. Mary.* **M2020. UMI 1235: 7.**

For a reference to Chaucer in a list of famous men of England, see MIEGE (1691); in this edition, the passage is found in part 2, 17.

864. MILLINGTON, EDWARD. *A Catalogue of Ancient and Modern Books.* **C1273. UMI 1647: 13.**

Millington offered a variety of books for sale by auction "for the Entertainment and Diversion of the Gentry and Citizens of Norwich" at Mrs. Oliver's house on Monday, 10 July 1693. In the catalogue, under the heading "Miscellanies in Folio," item number 40 is listed as "*Chaucers* Works (old Edit.) [no date or place of publication]," 28. On the same page we find listed "*Spencers* Fairy Queen," "*Montaigns* Essays," and "Mrs. *K. Phillips* Poems."

865. MONTAIGNE, MICHEL DE. *Essays.* **M2480. UMI 1816: 13a.**

For an echo of a line from *The Reeve's Tale*, see MONTAIGNE (1685); in this edition, the passage is found on 191.

866. RYMER, THOMAS. *A Short View of Tragedy.* **R2429. UMI 399: 12.**

Rymer (1641–1713) is identified on the title page as "Mr. Rymer, servant to their Majesties." As Spurgeon notes (1: 265), he mentions Chaucer in the table of contents for chapter 6: "Chaucer *refin'd our English*" (sig. A7r). In chapter 6, in a section about the poets of Provence, he notes Chaucer's contributions to the English language. Rymer writes:

> [T]hey who attempted verse in English, down till *Chaucers* time, made an heavy pudder, and are always miserably put to't for a word to clink: which commonly fall so awkard [*sic*], and unexpectedly as dropping from the Clouds by some Machine or Miracle.
> *Chaucer* found an Herculean labour on his Hands; And did perform to Admiration. He seizes all Provencal, French or Latin that came in his way, gives them a new garb and livery, and mingles them amongst our English: turns out English, gowty, or superannuated, to place in

their room the foreigners, fit for service, train'd and accustomed to Poetical Discipline.

But tho' the Italian reformation was begun and finished well nigh at the same time by *Boccace*, *Dante*, and *Petrarch*. Our language retain'd something of the churl; something of the Stiff and Gothish did stick upon it, till long after *Chaucer*.

Chaucer threw in Latin, French, Provencial, and other Languages, like new Stum to raise a Fermentation; In Queen *Elizabeth*'s time it [poetry] grew fine, but came not to an Head and Spirit, did not shine and sparkle till Mr. *Waller* set it a running. (78–79)

867.   SAUNDERS, FRANCIS. "A Catalogue of Books," in *A Collection of Poems by Several Hands. Most of Them Written by Persons of Eminent Quality*. C5174. UMI 1122: 4.

At the end of this anthology, there is *"A Catalogue of Books Printed for, and Sold by* Francis Saunders." Under the heading "Folio" Saunders lists "Mr. *Chaucer*'s Works" (sig. T3v).

868.   SAUNDERS, FRANCIS. "A Catalogue of Books" in Nahum Tate's *A Present for the Ladies. The Second Edition Corrected*. T213. UMI 1579: 35.

At the end of this work is found "A Catalogue of Books Sold by F. Saunders in the New Exchange in the Strand." Under the heading "Poetry and Plays. Folio's," number 8 is listed as *"Chaucer*'s Works." (no pagination; no signature)

869.   *The Secret History of the Four Last Monarchs of Great Britain*. C7347. UMI 1001: 10.

For a reference to an unnamed bishop who bragged that he had never read a line of Chaucer because he was linked (in the bishop's mind) with Luther and Calvin, see *The Secret History* (1690); in this edition, the passage is found on 7.

870.   SHADWELL, THOMAS. *The Works of Tho. Shadwell, Esq; Late Poet Laureat, and Historiographer Royal*. S2834. UMI 296: 8.

For a reference to "old Chaucer" in *The Woman Captain*, see SHADWELL (1680); in this collection, the comedy is the twelfth play 12 (sig. C2v).

871.   TONSON, JACOB. "Catalogue of Books" in Aphra Behn's *Love Letters Between a Noble-Man and his Sister*. B1742. UMI 1376: 17 and 1495: 11.

This edition of Mrs. Behn's work was "Printed for Jacob Tonson, at the Judge's Head in Chancery-Lane, and Joseph Hindmarsh, at the Golden Ball in Cornhill" (from the title page of the second part). At the end of volume 2 (following page 405), we find a catalogue headed: "Books Printed for Jacob Tonson, at the

Judges Head in Chancery Lane near Fleet-street." In the catalogue, under the heading "Poetry," the first work listed is "The Works of our Ancient, Learned, and Excellent *English* Poet *Jeoffery Chaucer*, as they have been lately compared by the best Manuscripts, and several things added never before in Print. Top which is adjoin'd, The Story of the Siege of *Thebes*. By John Lidgate, Monk of *Bury*: Together with the Life of *Chaucer*; with a Dictionary explaining the obsolete Words" (no signature; no pagination). The next work advertised is Spenser's *Works*, followed by the works of Davenant, Milton's *Juvenile Poems*, *Paradise Lost* and *Paradise Regained*, and Cowley's *Works*.

872. Tonson, Jacob. "Catalogue of Books" in *The Fourth Volume of Plutarch's Lives*. P2639A. UMI 1977: 3.

At the end of Plutarch's *Lives*, under the heading "Books Printed for Jacob Tonson at the Judge's Head in Chancery Lane near Fleetstreet," in a section headed "Poetry," Chaucer's works are listed first and are followed by those of Spenser and Milton. The entry reads: "The Works of *Jeffrey Chaucer* with his Life, and a Dictionary explaining the obsolete words" (unnumbered page, following 822).

873. WALLER, EDMUND. *Poems, &c. Written upon Several Occasions*. W518. UMI 950: 8; UMI 1079: 7.

For a reference to the difficulty of Chaucer's language for modern readers, see WALLER (1668); in this edition, the passage is found on 236–38.

874. WESLEY, SAMUEL. *The Life of our Blessed Lord & Saviour Jesus Christ*. W1371. UMI 1162: 8.

Wesley (1662–1735) is identified on the title page as "rector of South-Ormsby in the county of Lincoln." In "Notes to the First Book," Wesley speaks of his fondness for antique phrases and language: "Here once for all I tell the Reader, that 'tis not out of necessity I make use now and then of some of those *old Words*, whether out of a *vitious Imitation* of *Milton* and *Spencer*, I amn't so proper a Judge. All I'll say of 'em is, That I own I've ever had a *fondness* for some of 'em, they *please* me, and sound not disagreeably to my *Ear*, and that's all the Reason I can give for using 'em" (sig. E2r).

In "Notes to the Second Book," in an annotation for his choice of words in line 668, Wesley credits Chaucer for a phrase:

> *Lowting low*. One of *Spencer*'s and I think *Chaucer*'s Phrases, signifying no more than a *rustic* sort of a *Bow*. (sig. K2v)

In point of fact, if we turn back to the line in the text, we discover that Wesley (or perhaps the printer) changed his mind and substituted "bowing low" for the older locution that Chaucer uses in *Troilus and Criseyde*, *The House of Fame*, *The Romaunt of the Rose*, and elsewhere.

Other editions: W1372 (1694), sig. K2v; W1373 (1697), sig. K3v; W1373aA (1697), sig. K2v.

875.   WILSON, JOHN. *The Cheats. A Comedy.* W2919. UMI 970: 10.

For a reference to *The Canon's Yeoman's Tale* as the source and inspiration for Erasmus's *Alcumistica* and Jonson's *Alchemist*, see WILSON (1664); in this edition, the passage is found on sig. A3r.

Another edition in 1693: W2920, sig. A3r.

876.   WRIGHT, THOMAS. *The Female Vertuosos.* W3711. UMI 1082: 11.

Wright (*fl.* 1693) adapted parts of Molière's *Les femmes savantes* for this comedy that was "acted at the Queen's Theatre, by Their Majesties Servants." As Harris notes (*PQ*), Sir Timothy Witless, a country gentleman, is struck on the side of his head by Sir Maggot Jingle, a knight who claims to be a poet. Jingle then challenges Witless to write a madrigal on the subject of a "Box o' the Ear" (18). Witless produces the rhymes, but Jingle greets his poetic efforts with hoots of laughter. Witless responds by invoking the skull of Chaucer:

> What? do you Laugh? you Chimney-Sweeper of *Parnassus*!—Tho' I
> take a Box o'th'Ear; I have too much Honour to put up a Jeer: By the
> Scull of *Chaucer*, I'll Rhime thee Black and Blue.—Come if you dare!
> you Poet Laureat of *Bedlam*. (18–19)

877.   YALDEN, THOMAS. "To Mr. Congreve. An Epistolary Ode. Occasion'd by his late Play" in *Examen poeticum: Being the Third Part of Miscellany Poems.* Ed. John Dryden. D2277. UMI 489: 10.

As Spurgeon notes (1: 266), Yalden (1670–1736) writes of "neglected Spencer" and the trials and tribulations to which all poets are subject:

> Thus did the World thy great Fore-Fathers use,
> Thus all the inspir'd *Bards* before,
> Did their hereditary Ills deplore:
> From tuneful *Chaucer's*, down to thy own *Dryden's* Muse. (347)

1694

878. ADDISON, JOSEPH. "An Account of the Greatest English Poets" in *The Annual Miscellany for the year 1694. Being the Fourth Part of Miscellany Poems.* John Dryden, ed. D2237. UMI 92: 13.

As Spurgeon notes (1: 266), Addison (1672–1719) includes Chaucer among the greatest English poets in a poem dedicated to Henry Sacheverell and dated 3 April 1694. Addison adds that Chaucer's language is rusty:

> *Since, Dearest* Harry, *you will needs request*
> *A short Account of all the Muse possest;*
> *That, down from* Chaucer's *days to* Dryden's *Times,*
> *Have spent their Noble Rage in* Brittish [*sic*] *Rhimes;*
> *Without more Preface, wrote in Formal length,*
> *To speak the Undertakers want of strength,*
> *I'll try to make they're* [*sic*] *sev'ral Beauties known,*
> *And show their Verses worth, tho' not my Own.*

>   Long had our dull Fore-Fathers slept Supine,
> Nor felt the Raptures of the Tuneful Nine;
> Till *Chaucer* first, a merry *Bard*, arose;
> And many a Story told in Rhime and Prose.
> But Age has Rusted what the *Poet* writ,
> Worn out his Language, and obscur'd his Wit:
> In vain he jests in his unpolish'd strain,
> And tries to make his Readers laugh in vain.
>   Old *Spencer* next, warm'd with Poetick Rage,
> In Antick Tales amus'd a Barb'rous Age [etc.] (317–18)

879. BATEMAN, CHRISTOPHER. *A Catalogue of the Library of a Person of Honour.* Not in Wing. UMI Early English Books: Tract Supplement: D7: 2 (S.C.921.[2]).

Bateman's auction of "curious" books and nearly a thousand manuscripts from the library of Henry Hyde, Earl of Clarendon, was held at the Sign of the Bible and Crown in Pater-Noster Row in 1694. In the catalogue, under the heading "Libri in Folio," number 207 is listed as "*Chaucer's* Works. Ms." (5; sig. C1r); lot 221: as "*Chaucer's* Tale, and several Tracts of *Lydgate*" (6; sig. C1v); and number 355 as "*Chaucer*, on Vellum. *Ms.*" (9; sig. D1r).

STC online erroneously catalogues this work with a date somewhere between 1701 and 1703.

880. BLOUNT, THOMAS POPE. *De re poetica: or, Remarks upon Poetry. With Characters and Censures of the Most Considerable Poets.* B3347. UMI 123: 2.

Blount (1649–1697) is identified on the title page as "Sir Thomas Pope Blount." In a section headed "Concerning the English Poetry; and their Language in relation to Poetry," he notes the difficulty of Chaucer's language for his contemporaries:

> It would mortifie an *English* Man, to consider, that from the time of
> *Boccace,* and of *Petrarch,* the *Italian Language* has varied very little: And
> that the *English* of *Chaucer* their Contemporary, is not to be understood
> without the help of an old *Dictionary.* (92)

As Spurgeon notes (1: 267), in the second part of this work, "Characters and Censures," there is a section headed "Geoffry Chaucer":

> Three several Places contend for the Birth of this Famous *Poet. First,*
> *Berkshire,* from the words of *Leland,* that he was born in *Barocensi Pro-*
> *vinciâ;* and Mr. *Cambden* affirms, that *Dunington-Castle,* nigh unto
> *Newbury,* was Anciently his Inheritance. *Secondly, Oxfordshire,* where,
> *John Pits* is positive, that his Father (who was a Knight) liv'd, and that
> he was born at *Woodstock. Thirdly,* The Author of his Life, Printed 1602.
> Supposes him to be *born* at *London.* But though the place of his Birth
> is not certainly known, yet this is agreed upon by all hands, that he was
> counted the chief of the *English Poets,* not only of his time, but contin-
> ued to be so esteem'd till this Age; and as much as we despise his old
> fashion'd Phrase, and Obsolete Words, *He* was one of the first Refiners
> of the *English* Language.
>
> Of how great esteem he was in the Age wherein he flourish'd, *viz.*
> the Reigns of *Henry* the IV. *Henry* the V. and part of *Henry* the VI.
> appears, besides his being Knighted, and made *Poet Lauriate* by the
> Honour he had to be ally'd by Marriage to the great Earl of *Lancaster,*
> *John* of *Gaunt.*
>
> We have several of his Works yet extant, but his *Squires Tale,* and
> some other of his Pieces are not to be found. [Spurgeon's transcription
> ends here.]
>
> *John Pits,* in his *De Illustribus Angliæ Scriptoribus,* says, That *Chau-*
> *cer* so illustrated the *English* Poetry, that he may justly be esteem'd our
> *English Homer.*
>
> *He* likewise tells us, that he was an Excellent *Rhetorician,* a skillful
> *Mathematician,* an acute *Philosopher,* and no contemptible *Divine.*
>
> *Winstanley,* in the Lives of the *English Poets,* compares *Chaucer* for
> the sweetness of his *Poetry,* to *Stesichorus;* And *(saith he)* as *Cethegus*

was call'd *Suadæ Medulla*, so may *Chaucer* be rightly call'd the Pith and Sinews of Eloquence, and the very life it self of all Mirth and pleasant Writing. Besides, one gift he had above other Authors, says *Winstanley*, and that is, by the Excellencies of his Descriptions, to possess his Readers with a stronger Imagination of seeing that done before their Eyes which they Read, than any other that ever Writ in any Tongue.

But above all, *He tells* us, *Chaucer's Canterbury Tales*, is most valu'd and esteem'd of.

The Learned and Ingenious Mr. *Roger Ascham* calls *Chaucer*, The *English Homer*; adding also, That he values his Authority equal to that of *Sophocles* or *Euripides* in *Greek*.

Sir *Philip Sidney*, in his *Defence of* Poesie, gives him this Character; Chaucer *undoubtedly did excellently in his* Troilus *and* Crescid, *of whom truly I know not whether to marvel more, either that* He *in that misty time could see so clearly, or* We *in this clear Age walk so stumblingly after him.*

This agrees with the following Verses, made by Sir *John Denham*:

Old Chaucer, *like the Morning Star,*
To us discovers Day from far;
His light those Mists and Clouds dissolv'd,
Which our dark Nation long involv'd;
But he descending to the Shades,
Darkness again the Age invades.
    J. Denham. *The* 3d. *Edit.* 1684. *pag.* 89.

Sir *Henry Savil*, in his *Preface* to *Bardwardin's* Book against *Pelagius*, says, that *Chaucer* was the chief of our *English* Poets, and that he had a sharp Judgment, and a pleasant Wit; and that he was also well skill'd both in Philosophy and Divinity.

Sir *Richard Baker*, in the Reign of *Edward* the *Third*, stiles Sir *Geoffry Chaucer*, the *Homer* of our Nation; adding, That he found as sweet a Muse in the Groves of *Woodstock*, as the *Ancients* did upon the Banks of *Helicon*.

Cambden also, in his *Britannia*, tells us, That it is the only thing the Town of *Woodstock* hath to brag of, That she gave Birth to *Geoffrey Chaucer*, our *English Homer*; of whom, in his Opinion, may truly be said, that which an *Italian Poet* once apply'd to *Homer*:

— *Hic ille est, cujus de gurgite Sacro*
Combibit arcanos vatum omnis turba furores.

Dr. *Sprat*, in his *History* of the *Royal Society*, *pag.* 42. says, That till the time of King *Henry* the *Eighth*, there was scarce any man regarded the *English Language*, but *Chaucer*; and that nothing was Written in it, which one would be willing to read twice, but some of *his* Poetry; But that then it began to raise it self a little, and to sound tolerably well.

Tho' *Verstegan* commends *Chaucer*, as an excellent Poet for his time; yet he wholly differs from those, who are of opinion, that *he* did so mightily refine the *English Language*. Indeed, he rather condemns *Chaucer* for adulterating the *English Tongue*, by the mixture of so many *French* and *Latin* Words.

This our *Poet*, lies buried in *Westminster* Abby, with the following Inscription:

Qui fuit Anglorum *vates ter maximus olim*,
    Galfridus Chaucer, *conditur hôc Tumulo*.
Annum si quæras Domini, si tempora Mortis,
    Ecce notæ subsunt, quæ tibi cuncta notant;
25 Octobris 1400.
    Ærumnarum requies Mors.
Nicolaus Brigham *hos fecit* Musarum *nomine sumptur.* (41–44)

In the section on Edmund Spenser, Blount notes that Spenser was buried near Chaucer:

The Expence of his Funeral and Monument was defray'd at the sole charge of *Robert*, first of that Name, Earl of *Essex*. He lies buried in *Westminster-Abbey*, near *Chaucer*, with this *Epitaph*:. . . . (216).

The entry for Chaucer is a slightly edited version of Blount's Latin *Censura celebriorum authorum* (1690), B3346. The passage on Chaucer is found on 312–13; Spencer is not included in this collection of literary biographies.

881.   BOHUN, EDMUND, in Louis Moréri's *Great Historical, Geographical, and Poetical Dictionary.* M2725. UMI 1447: 1.

Moréri (1643–1694) published several editions of *Grand dictionaire historique*, "a curious miscellany of sacred and prophane history," and it was enlarged by Jean Le Clerc (1657–1736). The sixth edition was translated by Edmund Bohun (1645–99) and augmented to include "the lives . . . [of the] most famous men of all arts and sciences" in England, Scotland, and Ireland. Bohun includes no main entry for Chaucer; he does, however, mention him in the one for Spenser:

Spenser (*Edmund*) born in *London*, was brought up at *Pembroke Hall* in *Cambridge*, where he became very learned, but especially noted for his *English* Poetry and Imitation of *Chaucer.* . . . At his return from *Ire-*

land he was robb'd of the little he had, and falling into want it broke his Heart, so that he died *An.* 1598, and was honorably interr'd at the Charges of *Robert* Earl of *Essex*, near *Chaucer.* (sig. N3r)

882.   BULLORD, JOHN. *Bibliotheca Belwoodiana.* B1863. UMI 408: 7.

Bullord auctioned the library of the lately deceased Roger Belwood, Serjeant at Law of the Middle Temple, on 4 February 1694. In the catalogue, under the heading "Miscellany in Folio," lot 123 is listed as "Jeffr. Chaucer's Works, with his Life—1687" (15).

883.   BULLORD, JOHN. *An Excellent Collection of Books.* E3797. UMI 1758: 52

Bullord began auctioning the library of "an eminent Serjeant at Law, lately deceased" at Toms Coffee-House on Monday, 2 July 1694. In the catalogue, under the heading "English Divinity, History and Miscellany in Folio," number 99 is listed as "*Geofrey Chaucer's* works compleat, with his life—1678" (11); the date should probably read 1687.

884.   BULLORD, JOHN. *The Library of Mr. Tho. Britton, Smallcoal-man.* B4828. UMI 1826: 10.

Thomas Britton (1654?–1714),[46] a coal dealer, concert promoter, and bibliophile, disposed of a portion of his collection using the services of Bullord who began the auction at Tom's Coffee-House on Thursday, 1 November 1694. In the sales catalogue, under the heading "Bundles of Pamphlets in Quarto," lot number 48 is listed as "Bundel of poetical Tracts," one of which was: "*Chaucer*s Ploughmans Tale with an exposition, 1606" (31).

885.   *A Catalogue of Excellent Books, in Greek, Latin and English.* C1326. UMI 1774: 14.

An auction was held at Toms Coffee-House on 15 October 1694. In the catalogue, under the heading "English Divinity, History, &c. In Folio," number 71 is listed as "Chaucers Works last edition [no date]" (5, second pagination).

886.   DARE, JOSIAH. *Counsellor Manners, His Last Legacy to His Son.* D248. UMI 1255: 5.

For a paraphrase of a couplet from *The Wife of Bath's Tale* and a precis of an incident related by Chauntecleer in *The Nun's Priest's Tale*, see DARE (1673); in this edition, the passages are found on 3–4, 144–45.

---

[46] See Douglas A. Reid's article in *Oxford DNB.*

887.   DRYDEN, JOHN. *The Works of Mr. John Dryden.* D2209. UMI 1549: 1.

For references to the difficulty of Chaucer's language for Dryden's contemporaries and to Chaucer's translation of *Troilus and Criseyde* from the Latin of "one Lollius a Lombard," see DRYDEN (1679); in this collection, the play is in vol. 2.

For an allusion to *The Nun's Priest's Tale* in *Amphitryon*, see DRYDEN (1690); in this collection, the play is in vol. 3

For an allusion to *The Nun's Priest's Tale* in *The Hind and the Panther*, see DRYDEN (1687); in this collection the poem is in vol. 4.

888.   DUTTON, JOHN. *John Dutton's, Alias Prince Dutton's Farewel to Temple-Bar.* D2909B. UMI 2513: 12.

This work is cast as a letter addressed to "Neighbors, and Fellow-Mechanicks" and comes "From amongst the Lunaticks at Dr. Adam's House, over-against the Kings Head in Marybone, April 26. 1694." Dutton (*fl.* 1694) purports to explain to one and all why he has withdrawn from his wife and six children to spend two months in confinement "amongst distempered People" (1). In a valedictory poem, Dutton calls Chaucer old fashioned:

> *Then farewel all you old Ingenious,*
> *This ungrateful Age is so Abstenious* [*sic*],
> *That old Fashion'd* Chaucers English,
> *Charmingly like Oracle spoke; Pish,*
> *'Tis all Time and Labour lost, I could*
> *Wish our Genius were not so cold,*
> *In not considering well our Future State,*
> *But leave all Holy Practise till too late.*
> *Our Learned* Hudibras *did fortel many*
> *Accidents, that are our present Destiny;*
> *In giving way to Swearing, Lying, Evil*
> *Habits that are encourag'd by the Devil.* (sig. E1r)

889.   EDWARDS, JOHN. *A Discourse Concerning the Authority, Stile, and Perfection of the Books of the Old and New-Testament.* E202A. UMI 1422: 26b and UMI 2389: 4.

For a discussion of the meaning of *dulcarnon* (an allusion to *Troilus and Criseyde* 3: 931, 933), see EDWARDS (1693); in this edition, the passage is found on 247.

890.   GADBURY, JOHN. Εφημερις [Ephemeris], *or a Diary Astronomical* [for 1694]. A1773. UMI 705: 32.

Gadbury (1627–1704) is identified on the title page as a "student in physick and astrologie." In a section headed "A brief Discourse of the Planetary Hours," he cites Chaucer and alludes to *Treatise of the Astrolabe*:

I spare to mention a great number of Learned Authors that have defended this Doctrine, both Ancient and Modern; but cannot omit to take notice, That the Venerable *Chaucer* (tho an Enemy to the Frauds of Astrologers (as what Honest Man is not? yet) hath approved of, and taught this Doctrine of the *Planetary Hours.* (sig. C5r)

891.   H., N. *The Ladies Dictionary; Being a General Entertainment for the Fair-Sex: A Work Never Attempted Before in English.* H99. UMI 667: 1.

As Harris notes (*PQ*), the author writes of "Promises and Vows" in matters of love. When he turns to promises made by women, he quotes a modernized couplet from *The Wife of Bath's Prologue* (lines 227–28):

They [women] can also, upon occasion, so weep that one would conclude their very hearts would dissolve within them, and flow from them in Tears from their Eyes, when we perceive them like Rocks droping Water; and yet all this is but in Jest; for they can wipe away their tears like Sweat; weep with one Eye, as the saying is, and laugh with the other; or like some Children, who cry and laugh both at a time, and Old Chaucer, in his home-spun Rhythms, says,
> For half so boldly there can none
> Swear and Lie as Women can.

But this must not reflect upon all Women; for some are Religiously Conscientious to a miracle. (382)

892.   HOWELL, WILLIAM. *Medulla historiæ anglicanæ.* H3142A. UMI 2031: 13.

For a reference to Chaucer as England's poet laureate in the reign of Richard II, see HOWELL (1679); in this edition, the passage is found on 164.

893.   MIEGE, GUY. *The New State of England under Their Majesties K. William and Q. Mary.* M2021. UMI 2869: 22.

For a reference to Chaucer in a list of famous men of England, see MIEGE (1691); in this edition, the passage is found in part 2, 17.

894.   MILLINGTON, EDWARD. *Bibliotheca Ashmoliana.* A3981. UMI 1582: 23.

Millington auctioned the library of "the Learned and famous Elias Ashmole, Esq" on 22 February 1694 at Rolls's Auction House in Petty-Cannon-Alley (title page). In the catalogue, under the heading "English Miscellanies in Folio," number 2 is listed as "The Works of our Learned Poet *Jeffrey Chaucer*, with his Life —1598" (5); number 139 as "Works of *Geffery Chaucer*, with the works of *J. Lydgat*, Monk of *Bury*—[no date]" (8). In another grouping, also headed "English Miscellanies in Folio," lot 109 is listed as "Works of *Geof. Chaucer*, with his Life—1602" (14).

895.   MILLINGTON, EDWARD. *Bibliotheca Cogiana.* C4890. UMI 1774: 40.

Millington began auctioning the entire library of the Reverend and Learned Dr. Nathaniel Coga, "Nuperrime Magist. Aulæ Pembrok, in Acad. Cantab. Defuncti" (title page) on 27 November 1694 at the Falcon Inn in Petty-Cury. In the catalogue, under the heading "Miscellany Books in Folio," number 29 is listed as "The Works of our English Poet Jeffr. Chaucer, with his Life—1687"; lot 37 as "Jeffr. Chaucer's Works, a very antient [*sic*] Edition. Wants Title, &c. —[no date]" (23, really 32; sig. I2v).

896.   MILLINGTON, EDWARD. *A Catalogue of Ancient and Modern Books.* C1273a. UMI 2308: 11.

Millington held an auction on 26 March 1694 at Mr. Ferrour's Coffee-House at the Sign of the Turks-Head in Kings-Lynn for the diversion and entertainment of all and sundry in the environs. In the catalogue, under the heading "Miscellanies in Folio," number 31 is listed as "Chaucers Works an Ancient and Learned English Poet—1687" (24).

897.   PERO, JOHN. *A Catalogue of Choice Latin and English Books.* C1304. UMI 1774: 13.

Pero's auction was held at the Sign of the Crown, next door to his book shop at the Sign of the White Swan in Little-Britain, on 28 November 1694. In the catalogue, under the heading "Divinity, History, &c. In Folio," lot number 1 is listed as "The Works of our Learned English Poet, Jeffrey Chaucer—Lond. 1687" (1).

898.   PRESTON, RICHARD GRAHAM. *The Moral State of England, with the Several Aspects It Beareth to Virtue and Vice.* P3313. UMI 2213: 20.

For a reference to Chaucer linked with Spenser, see PRESTON (1670); in this edition, the passage is found on 67.

899.   RABELAIS, FRANÇOIS. *Pantagruel's Voyage to the Oracle in the Bottle Being the Fourth and Fifth Books of the Works of Francis Rabelais, M. D.* R107. UMI 224: 11.

In this translation by Peter Anthony Motteux of *Gargantua et Pantagruel* (books 4 and 5), he echoes a line from *The Manciple's Prologue*: "Sires, what! Dun is in the myre!" (line 5). In chapter 63, Motteux translates:

> With this accident we were all out of sorts, moping, drooping, metagrabolized as dull as *Dun* in the Mire. . . . (249)

900. RAMSAY (or RAMESEY), WILLIAM. *Conjugium conjurgium: or, Some Serious Considerations on Marriage.* R230A. UMI 2357: 22.

For a spurious quotation attributed to Chaucer and genuine quotations from *The Knight's Tale*, *The Wife of Bath's Prologue*, and *The Romaunt of the Rose*, see RAMSAY (1673); in this edition the passages are found on 51 (*sic*, really 49), 74–75, 77–78, 80.

901. R[OGERS], T[HOMAS]. *A Posie for Lovers: or, The Terrestrial Venus Unmaskt.* R1842E. UMI 799: 26 (identified as R1840).

In "The Luscious Penance: or The Fasting Lady," Rogers (1660–1694) refers to patient Griselde, perhaps an allusion to the *Clerk's Tale*:

> At *Dido's* Fate I've often wept, and bled;
> Nor can I Patient *Grisle's* Story read
> Without a Sigh. (12)

902. RYMER, THOMAS. "Preface of the Translator" in René Rapin's *Reflections on Aristotle's Treatise of Poesie.* R271. UMI 398: 3 and UMI 2236: 1.

For a reference to Chaucer and the parlous state of the English language in his day, see RYMER (1674); in this edition, the passage is found on sig. A5v.

903. SCARRON, PAUL. *Scarron's Novels.* S835. UMI 2272: 9

For an echo of a line from *The General Prologue*, see SCARRON (1665); in this edition, the passage is found on 19.

904. SOUTH, ROBERT. *Twelve Sermons Preached upon Several Occasions. The Second Volume.* S4746. UMI 1131: 2.

South (1634–1716) is identified on the title page as "Robert South, D.D." In this collection, in a sermon headed "An Account of the Nature and Measures of Conscience" that was "Preached Before the University at Christ-Church, Oxon" on 1 November 1691, South appears to echo a line from *The Reeve's Tale*: "The gretteste clerkes been noght wisest men" (line 4054). In a passage about the possibility of any "Casuist or Learned Divine" being mistaken in his judgement of "the Estate of a man's Soul," South writes:

> If he does judge right, yet the Man cannot be sure that he will declare that Judgment sincerely and impartially, (the *greatest Clerks* being not always the *honestest*, any more than the *wisest Men*,) but may purposely sooth a man up for Hope or Fear, or the Service of some sinister Interest. (536)

Other editions: S4748 (1697), 472–73.

905.   URQUHART, THOMAS. "Preface" in *The Works of F. Rabelais, M.D.: or, The Lives, Heroic Deeds and Sayings of Gargantua and Pantagruel.* R104. UMI 1429: 6.

Urquhart (1611–1660) is identified on the title page as "Sir Tho. Urchard, Kt." This augmented edition of Urquhart's translation contains a preface that is not found in either the 1653 or the 1664 editions. Urquhart writes of the difficulty of Rabelais' language, compares it to Chaucer's:

> [W]hen a Reader meets with many words that are unintelligible (I mean to him that makes it not his business to know the meaning of dark and obsolete Expressions) the Pleasure which what he understands yields him, is in a greater measure allay'd by his disappointment; of which we have Instances when we read *Chaucer*, and other Books, which we do not thoroughly understand. (xlii)

906.   WALLER, EDMUND. *Poems, &c. Written upon Several Occasions.* W519. UMI 588: 7.

For a reference to the difficulty of Chaucer's language for modern readers, see WALLER (1668); in this edition, the passage is found on 236–38.

907.   WESLEY, SAMUEL. *The Life of our Blessed Lord & Saviour Jesus Christ.* W1372. UMI 906: 18.

For a reference to Wesley's fondness of antique language and his use of a Chaucerian word, see WESLEY (1693); in this edition, the passages are found on sigs. E2r and K2v.

1695

908.   B., T. "A Dedication" in Michael Drayton's *England's Heroical Epistles.* D2145. UMI 314: 3.

For a reference to Chaucer in a commendatory poem, see B., T. (1689); in this edition, the passage is found on sig. A4r.

909.   BARNARD, JOHN AUGUSTINE, and BOHUN, EDMUND. *A Geographical Dictionary.* B3455. UMI 1564: 14.

For an allusion to *The Reeve's Tale*, see BARNARD (1693); in this edition, the passage is found on 376.

910. BULLORD, JOHN. *Bibliotheca Littletoniana.* **L2559. UMI 1797: 10.**

Bullord began auctioning the library ("A Curious Collection of Books") of Adam Littleton, D.D., Prebendary of Westminster, on Monday, 15 April 1695, at Tom's Coffee House. In the catalogue, under the heading "English Divinity, History, Miscellany, Law, &c. in Folio," number 37 is listed as "*Chaucers* Works *Roberts* map of commerce — [no date]" (²1); and lot 55 as "*Chaucers* Works last edition [no date]" (²2).

Alderson & Henderson cite the second edition (1719), sig. A8v.

911. BULLORD, JOHN. *A Curious Collection of Books.* **C7623. UMI 1757: 13.**

Bullord held an auction of books in divinity, history, and philology in a variety of languages on 11 June 1695 at Tom's Coffee-House. In the catalogue, in the second section, under the heading "English Divinity, &c. In Folio," number 112 is listed as "*Chaucers* Works [n.p., n.d.]"; and lot 123 as "*Chaucers* Works best edition [n.p., n.d.]" (²3).

912. COLVIL, SAMUEL. *Whiggs Supplication.* **C5429. UMI 660: 12.**

For a reference to cockscombs who pay insufficient attention when they read Chaucer, see COVIL (1681); in this edition, the passage is found on 42. Harris (*PQ*) cites this edition rather than the first.

913. DRYDEN, JOHN. *Troilus and Cressida: or, Truth Found Too Late.* **D2391. UMI 688: 14.**

For references to the difficulty of Chaucer's language for Dryden's contemporaries and to Chaucer's having translated *Troilus and Criseyde* from the Latin of Lollius, see DRYDEN (1679); in this edition, the passages are found on sig. A3v, A4v.

914. DRYDEN, JOHN. *The Works of Mr. John Dryden.* **D2210. UMI 2495: 4.**

For references to the difficulty of Chaucer's language for Dryden's contemporaries and to Chaucer's having *Troilus and Criseyde* from the Latin of "one Lollius a Lombard," see DRYDEN (1679); in this collection, the play is the ninth play in the second volume.

For an allusion to *The Nun's Priest's Tale* in *Amphitryon*, see DRYDEN (1690); in this collection, the play is the fourth play in the third volume.

For an allusion to *The Nun's Priest's Tale* in *The Hind and the Panther*, see DRYDEN (1687); in this collection, the poem is ninth work in the fourth volume.

Another collection in 1695: *The Dramatic Works of Mr. John Dryden*, D2211, does not include *The Hind and the Panther*.

915.   *A Fair Character of the Presbyterian Reformling's Just and Sober Vindication*. F94A. UMI 2687: 21.

The author of this pamphlet writes in response to articles in the *Weekly Reformer* of 30 January and 29 May. He attributes a quotation Chaucer:

> I never push home a Topick with the *Rhetorick of the Sword*: I write with such *Ink* as He does, not with *Blood*. . . . Indeed to be called so many Names, would make a Man scratch where it does not itch, as CHAUCER has it upon *another Account*: I care not what the *Italians* say [in a shoulder note: "*To see Men live poor to dye rich.*"]; but I wonder he should travel so far for an *Itch of a Popish Expression*. (17)

916.   FARIA Y SOUSA, MANUEL DE. *The Portugues Asia: or, The History and Discovery and Conquest of India by the Portugues. Written in Spanish*. F428. UMI 93: 16.

The author is identified on the title page as Manuel de Faria y Sousa, of the Order of Christ. In this translation by Capt. John Stevens (d. 1726) of *Asia Portuguesa*, in a passage about Count de Redondo's response to Malabar pirates in the early 1560s, Stevens appears to echo the description of the shipman in *The General Prologue*: "Of nyce conscience took he no keep" (line 398). He writes:

> The Vice-Roy dispatched . . . *Dominick de Misquita*, a Man of Valour and no nice Conscience, as was requisite for such an Action. (220).

917.   GADBURY, JOHN. Εφημερις: *or, A Diary Astronomical, Astrological, Meteorological, for the Year of Grace, 1695*. A1774. UMI 1392: 47.

As Harris notes (*PQ*), at the end of his almanac for 1695, Gadbury (1627–1704) appended a learned essay entitled "A Brief Enquiry into the Copernican Astrology, which Respects the Sun as Center of the World." Gadbury begins: "The Doctrine of *Copernicus* touching the System of the World, is no New or Upstart Opinion, but an Antiquated Verity, more happily in this Age by him revived" (sig. C1r). He concludes by attempting to reconcile the disciplines of astrology and astronomy, and he buttresses his argument with a quotation from *The Parliament of Fowls* (lines 22–25):

> And the Excellent *Chaucer* wrote an Immortal Truth in his *Assembly of Fowles*, in these Verses, *viz.*
> For out of the Old Fields, as men saith,
> Commeth all this new Corne, fro Yere to Yere;
> And out of Old Bookes, in good Faith,
> Commeth all this New Science that men Lere. (sig. C7v)

918.   Gibson, Edmund, *trans. Camden's Britannia, Newly Translated into English: With Large Additions and Improvements.* C359. UMI 132: 2.

For references to Chaucer's association with Woodstock in Oxfordshire and his burial in Westminster, see Camden (1586), Boswell & Holton No. 439, and Camden (1610), Boswell & Holton No. 811.

For a quotation of lines from *The General Prologue* that describes the Franklin, see Camden (1610) in the Appendix; in this edition, the passage is found on clxxviii.

In this new translation, Gibson (1669–1748) is identified on the title page as being "of Queens-College in Oxford." In the chapter headed "Barkshire," Gibson writes:

> [T]he little river *Lamborn* . . . runs beneath *Dennington*, call'd also *Dunnington*, a little but very neat castle, seated on the brow of a woody hill, having a fine prospect, and windows on all sides very lightsome. They say . . . it was the residence of *Chaucer* . . . [In a footnote: "It was the house of *Jeoffery Chaucer*, and there under an Oak (commonly call'd *Chaucer's Oak*) he is said to have penn'd many of his famous Poems. The Oak till within these few years was standing."] (col. 142)

In the chapter headed "Kent," Gibson alludes to *The Prologue of the Canon's Yeoman's Tale*, "At Boghtoun under Blee, us gan atake | A man that clothed was in clothes blake" (lines 556–57).

> And Chaucer [in a shoulder note: "Poems. pag. 54"] going in Pilgrimage to St. Thomas, pass'd thro' *Boughton* to Canterbury; as they still do. (col. 218)

In the chapter about Oxfordshire, Gibson notes Chaucer's connection with Woodstock and recalls Camden's epithet for Chaucer, "our English Homer." Gibson writes:

> The town having now nothing else to be proud of, does boast of the honour of being the birth place of our English *Homer, Jeffrey Chaucer*: To whom, and some other of our English Poets, I may apply what the learn'd Italian sung of *Homer* and other Greeks.
> —*Hic ille est, cuius de gurgite sacro*
> *Combibit arcanos vatum omnis turba furores.*
> This is he, to whose immortal spring of wit
> Each water Poet ows [*sic*] his rivulet.
> For he defying every rival in wit, and leaving all our Poetasters at a long distance from him,

—jam monte potitus,
Ridet anhelantem dura ad fastigta turbam.
Sits down in triumph on the conquer'd height,
And smiles to see unequal Rivals sweat. (col. 255)

The passage is marked with a shoulder note: "Alumnus suus. Jeffrey Chaucer."
Under the heading "Middlesex," Gibson writes of notable persons buried in Westminster:

> *Geoffrey Chaucer,* who being Prince of the English Poets, ought not to
> be pass'd by; as neither *Edmund Spencer,* who of all the English Poets
> came nearest him in a happy genius, and a rich vein of Poetry. (col. 319)

"Chaucer, Jeoffr." and "Chaucer's Oak" are noted in the index, sig. f2v.

919.   HOWARD, EDWARD. *Caroloiades redivivus: or, The War and Revolutions in the Time of King Charles the First. An Heroick Poem.* H2968. UMI 1287: 6.

For a reference to Chaucer and Spenser as "Powerfull Sons of Phebus," see HOW-ARD (1689); in this edition, the passage is found on 137.

920.   HUME, PATRICK. *Annotations on Milton's Paradise Lost.* H3663. UMI 358: 10.

Hume, a London schoolmaster, identifies himself on the title page as "Φιλοποιήτης" [Philopoietes]. He also advises readers that within his work "The Texts of Sacred Writ, relating to the POEM, are Quoted; The Parallel Places and Imitations of the most Excellent *Homer* and *Virgil,* Cited and Compared; All the Obscure Parts render'd in Phrases more Familiar; The Old and Obsolete Words, with their Originals, Explain'd and made Easie to the *English* Reader" (title page).

In his comments on *Paradise Lost* 2.5.704, Hume cites Chaucer's use of the *grieslie,* a word he used a dozen or so times. Hume writes:

> *The Grieslie Terrour;* Thus spake grim Death, that ghastly dreadly King.
> *Grieslie,* an old Word for Ugly, used by *Chaucer* and *Spencer.* . . . (81)

As Alderson & Henderson note, Hume also cites Chaucer's use of *buxomness,* perhaps an allusion to *Truth* (line 15) in his annotation of *Paradise Lost* 2.5.842:

> *Wing silently the buxom Air;* Fly unperceiv'd through the yielding Air:
> *Buxom,* plyable, yielding . . . *Buxomness* in *Chaucer* is put for Lowliness,
> Humility. *Spencer* makes it the Epithete of the Air. . . . (86)

As Alderson & Henderson also note, Hume quotes a modernized couplet from *The Wife of Bath's Prologue* (lines 59–60) in his annotation of Milton's use of the word *defended*:

> [I]n the Law sense, *to Prohibit*, so used by *Chaucer*:
> *Where can you say in any manner Age,*
> *That ever God defended Marriage.* (292)

Another edition in 1695 with a different title: *Paradise Lost. To Which Is Added, Explanatory Notes upon Each Book. The Sixth Edition*, M2151, same pagination.

921.   J., W. "Preface" in Renè Le Bossu's *Treatise of the Epick Poem*: . . . *Done into English from the French, with a New Original Preface upon the Same Subject, by W. J.* L804. UMI 74: 9.

As Alderson & Henderson note, in his preface, W. J. cites Thomas Rymer's critique of René Rapin's *Reflections* and his opinions about early English poets.

> He [Rapin] has not indeed made any Reflections on our *English* Poets, and this *Rymer* presumes proceeded from his ignorance of our Language, which he did not understand so well, as to pass a Judgment on what was writ in it. Whereupon *Rymer* himself has undertook to Criticise [*sic*] upon them. *Chaucer*, he will not allow for an *Epick* Poet, the Age he lived in not being sufficient for a great design; being an Age of Tales, Ballads and Roundelays. (sig. a2r)

922.   JEVON, THOMAS. *The Devil of a Wife: or, A Comical Transformation.* J732. UMI 1425: 9.

For a reference to Chaucer and the Wife of Bath, see JEVON (1686); in this edition, the passage is found on 21–22. See also *The Wanton Wife of Bath* (1641).

923.   KENNETT, WHITE. *Parochial Antiquities.* K302. UMI 1288: 4.

White Kennett (1660–1728) is identified on the title page as "Vicar of Ambrosden." As Alderson & Henderson note, Kennett cites Chaucer several times in a section headed "A Glossary to Explain The Original, the Acceptation, and Obsoleteness of Words and Phrases. And to shew the Rise, Practice and Alteration of Customs, Laws, and Manners."

In his definition of *baius* Kennett quotes a line from *The Canon's Yeoman's Tale* (line 1413):

> Baius *Equus*. A bay horse. . . . Hence *Baiard* an appellative for horse.
> Prov. *None so bold as Blind Bayard.* — Or in *Chaucer's* phrase,
> Ɏe ben as bold as is Bayard the blind. (sig. Bbbbb2v)

In his definition of *bordel*, Kennett cites Chaucer's use of *burel man*, an allusion to *The Franklin's Tale* (line 716):

> Bordel . . . a lew'd publick house, a Stews, from which *femme bordelier* a common whore. Hence in *Chaucer* a *Borel-Man* a loose idle fellow, and *Borel-folk* Drunkards and Epicures, (which the *Scotch* now call *Bureil-folk*)
>> 𝕲𝖔𝖉𝖉𝖊𝖘 𝖍𝖔𝖚𝖘 𝖎𝖘 𝖒𝖆𝖉𝖊 𝖆 𝖙𝖆𝖛𝖊𝖗𝖓 𝖔𝖋 𝖌𝖑𝖚𝖙𝖙𝖔𝖓𝖘, 𝖆𝖓𝖉 𝖆 𝖇𝖔𝖗𝖉𝖊𝖑 𝖔𝖋 𝕷𝖞𝖈𝖍𝖔𝖚𝖗𝖘. (sig. Ccccc1v)

In his definition of *cock-boat*, Kennett quotes couplet from *The Legend of Good Women* (lines 1480–81):

> Cock-boat. A small boat that waits upon a larger vessel. . . . [W]hat we now call a *Cock*-boat, was formerly a *Cogge*-boat, and simply a *Cogge*. As . . . *Chaucer*
>> 𝕳𝖊 𝖋𝖔𝖚𝖓𝖉 𝕵𝖆𝖘𝖔𝖓 𝖆𝖓𝖉 𝕳𝖊𝖗𝖆𝖈𝖑𝖊𝖘 𝖆𝖑𝖘𝖔
>> 𝕾𝖍𝖚𝖙𝖙𝖊 𝖎𝖓 𝖆 𝕮𝖔𝖌𝖌𝖊 𝖙𝖔 𝖑𝖔𝖓𝖉 𝖜𝖊𝖗𝖊 𝖞𝖌𝖔𝖊. (sig. Ddddd4r)

In his definition of *computum*, Kennett quotes a couplet from *The General Prologue* (lines 359–60):

> Computum . . . To give up *accounts*. Hence the old word a *Count* or Declaration in Law. The *Contours* or *Counters* were the Serjeants at Law retain'd to plead a cause, as *Chaucer*,
>> 𝕬 𝕾𝖍𝖊𝖗𝖎𝖋𝖋 𝖍𝖆𝖉 𝖍𝖊 𝖇𝖊𝖊𝖓, 𝖆𝖓𝖉 𝖆 𝕮𝖔𝖓𝖙𝖔𝖚𝖗
>> 𝕸𝖆𝖘 𝖓𝖔 𝖜𝖍𝖊𝖗𝖊 𝖘𝖚𝖈𝖍 𝖆 𝖜𝖔𝖗𝖙𝖍𝖞 𝖁𝖆𝖛𝖆𝖘𝖔𝖚𝖗. (sig. Eeeee1v)

In his definition of *coppire domum*, Kennett cites Chaucer as his authority for use of the word *cope*:

> Coppire . . . A *cope* or upper garment, as the outer vest of a Priest, and the Cloak or Surtout of any other person, as in *Chaucer* a *cope* is us'd for a Cloak. (sig. Eeeee2r)

In his definition of *draw-gere*, Kennett quotes a line from the fourth book of *Troilus and Criseyde* (line 286):

> Draw-Gere. Any furniture of cart-horses for drawing a waggon or other carriage . . . well habited or well fitted with arms, as in *Chaucer*, *Troilus*,1. 4. *f.* 167. 𝕿𝖔 𝖕𝖗𝖊𝖛𝖊 𝖎𝖓 𝖙𝖍𝖆𝖙 𝖙𝖍𝖞 𝖌𝖎𝖊𝖗𝖋𝖚𝖑𝖑 𝖛𝖎𝖔𝖑𝖊𝖓𝖈𝖊. (sig. Fffff2r)

In his definition of *duarium*, Kennett quotes a line from the fifth book of *Troilus and Criseyde* (line 230):

> Duarium. The dowry of a wife settled on her in marriage to be enjoy'd after her husband's decease. The English *Dowrie* . . . to *dowe*, i.e. to give, as *Chaucer* 𝕿𝖔 𝖜𝖍𝖔𝖒 𝖋𝖔𝖗 𝖊𝖇𝖊𝖗𝖒𝖔𝖗𝖊 𝖒𝖎𝖓𝖊 𝖍𝖆𝖗𝖙 𝕴 𝖉𝖔𝖜𝖊. . . . (sig. Fffff2v)

In his definition of *haia*, Kennett quotes a snippet of a line from *The Romaunt of the Rose* (line 54):

> Haia. A hedge . . . Proverb in *Chaucer*, 𝕹𝖊𝖙𝖍𝖊𝖗 𝖇𝖚𝖘𝖐 𝖓𝖔𝖗 𝖍𝖆𝖞, i.e. Neither wood nor hedge. . . . (sigs. Gggggg4v–Hhhhh1r)

In his definition of *husebote*, Kennett cites Chaucer as his authority and quotes a partial line from *The Canon's Yeoman's Tale* (line 1481):

> Husebote. . . . *Bote*, a remedy, as *Chaucer*, *Bote of his bale*, i.e. remedy of his grief. (sig. Hhhhh3r–4r)

In his definition of pullanus, Kennett cites the authority of Chaucer and alludes to *The General Prologue*, "This Reve sat upon a full good stot" (line 615):

> Pullanus, *Pullus*. A colt or young horse, by *Chaucer* call'd a *Stod*. . . . (sig. L11112v)

In his definition of *swanemotum*, Kennett cites Chaucer as his authority for the word *swinker* and thus alludes to *The General Prologue of The Canterbury Tales* (line 531) or *The Romaunt of the Rose* (line 6857):

> Swanemotum . . . a *swain*, as *Country-swain*, *Boot-swain* . . . a labourer, whom *Chaucer* calls a *swinker* . . . in *Kent* a hard labourer is said to *swink it away*. (sig. Nnnnn2r)

In his definition of *thassare*, Kennet quotes *The Knight's Tale* (line 1005):

> Thassare . . . In old Eng. *Taas* was any sort of heap. As *Chaucer*, — 𝕿𝖔 𝖗𝖆𝖓𝖘𝖆𝖐𝖊 𝖎𝖓 𝖙𝖍𝖊 𝖙𝖆𝖆𝖘 𝖔𝖋 𝖇𝖔𝖉𝖎𝖊𝖘 𝖉𝖊𝖆𝖉. And *Lidgate Troi 1.1.* 4. c. 30.
> 𝕬𝖓 𝖍𝖚𝖓𝖉𝖗𝖊𝖉 𝖐𝖓𝖞𝖌𝖍𝖙𝖘 𝖘𝖑𝖆𝖎𝖓 𝖆𝖓𝖉 𝖉𝖊𝖆𝖉 𝖆𝖑𝖆𝖘
> 𝕿𝖍𝖆𝖙 𝖆𝖋𝖙𝖊𝖗 𝖜𝖊𝖗𝖊 𝖋𝖔𝖚𝖓𝖉 𝖎𝖓 𝖙𝖍𝖊 𝕿𝖆𝖆𝖘. (sigs. Nnnnn3v–4r)

In his definition of *tremuta*, Kennett quotes *The Reeve's Tale* (line 4039):

Tremuta . . . The Hooper or Hopper in a Mill. . . . Our *Hopper* seems from the *Sax* . . . to *hop*, dance, or turn about, to *hobble*, &c. as is implied by Chaucer, The hopper waggeth to and fro. (sig. OOOOO1r–v)

924. MILLINGTON, EDWARD. *Bibliothecæ nobilissimæ pars tertia & ultima.* B2863. UMI 2549: 9.

Millington says the books he offers for sale at this auction were "*Collected at prodigious Expence, and with incomparable Judgment*" (fol. 2r). He adds: "*The Sales that of late have been made by different ways, have begot such a commendable Itch in the Minds of several Worthy and Learned Noblemen, Gentlemen, &c. after the finest Copies of the Choicest Books in all Faculties, that I must frankly own, that to oblige these more especially, I sell this Noble Library.*" He promises that the copies are "*all clean, many extreamly beautiful, richly Bound, large Paper,* Turkey-*Leather, &c. the rest generally Filleted, Gilt, and Letter'd* A la mode Angleterre, A la mode Francois [*sic*]." The sale was scheduled to begin on Thursday, 20 June 1695 at Millington's Auction-House in St. Bartholomew Close at 4 o'clock every afternoon exactly to 8 o'clock in the evening. Sales would continue until all books were sold.

In the catalogue, under the heading "Divinity, &c. in Folio," number 30 is listed as "*Chaucer's* Works, a famous English Poet — 1602" (37).

925. MILLINGTON, EDWARD. *Catalogus variorum librorum.* C1461. UMI 2552: 2.

Millington held an auction at Rolls's Coffee-House in St. Paul's Church-Yard on 21 January 1695. In the catalogue, under the heading "Miscellanies, History, and Travels, &c. in Folio," lot number 23 is listed as "The compleat Works of Sir *Jeffery Chaucer*, with his Life *Lond.* 1687" (20).

926. MILTON, JOHN. *Poems of Mr John Milton.* M2162. UMI 155: 10.

For an echo of a line from *The Wife of Bath's Tale* and an allusion to *The Squire's Tale* in "Il Pensero" and an allusion to Chaucer in "Mansus," see Milton (1645); in this edition, the passages are found on 4, 5, 54.

Also collected in *The Poetical Works of Mr. John Milton* (1695), M2163 (the fourth work), same pagination.

927. NICHOLSON, JOHN. *A Catalogue of Excellent Books.* T2117b. UMI 2067: 13.

Nicholson auctioned the libraries of the Right Hon. Sir John Trenchard and that of an eminent divine of the Church of England on 25 November 1695. In the catalogue, under the heading "Divinity, History, &c. English, in Folio," number 49 is listed as "Chaucer's Works, the best Edit. with the Life — 1602" (26).

928.   OLDHAM, JOHN. *The Works of Mr. John Oldham.* O230. UMI 1022: 20.

For a reference to Chaucer's penchant for coining new words in "Horace His Art of Poetry" and a reference to the diminished appreciation of Chaucer's poetry in a tribute to the Earl of Rochester, see OLDHAM (1681); in this collection, the passages are found on 5, 82–83 (second pagination).

929.   P., L. *Two Essays Sent in a Letter from Oxford.* P77. UMI 363: 21.

The author is described on the title page as "L. P. Master of Arts." As Dobbins notes (*MLN*), in the second essay "Concerning the Rise, Progress, and Destruction of Fables and Romances," the author cites Chaucer:

> The most early strokes, we meet with, are in *Dante*, *Petrarch*, and *Boccace*, in *Chaucer*, and *Wiclef* . . . . (36)

930.   PARTRIDGE, JAMES. *An Excellent Collection of English Books.* P614. UMI 1211: 2. And *An Appendix to the Catalogue.* P613. UMI 1388: 18.

James Partridge's large library was auctioned in two sessions; the first of these began on 25 November 1695 at the Sign of the Naked Boy at the corner of Paternoster Row and Warwick Lane. In the catalogue, under the heading "English Books. Folio," lot 37 is listed as "Chaucer's Canterbury Tales—[no date]" (2), and in a second lot of folios, number 202 as "Chaucer's Works—1687" (11).

The second auction was scheduled to begin on 16 December. In the catalogue appendix, under the heading "Books in Folio," lot 32 is listed as "*Chaucers* works, with his Life, and Explanation of difficult words—[no date]" (2).

931.   PRESTON, RICHARD GRAHAM. Epistle in Boethius's *Of the Consolation of Philosophy.* B3433. UMI 126: 6.

In an epistle addressed "To the Reader," Lord Preston (1648–1695) comments on Chaucer's translation of Boethius and how difficult Chaucer's language is for the modern reader:

> Chaucer, *the ancient Poet of our Nation, was the first whom I find to have attempted a Translation of this Book into our Tongue: but that is now almost as unintelligible to the English Reader as the Original is; the Alterations of our Language, which he is said, before any of our Countrymen, to have endeavoured to refine, having been very many and great since the times in which he flourished.* (sig. A2r)

932.   S., W., in John Bullokar's *An English Expositor: Teaching the Interpretation of the Hardest Words Used in Our Language*. B5435a. UMI 1545: 15.

For a reference to Chaucer and *The Prologue to the Squire's Tale* in the definition of *Chivancy*, see S., W. (1654); in this edition, the passage is found on sig. B12r.

For a reference to Chaucer and allusion to *The Nun's Priest's Tale*, see S., W. (1663); in this edition, the passage is found on sig. B11r.

933.   SAUNDERS, FRANCIS. "A Catalogue of Books" in *The Temple of Death*. T663. UMI 1580: 2.

At the end of this work is found "A Catalogue of Books Sold by F. Saunders in the New Exchange in the Strand." Under the heading "Poetry and Plays. Folio's," number 8 is "*Chaucer*'s Works" (no pagination; no signature).

934.   SHAKESPEARE, WILLIAM. *Othello, the Moor of Venice*. S2939. UMI 297: 33.

For possible similarities to *Troilus and Criseyde*, see SHAKESPEARE (1622), Boswell & Holton No. 1035.

935.   SHAKESPEARE, WILLIAM. *The Tragedy of Hamlet Prince of Denmark*. S2954. UMI 1578: 24.

For verbal parallels and contextual similarities that may indicate the influence of *The Legend of Good Women* and *The Monk's Tale*, see SHAKESPEARE (1604), Boswell & Holton No. 693.

Another edition in 1695: S2955.

936.   TALLENTS, FRANCIS. *A View of Universal History* (1685). T129A. UMI 2373: 13 and UMI 1558: 14 (as T130).

In his chart of historical events from the creation down to the year 1680, Tallents (1619–1708) includes a list of eminent writers for the modern periods. In the period of 1300–1400, he includes "Dantes," "Fra: Petrarch," and "Boccace," and notes that the latter "reforms ye Italian." At the end of the century he lists "Geffr. Chaucer p[oet]" and "Joh. Gower p[oet] &c." (no pagination; no signatures)

1696

937.   AUBREY, JOHN. *Miscellanies*. A4188. UMI 856: 20.

As Spurgeon notes (1: 267), but does not transcribe, Aubrey (1626–1697) refers to Chaucer twice. In a passage about the Gawen family of Wiltshire, Aubrey writes of William Thinne and *The Squire's Tale*:

Mr. *Thinne* in his Explanation of the hard words in *Chaucer*, writes thus, 𝔊𝔞𝔴𝔶𝔫. . . . This *Gawyn* was Sisters Son to *Arthur* the Great. . . . In the Year 1082 in a Province of *Wales* called *Rose* was his Sepulchre found. *Chaucer* in the Squires Tale.

𝕿𝖍𝖎𝖘 𝖘𝖙𝖗𝖆𝖚𝖓𝖌𝖊 𝕶𝖓𝖎𝖌𝖍𝖙 𝖙𝖍𝖆𝖙 𝖈𝖆𝖒𝖊 𝖙𝖍𝖚𝖘 𝖘𝖔𝖉𝖊𝖓𝖑𝖞
𝕬𝖑𝖑 𝖆𝖗𝖒𝖊𝖉, 𝖘𝖆𝖛𝖊 𝖍𝖎𝖘 𝖍𝖊𝖆𝖉, 𝖋𝖚𝖑𝖑 𝖗𝖔𝖞𝖆𝖑𝖑𝖞
𝕾𝖚𝖑𝖚𝖊𝖉 [*sic*] 𝖙𝖍𝖊 𝕶𝖎𝖓𝖌, 𝖆𝖓𝖉 𝕼𝖚𝖊𝖊𝖓, 𝖆𝖓𝖉 𝕷𝖔𝖗𝖉𝖘 𝖆𝖑𝖑
[. . . . . 5 lines . . . .]
𝕹𝖊 𝖈𝖔𝖚𝖑𝖉 𝖍𝖎𝖒 𝖓𝖔𝖙 𝖆𝖒𝖊𝖓𝖉 𝖔𝖋 𝖓𝖔 𝖜𝖔𝖗𝖉. (28–29)

938. Axe, Thomas. *A Catalogue of English Books.* C1320. UMI 1756: 15.

Axe's auction was held at the Exchange Coffee-House and began on 3 December 1696 at 5 o'clock in the afternoon. In the catalogue, under the heading, "Books in Folio," number 145 is listed as "*Geofrey Chaucer's* Works, the last Edition—*Lond.* 1688" (sig. A2v); the date should probably read 1687.

939. Baker, Richard. *A Chronicle of the Kings of England.* B510. UMI 1754: 20.

For references to Chaucer as John of Gaunt's brother-in-law, "the Homer of our nation," his association with Woodstock, his translation of *The Romaunt of the Rose*, and his burial place in Westminster, see Baker (1643) and (1653); in this edition, the passages are found on 132, 134, 155, 167, and sig. L11113v.

940. Bunyan, John. *The Pilgrim's Progress. The Second Part.* B5580. UMI 1248: 9.

For an echo of *Troilus and Criseyde* 5: 1786, in "The Author's Way of Sending forth his Second Part of the Pilgrim," see Bunyan (1684); in this edition, the passage is found on sig. A2r.

941. Clavel, Robert. *A Catalogue of Books Printed in England Since the Dreadful Fire of London in 1666. to the End of Michaelmas Term, 1695. The Fourth Edition.* C4599. UMI 135: 18.

In this catalogue, in alphabetical order (more or less), under the heading "Poetry," Clavel lists: "𝕮𝖍𝖆𝖚𝖈𝖊𝖗 (*Jeffery*) his Works, fol." (103).

942. Coles, Elisha. *An English Dictionary.* C5075. UMI 412: 8.

For references to Chaucer in Coles's epistle to the reader and in various definitions, see Coles (1676); in this edition, the passages are found on sigs. A3r, H4r, I4v, N1v.

943.   DELONEY, THOMAS. *The Garland of Good-Will.* D951. UMI 1548: 18.

For what may be a faint allusion to *The Clerk's Tale*, see DELONEY (1628) in Boswell & Holton No. 1116. In this edition, the passage is found in the second part, where part 2, number 4, is headed "Of Patient Grissel and a Noble Marquis" (sig. D6r–8v).

944.   EDWARDS, JOHN. *A Discourse Concerning the Authority, Stile, and Perfection of the Books of the Old and New-Testament.* E203. UMI 1569: 1.

For a discussion of the meaning of *dulcarnon* (an allusion to *Troilus and Criseyde* 3: 931, 933), see EDWARDS (1693); in this edition, the passage is found on 247.

945.   HOWELL, JOHN. *Catalogus Librorum.* A3993. UMI 1414: 48.

Howell conducted an auction of the library of Rev. George Ashwell, formerly Fellow of Wadham College, on 5 May 1696 at the Auction House in Ship Lane. In the catalogue, under the heading "English Miscellanies in Folio," lot number 13 is listed as "*Chaucer (Jeffery)* Works of that Incomparable Poet—1687" (sig. O1r).

946.   JOHNSON, RICHARD. *The Famous History of the Seven Champions of Christendom. The Third Part.* J804. UMI 1387: 16.

For a reference to changes in the English language since Chaucer's eloquent lines were in vogue, see JOHNSON (1686); in this edition, the passage is found on sig. A3r–v.

947.   LINDSAY, DAVID. *The Works of the Famous and Worthy Knight, Sir David Lindsay of the Mount.* L2320. UMI 964: 8.

For a reference to Chaucer's skill as a poet in the prologue of *The Testament of Papingo*, see LINDSAY (1538) in Boswell & Holton No. 146; in this edition, the passage is found on sig. G7v.

For a passage that mentions the fable of *Troilus and Criseyde* in an epistle to the king that is set before the prologue to "The Dreme of Sir David Lindsay," see LINDSAY (1558) in Boswell & Holton No. 209; in this edition, the passage is found and appears on sig. H11r.

948.   MILLINGTON, EDWARD. *Bibliotheca Prestoniana.* P3311. UMI 2038: 9.

Millington (ca. 1636–1703), London bookseller, prepared a catalogue of the library of Richard Graham, Viscount Preston, which was offered for sale by auction on 9 November 1696 at Rolls's Auction House in Petty Canon's Alley near St. Paul's.

In a foreword to the catalogue, Millington advises would-be buyers that Lord Preston's English books are "the best and largest Collection of all Subjects, that has been printed in any Catalogue . . . the Books are generally Gilt and Letter'd, sufficiently inviting of all Persons to an antecedent View, at the usual Hours before the time of Sale" (sig. [A]2r). In the sales catalogue, under the heading "English in Folio," number 165 is listed as "*Chaucer's* (G.) Works compar'd with the best Manuscripts with the Au L.—1687" (28); and lot 178 as "Works of that renoun'd English Poet *G. Chaucer.* Printed by *R. Toye*—[no date]" (29).

949.　MILLINGTON, EDWARD. *Collectio multifaria diversorum librorum plurimis facultatibus maxime insignium.* C5104. UMI 1756: 42.

Millington writes that "The Sale will begin on Thursday the Sixth of February 1695/6 at Four of the Clock in the Afternoon exactly, as Rolls's Auction-house in Petty-Canon-Hall in Petty Canon-Alley in St. Paul's Church-yard, continuing to Eight in the Evening daily till all the Books are sold" (title page). In the catalogue, under the heading "Divinity, History, &c. in Folio," lot number 138 is listed as "*Jeffey* [*sic*] *Chaucer's* entire Works, with an explanation of Words —1662" (15); the date should probably read 1602.

950.　MONRO, ALEXANDER. *A Letter to the Honourable Sir Robert Howard.* M2441. UMI 392: 3.

Monro's letter to Howard was "occasioned by a late book entituled, A two-fold vindication of the late Archbishop of Canterbury [i.e., John Tillotson]." In a passage about Scottish dialect, he writes:

> We of *Scotland*, (besides a different Accent) retain a great many of the Old *Saxon* words, which are not now us'd in *England*: But they that understand the *English* Language accurately, understand also those *Saxon* words, some of which may be met with, in the Old Version of the Psalms, daily read in the Churches. And . . . he may read *Milton's* Poems, and *Chaucer's* Works where he may see many of those words that distinguish the *Scottish* Idiom, from that which is now us'd in *England*. (8)

951.　MOTTEUX, PETER ANTHONY. *Love's a Jest.* M2953. UMI 1153: 6.

This comedy written by Motteux (1660–1718) was "acted at the New Theatre in Little-Lincolns Inn-Fields" (title page). In 5.1, Gaymood, speaking to Plot, refers to Sir Pandarus, perhaps alludes to *Troilus and Criseyde*:

> *Plot,* [*sic*] Here's *Fanny* shall act my Niece, and Wed Squire *Ilbred*; be sure the Parson and you whisper all the while. As soon as you have done, we'll all come in and be Witnesses. But hark you, Sir *Pandarus*; if you offer to be familiar, take notice, I'll make a Capon of a Craven. (66)

952.   NICOLSON, WILLIAM. *The English Historical Library: or, A Short View and Character of Most of the Writers Now Extant.* N1146. UMI 722: 5.

Nicolson (1655–1727) is identified on the title page as "Arch-Deacon of Carlisle"; later he became Bishop of Carlisle (1702–1718) and Bishop of Derry (1718–1727). As Dobbins notes (*MLN*), Nicolson mentions Chaucer in part 1, chapter 6, "Of the Writers of Particular Lives of our Kings since the Conquest." In a passage about the unlucky reign of Richard II, Nicolson writes:

> I have not heard of any who have thought it worth their while to write his Life; except only a poor Knight of *John Pits*'s Creation. That Author says, That one Sir *John Gower* (a *Yorkshire* Knight, and Cotemporary [*sic*] with the Famous *Chaucer*) died in the Year 1402. leaving behind him a deal of Monuments of his Learning. . . . (214)

For a reference in Pt. 3, see NICOLSON (1699).

Another edition: N1146A (1697), 214.

953.   OLDHAM, JOHN. "A Pastoral" in the Earl of Rochester's *Poems, &c. On Several Occasions.* R1757. UMI 1577: 15.

For a reference that says Rochester will be mourned more than Chaucer, see OLDHAM, *Some New Pieces* (1681); in this edition, the passage is found on x–xi (sig. a2v–3r).

954.   PHILLIPS, EDWARD. *The New World of Words: or, A Universal English Dictionary.* P2073. UMI 1237: 1.

For a pictorial representation of Chaucer on an engraved title page, see PHILLIPS (1658), (1662), (1671), and (1678); in this revised edition, a reference to Chaucer is found in the preface, sig. a2v. References to Chaucer from earlier editions are also found in definitions of *Adventaile*, previously spelled *Advenale* (sig. B1r), *Amalgaminge* (sig. C1r), *Amortize* (sig. C2r), *Arblaster* (sig. D3r), *Argoil* (sig. D3v), *Arret* (sig. D4r), *Arten* (sig. D4v), *Assoyle* (sig. E1v), *Asterlagour* (sig. E1v), *Autremite* (sig. E4r), *Barm-cloth* (sig. F1v), *Bay* (sig. F2v), *Bend* (sig. F3v), *Burnet* (sig. H1r), *Caitisned* (sig. H2v), *Chas teleyn* (sig. K2v), *Chekelaton* (sig. garbled), *Chelandri* (sig. garbled), *Chertes* (sig. garbled), *Chevesal* (sig. garbled), *Chimbe* (sig. garbled), *Chincherie* (sig. garbled), *Cierges* (sig. garbled), *Citriale* (sig. garbled), *Clergion* (sig. Aa1r), *Clicket,* (sig. Aa1r), *Clinket* (sig. Aa1r), *Curebulli* (sig. Dd1r), *Dennington* (sig. Ee1v), *Desidery* (sig. Ee2v), *Deslavy* (sig. Ee2v), *Digne* (sig. Ee4v), *Discure* (sig. Ff1v), *Divine* (sig. Ff2v), *Dowtremere* (sig. Ff4r), *Ebrack* (sig. Gg2r), *Fonne* (sig. Kk3v), *Gibsere* (sig. Aaa1r), *Giglet* (sig. Aaa1r), *Gourd* (sig. Aaa2v), *Haketon* (sig. Bbb1r), *Hanselines* (sig. Bbb1v), *Jewise* (sig. Ddd1r), *Losenger* (sig. Hhh4r), *Mangon* or *Magonel* (sig. Iii3r), *Miswoman* (sig. Aaaa3v), *Rebeck* (sig. Iiii2v), *Woodstock* (sig. Hhhhh4r).

In this revised edition, Chaucer references are also found in other definitions:

> *Abawed, Chaucer.* Daunted, Abashed. (sig. A1v) [Chaucer uses *abawed* once, in *The Romaunt of the Rose* (line 3646).]
>
> *Acale, Chaucer,* Cold. (sig. A2v) [*Acale* is not found in Tatlock & Kennedy, but Chaucer uses *accolde* once, in *The Romaunt of the Rose* (line 2658).]
>
> *Achecked, Chaucer,* cloaked. (sig. A3r) [Chaucer uses *achekked* once, in *The House of Fame* (3: 1003).]
>
> *Acloyed, Chaucer,* overcharg'd. (sig. A3r) [Chaucer uses *acloyeth*, a variant, once, in *The Parliament of Fowls* (line 517).]
>
> *Agilted,* offended. *Chaucer.* (sig. B2v) [Twelve references in Tatlock & Kennedy.]
>
> *Agredge. Chaucer.* to gather together. (sig. B2v) [Several reference to *agregge* (and variants) in Tatlock & Kennedy.]
>
> *Agroted,* swell'd, made big. *Chaucer.* (sig. B2v) [Chaucer uses *agroted* once, in *The Legend of Good Women* (line 2454).]
>
> *Agrutched,* Abridg'd. *Chaucer.* (sig. B2v) [Not found in Tatlock & Kennedy.]
>
> *Aledge, Chaucer,* ease. (sig. B4r) [Chaucer uses *allege* five times: *The Knight's Tale* (line 3000); *The Merchant's Tale* (line 1658); *Troilus and Criseyde* (3: 297); *The House of Fame* (1: 314); and *The Romaunt of the Rose* (line 6626).

Apparently either Phillips grew weary of searching for words with a Chaucerian connection or his publisher grew impatient, for there are no other new references to Chaucer in this edition.

955.   S., J. *The Case of the Quakers Relating to Oaths Stated.* S48A. UMI 2317: 17.

For a reference to Chaucer's Jack Upland, to Chaucer as "the dad of English Poets," and to Chaucer's "Romance," see S., J. (1674); in this edition, the passage is found on 39.

956.   *The Session of the Poets, Holden at the Food of Parnassus-Hill. July the 9th, 1696.* S2646a. UMI 1269: 4.

As Spurgeon notes (1: 268), there is a reference to "old Chaucer" in this satire. Mr. Welbred is called on to give an account to the court regarding T. B.'s pretentions to poetry; he says T. B. composes ballads in the vein of Chaucer, refers to "The Ballad of our Lady" ("Prier a Nostre Dame") and perhaps alludes to *The Nun's Priest's Tale*:

Indeed his chiefest Talent lies in composing such sort of Ballads, as
Patient Grissel, or old *Chaucer*'s goodly Ballad of our Lady, whose Title
is usually a most lamentable Example of the doleful Desperation of a
miserable Wordling. (37)

957.   SMITH, THOMAS. *Catalogus librorum manuscriptorum bibliothecæ Cottonianæ.* S4233. UMI 548: 17.

Smith (1638–1710) is described on the title page as "ecclesiæ anglicanæ presby-
tero." As Spurgeon notes (1: 268), there are two (?) manuscripts relating to Chaucer in the collection of Sir Robert Cotton (1571–1631).

Under the rubric "Galba," Smith catalogues: "IX. Chaucer. Exemplar emen-
date scriptum" (65).

Under the rubric "Otho," Smith records a clutch of works (items XVIII:
24–28) relating to Chaucer:

24. A Ballade made by Geffrey Chaucer upon his death-bed, lying in
his anguish.
25. Ballad ryall [*sic*], made by Chaucer.
26. Chaucer's ballade to his purse.
27. Cantus Troili.
28. Pictura Galfridi Chauceri. (69).

958.   WINSTANLEY, WILLIAM. *The New Help to Discourse: or, Wit, Mirth, and
Jollity, Intermixt with More Serious Matters.* W3071A. UMI 2183: 6.

For two quotations from *The General Prologue*, see WINSTANLEY (1668); in this
revised edition, the first passage has been deleted through revision and the second is found on 160.

1697

959.   B., T. "A Dedication" in Michael Drayton's *England's Heroical Epistles.*
D2146. UMI 2788: 2.

For a reference to Chaucer in company with Spenser and Jonson in a commendatory poem, see B., T. (1689); in this edition, the passage is found on sig. A4r.

960.   *Bibliotheca Curiosa: or, A Choice Collection of Books.* B2820. UMI 1349: 14.

The "Library of an Eminent Merchant (Deceased,) in the City of London, and
many of them Collected in this Travels" was offered for sale by auction on 15
November 1697. In the second part of the catalogue, under the heading "English
Miscellanies in Folio," number 153 is listed as "*Chaucer* (Sir *Ge.*) His Works, best
Edit. [no date]" (10; sig. D1v).

961.   BRITAINE, WILLIAM DE. *Humane Prudence.* B4807. UMI 732: 6.

For a spurious quotation attributed to Chaucer, see BRITAINE (1686); in this edition, the passage is found on 99.

962.   BULLORD, JOHN. *A Catalogue of Theological, Philosophical, Historical,
Philological, Medicinal & Chymical Books.* R1448A. UMI 2217: 22 (identified as
R2210).

Bullord began auctioning the library of the late Dr. Rugeley at his former dwelling near Southampton House in Bloomsbury on "Tuesday the 19th instant" (no
month or year on title page). In the catalogue, under the heading "Divinity, History, Geography, & Poetry, in Folio," number 21 is listed as *"Geofrey Chaucers*
works the best edition – –1682" (34); the date is puzzling and should probably be
read as 1602.

963.   BULLORD, JOHN. *The Library of the Right Reverend Robert, late Lord
Bishop of Chichester.* G2150b. UMI 1794: 13.

Bullord began auctioning the extensive library of the late Right Rev. Robert
Grove, Lord Bishop of Chichester, on 27 April 1697, at Tom's Coffee House
near Ludgate. Grove had died from injuries incurred when he jumped from his
coach after his horses became uncontrollable. His widow and five children were
in financial straits because he had failed to provide for their future, and no doubt
the library was auctioned in order to alleviate their plight. In the sales catalogue,
under the heading "English Books in Divinity, History, Geography, Poetry, &c.
in Folio," lot 23 is listed as *"Chaucers* Works — ib. [i.e., London] 1598" (29; sig.
I1r).

**964.   *Catalogi librorum manuscriptorum Angliæ et Hiberniæ in unum collecti,
cum indice alphabetico.* C1253. UMI 449: 7 and UMI 449: 8.

Although this monumental work is commonly known as Edward Bernard's
(1638–1697) *Catalogue of Manuscripts*, Humphrey Wanley (1672–1726) compiled
four of the catalogues included, and Thomas Tanner (1674–1735) did others.

Spurgeon (3: 4.81) notes that there are a dozen Chaucerian manuscripts
listed in this catalogue, but apparently she misread the index, for there are many
more.

In volume 1, part 1, "Librorum Manuscriptorum Bibliothecæ Bodleianæ,"
under the running head "Codices Manuscripti Var. Ling. Guilielmi Laudi,"
number 1234.69 is "Jeffrey *Chaucer* his Canterbury *Tales*" (68); and number
1476.50 is "Geoffrey *Chaucer* His Canterbury Tales, except the Plowman's Tale.
v.G.69" (72).

Under the running head "Codices Manuscripti Latini Kenelmi Digbæi,"
number 1673.72 is "A Treatise of *Chaucer* to his Son touching the Astrolabe to
the latitude of Oxford" (80).

Under the running head "Codices Manuscripti Thomæ Bodleii," number 2151.16 is "*Chaucer* of the Astrolabe" (112); number 2527.32 is "*Chaucer*'s Tales" (132).

Under the running head "Codices Manuscripti Joannis Seldeni," number 3354.24 is "Geoffrey *Chaucer*'s Troylus, with other Poems of that Age and perhaps Author" (162); number 3360.30: "*Chaucer*'s Tales" (162); number 3444.56 is "Troilus and Cressida by *Chaucer* An. 1441. 19. Regis *Hen. VI*" (165); and number 3488.100 is "*Chaucer*'s Works printed by Rich. Pynson" (167).

Under the running head "Codices Manuscripti in Hyperoo Bodleiano," number 3554.64 is "Geoffrey *Chaucer* his tract concerning the use of the Astrolabe" (170).

Under the running head "Codices Manuscripti Thomæ Bodleii," under the heading "Codices Manuscripti XXIX. Ex dono Illustrissimi Domini Thomæ Fairfax Baronis Cameronii," number 3896.16 is "A Book of old English Poëtry, by Tho. *Hoclove* [*sic*], *Lydgate*, *Chaucer*, &c." (180); and under the heading "Tres libri scripti manu quos in hoc Gazophylacium conject vir eruditione, pietate ac genere insignissimus Carolus Hattonus," number 4138.1 is "*Chaucer* veteris Poëtæ Angli Opera" (186).

Under the running head "Joaanis Lelandi Collectanea," volume 3, number 5104.39 is "Epitaphium Chauceri & sepultura Jo. Goweri, 48" (240); number 5105.211 is "De Galfrido Chaucero, 300" (245).

Under the running head "Codices Manuscripti Francisci Junii," number 5118.9 (really 5121.9) is "The works of Geffrey Chaucer, fol. Lond. 1598. Cui ad marginem plurimi F. Junii notæ adscribuntur, & ad finem Chartæ quædam solutæ ejusdem naturæ" (248).

Under the running head "Codices Manuscripti Ashmoleani," under the heading "Poems English," number 6928 is "The Cook's Tale. Manu Ashmol. 43.4" (320); number 6937: "Chaucer's Piller, or the Squires Tale found out by John Lane, 1630. 4to. 53" (320); number 6943: "The Tragedy of Rome, and diverse other Miscellanies, by Lydgate, Gower, and Chaucer, fol. 59. 2 &c." (320); number 6986: "Chaucer's Prophesy" (320).

In the catalogue for the various colleges in Oxford, there are five references. Under the running head "Codices Manuscripti Collegii Novi," number 1278.314: "*Chaucer*'s Works" (38).

Under the running head "Codices Manuscripti Collegii Corporis Christi," number 1665.198: "Sir *Jeffry Chaucer*'s Canterbury Tales. Fol. Membr." (56); in a section headed "Briani Twyne, S. T. B. & C.C.C.," number 1730.263: "Notes out of Sir *Philip Sidney*, *Chaucer*, and *Erasmus*" (57).

Under the heading "Librorum Manuscriptorum Colegii S. Trinitatis in Oxonia Catalogus," number 1991.54: "*Jeffry Chaucer*'s Works" (65).

In a section headed "Libri Omissi," number 2365: "Sir *Jeffry Chaucer*'s Works. C.2.9 Art. *Mert. Coll.*" (78).

In the catalogue for Cambridge colleges, there are five entries related to Chaucer. In the catalogue of manuscripts in Trinity College, number 270.15: "Chauceri opera" (95); number 532.7: "Chauceri opera" (100).

In the catalogue of manuscripts in St. Benedict college, number 1293.17: "Troylus Chauceri, Anglice, cum Pictura suavissima" (132); number 1471.194.1: "Tractatus Astrolabii, Anglice, secundum Chaucerum factus, in gratiam filii sui Ludowici" (138).

In volume 2, in a section on English cathedral libraries, we find the all entries noted by Spurgeon. In the catalogue of manuscripts in Lichfield Cathedral library, number 1382.2: "An ancient *Chaucer*, with gilt Letters. Fol." (32).

In the catalogue of manuscripts in Coventry Cathedral library, number 1457.12: "A Preiour to our Ladye, made by *Geffreie Chaucer*, after the order of the *A.B.C.*" (33).

Under the heading "Codices Manuscripti Bibliothecæ Norfolcianæ," number 3038.139: "A piece of Divine Poetry, in old English Sir *John Mandevile's* Travels. *Chaucer's Melibee*" (77).

In the catalogue of manuscripts in the library of Francis Bernard, M. D., under the heading "Libri Miscellanei in Folio," number 3579.10: "*Geoffry Chawcer's* Works. Imperfect" (89).

In the catalogue of manuscripts in Sion College library, number 4091.27: "Part of Geoffrey Chaucer's Poem of his Canterbury Tale, 4to" (107).

In the catalogue of manuscripts in the library of Samuel Pepys, number 6786.67: "Pieces of Chaucer, written near his own time, some whereof never printed, fol." (209).

In the catalogue of manuscripts in the library of Henry Worseley, number 6891.43: "Geofrey Chaucer's tales, written on Paper, nigh as old as Chaucer himself. Imperfect towards the end" (213).

In the catalogue of manuscripts in the library of Robert Burscough, number 7703.84: "Troilus and Chryseis, by Jeffrey Chaucer" (235).

Under the heading "Librorum Manuscriptorum Cinnus," number 8729.20: "Chaucer's Works. Penes Samuelem Hodley, Scholæ Grammat. apud Hackney prope Londinium Moderatorem" (250).

In the collection of Abraham Pryme, number 9185.6: "All the Works of Old Chaucer in long folio. This Vol. belong'd to the Monastery of Canterbury. Penes D. Edmund. Canby de Thorn, in Com. Ebor." (360).

Under the heading "Librorum Manuscriptorum Admodum Reverendi in Christo Patris D. D. Joannis More Episcopi Norvicensis Catalogus," number 9195.9: "Codex membrancenus in fol. Continet formulas bene multas Literarum escambii & alias plurimas de rebus & negotiis Ecclesiasticis, Latine quasdam, quasdam Gallice. Item Tractatum de Astrolabio compilatum per Galfridum Chaucer in usum filii sui Ludovici lingua Anglicana. In fine: Explicit tractatus de conclusionibus Astrolabii compilatus per Galfridum Chaucer ad filium suum Scholarem tunc temporis Oxoniæ ac sub tutela illius nobilissimi philosophi

Magistri N. Strode" (361); number 9211.25: "Chauceri opera eleganti manu. Codex membr. in fol." (362).

In an appendix to volume 2, there are others missed by Spurgeon. In a catalogue of manuscripts in the library of Henry Hyde, Earl of Clarendon, number 81.81: "Sir Geoffrey Chaucers' [sic] Works, fol." (14).

Under the heading "Codices Manuscripti Collegii S. Trinitatis," number 762.622.5: "Geoffrey Chaucer's work of Chymistry, 4to. F.123" (44).

965. *A Catalogue of Latin and English Books, Both Antient [sic] and Modern.* **C1343. UMI 1774: 17.**

Among the books scheduled to be sold by auction at Walsal's Coffee-House on 12 July 1697, under the heading "Books in Folio, English," lot 41 is listed as "The Works of our Antient [sic] Poet *Jeffery Chaucer*, with his Life, and a Key to the difficult words—[no date]" (9; sig. D1r).

966.   DRYDEN, JOHN. "Dedicatory Epistle" in *The Satires of Decimus Junius Juvenalis. Translated into English Verse. By Mr. Dryden, and Several Other Eminent Hands.* J1289. UMI 1012: 19; UMI 1444: 27.

For references to Spenser's imitation of Chaucer's language, see DRYDEN (1693); in this edition, the passage is found on xiii–xiv.

A reissue in 1697: J1290 (UMI 1444: 27), xiii–xiv.

967.   DRYDEN, JOHN. "Dedicatory Epistle" in *The Works of Virgil. Translated into English Verse by Mr. Dryden.* V616. UMI 1319: 1.

As Spurgeon notes (1: 269), Dryden refers to Chaucer in his dedicatory epistle to Hugh, Lord Clifford of Chudleigh. Dryden writes that *"the Shepherd's Kalendar of* Spenser, *is not to be match'd in any Modern Language."* He continues:

> Spencer *being Master of our Northern Dialect; and skill'd in* Chaucer's *English, has so exactly imitated the* Doric *of* Theocritus, *that his Love is a perfect Image of that Passion Which God infus'd into both Sexes, before it was corrupted with the Knowledge of Arts, and the Ceremonies of what we call good Manners.* (sig. A2r)

Spurgeon notes (1: 269) another reference in Dryden's "Postscript to the Reader":

> [A]ll our Poets, even those in who being endu'd with Genius, yet have not Cultivated their Mother-Tongue with sufficient Care; or relying on the Beauty of their Thoughts, have judg'd the Ornament of Words, and sweetness of Sound unnecessary. One is for raking in *Chaucer* (our *English Ennius*) for antiquated Words, which are never to be reviv'd, but

when Sound or Significancy is wanting in the present Language. (621; sig. Hhhh1r)

Another edition: V617 (1698), sig. A2r, 671 (sig. Qqqq3r).

968.   Evelyn, John. *Numismata. A Discourse of Medals, Antient and Modern.* E3505. UMI 276: 6.

In chapter 8, "Of Heads and Effigies in Prints and Taille-douce: Their Use as they Relate to Medals," in a section devoted to those "Names of the most Renowned, Famous and Illustrious of our own, and other Nations worthy the Honor of Medal, or at least of some Memory," in a collection of "Poets and Great Wits," Evelyn (1620–1706) includes: *"Chaucer"* (262).

969.   Hartley, John, and George Huddleston. *A Catalogue of the Library of the Reverend and Learned Dr. Scattergood, Deceas'd.* S840. UMI 291: 6.

Hartley and Huddleston conducted an auction at Hartley's bookshop near Gray's-Inn in Holborn on 26 July 1697. In the catalogue, under the heading "English Miscellanies in Folio," number 47 is listed as *"Chaucer's* Works – – ibid. [i.e., London] 1602" (54).

970.   Millington, Edward. *Bibliotheca Bassetiana.* B1050. UMI 1376: 14.

Millington auctioned the library of William Bassett, late rector of St. Swithin's in London, on 4 February 1697 at Rolls's Auction House. In the catalogue, under the heading "English Miscellanies in Folio," lot 104 is listed as "Chaucers Works last Edition [no date]" (30).

Another edition: B1049b (undated), same pagination.

971.   Millington, Edward. *Bibliotheca selectissima: sive, catalogus variorum librorum antiquorum & recentiorum variis facultatibus clarissimorum.* H700. UMI 1424: 18.

Millington began auctioning the library of Michael Harding of Trinity College (Oxford) on 8 November 1697. In the catalogue, under the heading "English Miscellanies in Folio," item number 65 was "Chaucer's Works—ibid. [i.e., London] 1687" (sig. G1r).

972.   Milton, John. *The Works of Mr. John Milton.* M2086. UMI 111: 14.

For a quotation from *The General Prologue* (a reference to the Frere) and quotations from the spurious *Ploughman's Tale*, and "our renowned Chaucer," see Milton, *Of Reformation Touching Church-Discipline in England* (1641); in this collection of Milton's prose works, the passages are found on 181, 184–85, 188, 194.

For a reference to "learned" Chaucer's orthography and possible allusions to *The Man of Law's Tale*, *The Parliament of Fowls*, *The Legend of Good Women*, *The Book of the Duchess*, *The Wife of Bath's Prologue*, *The Complaint of Fair Anelida and False Arcite*, and *Troilus and Criseyde*, see MILTON, *Animadversions upon the Remonstrants Defence, against Smectymnuus* (1641); in this collection, the passage is found on 297.

973. *Poems on Affairs of State from the Time of Oliver Cromwell.* P2719. UMI 1337: 42.

For a reference to Chanticlere and Pertelot, an allusion to *The Nun's Priest's Tale*, see MARVELL (1667); in this edition, the passage is found on 81.

For an allusion to *The House of Fame*, see "Rochester's Farewel" [*sic*] in *The Third Part of Poems on Affairs of State* (1689); in this edition, the passage is found on 159.

974. POLSTED, EZEKIEL. ΚαλäÂ Τελωνήσανται [Kalos Telonesantai]: *or, The Excise Man. Shewing the Excellency of His Profession.* P2780B. UMI 2012: 8.

Polsted is identified on the title page as "Ezekiel Polsted, A.B." In chapter 8, in a passage about the excise man's obligation to be upright in behavior, impervious to bribery, and completely impartial, he attributes a proverb to Chaucer. He writes:

[The excise *man*] knows if he should once prove false . . . the odds are very unequal [i.e., likely], but they [i.e., those who owe taxes] will [prove false] too . . . so that if that Theological Maxim, That things wrong-fully got, have a very uncertain Assurance, convinces him not; yet that Political one of *Seneca* is absolutely prevalent, That it is a great Fault to believe every one, and a great one too to trust One, which makes him in this Case to acquiesce with *Chaucer*, when he tells us,
    —As Proverbs do say,
Three may keep Counsel, if Twain be away. (32)

975. SOUTH, ROBERT. *Twelve Sermons Preached upon Several Occasions. The Second Volume.* S4748.

For an echo a line from *The Reeve's Tale*, see SOUTH (1694); in this edition, the passage is found on 472–73.

976. *State-Poems; Continued From the Time of O. Cromwel, to the Year 1697. Written by the Greatest Wits of the Age.* S5325a. UMI 1876: 2.

In "Cæsar's Ghost," there is a reference to January and May, perhaps an allusion to *The Merchant's Tale*. Great Cæsar appears to the writer to be in a dream:

Here an old batter'd *Tangieren* he beheld,
More mawl'd by Love than e're he was in Field;
Yet wondrous Amorous still, and wondrous gay,
Old *January* dizen'd up in *May*. (166)

977. TATE, NAHUM. "Preface" in Sir John Davies' *The Original, Nature, and Immortality of the Soul.* **D405. UMI 24: 19.**

As Bond notes (*SP* 28), Nahum Tate (1652–1715) quotes Sir Philip Sidney on Chaucer. In the unsigned preface to Davies' work, Tate writes:

[A]s Sir Philip Sidney *said of* Chaucer, *That he knew not which he should most wonder at, either that He in his dark Time should see so distinctly, or that We in this clear Age should go so stumblingly after him; so may we marvel and bewail the low Condition of Poetry now.* (sig. A8v)

978. *The Trial and Determination of Truth.* **T2166. UMI 554: 2.**

This work was written in answer to *The Best Choice for Religion and Government.* In "The Preface to the Reader, Gentle or Simple," the author attributes an aphorism to Chaucer (but may allude to *The Squire's Tale*, lines 220–24):

There's no Ear so deaf, as that which Interest has stopp'd; and none so miserably blind, as those that resolvedly shut their Eyes against the plainest Demonstrations of Truth. The Words of an old Author are at this day verified of the English,
  "What they like not, they never understand.["]
      JEOF. CHAUCER. (sig. A2v)

979. TRYON, THOMAS. *A Way to Health, Long Life and Happiness: or, A Discourse of Temperance.* **T3202.**

For an echo of a line from *The Reeve's Prologue*, see TRYON (1683); in this edition, the passage is found on 416.
  Other editions in 1697: T3202A (1697), 416; T3202B (1697), 416.

980. WESLEY, SAMUEL. *The Life of our Blessed Lord & Saviour Jesus Christ.* **W1373aA. UMI 906: 19 (identified as W1373).**

For a reference to Wesley's fondness of antique language and his use of a Chaucerian word, see WESLEY (1693); in this edition, the passages are found on sig. K2v.
  Another edition in 1697: W1373, sig. K3v.

981.   *A Word in Season: or, An Essay to Promote Good-Husbandry in Hard and Difficult Times.* W3547C. UMI 2539: 10.

This little work is cast in the form of a letter "Being, in part, Advice from a Gentleman, to his Son a Tradesman in London" (title page). In a discussion of piety, honesty, and religiosity, after citing "Monsieur Charron"[47] and Dr. Stillingfleet,[48] the writer mentions Chaucer and attributes an aphorism to him (but may allude to *The Squire's Tale*, lines 220–24):

> Dr. *Stillingfleet*, when Dean of St. *Pauls*, in one of his printed Sermons tells us; That no Man will sooner affirm a thing to be false, than he that knows it to be against his Interest to believe it to be true. And even Old *Geofry Chaucer* long since hath told us; That *English men*, what they not like, they will never understand. (10)

982.   WOTTON, WILLIAM. *Reflections upon Ancient and Modern Learning. The Second Edition, with Large Additions.* W3659. UMI 1602: 57.

Wotton (1666–1727) is identified on the title page as chaplain to the Earl of Nottingham. As Alderson & Henderson note, in this augmented edition, in the fifth chapter, "Of Ancient and Modern Grammar," Wotton alludes to the evolution of the English language since the days of Chaucer:

> [T]he *Grammar* of *English* is so far our own, that Skill in the Learned Languages is not necessary to comprehend it. *Ben. Johnson*[49] was the first Man, that I know of, that did any Thing considerable in it: but he seems to have been too much possessed with the Analogy of *Latin* and *Greek*, to write a perfect Grammar of a Language whose Construction is so vastly different; tho' he falls into a contrary Fault, when he treats of the *English Syntax*, where he generally appeals to *Chaucer* and *Gower*, who lived before our Tongue had met with any of that Polishing, which, within these last CC Years,[50] has made it appear almost entirely new. (60)

---

[47] Probably Pierre Charron (1541–1603), author of *De la sagesse*, translated into English as *Of Wisdom* (1608) and frequently reprinted.

[48] Edward Stillingfleet (1635–1699), a well-known London preacher, became Dean of St. Paul's in 1678 and then Bishop of Worcester in 1689.

[49] Ben. Johnson, i.e., Benjamin Jonson. For references to Chaucer in Jonson's *Grammar*, see JONSON (1640), Boswell & Holton No. 1363.

[50] CC Years, i.e., two hundred years.

1698

983.   BERNARD, FRANCIS, M. D. *A Catalogue of the Library.* B1992. UMI 1056: 15.

The immense library of Dr. Bernard (1627–1698), fellow of the College of Physicians and physician at St. Bartholomew's Hospital, was auctioned at the late doctor's dwelling in Little Britain on 4 October 1698. In the third part of the catalogue, under the heading "English Books in Divinity, History, &c. Folio," number 9 is listed as "*Chaucer*'s Works with his Life, best edition, *Lond.* 1602" (≟34); lot 62 as "*Chaucer*'s Works the best Edition, *Ib.* 1602" (≟35); number 142 as "*Chaucers* (*Geoff*) Tales, Imperfect [no date]" (≟37); lot 156 as "*Chaucers* (*Geoff.*) Works [no date]" (≟38). In octavo, number 56 is listed as "*Chaucers* (*Jeof*) Millers Tale, and the Wife of Baths Tale with a Commentary, Ib. [i.e., London] 1665" (≟57) and lot 671 is "*Chaucer*'s Ghost, 1672" (≟73).

984.   DARE, JOSIAH. *Counsellor Manners, His Last Legacy to His Son.* D248A. UMI 1944: 24.

For a paraphrase of a couplet from *The Wife of Bath's Tale* and a precis of an incident related by Chauntecleer in *The Nun's Priest's Tale*, see DARE (1673); in this edition, the passages are found on 3–4, 144–45.

985.   DENNIS, JOHN. *The Usefulness of the Stage to the Happiness of Mankind, to Government and to Religion.* D1046. UMI 140: 11.

As Spurgeon notes (1: 270), in responding to Jeremy Collier's screed against the stage, Dennis (1657–1734) places Chaucer as the first English author of merit. In part 1, chapter 4, he writes:

> It was first in the Reign of King *Henry* the Eighth that the Drama grew into form with us: It was establish'd in the Reign of Queen *Elizabeth*, and flourish'd in that of King *James* the First. And tho I will not presume to affirm, that before the Reign of King *Henry* the Eighth we had no good Writers, yet I will confidently assert, that, excepting *Chaucer*, no not in any sort of Writing whatever, we had not a first rate Writer. But immediately upon the establishment of the Drama, three prodigies of Wit appear'd all at once, as it were so many Suns of amaze the learned world. The Reader will immediately comprehend that I speak of *Spencer*, *Bacon* and *Raleigh.* . . . (39–40)

986.   DRYDEN, JOHN. "Dedicatory Epistle" in *The Works of Virgil. Translated into English Verse by Mr. Dryden.* V617. UMI 1581: 2.

For references to Spenser's imitation of Chaucer's language and to Chaucer as "our English Ennius," see DRYDEN (1697); in this edition, the passages are found on sig. A2r and 671 (sig. Qqqq3r).

987.   D'URFEY, THOMAS. *The Campaigners: or, The Pleasant Adventures at Brussels. A Comedy.* D2705. UMI 530: 2.

Along with the play, D'Urfey (1653–1723) includes a preface written in response to Jeremy Collier's abuses of poets. D'Urfey praises Chaucer, attributes a quotation to him, and quotes "Truth: Balade de Bon Conseyl":

> I must necessarily inform the Partial, as well as Impartial Reader, that I had once design'd another kind of Preface to my Comedy . . . but having in the interim been entertain'd with a Book lately Printed, full of Abuses on all our Antient as well as Modern Poets, call'd *A View of the Immorality and Prophaness of the English Stage*; and finding the Author [Jeremy Collier] . . . indecently, unmanner'd, and scurrilous in his unjust Remarks on me, and two of my Plays, *viz.* the first and second parts of the *Comical History of* Don Quixote. I thought I could not do better . . . than (instead of the other) to print a short Answer to this very Severe and Critical Gentleman. . . . (1)
>
> We find, for many Ages past, Poets have enjoy'd this Priviledge [of satirizing iniquity]; our Prince of Poets, *Chaucer*, had so much to do in this kind, that we find him weary himself, and loth to weary others with it.
>
>   Of Freers I have told before,
>   In making of a Crede,
>   And yet I could tell worse, or more,
>   But Men would werien it to read.
>
> This I think is pithy, but here again I think his Counsel to them is much better.
>
>   Fly fro the Prease and dwell with soothsasiness,
>   Suffice unto thy good, tho it be small,
>   For horde hath, and climbing tickleness,
>   Prease hath Envy, and wele is blent ore all;
>   Savour no more then thee beholde shall,
>   Rede wele thy self that other folk canst rede,
>   And trough thee shall deliver it is no drede.
>
> Now if he be Moral enough to take old *Chaucer*'s Advice I shall be glad; and so much for that subject. (15)

The first passage from "our Prince of Poets" is marked with a shoulder note: "Chaucer."

988.   D'URFEY, THOMAS. *Pendragon: or, The Carpet Knight His Kalendar.* P1142. **UMI 504: 18.**

In "October's Canto," D'Urfey (1653–1723) appears to allude to *The House of Fame*. In a passage in which Pendragon questions rampant rumors of overturning the government, he writes:

> *Pendragon* . . . saw no danger of Event
> To over-turn the Government:
> Nor did he think the Tales which flew
> About confus'd'ly, could be true.
> Yet that they well might understand too
> The *Quis, Quid, Quomodo, Cur, Quando,*
> of this bold Whisper, Both agreed
> To walk with all convenient speed
> To the next Coffee-house of Fame,
> To learn the Certainty o' th' same. (144).

As Bond notes (*SP* 28), D'Urfey closes "October's Canto" with a reference to Chaucer:

> ['T]is but reas'nable and fit
> That short-liv'd Pleasures should be sweet.
> *Mensis Octobris explicit.*
> So was Authentick *Chaucer* wont
> At a full Period or Point
> Of the same Tale, to close the Joint. (155)

989.   FERGUSON, ROBERT. *A View of an Ecclesiastick in His Socks & Buskins.* **F764. UMI 665: 13.**

Ferguson (d. 1714) takes it upon himself to reprimand Vincent Alsop "for his Foppish, Pedantick, Detractive and Petulant Way of Writing" (title page). In doing so, he mentions Chaucer's obsolete language:

> But to bestow some *Reflections* upon what I have rehearsed out of our Author, the first thing I would observe is, that the little *Wit* that appears in any thing he has said, is perfectly *Antiquated*, and out of *Date*. *Chaucer's obsolete* English would sooner be accounted Elegant and Rhetorical among the *Politest* Masters of our Refin'd and Modern Language, than these *Puns, Quibles* and *Drollings* of an Infantill [*sic*], unpolish'd

Age will pass, and be admitted for Schemes of Maturated, Adult, and Pregnant *Wit*. (31)

990. *The Golden Age: or, The Reign of Saturn Review'd*. G1011. UMI 1461: 49.

This work, ostensibly written by "Hortolanus, Junr." and "preserved and published by R. G." includes a long quotation from *The Canon's Yeoman's Tale*. In a passage about the stone that is essential to alchemical success:

> *Her name is* Magnetia, *few people her knowe,*
> *She is fownde in high places as well in lowe;*
> Plato knew her Property and called her by her name,
> And Chaucer *rehearseth how* Titanos *is the same,*
> *In the* Channons Yeomans Taile, *saying what is thus,*
> *But* Quid ignotum per Magis ignotius, (*&c.*) (38)

But to return to *Chaucer*, who calls it *Titanos*, in his Tale of the *Chanons Yeoman* . . . he writes thus.

> *Lo thus saith* Arnolde *of the new Toune,*
> *As his* Rosayre *maketh mencioune:*
> . . . .
> *Man to enspyre and eke for to defende,*
> *Whan that him lyketh, to this is his ende.* (41–43)

991. *Herodian's History of the Roman Emperors*. H1581. UMI 383: 16.

Herodian's *History* was "done from the Greek by a gentleman at Oxford." In book 2, in a description of Severus, the translator appears to echo the description of the shipman in *The General Prologue*: "Of nyce conscience took he no keep" (line 398). He writes:

> [N]o man in the World made professions of Kindness and Friendship with more Art and Address than *Severus*: He was no man of nice Conscience, but wou'd lye and falsifie without scruple to serve a Turn, and wou'd even stretch an Oath if his Affairs requir'd it. (116–17)

992. MERITON, LUKE. *Pecuniae obediunt omnia. Money Masters All Things: or, Satyrical Poems*. M1821B. UMI 642: 18

In this collection of poems "shewing the power and influence of money over all men" (title page) Meriton echoes Chaucer's description of the Miller in *The General Prologue*: "he hadde a thombe of gold, pardee" (line 563). In "On Millers," he writes:

When Corn is dear, the Miller often is
(To get great Gains) tempted to do amiss,
Not pleas'd with's due, excessive Toll he'll take,
And all the Country cheat for Money's sake;
And by this means the Adage does fulfill,
It is as sure as there's a Thief i'th' Mill.
And the old Saying is, as has been told,
An honest Miller has a Thumb of Gold. (77)

993. MILLINGTON, EDWARD. *Bibliotheca Levinziana.* L1826. UMI 1710: 31.

Millington began auctioning the library of Rev. William Levinz, late president of St. John's College (Oxford) and sometime Regius Professor of Greek, on 29 June 1698. In the catalogue, under the heading "Miscellanies, in Folio," number 62 is listed as "Jeffrey Chaucer's Works, with an Explication of Words—1687" (29).

994. OLDHAM, JOHN. *The Works of Mr. John Oldham.* O231.UMI 724: 2 (film is incomplete).

For a reference to Chaucer's penchant for coining new words in "Horace His Art of Poetry" and a reference to the diminished appreciation of Chaucer's poetry in a tribute to the Earl of Rochester, see OLDHAM (1681).

995. ORRERY, CHARLES BOYLE. *Dr. Bentley's Dissertations on the Epistles of Phalaris, and the Fables of Aesop Examin'd.* O469. UMI 431: 10.

Orrery is identified on the title page as "the Honourable Charles Boyle, Esq." He was raised to the Irish peerage as the fourth earl of Orrery in 1703. Here he writes in response to Richard Bentley (1662–1742). In a passage about the instability of languages, Orrery (1674–1731) mentions Chaucer:

> Does he [Bentley] take the *Greek* of *Lucian* to be as different from that of *Plato*, as our *English* Now is from that which was spoken soon after the Conquest? Are not *Homer* and *Oppian*[51] much nearer one another in their Language than *Chaucer* and *Cowly*, tho' in Time they are far more distant? (70)

996. S., W., in John Bullokar's *An English Expositor: Teaching the Interpretation of the Hardest Words Used in Our Language.* B5436. UMI 1545: 15.

For a reference to Chaucer and *The Prologue to the Squire's Tale* in the definition of Chivancy, see S., W. (1654); in this edition, the passage is found on sig. B12r.

---

[51] Oppian was a second century Græco-Roman poet.

For a reference to Chaucer and allusion to *The Nun's Priest's Tale*, see S., W. (1663); in this edition, the passage is found on sig. B11r.

997.   SPELMAN, HENRY. *Reliquiae Spelmaniae. The Posthumous Works Relating to the Laws and Antiquities of England.* S4930. UMI 335: 8.

Spelman (1564?–1641) is identified on the title page as "Sir Henry Spelman kt." Under the running head "The Original of the Terms," i.e., the terms of court, he uses *The House of Fame* to allude to Ovid's description of the roost of rumor (*Metamorphoses*, book 12). In chapter 3, "Why some Law business may be done on days exempted," Spelman writes:

> As for the *Star-chamber*, it . . . was necessary therefore that this Session should not only be daily open, but (as it is said of the house of *Fame*) *Nocte dieque patens*; for an evil may happen in the night that would be too late to prevent in the morning. (94–95)

As Dobbins notes (*MLN*), Spelman quotes a modernized couplet from *The Reeve's Tale* (lines 4285–86) in a section headed "Icenia: sive Norfolciæ Descriptio Topographica." In a passage about Bronholm, Spelman writes of Chaucer's usage:

> Cœnobitis interea luculentus quæstus. Hujus meminit sub exitu quarti abhinc seculi *Galfridus Chaucer* in *Præpositi lasciva Fabula*:
>   *And with the falle out of her sleep she braide,*
>   *Help holy Cross of* Bromholme *she said.* (153).

Chaucer is also mentioned in "Index Authorum," sig. Ff1r.

998.   TRYON, THOMAS. *A Way to Health, Long Life and Happiness: or, A Discourse of Temperance.* T3203.

For an echo of a line from *The Reeve's Prologue*, see TRYON (1683).

999.   *The Wanton Wife of Bath.* W723A. UMI 2124.4: 31 (identified as W720).

For a reference to Chaucer's writing of a wanton wife of Bath, see *The Wanton Wife of Bath* (1641). Here Chaucer's name is spelled correctly.

1000.   WARE, JOHN. *A Catalogue of Books.* S2134A. UMI 2885: 21.

Ware began auctioning the library of "that Learned and Ingenious Gentleman Thomas Scudamore, Esq; Deceased" on 14 November 1698 at Dick's Coffee House in Skinner Row, Dublin. In the catalogue, under the heading "Libri in Folio," number 1 is listed as "*Chaucer*'s Works" (2).

1001. WHARTON, GEORGE. "To my Very Honoured Friend," in Gaultier de Coste, Seigneur de La Calprenède's *Hymen's Præludia: or, Love's Master-Piece. Now Rendred into English, by Robert Loveday.* L124A. UMI 1780: 10.

For a reference to Chaucer and Gower as a pair who refined the English language, see WHARTON (1652); in this edition, the passage is found on sig. A4v.

1699

1002. A., J. "Commedatory Poem" in *Titus Lucretius Carus, His Six Books of Epicurean Philosophy, Done into English Verse, with Notes* [by Thomas Creech]. L3449C. UMI 1063: 11.

For a reference to Chaucer's connection to Cambridge and his having been inspired by the River Cam, see A., J. (1683); in this edition, the passage is found on sig. C4v.

1003. BARON, WILLIAM. *A Just Defence of the Royal Martyr.* B897. UMI 10: 19.

Writing to defend Charles I "from the many false and malicious aspersions in Ludlow's Memoirs and some other virulent libels of that kind," Baron (b. 1636) mentions Chaucer and attributes an aphorism to him (but may allude to *The Squire's Tale*, lines 220–24). In chapter 5 "Of the King's Murder," Baron writes:

> When his *Majesty* we are now discoursing of, had so far baffled *Henderson*[52] . . . the peevish old Fellow in the end would not vouchsafe him a *Reply*, He pleasantly tells him, you may have something of that which *Chaucer* saith belongs to the *People* of England, *What they not like they never Understand*; the common Practice of *Fools* and *Knaves* . . . (209)

1004. BEHN, APHRA. Interpolation in *History of Oracles, and the Cheats of the Pagan Priests.* F1413A. UMI 1700: 46.

For a reference to Chaucer's tales, see BEHN (1688); in this edition, the passage is found on 134.

1005. *A Catalogue of Valuable and Choice Books.* C1413. UMI 1611: 23.

The libraries of a "person of eminent quality, and a learned divine deceased" were auctioned at Howson's Coffee-House in Devereaux Court without Temple-Bar on the 17th [no month on title page] 1699. In the catalogue, under the heading "English Miscellanies in Folio," lot 23 is listed as "*Chaucer*'s Works, with an explan. of his hard words of Decla. &c. [no date]" (42).

---

[52] Alexander Henderson. See Boswell & Holton No. 1454.

1006. CLEVELAND, JOHN. *The Works of Mr. John Cleveland.* C4655. UMI 1032: 9.

For an echo of a line from *The Manciple's Prologue*, see CLEVELAND (1644); in this edition, the passage is found on 67.

For a reference to Chaucer and an allusion to *The Pardoner's Prologue* in "A Letter sent from a Parliament Officer at Grantham," see CLEVELAND (1658); in this collection, the passage is found on 95–96.

For Cleveland's citation of Chaucer and his reference to Jack Straw's riot in *The Nun's Priest's Tale*, see CLEVELAND (1654); in this collection, the passage is found on 424.

1007. DARE, JOSIAH. *Counsellor Manners, His Last Legacy to His Son.* D249. UMI 2479: 18.

For a paraphrase of a couplet from *The Wife of Bath's Tale* and a precis of an incident related by Chauntecleer in *The Nun's Priest's Tale*, see DARE (1673); in this edition, the passages are found on 3–4, 144–45.

1008. DEFOE, DANIEL. *The Compleat Mendicant or Unhappy Beggar, Being the Life of an Unfortunate Gentleman.* D830. UMI 179: 15.

The protagonist of this sad tale converses with an unfortunate stranger he has met on the road to Oxford. In chapter 3, in a passage about the necessity of cheerfulness and fortitude in the face of distress, Defoe (1661?–1731), or possibly Thomas Price, attributes a couplet to Chaucer:

> I quoted the old Verse to him: *Salamen miseris Socios habuisse doloris.*
> And he replied to me again out of Mr. *Chaucer.*
>> 'Tis vain to Sigh, and make great Moan,
>> For there is help, or there is none.
> And thus in a mutual Condolement of each others Misfortunes, we trudg'd on . . . (22)

1009. FINCH, CHARLES. "Bellositum" in *Musarum Anglicanarum analecta: sive, Poemata quædam melioris notæ.* M3135A. UMI UMI 2292: 5.

For a reference to Chaucer's association with Oxford, see FINCH (1692); in this edition, the passage is found on 14.

1010. HARTLEY, JOHN. *Catalogus universalis librorum.* H973. UMI 420: 4.

In this catalogue of books in the Bodleian Library in Oxford, Hartley (*fl.* 1697–1709) lists:

Chaucer [*Geffrey*] His Work. *Lond.* 1561.
—Tales only, the first Edit. with Prologues and Pictures, of an antient Fr. Charact.
—Works with sev. Additions. *Lond.* 1542.
—Id.with divers Additions, viz. 24 Sheets, with the Siege of *Thebes*, by *John Lidgate* Monck of *Bury*. *Ib.* 1561.
—Id. with the Addition of 7 Tracts, and a Brass Fig. of the Progeny of *Chaucer. Ib.* 1598
—Id. as they have lately been compar'd with the best Manuscripts, and several things added; to which is adjoyned, the Siege of *Thebes*, by *John Lydgate*, Monck of *Bury*; together with the Life of *Chaucer*, and a Table Explaining the old and obscure Words, *&c. Ib.* 1687 (1.4.145)

In a catalogue of books English in Folio:

Chaucer's (Sir *Geoff.*) Works of antient Poetry, (*best Edit.* 16 [*sic*] (2.8.10)

1011. HOLLES, DENZIL. *Memoirs of Denzil Lord Holles, Baron of Ifield in Sussex, from the Year 1641 to 1648.* **H2464. UMI 421: 8.**
Baron Holles (1599–1680) writes sardonically about parliament's tender regard for the rights of the citizens of London and alludes to *The Summoner's Tale*:

> [T]hey are not wanting in their expressions to the City of their tenderness of it, wherefore they would give good instance, coming against it with Banners display'd, Horse and Foot armed, Cannon loaden, and only take possession of their Works and of the Tower, change their Militia, take from them *Westminster* and *Southwark*, commit their Mayor and principal Aldermen, yet doing the City no hurt (like the Fryer in *Chaucer*, who would have but of the Capon the Liver, and of a Pig the head, yet nothing for him should be dead) then marching through it so innocently, only putting that scorn upon them which none of their Kings ever did whe most provok'd. . . . (195–96)

1012. LANGBAINE, GERARD, THE YOUNGER. *The Lives and Characters of the English Dramatic Poets. First Begun by Mr. Langbain, Improv'd and Continued Down to This Time by a Careful Hand.* **L375. UMI 189: 10.**
As Spurgeon notes (1: 270), the "careful hand" mentioned in the title is Charles Gildon. For references to Cowley and Spenser's burial near unto Chaucer in Westminster Abbey and to the Jonson's placement of the *Masque of Queens* in *The House of Fame*, see LANGBAINE (1691); in this edition, the passages are found on 27, 47, 79. In this edition, the passage regarding Dryden's *Troilus and Cressida* has been altered, whether by Langbaine or Gildon is unclear:

Troilus and Cressida, or Truth found out too late, a Tragedy . . . Acted at the Duke's Theatre. One of Mr. *Shakespear's*, altered by Mr *Dryden*. The Story is to be found . . . in our old *Chaucer* in ancient *English*. (47)

In a section on Shakespeare, the author writes:

Troilus and Cressida . . . was reviv'd with Alterations, by Mr. *Dryden*; who added divers new Scenes. Plot from *Chaucer's Troilus and Cressida*. (129).

Other editions in 1699: L376, 27, 47, 79, 129; L376A, 27, 47, 79, 129.

1013. MIEGE, GUY. *The New State of England, Under Our Present Monarch K. William III.* M2022. UMI 1531: 18.

For a reference to Chaucer in a list of famous men of England, see MIEGE (1691); in this edition, the passage is found in part 2, 9–10.

1014. NICOLSON, WILLIAM. *The English Historical Library, Part III.* N1148. UMI 722: 7.

As Alderson & Henderson note, in the second chapter, "Of Acts, Ordinances, Journals, &c. of the Two Houses of Parliament," Nicolson refers to *The Canon's Yeoman's Tale*. In a section on printed statutes, Nicolson writes:

Our Acts of Parliament give often such fair Hints of the Humors most prevailing at the Time of their being enacted, as that many parts of our History may be recover'd from them, especially if compar'd with the Writers, either in Divinity or Morality, about the same Date. Thus, for Example, the Statute against Multiplication of Metals, discovers somewhat of the Ruinous Fancy (which had then seiz'd most of our Nobility) of trying Chymical Conclusions for the Attainment of the Philosopher's Stone; and he that reads *Chaucer's* Tale of the Canon's Yeoman, penn'd about the same time, will have a farther View of the Fashionable Vanity of those Days. (40)

For a reference in the first part, see NICOLSON (1696).

**1015. *The Patentee: or, Some Reflections in Verse on Mr. R– – –'s Forgetting the Design of his Majesty's Bear-Garden at Hockley in the Hole, and Letting Out the Theatre in Dorset-Garden to the Same Use, on the Day When Mr. Dryden's Obsequies Were Perform'd; and Both Play-houses Forbore Acting in Honour of His Memory.* P682. UMI 220: 5.

An unnamed poet addressed this verse epistle to the memory of John Dryden who had recently died and, as he notes, was buried near Chaucer:

Twas well perform'd, as it was well design'd
And Lords and Commons the Procession joyn'd;

· ·

Yet what avails it? That this Prince of Bards,
Has all just Honours paid, and due Regards;
That He in *Chaucer*'s Grave most Nobly sleeps,
And Fame around his Tomb her Vigils keeps:

· ·

As Noise, and Nonsense joyn'd together sit
And descecrates the Hallow'd Seat of WIT. (no pagination; [1])

1016. PHILLIPS, EDWARD. *The Beau's Academy.* P2064. UMI 2854: 35.

For a witty saying attributed to Chaucer, see PHILLIPS, *The Mysteries of Love and Eloquence* (1658); in this edition, the passage is found on 196.

1017. WARD, EDWARD. *The London Spy* **(Jan. 1699). Nelson and Seccombe 236. 103. Early English Newspapers 24: 1173. UMI English Literary Periodicals, reel 128.**

As Spurgeon notes (3: 4.82), in the issue for January 1699, the author recounts a recent trip to Jamaica with a "True Character of the People and Island." There he found plenty of women who were willing to keep him company. He paraphrases a couplet from *The Cook's Tale* (lines 4421–22), as he writes:

> Well, says my Friend, what do you think of all these pritty [*sic*] Ladys [*sic*]? I answer'd, I thought of them as I did of most of the Sex; I suppos'd they were all ready to obey the Laws of Nature, and answer the end of their Creation. Says he, This Place is a Nursery for Husbands, the Merchants Seraglio, for most that you see here, come under *Chaucer*'s Character of a Sempstriss, and so we'll leave them:
>
> > She keeps a Shop for Countenance,
> > And S — for Maintenance. (16)

1018. WARE, JOHN. *A Catalogue of Books in Several Faculties & Languages.* **C1285B. UMI 2751: 8.**

On 2 May 1699 at 3 o'clock in the afternoon, Ware began auctioning a "Choice Collection" of books at Dick's Coffee-House in Skinner Row in Dublin. In the sales catalogue, in the sixth session, among the books in folio, number 23 is listed as "*Chaucers* works" (14).

1700

1019.   A., J. "Commedatory Poem" in *Lucretius His Six Books of Epicurian Philosophy.* **L3450. UMI 1406: 1.**

For a reference to Chaucer's connection to Cambridge and his having been inspired by the River Cam, see A., J. (1683); in this edition, the passage is found on sig. C4v.

1020.   B., R. "On Our English Poetry," in Nahum Tate's *Panacea: A Poem upon Tea.* **T202. UMI 551: 8.**

In a commendatory poem headed "On our English Poetry, and this Poem upon Tea," R. B. mentions Chaucer:

> The *British* Lawrel by Old *Chaucer* worn,
> Still *Fresh* and *Gay*, did *Dryden*'s Brow Adorn:
> And that its Lustre may not fade on Thine,
> Wit, Fancy, Judgment, *Tate*, in thee combine. (sig. A6r)

1021.   BRITAINE, WILLIAM DE. *Humane Prudence.* **B4807A. UMI 2440: 9.**

For a spurious quotation attributed to Chaucer, see BRITAINE (1686); in this edition, the passage is found on 99.

1022.   BROWN, THOMAS. *A Description of Mr. D[ryde]n's Funeral. A Poem.* **B5056. UMI 271: 12.**

Spurgeon (1. 288) cites this satirical poem against Dryden but without attribution to Brown (1663–1704). Brown, perhaps stung with envy of Dryden's great fame and success when compared to his own miserable existence, concludes by citing Chaucer in company with Cowley and Spencer:

> And when on t'other Shoar he's landed safe,
> A Crowd of Fools attend him to the Grave,
> A Crowd so nauseous, so profusely lewd,
> With all the Vices of the Times endu'd,
> *That Cowley's Marble wept to see the Throng*,
> Old *Chaucer* laugh'd at their unpolish'd Song,
> And *Spencer* thought he once again had seen
> The Imps attending of his *Fairy Queen*. (8)

Other editions in 1700: B5057, *The Second Edition*, 8; B5058, *The Third Edition*, *with Additions*, 10.

1023. BULLORD, JOHN. *A Catalogue of the Libraries of Sr Andrew Henley and an Eminent Clergyman, Both Deceased.* H1449. UMI 2187: 10.

Bullard began auctioning two libraries "Consisting of Theological, Historical, Philological, Mathematical, and Medicinal Authors, in the Greek, Latin, Spanish, French, and English Tongues" and a number of prints by Italian and French masters at Tom's Coffee-House on "Monday the 12th instant" at 3 o'clock in the afternoon. The eminent clergyman is unknown and little is known of Henley other than that he was born around 1622 or 1623. In the sales catalogue, under the heading "English, Divinity, History, &c. in Folio," lot 36 is listed as "*Geffery Chaucers* Works 1542"; and number 75 as "*Jeffrey Chaucers* Works, the last Edit. With his Life 1687" (36).

1024. BULLORD, JOHN. *A Catalogue of the Library of Ralph Hough, Esq.* H2911. UMI 2868: 12

Bullord scheduled the sale of Hough's extensive library at Tom's Coffee House on "Tuesday the 16th instant [1700?]" at three in the afternoon. Under the heading "English Books in Folio," lot 79 is listed as "*Chaucers* Works 1687" (46).

1025. BULLORD, JOHN. *Catalogus libris exquisitissimis rarissimisque.* C1429. UMI 2474: 15.

On Monday, 20 June 1700, at 1 o'clock in the afternoon, with the express permission of Oxford's Vice-chancellor, Bullord began auctioning a large collection of books, mainly Latin works printed abroad ("*Typographos illustrissimos, elegantissime reperiuntur impressi*"), at the "Schola Moralis Philosophiæ." In the catalogue, under the heading "Libri Omissi in Folio," number 6 is listed as "*The Works of Geffrey Chaucer.* London 1561" (54). In the Folger Library copy of the catalogue, someone noted that the volume sold for 4s.

1026. COBB, SAMUEL. *Poetæ Britannici, a Poem Satyrical and Panegyrical.* C4773. UMI 1648: 9.

As Spurgeon notes (1: 271–72), Cobb (1675–1713) praises Chaucer with backhanded compliments:

> Sunk in a Sea of Ignorance we lay,
> Till *Chaucer* rose, and pointed out the Day.
> A Joking Bard, whose Antiquated Muse,
> In mouldy Words could solid Sence produce.
> Our *English Ennius* He, who claim'd his part
> In wealthy Nature, tho' unskill'd in Art.
> The sparkling Diamond on his Dung-hill shines,
> And Golden Fragments glitter in his Lines.
> Which *Spencer* gather'd, for his Learning known,

And by successful Gleanings made his own

. . . .

Mæonides and *Virgil* had been Thine!
Their finish'd Poems he exactly view'd,
But *Chaucer*'s Steps Religiously pursu'd.
He cull'd and pick'd, and thought it greater praise,
T' adore his Master, than improve his Phrase.
'Twas counted Sin to deviate from his Page;
So Sacred was th' Authority of Age!
The Coin must sure for currant Sterling pass,
Stamp'd with old *Chaucer*'s Venerable Face. (10)

1027. CONGREVE, WILLIAM. *The Way of the World.* **C5878. UMI 60: 10.**

This comedy by Congreve (1670–1729) was "acted at the theatre in Lincoln's-Inn-Fields by His Majesty's servants" (title page). In the first act, Congreve, following the example of Shakespeare, Dryden, and others in calling Pertelote *Partlet*, and thus alludes to *The Nun's Priest's Tale.* Having been told by a servant that he had witnessed a couple getting married, Mirabell responds:

> Do you go home again, d'ee hear, and adjourn the Consummation till
> further Order; bid *Waitwell* shake his Ears, and Dame *Partlet* rustle up
> her Feathers, and meet me at One a Clock by *Rosamond*'s Pond. (5)

1028. COWLEY, ABRAHAM. *The Works of Mr. Abraham Cowley.* **C6660. UMI 709: 23.**

For a reference to Cowley's burial place near Chaucer, see SPRAT (1668); in this edition, the passage is found on sig. b5v.

For a reference to Chaucer's "rich rhymes," see COWLEY (1656), C6683; in this edition, the passage is found on 96 (sig. Q4v).

1029. DRYDEN, JOHN. *Fables Ancient and Modern, Translated into Verse from Homer, Ovid, Boccace & Chaucer: With Original Poems.* **D2278. UMI 1503: 7.**

As Spurgeon notes (1: 272–85), Dryden pays homage to Chaucer throughout his preface (sigs. *A1r–*D2v). In a passage about the lineage of English poetry, Dryden writes:

> *Spencer* and *Fairfax* both flourish'd in the Reign of Queen *Elizabeth*:
> Great Masters in our Language . . . *Milton* was the Poetical Son of
> *Spencer*, and . . . *Spencer* more than once insinuates, that the Soul of
> *Chaucer* was transsus'd into his Body; and that he was begotten by him
> Two hundred years after his Decease. *Milton* has acknowledg'd to me,
> that *Spencer* was his Original; and many besides my self have heard our

famous *Waller* own, that he deriv'd the Harmony of his Numbers from
the *Godfrey of Bulloign*, which was turn'd into *English* by Mr. *Fairfax*. But
to return: Having done with *Ovid* for this time, it came into my mind,
that our old *English* Poet *Chaucer* in many Things resembled him, and
that with no disadvantage on the on the Side of the Modern Author, as I
shall endeavor to prove when I compare them: And as I am, and always
have been studious to promote the Honour of my Native Country, so
I soon resolv'd to put their Merits to the Trial, by turning some of the
Canterbury Tales into our Language, as it is now refin'd. . . . [T]o follow the Thrid[53] of my Discourse . . . from *Chaucer* I was led to think on
Boccace, who was not only his Contemporary, but also pursu'd the same
Studies. . . . He and *Chaucer*, among other Things, had this in common,
that they refin'd their Mother-Tongues, but with this difference. . . .
Chaucer (as you have formerly been told by our learn'd Mr. *Rhymer*) first
adorn'd and amplified our barren Tongue from the Provencall, which
was then the most polish'd of all the Modern Languages: But this Subject has been copiously treated by that great Critick, who deserves no
little Commendation from us his Countrymen. For these Reasons of
Time, and Resemblance of Genius, in *Chaucer* and *Boccace*, I resolv'd to
join them in my present Work. . . . (sig. A1r–v)

I proceed to *Ovid*, and *Chaucer*; considering the former only in
relation to the latter. With *Ovid* ended the Golden Age of the *Roman*
Tongue: From *Chaucer* the Purity of the English Tongue began. The
Manners of the Poets were not unlike: Both of them were well-bred,
well-natur'd, amorous, and Libertine, at least in their Writings, it may
be also in their Lives. Their Studies were the same, Philosophy, and
Philology. Both of them were knowing in Astronomy, of which Ovid's
Books of the *Roman* Feasts, and *Chaucer*'s Treatise of the *Astrolabe*, are
sufficient Witnesses. But *Chaucer* was likewise an Astrologer. . . . Both
writ with wonderful Facility and Clearness; neither were great Inven-
tors: For *Ovid* only copied the *Grecian* Fables; and most of *Chaucer*'s Stories were taken from his *Italian* Contemporaries, or their Predecessors:
Boccace his *Decameron* was first publish'd; and from thence our *Englishman* has borrow'd many of his *Canterbury* Tales: Yet that of *Palamon*
and *Arcite* was written in all probability by some *Italian* Wit, in a former
Age; as I shall prove hereafter: The Tale of *Grizild* was the Invention of
Petrarch; by him sent to *Boccace*; from whom it came to *Chaucer*: *Troilus*
and *Cressida* was also written by a *Lombard* Author;[54] but much amplified by our *English* Translatour, as well as beautified. . . . [But to return
to] *Ovid* and *Chaucer*, of whom I have little more to say. Both of them

---

[53] *Thrid*: thread.
[54] Lombard author is commonly known as Lollius.

built on the Inventions of other Men; yet since *Chaucer* had something
of his own, as *The Wife of Baths Tale, The Cock and the Fox*, which I have
translated, and some other, I may justly give our Countryman the Pre-
cedence in that Part. . . . Both of them understood the Manners; under
which Name I comprehend the Passions, and, in a larger Sence, the
Descriptions of Persons, and their very Habits: For an Example, I see
Baucis and *Philemon* as perfectly before me, as if some ancient Painter
had drawn them; and all the Pilgrims in the *Canterbury* Tales, their
Humours, their Features, and the very Dress, as distinctly as if I had
supp'd with them at the *Tabard* in *Southwark*: Yet even there too the
Figures of *Chaucer* are much more lively, and set in a better Light. . . .
The Thoughts and Words remain to be consider'd . . . [I acknowledge]
that *Ovid* liv'd when the *Roman* Tongue was in its Meridian; *Chaucer*,
in the Dawning of our Language: Therefore that Part of the Comparison stands not on an equal Foot, any more than the Diction of *Ennius*
and *Ovid*; or of *Chaucer*, and our present *English*. . . . The Vulgar Judges
. . . who call Conceits and Jingles Wit, who see *Ovid* full of them, and
Chaucer altogether without them, will think me little less than mad,
for preferring the *Englishman* to the *Roman*: Yet, with their leave, I
must presume to say, that the Things they admire are only glittering
Trifles. . . . *Chaucer* makes *Arcite* violent in his Love, and unjust in the
Pursuit of it: Yet when he came to die, he made him think more rea-
sonably: he repents not of his Love, for that had alter'd his Character;
but acknowledges the Injustice of his Proceedings, and resigns *Emilia*
to *Palamon*. What would *Ovid* have done on this Occasion? He would
certainly have made *Arcite* witty on his Death-bed. He had complain'd
he was farther off from Possession, by being so near, and a thousand
such Boyisms, which *Chaucer* rejected as below the Dignity of the Subject. . . . It remains that I say somewhat of *Chaucer* in particular.

In the first place, As he is the Father of English Poetry, so I hold
him in the same Degree of Veneration as the Grecians held Homer, or
the Romans Virgil: He is a perpetual Fountain of good Sense; learn'd in
all Sciences; and therefore speaks properly on all Subjects: As he knew
what to say . . .

As Spurgeon also notes (1: 284–85), Dryden places Chaucer in the company of
Homer and Virgil in an epistolary poem addressed "To Her Grace the Dutchess
of Ormond":

The Bard who first adorn'd our Native Tongue
Tun'd to his *British* Lyre this ancient Song:
Which *Homer* might without a Blush reherse,
And leaves a doubtful Palm in *Virgil*'s Verse:

He match'd their Beauties, where they most excell;
Of Love sung better, and of Arms as well.
Vouchsafe, Illustrious *Ormond*, to behold
What Pow'r the Charms of Beauty had of old;
Nor wonder if such Deeds of Arms were done,
Inspir'd by two fair Eyes, that sparkled like your own.
If *Chaucer* by the best Idea wrought,
And Poets can divine each others Thought,
The fairest Nymph before his Eyes he set;
And then te fairest was *Plantagenet*;
. . . .
O true *Plantagenet*, O Race Divine,
(For Beauty still is fatal to the Line,)
Had *Chaucer* liv'd that Angel-Face to view,
Sure he had drawn his *Emily* from You.
Or had You liv'd, to judge the doubtful Right,
Your Noble *Palamon* had been the Knight:
And Conqu'ring *Theseus* from his Side had sent
Your Gen'rous Lord, to guide the *Theban* Government.
Time shall accomplish that; and I shall see
A *Palamon* in Him, in You an *Emily*. (sig. A1r–2r)

As Spurgeon notes (1: 285), Dryden's versions of various of Chaucer's works are found herein: *The Knight's Tale*, headed "Palamon and Arcite, or the Knight's Tale from Chaucer," (1–99); *The Nun's Priest's Tale*, headed "The Cock and the Fox; or The Tale of the Nun's Priest from Chaucer," (223–53); *The Flower and the Leaf*, headed "The Flower and the Leaf; or The Lady in the Arbour. A Vision," (383–405); *The Wife of Bath's Tale*, headed "The Wife of Bath Her Tale," (477–99), *The Parson's Tale*, headed "The Character of a Good Parson. Imitated from Chaucer and Inlarg'd," (531–36). Chaucer's original versions of these tales are found on 567–646.

1030. *An Epistle to S*ʳ *Richard Blackmore, Occasion'd by the New Session of the Poets.* E3167. UMI 28: 10.

This anonymous verse epistle is addressed to Sir Richard Blackmore (d. 1729) in commiseration for his having been attacked by unkind critics. The poet laments the corruption of modern times, cites Chaucer as an example of old-time virtue:

The former Times produc'd prodigious Men
During the Reigns of *Chaucer* and of *Ben*,
Who show'd a Virtuous and exalted Mind,
Which from that time has ever since declin'd.

Cowley indeed endeavor'd to retrieve
The Fame of Verse, and Life to Virtue give;
But that vile Age was in League with Hell,
And he in the Attempt successless fell. (9)

1031.   *Familiar and Courtly Letters*. V682. UMI 1077: 14.

"Mr. B—," a resident of Covent Garden, writing in response to a lady's note, laments the lack of wit in contemporary poetry and notes that things were different in Chaucer's day:

> *Poetasters* are grown as numerous in this *Town* as *Quack-Doctors* at *London*, and every one so applies himself to the *Stage*, that the *White-fryars Printers* are quite beggar'd for want of *Balads* [*sic*]: Yet *Wit*, I observe, is as scarce as 'twas in the time of *Jeffry Chaucer*, when a *Distich* of *Verses* were worth a *Page* of *Prose*, and a *Song*, with a *Fa-la-la Chorus*, was much more listen'd to than a *Sermon*. (259)

1032.   FLAVEL, JOHN. *Husbandry Spiritualized: or, The Heavenly Use of Earthly Things. The Sixth Edition*. F1168.

For an echo of a line from *The Reeve's Prologue*, see FLAVEL (1669); in this edition, the passage is found on 330–31.

1033.   *The Flying Post: or, The Post-Master*. Nelson and Seccombe 156.782.

As Spurgeon notes (1: 286), but does not transcribe, there is an account of Dryden's funeral in the issue covering events of 14 May 1700. A reporter writes:

> Yesterday the corps [*sic*] of Mr. *Dryden*, the Poet, was honourably attended from the College of Physicians to the place of interment in *Westminster-Abby*, near the two famous poets, *Cowley* and *Chaucer*.[55] (verso)

1034.   H., N. "[In obitum celeberrimi Joannis Dryden]" in *Luctus Britannici: or, The Tears of the British Muses for the Death of John Dryden*. L3451. UMI 216: 8.

As Spurgeon notes (1: 288), but does not transcribe, a poet modestly identifies himself by his initials only in Latin verses written in memory of Dryden. He writes:

> Mamora Chauceri lacrymas, Couleiaq[ue] [illegible]
> Dum Drydene pium perficis Arte Chorum.

---

[55] This transcription is taken from Edmond Malone's edition of *The Critical and Miscellaneous Prose of Works of John Dryden* (London: H. Baldwin and Son, 1800), vol. 1, pt. 1, 379.

Dormis? an Moreris? non dormio: Musa Poëtis
Vix dormire dedit; sed minùs illi mori. (²15)

1035. HALL, HENRY. "To the Memory of John Dryden, Esq." in *Luctus Britannici: or, The Tears of the British Muses for the Death of John Dryden*. L3451. UMI 216: 8.

As Spurgeon notes (1: 286–87), a poem by Hall (ca. 1656–1707) is included in this collection of poems "By the Most Eminent Hands in the two Famous Universities, and by several Others" that commemorated the death of Dryden. Hall alludes to Dryden's "translation" of some of Chaucer's *Tales*, to his interment in Westminster Abbey near Chaucer, to Chaucer's influence on Spenser's poetry, and to Chaucer as the progenitor of the English literary tradition. He writes:

> *Greece* had a *Homer*; *Rome* a *Virgil* lost,
> And well *Britannia* do's her *Dryden* Boast:
> And still shall Boast the Beauties of the Dead,
> And with the freshest Bays adorn his Head.
> . . . .
> New Cloath'd by You, how *Chaucer* we esteem;
> When You've new Polish'd it, how bright the Jem!
> And lo, the Sacred Shade for thee mak's room,
> Thô Souls so like, should take but up one Tomb.
> . . . .
> Let us look back, and Noble Numbers trace
> Directly up from Ours, to *Chaucer*'s days;
> *Chaucer*, the first of Bards in Tune that Sung,
> And to a better bent reduc'd the stubborn Tongue.
> *Spencer* upon his Master much refin'd,
> He Colour'd sweetly, tho he ill Design'd;
> Too mean the Model for so vast a Mind.
> Thus while he try's to make his Stanza's Chime,
> Good *Christian* Thoughts turn *Renegade* to Rhime. (16–20)

1036. HARRINGTON, JAMES. *The Oceana of James Harrington, and His Other Works*. H816. UMI 533: 19.

For an echo a line from *The Reeve's Tale*, see HARRINGTON (1656); in this edition, the passage is found on 181–82.

1037. HIGGONS, BEVILL. "In celeberrimum Joannem Dryden Chauceri Sepulchro Intectum" in *Luctus Britannici: or, The Tears of the British Muses for the Death of John Dryden.* L3451. UMI 216: 8.

As Spurgeon notes (1: 288), but does not transcribe, Bevill Higgons (1670–1736) wrote some Latin verses in memory of Dryden:

> Suaviter hic longo dormi defuncte labore,
> Dum jungit socios una Caverna sinus;
> Dumq[ue] tuas canimus laudes, hæc accipe blanda
> Mente, minor Vatum quæ tibi turba damus.
> Galfridi exuvias quæ prisci incluserat olim
> Hospite lætetur Nobilis Urna novo:
> Drydeni cineres terrâ hac capiente repôstos,
> Chaucerus tumulo splendidiore jacet:
> O par fœlices! hac quis mercede srescuset
> Unâ vobiscum concubuisse, Mori? (28)

1038. *Luctus Britannici: or, The Tears of the British Muses for the Death of John Dryden.* L3451. UMI 216: 8.

As Spurgeon notes (1: 286–88), a number of poems commemorating the death of Dryden were collected and published by the booksellers Henry Playford (*vide supra*) and Abel Roper. An unsigned poem is headed "To the Memory of John Dryden, Esq." The poet writes:

> Celestial Muse, whose God-head could inspire
> The Bards of Old, with Rays of Genial Fire,
> And Teach 'em with Harmonious Tunes to raise,
> Immortal Structures, to their *Hero*'s praise;
> By whom ev'n late Posterity might know,
> How much the greatest Men to Poets owe.
> . . . .
> The Muse is fled,
> And there amongst the mighty Rivals, dead.
> Methinks I see the Reverend Shades prepare
> With Songs of Joy, to waft thee through the Air.
> And lead Thee o're the bright Ætherial Fields,
> To tast the Bliss which their *Elizium* yields.
> Where *Chaucer, Johnson, Shakespear,* and the rest,
> Kindly embrace their venerable Guest,
> Then in a Chorus sing an Ode of Praise,
> And Crown thy Temple with Eternal Bays.
> Whilst we in pensive Sables clad below

Bear hence in solemn Grief, and pompous Woe,
Thy sacred Dust to *Chaucer*'s peaceful Urn,
And round they awful Tomb profusely mourn. [Etc.] (34–36)

Another unsigned poem is headed "To Dr. Samuel Garth, occasioned by the much Lamented Death of John Dryden, Esq." A poet alludes to Dryden's modernization of some of Chaucer's *Tales* and the difficulty modern readers had with Chaucer's language:

Yet though his [Dryden's] Works are all sublimely Great,
And dare the Teeth of Time, and Rage of Fate;
. . . .
His latest Work, though in His last decays,
As far exceeds His former as Our Praise.
And *Chaucer* shall again with Joy be Read,
Whose Language with its Master lay for Dead,
'Til *Dryden*, striving His Remains to save,
Sunk in His *Tomb*, who *brought* him from his *Grave*. (55)

As Spurgeon also notes (1: 288), but does not transcribe, there are also a number of Latin poems with references to Chaucer that commemorate the life and talent of Dryden. Some are signed, but one is not.

In "Gallus" an unknown poet writes:

Nota tibi ante alios imprimis Fabula vates,
Virtutem arcanam, & morum Mysteria sacra
Intùs habens, qualem Chauceri sæpe canebat
Simplex munditie, & sine luxu culta Camœna. (25)

1039. MILLINGTON, EDWARD. *A Catalogue of Ancient and Modern Books.* **C1275. UMI 1647: 14.**

Millington held an auction for the entertainment and diversion of the gentry and citizens of Norwich and environs on 2 December 1700 at Mr. G. Rose's house. In the catalogue, under the heading "Miscellanies, in Folio," number 126 is listed as "*Chaucer*'s Works—1596" (20); the date is puzzling. Under the heading "Miscellanies, in Octavo, Twelves, &c.," lot 207 is listed as "*Chaucer*'s Ghost [no date]" (26).

1039a. MONTAIGNE, MICHEL DE. *Essays.* **M2481. UMI 795: 37 and UMI 796: 1.**

For an echo of a line from *The Reeve's Tale*, see MONTAIGNE (1685); in this edition, the passage is found on 191.

1040. *The New Wife of Beath* [*sic*], *Much Better Reformed*. N796. UMI 1783: 15.

Beath is a variant spelling of *Bath*, so the title carries an obvious allusion to Chaucer's good woman. As Spurgeon notes (1: 288), this work is an enlargement of *The Wanton Wife of Bath*, W719B (ca. 1641), q.v. There is, moreover, a clear reference to Chaucer in the opening lines:

> 𝔍n 𝔅eath, once dwelt a worthy 𝔚ife,
> 𝔒f whom brave 𝔆haucer mention makes
> 𝔖he lived a 𝔏icentious life,
> 𝔄nd namely in 𝔙enerial 𝔄cts. (2)

1041. OLDYS, ALEXANDER. *An Ode, By Way of Elegy, on the Universally Lamented Death of the Incomparable Mr. Dryden*. O267. UMI 218: 4.

Oldys gathers a mighty choir of poets—Rochester, Buckingham, Orrery, Davenant, Denham, Suckling, Shakespeare, Jonson, Beaumont, Fletcher, Spenser, and Drayton—to bewail the passing of Dryden. Chaucer then is introduced:

> Our *English Ennius*, He who gave,
> To *The Great Bard* kind welcom to his Grave,
> *Chaucer*, the *Mighty'st Bard* of yore,
> Whose Verse cou'd Mirth, to saddest Souls restore,
> Caress'd him next whil'st his delighted Eye,
> Express'd his Love, and thus his Tongue his Joy,
>   Was I, when erst Below (said he)
>   In hopes so Great a Bard to see:
> As *Thou my Son*, Adopted into *me*,
> And all this *Godlike Race*, some equal ev'n to Thee!
>   O! tis enough. — Here soft *Orinda* came,
>   And Sprightly *Astra*, Muses Both on Earth;
>   Both Burn'd here with a Bright Poetic flame,
>   Which to their happiness *above* gave birth;
>   Their Charming Songs, his entertainment close
> The *mighty Bard* then smiling, Bow'd and 'rose. (6)

In the Folger Library copy of this work, someone has underlined *Orinda* and *Astra* and written in the margin: "Mrs Phillips" and "Mrs Behn."

1042. OSBORNE, FRANCIS. *The Works of Francis Osborn. The Tenth Edition.* O507A. UMI 2838: 13.

For a reference to a bishop who boasted that he had never read a line of Calvin or Chaucer, see OSBORNE (1658); in this collection, the passage is found on 396.

1043. *The Patentee*. P682. UMI 220: 5.

The subtitle of this anonymous broadside is "Some Reflections in Verse on Mr. R—'s [Christopher Rich] forgetting the Design of his Majesty's Bear-Garden at Hockly in the Hole, and letting out the Theatre in Dorset-Garden to the same Use, on the Day when Mr. Dryden's Obsequies were perform'd; And both Play-houses forbore Acting in Honour to his Memory." As Bowyer notes (*SP* 28), in the body of the text, the unknown author places Dryden in company with Chaucer:

> Yet what avails it? That this Prince of Bards,
> Has all just Honours paid, and due Regards;
> That He in *Chaucer's* Grave most Nobly sleeps,
> And Fame around his Tomb her Vigils keeps.

1044. PHILLIPS, EDWARD. *The New World of Words*: or, *A Universal English Dictionary*. P2074. UMI 2729: 3.

For a pictorial representation of Chaucer on the engraved title page and for references to him in the preface (in this edition, no pagination or signature), see PHILLIPS (1658), (1662), (1671), (1678), and (1696). References to Chaucer in earlier editions are also found in definitions of *Abawed* (sig. A1v), *Acale* (sig. A2v), *Achecked* (sig. A3r), *Acloyed* (sig. A3r), *Adventaile* (sig. B1r), *Agilted* (sig. B2v), *Agredge* (sig. B2v), *Agroted* (sig. B2v), *Agrutched* (sig. B2v), *Aledge* (sig. B4r), *Amalgaminge* (sig. C1r), *Amortize* (sig. C2r), *Arblaster* (sig. D3r), *Argoil* (sig. D3v), *Arret* (sig. D4r), *Arten* (sig. D4v), *Assoyle* (sig. E1v), *Asterlagour* (sig. E1v), *Autremite* (sig. E4r), *Barm-cloth* (sig. F1v), *Bay* (sig. F2v), *Bend* (sig. F4v), *Burnet* (sig. H1r), *Caitisned* (sig. H2v), *Chasteleyn* (sig. K2v), *Chekelaton* (sig. garbled), *Chelandri* (sig. garbled), *Chertes* (sig. garbled), *Chevesal* (sig. garbled), *Chimbe* (sig. garbled), *Chincherie* (sig. garbled), *Cierges* (sig. K3r), *Citriale* (sig. K4r), *Clergion* (sig. Aa1r), *Clicket*, (sig. Aa1r), *Clinket* (sig. Aa1r), *Curebulli* (sig. Dd1r), *Dennington* (sig. Ee1v), *Desidery* (sig. Ee2v), *Deslavy* (sig. Ee2v), *Digne* (sig. Ee4v), *Discure* (sig. Ff1v), *Divine* (sig. Ff2v), *Dowtremere* (sig. Dd4r), *Ebrack* (sig. Gg2r), *Fonne* (sig. Kk3v), *Gibsere* (sig. Aaa1r), *Giglet* (sig. Aaa1r), *Gourd* (sig. Aaa2v), *Haketon* (sig. Bbb1r), *Hanselines* (sig. Bbb1v), *Jewise* (sig. Ddd1r), *Losenger* (sig. Hhh4r), *Mangon* or *Magonel* (sig. Iii3r), *Miswoman* (sig. Aaaa3v), *Rebeck* (sig. Iiii2v), *Woodstock* (sig. Hhhh4r).

1045. PIX, MARY. *To the Right Honourable Earl of Kent . . . This Poem*. P2332a. UMI 2504: 11.

In praising the Henry Grey, Earl of Kent (1671–1740), Mrs. Pix links Chaucer and Spenser with Homer and Virgil:

[T]he Sovereign Queen of Fame,
Whose tuneful Art Records each noble Name:
She Sings the illustrious Virtues of the Great,
And makes them dear to each succeeding State. (4)
. . . .
Hence 'tis we Poetry and Musick trace,
And find both of bright Immortal Race:
. . . .
I heard them sigh and long to sound your Name,
And write it large in the great Book of Fame.
. . . .
In her smooth hand an open Scrole she bore,
Inscrib'd with Names I oft had seen before;
Immortal *Homer, Virgil* most Divine,
The Poets of the *Greek* and *Latin* Line,
But turning quick I found the British Race,
A numerous Stock, and fill'd a glorious Space;
Chaucer and *Spencer* were preserv'd with care,
But *D R Y D E N* did in Capitals appear. (6)

1046. PLAYFORD, HENRY. "Advertisement" in *The Postboy*. **Tuesday, 7 May 1700. Nelson and Seccombe 554.792.**

As Spurgeon notes (1: 286), Playford mentions Dryden's interment near Chaucer. In an advertisement inviting submissions of poetry for a memorial volume (*Luctus Britannici*) in Dryden's honor, Playford writes:

> The Death of the famous John Dryden, Esq., . . . being a Subject Capable of Employing the Best Pens; and several Persons of Quality, and others having put a stop to his Interment, which is designed to be in Chaucer's Grave, in Westminster-Abbey; This is to desire the Gentlemen of the two famous Universities, and others, who have a Repect for the Memory of the Deceas'd, and are inclinable to such performance, to send what Copies they please, as Epigrams, &c., to Henry Playford . . . and they shall be inserted in a Collection. . . .

1047. *The Post Boy.* **Nelson and Seccombe 554.793.**

As Spurgeon notes (1: 286), but does not transcribe, in the issue for 4–7 May 1700, there is a notice of Dryden's impending funeral that observes that Dryden will be buried near Chaucer:

> The Corps [*sic*] of John Dryden, Esq; is to lye in State for some time, in the Colledge of Physicians, and on Monday next, he is to be Conveyed

from thence in a Hearse in great Splendor to Westminster Abbey, where he is to be Interred with Chaucer, Cowley, and the rest of the renowned Poets. . . . (verso)

1048. *The Post Boy.* **Nelson and Seccombe 554.795.**

In an account dated Tuesday 14 May 1700, a reporter writes:

The Corps [*sic*] of the great and Witty Poet, John Dryden . . . was yesterday carried in great state to Westminster-Abbey, where he was interred with Chaucer, Cowley, &c. (verso)

1049. *The Post Man.* **Nelson and Seccombe 555.319A.**

As Spurgeon notes (1: 286), but does not transcribe, there is an account of Dryden's funeral in the issue for 11–14 May 1700. A reporter writes of the obsequies of 14 May but does not mention interment near Chaucer in Westminster Abbey.

1050. SCARRON, PAUL. *Scarron's Novels.* **S836. UMI 2019: 12**

For an echo of a line from *The General Prologue to The Canterbury Tales*, see SCARRON (1665); in this edition, the passage is found on 24.

1051. SHAKESPEARE, WILLIAM. *King Henry IV. With the Humours of Sir John Falstaff. A Tragi-comedy. As It Is Acted at the Theatre in Little-Lincolns-Inn-Fields by His Majesty's Servants. Revived, with Alterations. Written Originally by Mr. Shakespear.* **S2928. UMI 297: 27.**

For verbal parallels and similarities to *The Nun's Priest's Tale*, see SHAKESPEARE (1598), Boswell & Holton No. 613.

1052. TONSON, JACOB. "Catalogue" in William Congreve's *The Way of the World.* **C5878. UMI 60: 10.**

At the end of this work, there is a list of books printed for Jacob Tonson and offered for sale at his establishment within Gray's Inn Gate by Gray's Inn Lane. In the second title, there is a reference to Chaucer: "*Fables Antient and Modern. Translated into Verse from* Homer, Ovid, Boccace, Chaucer, *with Original Poems by Mr.* Dryden" (sig. N2v).

1053. TROTTER, CATHERINE. "The Heroick Muse" in *The Nine Muses: or, Poems Written by Nine Several Ladies upon the Death of the Late Famous John Dryden, Esq.* N1159. UMI 218: 2.

As Bowyer notes (*SP* 28), Catherine Trotter (Mrs. Patrick Cockburn) (1674?–1749) alludes to Dryden's modernized version of Chaucer's tales. She yokes Chaucer with Virgil, and they team up to sing Dryden's praise. Trotter writes:

> Cease all my tuneful Sisters, now refrain
> Your sacred Fire, you lavish it in vain,
> At least no grateful Vows I e're shall hear again.
> *Dryden*'s no more!. . . . .
> . . . .
> With *Virgil, Chaucer* sings Great *Dryden*'s Name,
> Who gave new luster to his darkned Fame;
> Dispel'd the Clouds by which he was conceal'd,
> And to his native Isle the Bard reveal'd;
> Not blest enough in his own glorious State,
> Till he to them a part Communicate. (15–17)

1054. VERNON, HENRY. "In Memoriam Joannis Dryden," in *Luctus Britannici: or, The Tears of the British Muses for the Death of John Dryden.* L3451. UMI 216: 8.

As Spurgeon notes (1: 288), but does not transcribe, Vernon wrote Latin verses in memory of Dryden. Vernon writes of Dryden's interment near Chaucer:

> Nemo Poetarum sic scripsit, nemo Sepulchro
> Aut potuit moriens Nobiliore Tegi.
> Inde jacent cineres *Chauceri*, atque inde *Denhami*
> Unbraque dat socios dextra, sinistra sinus.
> Sed quod in Æternos jam vivis mortuus Annos,
> Insequiturque Tuos Assequa Famo rogos,
> Hoc tibi non totum dedes, dum *Garthus*[56] amicum
> Et *Montacutus* junxerit almus opem.
> Nec tibi defuncto sic grates solveret Ætas,
> Ni daret Hic *Laudes,* Hic *Momumenta* daret. (218)

1055. *The Wanton Wife of Bath.* W723B. No UMI.

For an allusion to Chaucer's wife of Bath, see *The Wanton Wife of Bath* (1641).

---

[56] Samuel Garth

1056. WARD, EDWARD, ed. *The London Spy.* **Nelson and Seccombe 236.206.**

As Spurgeon notes (1: 286), but does not transcribe, Ward (1667–1731) penned a poem titled "To the Pious Memory of the most Sublime and Accurate Mr. *John Dryden*" that mentions Chaucer more than once. In the second stanza, Ward writes:

> *May Envy let His Dust in Quite Sleep;*
> *And Fame Eternal in his Volumes dwell;*
> *Whilst* Chaucer's *Sacred Tomb his Ashes keep,*
> *Ages shall o'er his Golden Writings Weep;*
> *And thus the melting Force of his strong Lines shall feel.* (6)

> Chaucer *and Cowley, gladly would Receive*
> *Thy Frozen Clay, into their silent Tomb;*
> *Desiring their Applause with yours might Live,*
> *In hopes your Fame, Eternity might give*
> *To theirs, and that your Lawrels might together Bloom.* (8)

As Spurgeon notes (3: 4.82), there is a reference which refers to Dryden's funeral and his burial near Chaucer. Ward writes:

> [T]he nobility and gentry attended the hearse to Westminster-Abbey, where . . . the last funeral rites being performed by one of the Prebends, he [i.e., Dryden] was honourably interred between Chaucer and Cowley. . . . (422)

1057. WARD, EDWARD. *A Step to the Bath: With a Character of the Place.* **W758. UMI 1161: 20.**

As Bowyer notes (*SP* 28), Ward's narrator refers to "Chaucer's Sempstress," a faint allusion to *The Cook's Tale* (lines 4421–22), in a passage about the types of people who congregated at Bath to take the waters. He characterizes the resort as "a Valley of Pleasure, yet a sink of Iniquity; Nor is there any Intrigues or Debauch Acted at *London*, but is Mimick'd there" (16):

> In the Evening we took a Walk into the Meadows, much resorted to for pleasant Rivers, and delicate Walks; 'tis a second *Hide-Park* for Coaches, and a St. *James*'s for *Beau*'s and *Belsa*'s of all sorts; there was *Chaucer*'s Sempstress, my Lord *R*—Mantua-Makers dandled by Cringing Fops, Antick Beaus, and Blustering Bullies innumerable. . . . (16)

Another edition in 1700: W759, 16.

1058. WESLEY, SAMUEL. *An Epistle to a Friend Concerning Poetry.* W1370. UMI 1559: 20.

As Spurgeon notes (1: 289), Wesley (1662–1735) and his contemporaries had difficulty with Chaucer's verse. Wesley writes:

> Of Chaucer's Verse we scarce the *Measures* know,
> So *rough* the *Lines*, and so *unequal* flow;
> Whether by Injury of *Time* defac'd,
> Or *careless* at the *first*, and writ in *haste*;
> Or *coursly*, like old *Ennius*, he *design'd*
> What After-days have *polish'd* and *refin'd*.
> Spencer more *smooth* and *neat*, and none that He
> Could better skill of *English Quantity*;
> Tho by his *Stanza* cramp'd, his *Rhimes* less chast,
> And *antique Words* affected all disgrac'd;
> Yet *vast* his *Genius*, noble were his *Thoughts*,
> Whence equal Readers wink at *lesser* Faults. (12)

1059. WILLIAM WINSTANLEY. *The Protestant Almanack, for the Year 1700. By Philoprotest, a Well-willer to the Mathematicks.* A2240. UMI 1347: 14.

As Harris notes (*PQ*), "Philoprotest" quotes lines from the spurious work known as Chaucer's *Ploughman's Tale.* In an epistle addressed "To the Christian Reader," he writes:

> [By] matchless Labours both in the former and present Age . . . hath the Papal Crown attained to the Dignity it is now at; far different from the Condition of St. *Peter*, whose Successor they [i.e., Roman Catholics] brag themselves to be, who told the Cripple that expected Alms of him, *Gold nor Silver have I none*; they swimming in all manner of Wealth and Luxuriousness; as the ancient Poet *Geoffery Chaucer* thus expresseth in the *Plow-mans Tale.*

> *Popes, Bishops, and Cardinals,*
> *Cannons, Parsons, and Vicars,*
> *In God's Service I trow been false,*
> *That sacraments sellen here;*
> *And been as proud as* Lucifer,
> *Each Man look whether that I lye,*
> *Who so speaketh against her Power,*
> *It shall be holden Heresie.*

But I want room to anatomize them as I would do, being confined to a slender scantling of Paper. This therefore for this Year shall suffice. (sig. A3v–4r)

1060. *Wit and Mirth: or, Pills to Purge Melancholy. The Second Part.* W3134B. **UMI 1821: 19.**

In "An Ancient Song of Bartholomew-Fair," there is a reference to Patient Grizil, perhaps an allusion to *The Clerk's Tale.* The language indicates that the performance represents dialect or, perhaps, drunkenness.

> In Fifty-five, may I never Thrive,
> If I tell you any more than is true,
> To *London* che [*sic*] came, hearing of the Fame
> Of a Fair they call *Bartholomew*
> . . . .
> For a Penny you may zee a fine Puppet-play,
> And for Two-pence a rare piece of Art,
> And a Penny a Can, I dare swear a Man
> May put zix [*sic*] of 'em into a Quart.
> There Zights [*sic*] are so rich, is able to bewitch
> The Heart of a very fine Man-*a* [*sic*];
> Here's *Patient Grizil* here, and *Fair Rosamond* there,
> and [*sic*] the History of *Suzanna.* [&c.] (171)

The End.

Appendix of New References and Allusions 1500–1640

When Sylvia Holton and I were working on *Chaucer's Fame in England* back in the last years of the twentieth century, we agreed that many references to "the house of fame," "dun's in the mire," "spiced conscience," and such like were generic rather than Chaucerian. Later, however, we began to regret that we had not noted that many such references were, at the very least, Chaucerian echoes. Although many of the echoes in this collection are proverbial and, indeed, may have been proverbial in Chaucer's day, the references in this Appendix are not without interest.

In this Appendix I have not repeated every subsequent reference as it was reprinted in chronological order but have, instead, simply noted each occurrence in "other editions."

1476

1.   BURGH, BENEDICT, interpolation in Cato's *Paruus*. STC 4851. UMI 1342: 3.

Burgh is identified on the title page of the 1483 as "late Archedeken of Colchestre and hye chanon of saint stephens at westmestre." At the very end of this translation of Cato from the "frensshe" Burgh (d. in or before 1483) echoes the title of *The House of Fame*. In a farewell to the reader, he concludes:

Here have I fonde that shal you guyde & lede
Streight to gode fame & leve you in hir hous (no signatures or foliation)

Other editions: STC 4850 (1477), last page; STC 4852 (1483), last page.
    Also found in *The Godly Adverstisement or Good Counsell of the Famous Orator Isocrates. Whereunto Is Annexed Cato in Olde Englysh Meter*, STC 14275 (1557), last page.

1483

2.   GOWER, JOHN. *Confessio amantis: That Is to Say in Englysshe, The Confessyon of the Lover.* STC 12142. UMI 50: 7.

In addition to allusions noted by Boswell & Holton (No. 18), there may be others. In "liber primus," Gower (1325?–1408) echoes *The Wife of Bath's Tale*: "What thyng it is that wommen moost desire" (line 1007) and "What thyng that worldly wommen loven best" (line 1033). Gower writes:

> Al that to myn axyng longeth
> What al women moost desyre
> This wol I axe (fol. xviii v)
> She sayd treson wo the be
> That hast thus told the pryvyte
> Whiche al women most desyre (fol. xx r)

In "Liber secundus," Gower echoes a line from *Troilus and Criseyde*, "Unknowe, unkist, and lost, that is unsought" (1.809). He writes:

> And eche of them his tale affayteth
> Al to deceyve an Innocent
> Whiche wol not be of her assent
> And for men seyn unknown unkist
> Hyr thombe she helde in hyr fist (fol. xxxiii r)

In "Liber Quintus," Gower echoes lines from *The General Prologue* in the description of the Parson: "This noble ensample to his sheep he yaf, | That first he wroughte, and afterward he taughte" (lines 496–7). He writes:

> Cryst wrought fyrst/ & after taught
> Soo that the dede his word araught
> He yafe ensample in his persone
> And we the wordes have alone (fol. ci r)

In "Liber Octavus," Gower echoes a refrain from "Fortune": "For fynally, Fortune, I thee defye!" (lines 8, 16, 24). In a section about "Appollynus" Gower writes:

> Why shal I lyve & thou shalt dye
> Ha thou fortune I the defye (fol. clxxxxvii r)

Other editions: STC 12143 (1532), fols. 16r, 17r, 30r, 93v, 179v; STC 12144 (1554), fols. XVIr, XVIIr, XXXr, XCIIIv, CLXXIXv.

1494

3.   LYDGATE, JOHN, trans. *The Boke Calledde John Bochas Descrivinge the Falle of Princis, Princessis,* [and] *Other Nobles.* STC 3175. UMI 26: 8.

Lydgate (1313–1375) echoes the title of *The House of Fame* as he translates Giovanni Boccaccio's *De casibus illustrium virorum.* In "Prohemium libri quarti" in a passage in praise of "Petrarke in Rome laureate," Lydgate translates:

> And thus by writinge he gate him silf a name
> Perpetually to be in remembraunce
> Set and registred in the hous of fame
> And made epistles of full high substaunce (sig. n5r)

In book 5, chapter 6, in a passage about Duke Zantipas, Lydgate again echoes Chaucer's usage:

> To his noblenesse and famous chivalrye
> Whan he of knighthode sat hyest in his floures
> They of cartage by hatred and envye
> Maligned ageyn him cheef sonne of their socours
> Taclipsyd his light but ther ageyne auctours
> Have by writinge perpetuelly set his name
> And it regestred in the hous of fame (sig. r1v)

Near the beginning of book 6, Lydgate echoes the title of *The House of Fame*:

> [T]hou doest great diligence
> As they deserve to yeve them thanke or blame
> Settyst up one in royall excellence
> Within myn house called the house of fame
> The golden trumpet with blastys of gode name
> Enhaunceth one to full hye partyes
> Where Jupyter sitteth amonge the hevenly skyes (sig. t2v)

In a section headed "Hic loquitur Fortuna," Lydgate again echoes the title of *The House of Fame*:

> That thy name and also thy surname
> With poetys and notable olde auctours
> May be regestryd in the hous of fame
> By supportacion of my sodeyn favours
> By assitence also of my socours

Thy werke texplete the laurer for to wynne
At Saturnynus I wyll that thou begynne (sig. t5r)

Other editions: STC 3176 (1527), sig. R6v (no folio number), and fols. Cxxvi
verso, Cxliiii verso, Cxlvi recto; STC 3177.5 (1554?), fols. xciii recto, cxviii recto,
cxxxiiii verso, cxxvi verso.

1497

4.   LYDGATE, JOHN. [*The Siege of Thebes*. Begins] "Prologus Here begyn-
neth the prologue of the storye of Thebes." STC 17031. UMI 1: 18.

In addition to the references and allusions noted by Spurgeon (1: 26–31) and
Boswell & Holton (No. 34), there appears to be yet another in "Pars Tercis"
where Lydgate refers to Palamon and Arcite, and likely alludes to *The Knight's
Tale*. In a passage about Lycurgus, Lydgate writes:

And as I rede.In a nother [*sic*] place
He was the same myghty champyon
To Athens.that cam with palamon
Agaynst his brother. that was called Arcyte (sig. i1v–2r)

Also found in *The Workes of Geffrey Chaucer* (1561), STC 5075, fol. ccclxxii verso;
STC 5076 (1561), fol. ccclxxii verso; STC 5076.3 (1561), fol. ccclxxii verso; STC
5077 (1598), fol. 387v; STC 5078 (1598), fol. 387v; STC 5079 (1598), fol. 387v;
STC 5080 (1602), fol. 369v; STC 5081 (1602), fol. 369v; C3736 (1687), 650.

1504

5.   ATKINSON, WILLIAM. *A Full Devoute and Gostely Treatyse of the Imytacyon and Folowynge the Blessed Lyfe of Our Moste Mercyfull Savyour*. STC 23957.
UMI 2017:15.

Atkinson is identified on the title page as a "Doctor of divinitie." This *Treatyse* was "compyled in Laten by the right worshypful Doctor Mayster John Ger-
son" and "translate[d] into Englisshe" by Atkinson "at ye speciall request [and]
commaundement of the full excellent Pryncesse Margarete moder to our sover-
ayne lord Kynge Henry the .vii. and Countesse of Rychemount and Derby" (title
page). Under the running head "Parte. The thyrde," in chapter 61, "We ought to
forsake our selfe & folowe Cryste with our crosse," Atkinson echoes Chaucer's
"Truth. Ballade de Bon Conseyl": "And trouthe thee shal delivere, it is no drede"
(lines 7, 14, 21, 28). Atkinson writes:

If thou abyde in my way thou shalt knowe the very trouth and trouthe shall delyver the . . . . (sig. P4v)

Another edition: STC 23957 (1517), sig. P4v.

1510

6.   LYDGATE, JOHN. *The Proverbes of Lydgate.* STC 17026. UMI 1: 32.

In addition to references noted by Boswell & Holton (No. 66), there is another. Lydgate quotes Chaucer's ballad called "Fortune" entirely. It is headed "Ecce bonum consilium galfridi chaucers contra fortuna" (sig. a5r *et seq*. Signature "a" is irregular.).

Another edition: STC 17027 (1520?), sig. B1v.

1534

7.   LYDGATE, JOHN. *The Glorious Lyfe of Seint Albon Prothomartyr of England.* STC 256.UMI 21: 6

Lydgate calls this work is a translation, but it appears to be mostly his. He laments the lack of Petrarch's high style to trumpet the fame of Saint Alban of Verolame, a Christian martyr. Lydgate echoes the title of *The House of Fame*:

To call Clio my dulnesse to redresse
with all systers dwellyng at Elicon
what myght avayle to wryte the perfytenes
Of the holy martyr slayne full yore agone
For Christis fayth/ . . . .

I not acqueynted with muses of Maro
Nor with metris of Lucan/ nor . . .
. . . .
Of Fraunces Petrake the poete laureate

The golden trompet of the house of fame
with full swyfte wynges of the pegasee
Hath full farre the knyghtly mannes name
Borne in Verolame a famous olde citie
Knyghthode in Rome the cronycle who lyst se (sig. A2r)

8.   MEDWALL, HENRY. *Nature. A Goodly Interlude.* STC 17779. UMI 235: 4.

Medwall (*fl.* 1486) is identified on the title page as "chapleyn to the ryght reverent father in God Johan Morton somtyme cardynall and archebyshop of Canterbury." In a passage in which Mundus speaks with Innocencye, Medwall echoes Chaucer's description of the poor Parson, "Ne maked him a spiced conscience" (*The General Prologue*, line 526) or *The Wife of Bath's Prologue*, "Ye sholde been al pacient and meke, | And han a sweete spiced conscience" (lines 434–35).[1] Medwall writes:

> Alas have ye suche a spyced conscyence
> That wyll be entryked/ wyth every mery thought (sig. b3v)

And again later:

> Why have ye suche a spyced conscyence
> Now wythin your brest
> that chaungeth your mynde so sodenly (sig. c1v)

1535

9.   *The Dyaloge Bytwene Julius the Second, Genius, and Saynt Peter.* STC 14842. UMI 69: 18.

This work has been attributed to both Erasmus of Rotterdam and Publio Fausto Andrelinus, but neither the original title nor the translator is known. Whoever the translator was, he echoes Chaucer's description of the poor Parson, "Ne maked him a spiced conscience" (*The General Prologue*, line 526) or *The Wife of Bath's Prologue*, "Ye sholde been al pacient and meke, | And han a sweete spiced conscience" (lines 434–35). In a passage about critics of the "noughty lyvynge" of popes, bishops, and priests, the translator writes that Julius says to St. Peter:

> [A]s to our honour they regard not very much/ but maketh us theyr laughinge stockis, excepte some certeyne of spyced conscience/ which so moche feareth our thondrebolte & curse/ as thoughe it coude hurte them yt deserved it not. (sig. F1r)

St. Peter responds:

---

[1] See D. Biggins, "A Chaucerian Crux: *Spiced conscience*," *English Studies* 47 (1966), 169–80; and John C. Hirsh, "General Prologue 526: 'A Spiced Conscience'," *The Chaucer Review* 28.4 (1994), 414–17.

Yf they be so spyced conscyence: yet I do not well p*er* ceyve howe thou sholdst so sone styre the*m* up to so great warres, seing thou hast broken so many trucew with them. (sig. F1v)

Another edition: E3208B (1673), a different translation.

1538

10.   ELYOT, THOMAS. *The Dictionary of Syr Thomas Eliot Knyght.* STC 7659. UMI 36: 1.

Sir Thomas Elyot (1490?–1546) echoes Chaucer's description of the poor Parson, "Ne maked him a spiced conscience" (*The General Prologue*, line 526) and *The Wife of Bath's Prologue*, "Ye sholde been al pacient and meke, | And han a sweete spiced conscience" (lines 434–35). In his definition of scrupulous, Elyot writes:

It is also taken for moche sollicitude, also for dyfficultie, or spiced conscience. (sig. Z1v)

Other editions (with different titles): *Bibliotheca Eliotæ Eliotis Librarie* (1542), STC 7660, sig. Hh4r; *Bibliotheca Eliotæ Eliotis Librarie the Second Tyme Enriched by Thomas Cooper* (1552), STC 7662, sig. Rrr7v.

See also COOPER (1565).

1541

11.   ELYOT, THOMAS. *The Image of Governance.* STC 7664. UMI 36: 4.

In his dedicatory epistle addressed "To al the nobilitie of this flouryshynge royalme of Englande," Sir Thomas Elyot (1490?–1546) echoes a line from *The Reeve's Tale* (slightly modernized): "The gretteste clerkes been noght wisest men" (line 4054). He writes:

[M]any [men] being ignorant of good letters, do universally reprove all them that be studiouse in lerninge, alleginge this commune proverbe, The grettest clarkes be not the wisest men. (sig. a4r)

Other editions: STC 7665 (1544), sig. a4r; STC 7666 (1549), sig. A5v; STC 7666.2 (1552?), sig. A5v; STC 7667 (1556), sig. A5v.

1543

12.   HARDYNG, JOHN. *The Chronicle.* STC 12766.7. UMI 44: 1 (identified as STC 12767).

In addition to references noted by Boswell & Holton (No. 153), there are others. In chapter 9, "How Eneas exyled oute of Troye came to Cecyle and to Affrike to the cytee of Carthage," Harding echoes the title of *The House of Fame*. He writes:

> This worthy prince, kyng Eneas mortally
> Ended his lyfe that was of hye prowesse
> Where so God wyll to reigne eternally
> Within the house of fame . . . (fol. xiiv)

The next chapter is headed with another echo of the title of *The House of Fame*:

> Of the house of fame where knightes be rewarded after the merites of
> armes by Mars the God of armes . . . . (fol. xiir)

Another edition in 1643: STC 12767, same pagination.

1546

13.   HEYWOOD, JOHN. *A Dialogue.* STC 13291. UMI 134: 9.

In addition to the references noted by Boswell & Holton (No. 160), there appears to be another. In the second part, "The fourthe chapiter," a housewife and her husband conduct a dialogue that consists mainly of proverbs, and he echoes a line from *The Merchant's Tale*: "Old fish, and young flesh woll I haue full faine" (line 1418). Heywood writes:

> But my neighbours desyre rightly to measure, [quoth she]
> Cometh of neede, and not of corrupte pleasure,
> And my husbands more of pleasure, than of nede.
> Old fishe & yong flesh (quoth he) doth men best fede. (sig. G3r)

And in chapter 5 he echoes a line from *The Reeve's Tale*: "The gretteste clerkes been noght wisest men" (line 4054). Heywood writes:

> [F]or counsaile . . . I thought to have gon,
> To that cunnyng man, our curate sir John.
> But this kept me backe, I have herd now and then,
> The greatest clerkes be not the wysest men.

I think (quoth I) who ever that terme began,
Was neither great clerke, nor the greatest wise man. (sig. H1v)

Other editions: STC 13292 (1550), sig. D4v, D7r; STC 13293 (1556), sig. D4v, D7r; STC 13294 (1561), sig. D4v, D7r.

Also found in Heywood's *Woorkes*: STC 13285 (1562), sig. G1v, G3v; STC 13286 (1566), sig. G1v, G3v; STC 13287 (1577), sig. E1v, E3v; STC 13288 (1587), sigs. C8r, D2r; STC 13289 (1598), sigs. F4v, G2v.

1550

14.   BALE, JOHN. *The Apology of Johan Bale agaynste a Ranke Papyst.* STC 1275. UMI 484: 14.

Bale (1495–1563) echoes Chaucer's description of the poor Parson, "Ne maked him a spiced conscience" (*The General Prologue*, line 526) and *The Wife of Bath's Prologue*, "Ye sholde been al pacient and meke, | And han a sweete spiced conscience" (lines 434–35). In a passage about the "ranke papyst's" remarks about nuns who get married, Bale writes:

> The scrupul or spyced conscience that he hath in the matter, is concerning ye breake of her promyse made to God. (fol. 84v)

1552

15.   LYDGATE, JOHN. *The Cronycle of all the Kynges That Have Reygned in Englande.* STC 9983. UMI 384: 4.

In his account of Edward IV, Lydgate echoes the title of *The House of Fame*:

> Edward the .iii. of that name
> A noble prynce, a governoure most worthye
> Full excellent were his actes withouten blame
> And enrolled within the house of fame (one sheet, a fragment)

1555

16.   HEYWOOD, JOHN. *Two Hundred Epigrammes, upon Two Hundred Proverbs with a Thyrde Hundred Newely Added.* STC 13296. UMI 839: 8.

In "the thyrde hundreth" of his collection of proverbs, Heywood (1497?–1580?) echoes a line from *The Reeve's Tale*: "The gretteste clerkes been noght wisest men" (line 4054). In number 6, "Of greate Clarkes," he writes:

> The greatest clarkes be not the wysest men
> Be smaule lernd or unlernd fooles wysest then. (sig. D2v)

Also in Heywood's *Woorkes*: STC 13285 (1562), "Epigrams upon Proverbes," No. 206, sig. U4v; STC 13286 (1566), sig. U4v; STC 13287 (1577), sig. L8v; STC 13288 (1587), sig. P3r; STC 13289 (1598), sig. K4r.

1563

17.   BALDWIN, WILLIAM. *A Myrrour for Magistrates.* STC 1248. UMI 170: 4.

In addition to references noted by Boswell & Holton (No. 234), there may be another in "The Wilful Fal of black Smith, and the foolishe ende of the Lord Awdeley in June. Anno. 1496." There Baldwin echoes a line from *The Reeve's Tale*: "The gretteste clerkes been noght wisest men" (line 4054). He writes:

> The Hostler, Barber, Myller, and the Smyth,
> Heareof the sawes of such as wisedome ken,
> And learne some wit although they want the pith,
> The clarkes pretend and yet both now and then,
> The greatest clarkes prove not the wisest men:
> It is not right that men forbid should bee:
> To speake the truth al were he bond or free. (fol. 167v)

Other editions: STC 1249 (1571), fol. 152v; STC 1250 (1574), fol. 146r; STC 1251 (1575), fol. 146r; STC 1252 (1578), fol. 167v; STC 1252.5 (1578), fol. 167v.

Also found in John Higgins's *The Mirrour of Magistrates*: STC 13445 (1587), fol. 237r; STC 13446 (1610), 466.

Also found in Higgins's *The Falles of Unfortunate Princes*: STC 13447 (1619), 466; STC 13447.5 (1619), 466; STC 13448 (1620), 466; STC 13448.4 (1620), 466.

1565

18. THOMAS COOPER. *Thesarus linguæ Romanæ & Britannicæ.* STC 5686. UMI 205: 7

Cooper, identified on the title page as "Thomæ Cooperi Magdalenensis," recycles Sir Thomas Elyot's definition of *scrupulous* and thus alludes to *The Reeve's Tale.* See ELYOT (1538); here the passage is found on sig. TTTtt6r.

Other editions: STC 5687 (1573), sig. Xxxxx4v; STC 5688 (1578), sig. Xxxxx4v; STC 5678 (1584), sig. Xxxxx4v.

1567

19. PARKER, MATTHEW. *A Defence of Priestes Mariages.* STC 17519. UMI 434: 4.

Parker (1504–1575) echoes Chaucer's description of the poor Parson, "Ne maked him a spiced conscience" (*The General Prologue*, line 526) and *The Wife of Bath's Prologue*, "Ye sholde been al pacient and meke, | And han a sweete spiced conscience" (lines 434–35). Writing in response to a treatise by "a civilian, namyng hym selfe Thomas Martain doctour of the civile lawes" (title page), in an augmented version of an earlier edition, Parker writes:

> Forsooth his redy good wyll and accesse to the holy father of Rome, the supportation that he founde there, the spiced conscience he had in his wrong obedience unto that sea, esteemyng him so hyghly . . . made hym to esteeme his prince the lesse. (299)

20. TURBERVILLE, GEORGE. *Epitaphes, Epigrams, Songs and Sonets.* STC 24326. UMI 362: 7.

Turberville is characterized on the title page as a "Gentleman." In addition to a reference to Chaucer and allusions to *Troilus and Criseyde* noted in Spurgeon (3: 4.35) and Boswell & Holton No. 265, there may be others.

In "An Epitaphe on the death of Elyzabeth Arhundle," Turberville echoes the title of *The House of Fame*:

> Descending of a house of worthie fame
> Shee lincket at length with one of egall state,
> Who though did chaunge hir first & former name,
> Did not enforce hir vertues to rebate. (fol. 9r)

In a long poem headed "The Lover to Cupid for mercie, declaring how first he became his thrall, with the occasion of his defiyng Lover, and now at last what caused him to convert" there is a reference to Canace, perhaps an allusion to *The Squire's Tale*. The likelihood of this being an allusion is reinforced by Turberville's reference to Canace's incestuous relationship with her brothers—hinted at in *The Squire's Prologue* (as it is in Gower's version of the story). In a passage about those besotted with love, Turberville writes:

> What Canace enforcde
> to frie with frantick brands,
> In sort as up to yeeld hir selfe
> unto hir brothers hands?
> And others thousand mo
> of whome the Poets wright? (fol. 52v)

In "An Epitaph of Maister Win drowned in the Sea," Turberville again echoes the title of *The House of Fame*:

> O Neptune churlish Chuff . . . .
> . . . .
> Yet nathelesse his ever during name
> Is fast ingravde within the house of Fame. (fol. 128v)

In "The Lover in utter dispaire of his Ladies returne, in eche respect compares his estate with Troylus," Turberville appears to allude to *Troilus and Criseyde* and certainly alludes to Henryson's *Testament of Cresseid*, a work that was accessible only in an edition of Chaucer and was often attributed to Chaucer. He writes:

> My case with Troylus may compare,
> For as he felt both sorrow and care:
> Even so doe I most Miser Wight,
> That am a Troylus outright.
> As ere he could atchieve his wish,
> He fed of many a dolefull dish,
> And day and night unto the Skies
> The sielie Troian kest his cies [*sic*],
> Requesting ruth at Cresids hande
> In whome his life and death did stande:
> . . . .
> And as King Priams worthie Sonne
> For love of Cresid: so doe I
> All Venus Dearlings quight defie,

In minde to love them all aleeke,
That leave a Troian for a Greeke. (fols. 139r–140v)

In "An Epitaph on the death of Maister Arthur Brooke drownde in passing to New Haven," Turberville yet once more echoes the title of *The House of Fame*:

Let this suffice textall the life he led
And print his prayse in the house of Fame to stande. (fol. 144v)

Another edition: STC 24327 (1570), fols. 9r, 52v, 128v, 139r–140v, and 144v.

1570

21.   BILLINGSLEY, H. An annotation in *The Elements of Geometrie of the Most Auncient Philisopher Euclide of Megara*. **STC 10560. UMI 342: 5.**
Billingsley is described on the title page as a "citizen of London." In his annotation of Euclid's thirty-third theorum, "In rectangle triangles, the square whiche is made of the side that subtendeth the right angle, is equal to the squares which are made of the sides containing the right angle," Billingsley appears to allude to *Troilus and Criseyde* (3: 931–33). He writes:

This most excellent and notable Theoreme was first invented of the greate philosopher Pithagoras . . . And it hath bene commonly called of barbarous writers of the latter time Dulcarnon. (fol. 58r)

1573

22.   GASCOIGNE, GEORGE. *A Hundreth Sundrie Flowres*. **STC 11635. UMI 244: 2.**
In addition to the references noted in Boswell & Holton No. 310, there may be another. In "Gascoignes devise of a maske" for a double marriage in the family of Viscount Montacute, Gascoigne echoes the title of *The House of Fame*:

My father was a knight Mount Hermer was his name,
My mother of the Mountacutes, a house of worthy fame. (383)

Also found in *The Posies*, STC 11637 (1575), fol. xliiii; *The Whole Woorkes*, STC 11638 (1587), 44; and *The Pleasauntest Workes*, STC 11639 (1587), 44.

23.   PARTRIDGE, JOHN. *The Treasurie of Commodious Conceits & Hidden Secrets.* STC 19425.5. UMI 1755: 2.

In a commendatory poem headed "John Partridge to his Booke," Partridge (*fl.* 1566–1573) echoes Chaucer's line, "Go, litel bok, go litel myn tragedye" (*Troilus and Criseyde* 5: 1786):

> Goe foorthe my little Booke,
> That all on thee may looke . . . . (sig. A2v)

See also PARTRIDGE (1584), for a different poem with the same allusion.

1574

24.   FREAKE, EDMUND. "Epistle to the Reader" in *An Introduction to the Love of God. Accompted among the Workes of S. Augustine, and Set Forth in His Name.* STC 935. UMI 168: 8.

Freake signs his dedicatory epistle as "Edmund Roffen," i.e., as Edmund, bishop of Rochester. In an epistle addressed to the reader, in a passage about the art of translation, Freake (ca. 1516–1591) echoes Chaucer's description of the poor Parson, "Ne maked him a spiced conscience" (*The General Prologue*, line 526) and *The Wife of Bath's Prologue*, "Ye sholde been al pacient and meke, | And han a sweete spiced conscience" (lines 434–35). He writes:

> *I confesse me plainly that I have even wittingly used in this translation a certain fredome and libertie, and reduced the sense of the Author, to the consonancy, and Canon of the holy scripture. . . . This if any man either of spiced conscience, or wayward mynde, dislike or controle, I wish him more wyt, then fantastically to desire to have hurtfull thinges joyned to the wholesome as of necessity.* (sig. C1r-v)

Another edition: STC 936 (1581?), a different translation. See FLETCHER (1581). UMI 635: 18

25.   RICH, BARNABE. *A Right Exelent [sic] and Pleasaunt Dialogue betwene Mercury and an English Souldier Contayning His Supplication to Mars.* STC 20998. UMI 1332: 8.

In a passage about brave soldiers who have been conquered by love, Rich (1540?–1617) appears to allude to *Troilus and Criseyde*. He writes:

> Was not Hercules that noble conquerour, conquered him self by love with Dianayra . . . & Troilus with Cressid . . . . (sig. M3r)

26. SMITH, RICHARD. Commendatory poem in Richard Robinson's *The Rewarde of Wickedness*. STC 21121.7. UMI 351: 12.

In addition to the references noted in Boswell & Holton No. 321, there may be another. In a commendatory poem, Smith places Robinson in the house of Fame and echoes the title of *The House of Fame*:

> *Thou profered prise at* Olimpias, *and gotte the chiefest game,*
> *And through the schoole of cunning skill, hast scalde the house of Fame.* (sig. A4v)

1575

27. BEVERLEY, PETER. *The Historie of Ariodanto and Jenevra, Daughter to the King of Scottes*. STC 745.5. UMI 173: 6.

In this long narrative poem that draws heavily on Ariosto's *Orlando Furioso*, Peter Beverley of Staple Inn appears to allude to *Troilus and Criseyde*. In a passage about a knight who comes to court and entertains ladies with romances, Beverley writes:

> And now amongst the Scottishe Dames,
>   (as though he weare to chuse)
> He would discourse of histories,
>   and tell of forein newes.
> At first the siege of worthy Troy,
>   what knightes therein weare slayn:
> . . . .
> And how for falsing of her faith,
>   False Creseide fell uncleane. (sig. D8r)

1576

28. PETTIE, GEORGE. *A Petite Pallace of Pettie His Pleasure*. STC 19819. UMI 1390: 12.

Among the "pretie hystories . . . set forth in comely colours" (title page), Pettie (1548–1589) includes one headed "Cephalus and Procris." Therein twice he appears to allude to *Troilus and Criseyde*. In a passage in which Procris chides her would-be lover, Pettie writes:

> Were you so vaine to assure your selfe so surely of my vanity, that only thereupon you would undertake so great a journey? No, you are

conversaunt with no Cressid, you have no Helen in hande, wée women
will now learne to béeware of sutch guyleful guestes. (164)

In "Pigmalions friends, and his Image," the question is asked:

What constancy is to bée hoped for in kytes of Cressids kinde? may one
gather Grapes of thornes, Sugar of Thistels, or constancy of women?
Nay if a man sift the whole sexe thorowly, hée shall finde their wordes
to bee winde, their fayth forgery, and their déedes dissemblinge. (191)

Other editions: STC 19820 (1585), fols. 69v, 79v; STC 19821 (ca. 1590), no UMI;
STC 19822 (1608), sigs. S3r, X2r; STC 19823 (1613), sigs. S3r, X2r.

1577

29.   BULLINGER, HEINRICH. *Fiftie Godlie and Learned Sermons.* STC 4056.
UMI 183: 3.

Bullinger (1504–1575) is identified on the title page as "minister of the church of
Tigure in Swicerlande." In the second decade of sermons, the second sermon is
headed "Of Gods lawe, and of the two first commaundements of the first Table."
In his translation from the Latin, H. I., "student in divinitie," echoes Chaucer's
description of the poor Parson, "Ne maked him a spiced conscience" (*The General Prologue*, line 526) and *The Wife of Bath's Prologue*, "Ye sholde been al pacient
and meke, | And han a sweete spiced conscience" (lines 434–35). He translates:

[L]et no man thinke that before Moses time there was no lawe. . . .
Abraham in taking an oathe used alwayes a reverend feare, and a spiced
conscience, whereby it followeth that to him the name of the Lord was
holy and not lightly taken. (109–10)

Other editions: STC 4057 (1584), 109–10; STC 4058 (1587), 109–10.

30.   GRANGE, JOHN. *The Golden Aphroditis.* STC 12174. UMI 1380: 11.

Grange (*fl.* 1577) is identified on the title page as a gentleman and "student in
the common lawe of England." In addition to his references to Chaucer and to
Troilus noted in Boswell & Holton No. 354, there is another. In a section headed
"I.I. unto N.O.," in a passage about women who were untrue, he mentions that
Criseyde suffered from leprosy. Grange writes:

[W]hat should we thinke of . . . hir in England in the raigne of *Henry*
the eight, who havyng twelve sonnes, and lying sore sicke, confessed to

hir husbande that after the firste yeare shee was never true unto him? and was not *Cresida* turned unto a Lepre for hyr unconstancie? (sig. B2r)

1579

31. SPENSER, EDMUND. *The Shepheardes Calender.* STC 23089. UMI 354: 24.

In addition to references noted by Boswell & Holton (No. 384), there may be an allusion to *The Squire's Tale* (lines 115–31) in "Julye," where Spenser writes of a steed of brass:

> But shepheard mought be meeke and mylde,
> > well eyed, as *Argus* was,
> With fleshly follyes undefyled,
> > and stoute as steede of brasse. (fol. 28r–v)

Other editions: STC 23090 (1581), fol. 28r–v; STC 23091 (1586), fol. 28r–v; STC 23092 (1591), fol. 28r–v; STC 23093 (1597), 53; STC 23094 (1617), 31.

1580

32. LYLY, JOHN. *Euphues and His England.* STC 17070. UMI 477: 6.

In addition to the references noted by Spurgeon (1: 119, 3: 4.41, and 4: 1457–58) and Boswell & Holton (No. 393), there is another. Lyly (1554?–1606) echoes a line from *The Reeve's Tale*: "The gretteste clerkes been noght wisest men" (line 4054). In a passage in which a father reproves his sons who have "lived wantonly," he writes:

> [K]nowing that those that give themselves to be bookish are oftentimes so blockish that they forget thrift: Where-by the olde Sawe is verified, that the greatest Clearkes are not the wisest men, who digge still at the roote, while others gather the fruite . . . . (fol. 7v)

Other editions in 1580: STC 17068, fol. 8r; STC 17069, fol. 8r.

Other editions: STC 17071 (1581), fol. 7v; STC 17072 (1582), fol. 7v; STC 17072.5 (1584); STC 17073 (1586), sig. C3v; STC 17074 (1588), sig. C3v; STC 17074.5 (1592), sig. C4r; STC 17075 (1597), sig. C4r; STC 17076 (1601), sig. C4r; STC 17077 (1605), sig. C4r; STC 17078 (1606), sig. C4r; STC 17079 (1609), sig. C4r.

Also found in *Euphues the Anatomy of Wit*, STC 17064 (1617), sig. M4r; STC 17065 (1623), sig. M4r; STC 17066 (1631), sig. M4r; STC 17067 (1636), sig. M4r.

33.   SAKER, AUSTIN. *Narbonus. The Laberynth of Libertie.* STC 21593. UMI 1005: 06.

Saker is identified on the title page as "Austin Saker, of New Inne." He writes of "the discommodities that issue, by following the lust of mans will, in youth" (title page). In a passage advising young men to choose their friends carefully, he appears to allude to *Troilus and Criseyde*. Saker writes:

> [As you] walke the Cittie, and treade the streats . . . use the fellowshippe
> of faithfull freendes: and so make your choice, as you rue not your losse,
> nor repent your bargaine: for all sortes of freendes are here to be found,
> both good and bad: both honest and disloyall, both trusty and faithles:
> as wel the Spider as the Bee . . . as well Cressid forsworne, as Troylus
> most just of his worde. (8)

1581

34.   FLETCHER, ROBERT. Epistle in *An Introduction to the Loove of God*. STC 936. UMI 635: 16.

In an epistle addressed "To the Christian Readers," Fletcher (*fl.* 1581-1606) defends his verse translation of a work attributed to Saint Augustine. He writes:

> I know . . . meter is more acceptable to some than prose, & may with
> lesse capacitie be comprehended, as of children, young men and maides,
> &c. which mooved me also to take this paines therein, and the rather to
> suppresse that huge heape, & superfluous rable of balde Ballads, Rimes
> & Ridles, Song & Sonnets, yea, and whole volumes of vanity . . . for
> he that eyther Prose or Rime wyll be in print, if his Pen can but blotte
> foorth a Bable, it shall be a Ballad, with Finis, &c. at the ende. They
> be all Chaucers and Gowers, Lidgatges, and Bocases, and he is a foole
> that is not five Skeltons for cunning: these write woonders, newes never
> seene before, no, nor never heard of, but at Billings gate, or in Gra-
> vesende Barge. (sig. A5r-6r)

35.   HOWELL, THOMAS. *H. His Devises, for His Owne Exercise, and His Friends Pleasure.* STC 13875. UMI 467: 7.

In addition to an allusion to *Troilus and Criseyde* noted by Boswell & Holton (No. 399), there are two others in "Ruine the rewarde of Vice." Howell writes:

Then shake of Vice ye Nymphes of *Cressids* Crue,
And Vertue seeke, whose praise shall never die
. . . .
Loe here of Vice the right reward and knyfe,
That cuttes of cleane and tumbleth downe in heapes,
All such as treat Dame *Cressids* cursed steppes,
Take heede therfore how you and your pryme do spende,
For Vice brings plagues, and Vertue happy ende. (sig. B4r)

1582

36. PARTRIDGE, JOHN. *The Treasurie of Commodious Conceits and Hidden Secrets.* STC 19426. UMI 2207: 6.

In a commendatory poem headed "The Authour to his Booke, concerning his freend, whose importunate sute procured him to publish the same," Partridge again echoes Chaucer's line, "Go, litel bok, go litel myn tragedye" (*Troilus and Criseyde* 5: 1786):

Go little Booke of profite and pleasance,
Unto thy good Mistresse, without delay:
And tell her I send thee for the performance
Of her earnest sute, sith she would have no nay. (sig. A3v)

For a different poem with the same allusion, see PARTRIDGE (1573). By 1589, however, the poet may be echoing Spenser's prelude to *The Shepheardes Calender*, published in 1579 (see Boswell & Holton No. 384); and of course the same holds true for all subsequent similar references.

Other editions: STC 19427 (1584), sig. A3r; STC 19428 (1586), sig. A3r; STC 19429 (1591), sig. A3v.

With a new title, *The Treasurie of Hidden Secrets*: STC 19429.5 (1596), sig. A2v; STC 19430 (1600), sig. A2v; STC 19430.5 (1608), sig. A2v; STC 19431 (1627), sig. A2v; STC 19431.5 (1627), sig. A2v; STC 19432 (1633), UMI 1355: 18, sig. A2v; STC 19433 (1637), UMI 1458: 4, sig. A2v; P628 (1653), UMI 1533: 12, sig. A2v.

1583

37.   DES PÉRIERS, BONAVENTURE. *The Mirrour of Mirth and Pleasant Conceits.* STC 6784.5. UMI 1893: 7.

Des Périers (1500?–1544?) is characterized on the title page as "that worshipfull and learned gentleman." In this translation by Thomas Deloney (1543?–1600) of *Nouvelles récréations et joyeux devis*, there is an echo of the title of *The House of Fame*. In a section headed "Of a young-man of Parys newely marryed," Deloney translates:

> [S]he [i.e., the Parisian's young wife] was brought up & nourished in a house of fame. . . . (sig. F1v)

Another edition: STC 6784.7 (1592), sig. E1v.

1584

38.   COGAN, THOMAS. *The Haven of Health.* STC 5478. UMI 193: 17.

Cogan (1545?–1607) is described on the title page as "master of Artes, & Bacheler of Phisicke." Twice he appears to allude to *The Merchant's Tale*: "Old fish, and young flesh woll I haue full faine" (line 1418). In chapter 133, "Of Goates flesh," he writes:

> For most true is that English proverbe, young flesh & old fish doth men best feede. (119)

And in chapter 176, "The Preface to Fish," Cogan again echoes a line from *The Merchant's Tale*:

> And here occasion is offered to speake somewhat of the olde English proverbe touching the choise of fish, which is: That yong flesh and olde fish doth men best feede. (141)

Other editions: STC 5479 (1588), 119–20, 141; STC 5480 (1589), 119–20, 141; STC 5481 (1596), 118, 140; STC 5482 (1605), 118, 140; STC 5483 (1612), 118, 140; STC 5484 (1636), 136, 161–62.

39.   GREENE, ROBERT. *Arbasto. The Anatomie of Fortune.* STC **12217.** UMI **568:13.**

Greene (1558?–1592) is described on the title page as "Master of Arte." In a passage about men who flatter women, he appears to allude to *Troilus and Criseyde.* He writes:

> Polixena counted Achilles a flatterer, because he continued the siege against Troy. Cressid therfore forsooke Troilus, because hee warred against the Grecians, & we cannot count him our privy friende which is our open fo [*sic*]. (sig. D2v)

Other editions: STC 12219 (1589), sig. C4r; STC 12220 (1594), sig. C4r.
    Other editions with a different title: *The History of Arbasto King of Denmarke. Describing the Anatomy of Fortune,* STC 12221 (1617), sig. C2r; STC 12222 (1626), sig. C2r.

40.   PEELE, GEORGE. *The Araygnement of Paris.* STC **19530.** UMI **348: 05.**

This pastoral play was "Presented before the Queenes Majestie, by the Children of her chappell" (title page). At the end of the first act, Peele (1556–1596) echoes a line from *Troilus and Criseyde,* "Unknowe, unkist, and lost, that is unsought" (1: 809). Paris says to Oenone:

> My vowe is made and witnessed . . . .
> . . . .
> I will goe bring the one thy way, my flocke are here behinde,
> And I will have a lovers fee: they saie unkist, unkinde. (sig. B2v)

As Spurgeon (1: 142) notes, the line was also echoed in E. K.'s prefatory epistle to Spenser's *Shepheardes Calendar* (1579); see SPENSER, Boswell & Holton (No. 384). Spenser's work was very influential, so this and subsequent references may be echoes of Chaucer at a remove.
    Later in the play, Peele echoes the title of *The House of Fame.* In a passage in which Diana describes the Nymph Eliza, a stand-in for Queen Elizabeth, Peele writes:

> Her auncestors live in the house of fame,
> Shee giveth armes of happie victorie,
> And flowers to decke her lyons crowned with golde. (sig. E3r)

41.   RAINOLDS, JOHN, and JOHN HART. *The Summe of the Conference Betweene John Rainolds and John Hart Touching the Head and the Faith of the Church.* STC 20626. UMI 391: 4.

In the course of the dialogue between Rainolds (1549–1607) and Hart, Hart observes that "Waldensis" (probably a reference to Thomas Netter of Saffron Walden, sometimes called the last great medieval theologian) was "a great Clerke in the time he lived." In chapter 4, Rainolds responds with a "proverbe" that echoes a line from *The Reeve's Tale*: "The gretteste clerkes been noght wisest men" (line 4054):

> It may bée: such a one as gave occasion to the proverbe, that the greatest Clerkes are not the wisest men. (162)

Other editions: STC 20627 (1588), 121; STC 20628 (1598), 121; STC 20629 (1609), 121.

42.   SCOTT, REGINALD. *Scot's Discovery of Witchcraft Proving the Common Opinions of Witches Contracting with Divels, Spirits, or Familiars to Be but Imaginary, Erronious Conceptions and Novelties.* STC 21864. UMI 1116: 7.

For references to Chaucer and quotations from *The Wife of Bath's Tale*, and *The Canon's Yeoman's Prologue* and *Tale*, see SCOTT (1584) in Boswell & Holton No. 427.

In book 16, chapter 5, Scott echoes a line from *The Reeve's Tale*: "The gretteste clerkes been noght wisest men" (line 4054). He writes:

> To passe over all the fables, which are vouched by the popish doctors . . . whose zeal and learning otherwise I might justly commend . . . [in a shoulder note: "The greatest clarkes are not the wisest men."] (477)

In his bibliography of "[English] Authors used in this Book," Scott (1538?–1599) lists "Geffrey Chaucer" (sig. B6v).

Other editions: S944 (1654), sig. B4v and p. 344; S945A (1665), sig. (b4)v and p. 205; S945 (1665), sig. (b4)v and p. 205; S943 (1651), sig. B4v and p. 344; S943A (1651), sig. B4v and p. 344; S944 (1654), sig. B4v and p. 253; S945A (1665), sig. (b4)v and p. 205; S945 (1665), sig. (b4)v and p. 205.

1585

43. PEELE, GEORGE. *The Device of the Pageant Borne before the Woolstone Dixi Lord Mayor of the Citie of London.* STC 19533. UMI 1526: 11.

In a passage spoken by "London" in praise of Queen Elizabeth, Peele echoes the title of *The House of Fame.* He writes:

> Then let me live to carroll of her name,
>   that she may ever live and never dye:
> Her sacred shrine set in the house of fame,
>   consecrate to eternall memorie. (sig. A3r)

1587

44. BRIDGES, JOHN. *A Defence of the Government Established in the Church of Englande for Ecclesiastical Matters.* STC 3734. UMI 179: 1.

Bridges (d. 1618) is identified on the title page as the "Deane of Sarum." In book 1, he echoes a line from *The Reeve's Tale*: "The gretteste clerkes been noght wisest men" (line 4054). Bridges writes:

> What now shall we saye to the gifte or office of them that had the worde of wisedome given unto them? Was that . . . the gifte of knowledge or learning. For these are distinguished heere the one from the other, (as we commonlie say: The greatest clearkes are not alwayes the wisest men) . . . . (70)

45. GREENE, ROBERT. *Euphues His Censure to Philautus.* STC 12239. UMI 1174: 1.

In addition to the allusion to *Troilus and Criseyde* noted by Boswell & Holton (No. 454), there is another. In a passage under the heading "Hectors Tragedie," Greene echoes a line from *The Reeve's Tale*: "The gretteste clerkes been noght wisest men" (line 4054). He writes:

> [T]hou arte wise and learned, but beware thou soare not too high in selfe conceipt. . . .[L]et not the olde proverbe tread on thy heele, that the greatest clarkes are not the wisest men . . . . (sig. I4r)

Another edition: STC 12240 (1634), sig. H3r.

46.   KNOX, JOHN. *The History of the Reformation of Relgion in the Realm of Scotland.* STC 15071. UMI 253: 10

Knox (1505–1572) echoes a line from *The Reeve's Tale*: "The gretteste clerkes been noght wisest men" (line 4054). In an essay headed "He that thinketh to be saved by his works, calleth himself Christ," he writes of a Friar who came to a tavern and called for a drink. Before it was forthcoming, a woman asked him to resolve an argument that she and her friends were having before he arrived. Knox writes:

> [She said that the conundrum was] What honest man wil do greatest service for least expences. And while I was musing (said the Frier) what that should mean, she said, *I see, father, that the greatest Clerks are not the wisest men.* (17)

Another edition with a different title: *The Historie of the Reformation of the Church of Scotland* (1644), K739, 17.

1588

47.   FRAUNCE, ABRAHAM. *The Lawiers Logike.* STC 11344. UMI 1137: 12.

In addition to the reference to the obsolescence of the language used in Chaucer's day noted by Boswell & Holton (No. 464), there is another to *The Squire's Tale* that comes by way of Spenser's *Shepheardes Calender* (see No. 22 above). In the fifth chapter, "Of the congregative Axiome," Fraunce writes:

> The congregative is eyther copulative, or connexive: copulative is that, whose coniunction is copulative, as that of Thornalyn in July.
>   But shepheard mought be meeke and milde,
>   well eyed, as *Argus* was:
>   With fleshly folly undefilde,
>   and stout, as steed of brasse. (fol. 93r)

Other editions in 1588: STC 11343, fol. 93r; STC 11345, same pagination.

1589

48.   GREENE, ROBERT. *Ciceronis amor. Tullies Love.* STC 12224. UMI 344: 10.

Greene is described on the title page as "in Artibus Magister." In a passage in which Tullie chides Terentia because of the ill-treatment she has given Lentulus, Greene appears to allude to *Troilus and Criseyde.* He writes:

> The crueltie of *Cresida* never amated so the hardy *Troilus* as the frowne of *Terentia* hath pierst *Lentulus* . . . . (47)

Other editions: STC 12225 (1597), 46; STC 12226 (1601), sig. G2r; STC 12227 (1605), sig. G2r; STC 12228 (1609), sig. G2r; STC 12229 (1611), sig. G2r; STC 12230 (1616), sig. G2r; STC 12231 (1628), sig. G2r; STC 12232 (1639), sig. G2r.

49.   NASH, THOMAS. *Mar-Martine.* STC 17461. UMI 433: 11/12.

Nash (1567–1601) echoes a line from *Troilus and Criseyde,* "Unknowe, unkist, and lost, that is unsought" (1: 809). He writes:

> *Thou caytif kerne, uncouth thou art, unkist thou eke sal bee.* (sig. A2v)

As Spurgeon (1: 142) notes, the line also echoes E. K.'s prefatory epistle to Spenser's *Shepheardes Calendar* (1579); see SPENSER, Boswell & Holton No. 384. *Another edition* in 1589: STC 17462a, UMI 1731: 32

50.   ROBINSON, RICHARD. *A Golden Mirrour.* STC 21121.5. UMI 1840: 5.

In a passage headed "Verses pend upon the Etimologie of the name of the right honorable, Fardinando, Lord Strange," Robinson (*fl.* 1574) extolls the virtues of Lord Strange and echoes the title of *The House of Fame.* The poet dreams that Fame commands him to write:

> Fame in her flight, by chance found me
> Asléepe upon a banke,
>
> . . . .
> . . . . . . I (said she) wilt now indite
>
> . . . .
> Recorded is his life by mée,
> Within my house of fame:
> From age to age his memorie
> Shall still advance his name. (sig. C3v–4r)

51.   WARNER, WILLIAM. *Albions England.* STC 25080. UMI 370: 4.

In addition to allusions noted by Boswell & Holton (No. 444), there appears to be another in this revised and augmented edition. In book 1, chapter 31, Warner (1558?–1609) appears to allude to a line from *Troilus and Criseyde*, "Unknowe, unkist, and lost, that is unsought" (1: 809). Warner writes:

> I Entring Guest-wise on a time the frolicke Thæban Court,
> Mine eye presented to mine heart a Nymph of lovelie Port.
> Her knew I not, nor knew she me, unknowne therefore unkist
> I loyter on the Earth, meane while in Heaven not unmist. (137)

As Spurgeon (1: 142) notes, the line was also echoed in E. K.'s prefatory epistle to Spenser's *Shepheardes Calendar* (1579); see SPENSER, Boswell & Holton No. 384.
    Other editions: STC 25081 (1592), 137; STC 25082 (1596), 154; STC 25082a (1597), 154; STC 25083 (1602), 154; STC 25084 (1612), 139 (really 154).

1590

52.   GREENE, ROBERT. *Greenes Never Too Late: or, A Powder of Experience.* STC 12253. UMI 1238: 16.

In addition to several references to Troilus and Criseyde noted by Boswell & Holton (No. 481), there is another. In a section headed "Mullidor the malecontent, with his pen clapt full of love, to his Mistris Mirimida," Greene seems to echo *The Wife of Bath's Tale*: "What thyng it is that wommen moost desire" (line 1007), "What thyng that worldly wommen loven best" (line 1033), and "Women desiren have sovereynte" (line 1038).

> I am content . . . rather to holde you for my Mistris than my wife. Then seeing you shall have the soveraintie at my hands, which is the thing women desire. (sig. K1v)

53.   LODGE, THOMAS. *Rosalynde. Euphues Golden Legacie.* STC 16664. UMI 2169: 4.

Lodge (1558?–1625) is identified on the title page as "T. L. Gent." In a section headed "Rosalyndes description," Lodge appears to allude to *The Wife of Bath's Tale*: "Women desiren have sovereyntee" (line 1038). Lodge writes:

> Oh Mistress quoth Ganimede, hold your peace, for you are partiall: Who knowes not, but that all women have desire to tye soveraintie to their petticotes . . . . (sig. I1v)

Other editions: STC 16665 (1592), UMI 476: 01, sig. H1v; STC 16666 (1596), sig. G3v; STC 16667 (1598), sig. G3v; STC 16668 (1604), sig. G3v; STC 16669 (1609), sig. G3v; STC 16670 (1612), sig. G3v; STC 16672 (1623), sig. G3v; STC 16673 (1634), sig. G3v; STC 16673.5 (1634), sig. G3v.

1591

54. AGGAS, EDWARD. *An Answeare to the Supplication against Him*. STC 664. UMI 907: 11.

In this work "faithfully translated out of French by E. A." (title page), Aggas (b. in or before 1549, d. 1625?) echoes the description of the Parson in *The General Prologue*: "That first he wroughte, and afterward he taughte" (line 497). He writes/translates:

> Our L. Jesus Christ, to winne the Jewes hearts, began first by well doing, and afterward he taught. (sig. D4r)

55. BARROW, HENRY. *A Brief Discoverie of the False Church*. STC 1517. UMI 172: 10.

In a 1707 edition of this work, Barrow is described on the title page as "a member of the honourable society of Grays-Inn, who suffered deaths for his non-conformity to the Church of England." Here, in a passage about learned but "grosly popish" divines, Barrow (1550?–1593) echoes a line from *The Reeve's Tale*: "The gretteste clerkes been noght wisest men" (line 4054). He writes:

> I perceave now the greatest clarkes are not alwaies the wisest men. (85)

1593

56. DRAYTON, MICHAEL. *Idea. The Shepheards Garland*. STC 7202. UMI 381: 3.

In addition to the references noted by Boswell & Holton (No. 518), there may be another in "The Fifth Eglog," where Drayton places "Mother of Muses, great Apollos bride" in the House of Fame and echoes the title of *The House of Fame*:

> Earths heaven, worlds wonder, hiest house of fame,
> > Reviver of the dead, eye-killer of the live,
> Belov'd of Angels, Vertues greatest name
> > Favours rar'st feature, beauties prospective,
> > Oh that my Verse thy vertues could contrive. (33)

57.   GREENE, ROBERT. *Greenes Mourning Garment.* STC 12251. UMI 1101: 15.

Greene (1558?–1592) is identified on the title page as "R. Greene. Utriusq[ue] academia in artibus magister." In addition to the reference to Chaucer noted by Spurgeon (1: 131) and Boswell & Holton No. 480, Greene appears to allude to *Troilus and Criseyde.* In a passage about fickle women, he writes:

> [W]hat are their loves? like the passage of a Serpent over a stone, which once past can never be seene. They will promise mountaines and performe moulhilles, say they love with Dido, when they fayne with Cresida . . . . (41)

Another edition: STC 12252 (1616), sig. D4v.

58.   P., G. "The Praise of Chastitie" in *The Phœnix Nest.* STC 21516. UMI 1033: 18.

G. P. is characterized in the heading of this poem as "Master of Arts," and here he echoes the title of *The House of Fame.* He writes:

> The Phrygian knights, that in the house of fame,
> Have shining armes of endles memorie,
> By hot and fierce repulse did win the same,
> Through Helens rape, hurt Paris progenie. (12)

59.   PEELE, GEORGE. *The Honour of the Garter.* STC 19539. UMI 384: 12.

In addition to those general allusions noted by Spurgeon (1: 140) and Boswell & Holton (No. 532), Peele echoes the title of *The House of Fame.* In a passage about King Edward, Peele writes:

> I found at last King *Edward* was the man,
> Accompanyed with Kings and Conquerours,
> That from the spacious aerie house of *Fame*,
> Set forward royally to solemnize,
> Th' installment of some new created knights. (sig. B4r)
> . . . .
> For in the house of *Fame* what famous man,
> What Prince but hath his Tropie and his place? (sig. C1v)
> . . . .
> Yet in the house of *Fame* and Courtes of Kings,
> Envy will bite, or snarle and barke at least . . . . (sig. C3v)

Also found in *Great Brittaines General Joyes. Londons Glorious Triumphs* (1613), q.v., attributed to Antony Nixon and considerably revised.

1594

60.   GREENE, ROBERT. *The Historie of Orlando Furioso.* STC 12265. UMI 344: 13.

The title page advises readers that this play "was plaid before the Queenes Majestie." In a scene about midway in the play, "a clown" (dressed as Angelica) pretends that Orgalio gave her eighteen pence and let her go, but Orlando does not believe her and compares her to "faithles Cresida." Greene (1558?–1592) probably alludes to *Troilus and Criseyde.* He writes:

> Orl: Why strumpet, worse than Mars his trothlesse love.
> Falser than faithles Cresida: strumpet thou shalt not scape. (sig. F2r)

Another edition: STC 12266 (1599), sig. F1r.

61.   LEWKENOR, LEWIS. Interpolation in *The Resolved Gentleman.* STC 15139. UMI 1177: 23.

The Resolved Gentleman is Lewkenor's translation of *Chevalier délibéré* by Oliver de La Marche (ca. 1426–1502). At the end of that work Lewkenor added "A short discourse of the Princes of Burgundie," at the end of which he echoes the title of *The House of Fame.* In an interpolation about Queen Elizabeth, he writes:

> [H]er Majestie [in a shoulder note: "*Queene Elizabeth.*"] whose Princely name . . . will leave the glorious storie of her happie reigne, to those golden pennes, that being dipped in the licour of the Muses, may like *Ariosto* his silver Swannes, with a cleere flight beare up her sacred name, and in dispite of Time, fasten the same to the faire pillars of Eternitie, in the highest turret of the house of Fame. (73–73)

1596

62.   BUREL, JOHN. "An Application Concerning Our Kings Majesties Persoun," in *To the Richt High, Lodwik Duke of Lenox.* STC 4105. UMI 412: 12.

In a poem in praise of James VI of Scotland, Burel echoes the title of *The House of Fame:*

This valiant King, justly deservis the croun,
Lang mot he live, with sick a worthy name,
His ventrous acts, and royhall hie renoun,
Ingravit is, within the house of fame,
But ony spot, infirmitie or blame:
O God, gif it, a gret rejoysing be,
Sick properties, intill a Prence to se. (sig. K2v)

63.   Le Sylvain, Alexandre. *The Orator*. STC 4182. UMI 413: 2.

In this translation by "L. P." (sometimes attributed to Anthony Munday) of Le Sylvain's *Epitomes des cent histoires tragicques*, there appears to be an echo of *The Wife of Bath's Tale*: "What thyng it is that wommen moost desire" (line 1007), "What thyng that worldly wommen loven best" (line 1033), and "Women desiren have sovereyntee" (line 1038). L. P. translates an answer to "Declamation 11":

[Y]ou must remember my Princesse, that he is her son who hath made the zeale of her countrie strive and triumph over the name of a Princess . . . over soveraigntie so greatly desired of women . . . . (76)

1597

64.   Gry., Hu. "Upon the Authors Muse," in *Sinetes Passion uppon His Fortunes*. STC 19338. UMI 550: 5.

In a commendatory poem for Robert Parry (*fl.* 1540–1612), "Hu. Gry." echoes the title of *The House of Fame*. He writes:

If Poets with penne doe purchase praise,
Let Parrie then possesse his parte:
Whose Posies rate, report doeth raise,
To Pernasse Mount of due desarte.
    In house of Fame he ought have place,
    Yf Ovid ev'r deserved that grace. (sig. A3v)

65.   Shakespeare, William. *Romeo and Juliet*. STC 22322. UMI 353: 11.

In addition to other allusions noted by Boswell & Holton (No. 592), there may be another. In the first act, Mercutio attempts to entice Romeo to go dancing and echoes a line from *The Manciple's Prologue*: "Sires, what! Dun is in the myre!" (line 5). Shakespeare writes:

Tut, duns the Mouse, the Constables owne word,
If thou art dun, weele draw thee from the mire. (sig. C1r)

Other editions: STC 22323 (1599), sig. C1v; STC 22324 (1609), sig. C1v; STC 22325a (1622), sig. B4v; STC 22326 (1637), sig. B4v.

Also found in Shakespeares *Comedies, Histories, & Tragedies*, STC 22273 (1623), ³57; STC 22274 (1632), ³86; S2913 (1663), 646; S2914 (1664), 646; S2915 (1685), ²308.

1598

66.   GREENE, ROBERT. *The Scottish Historie of James the Fourth, Slaine at Flodden*. STC 12308. UMI 344: 22.

In the third act, in a scene featuring Lord Ateukins and his servant Andrew, Greene echoes a line from *The Reeve's Tale*: "The gretteste clerkes been noght wisest men" (line 4054). He writes:

> [T]he greatest Clarkes are not the wisest, and a foole may dance in a hood, as wel as a wise man in a bare frock. . . . (sig. F2r)

ca. 1599

67.   DAVIES, SIR JOHN. *Epigrammes*. STC 6350.5. UMI 1750: 3.

"Epigrammata prima" is addressed "Ad Musam," and there Davies (1596–1626) echoes the title of *The House of Fame*. He writes:

> Flie merry Muse unto that merry towne,
> where [*sic*] thou mayst playes, revels, and triumphes see
> The house of fame, & Theatre of renowne,
> Where all good wits & spirits be. (sig. A3r)

Also found in *Ovid's elegies: Three Books by C. M. Epigrames by J. D.*, STC 6350 (n.d.; after 1602), sig. F4r; STC 18932 (n.d.; ca. 1630), sig. E8v; STC 18933 (n.d.; ca. 1640), sig. E8v.

68.   MORTON, THOMAS. *A Treatise of the Nature of God*. STC 18198. UMI 1389: 2.

In the third section of chapter 3, "Of the faculties of mans soule attributed to God," in a dialogue between a gentleman and a scholar, Thomas Morton of Berwick echoes a line from *The Reeve's Tale*: "The gretteste clerkes been noght wisest men" (line 4054). He writes:

[A]s it is usually said of your schollers, that the greatest Clarkes are not the wisest men. . . . (109)

1601

69.   WEEVER, JOHN. *The Mirror of Martyrs: or, The Life and Death of Sir John Old-Castle.* STC 25226. UMI 1224: 5.

In a passage in which "Old-Castle" speculates on his fame after death, Weever (1576–1632) echoes the title of *The House of Fame*. The knight imagines that some poet will hear a voice commanding him to set forth in "immortal verse" his "entomblesse worth." Weever writes:

> Then should the world on brasen pillers view me
> with [*sic*] great *Achilles*, in the house of Fame;
> His Tutor'd pen with Tropheis would renew me,
> And still repaire the ruin of my name . . . . (sig. F2v)

1602

70.   DEKKER, THOMAS. *Satiro-Mastix: or, The Untrussing of the Humorous Poet.* STC 6521. UMI 881: 9.

In a scene featuring Horace and Asinus, Dekker (ca. 1572–1632) echoes a line from *The Reeve's Tale*: "The gretteste clerkes been noght wisest men" (line 4054). Horace suggests that Asinius read a good book, and he replies:

> Leave have you deare Ningle, marry for reading any book. . . tis out my Element: no faith, ever since I felt one hit me inth teeth that the greatest Clarkes are not the wisest men, could I abide to goe to Schoole. . . . (sig. C3r)

71.   NICHOLSON, SAMUEL. *A Sermon, Called Gods New Yeeres-Guift Sent unto England.* STC 18547. UMI 1551: 15.

In a passage about the mystery of God's love for sinners, Nicholson echoes a line from *The Reeve's Tale*: "The gretteste clerkes been noght wisest men" (line 4054). He writes:

> Thus did our Saviour shake up this foolish shadow of a Prophet . . . this emptie vessell contayning nothing but ye bare name of a Doctor . . . whose example if we moralize, it teacheth us, That (in Gods matters) the greatest Clarkes are not the wisest men. (sig. A7v–8r)

1603

72.　Crosse, Henry. *Vertues Common-wealth: or, The High-way to Honour.* STC 6070. UMI 2039: 11.

In addition to a reference to Chaucer's decorum noted by Boswell & Holton (No. 685), Crosse also echoes the title of *The House of Fame.* In a passage contrasting the paths of pleasure and virtue, he writes:

> [T]he pathe leading to *Vertue*, though it be toylesome, laborious, difficult, a way uneasie to be trackt, hard to finde, craggie, stonie, thorny, and a sweating turmoyle . . . [yet he that] goeth streight to his journies ende, shall arrive at the house of Fame, be crowned with honor . . . for though the rootes of *Vertue* be bitter, yet the fruites be sweete. (sig. G1r)

Another issue in 1603: STC 6070.5, sig. G1r.
　　Another edition with a different title: *The Schoole of Pollicie,* STC 6071 (1605), sig. G1r.

73.　Dowland, John. *The Third and Last Booke of Songs and Aires.* STC 7096. UMI 882: 2.

In his epistle addressed to the reader, Dowland echoes the title of *The House of Fame.* He writes:

> *The applause of them that judge, is the incouragement of those that write.* . . .
> *As in a hive of bees al labour alike to lay up honny opposing themselves against none but fruitles drones; so in the house of learning and fame, all good indevours should strive to ad somewhat that is good* . . . . (sig. A2v)

1605

74.　Jonson, Benjamin. *Sejanus His Fall.* STC 14782. UMI 757: 22

Jonson (1573?–1637) echoes Chaucers description of the poor Parson, "Ne maked him a spiced conscience" (*The General Prologue*, line 526) and *The Wife of Bath's Prologue,* "Ye sholde been al pacient and meke, | And han a sweete spiced conscience" (lines 434–35) in *Sejanus,* act 5, where Sejanus says to Flamen:

> Be thou dumbe, scrupu'lous Priest:
> . . . .
> Avoid these fumes, these superstitious Lights,
> And all these coos'ning *Ceremonies*; You.
> Your pure, and spiced conscience. (sig. K4r–v)

444JACKSON CAMPBELL BOSWELL

Also found in *The Workes of Benjamin Jonson* (1616), STC 14752, 420; and J1006 (1692), 145–46.

1606

75.   BRYSKETT, LODOWICK. *A Discourse of Civill Life*. STC 3958. UMI 916: 5.

In a passage about "men of great learning" behaving rudely, Bryskett echoes a line from *The Reeve's Tale*: "The gretteste clerkes been noght wisest men" (line 4054). He writes:

[I]t hath bin fitly used for a proverbe among us, that the greatest clerkes are not alwayes the wisest men. (14)

1607

76.   BEAUMONT, FRANCIS, and JOHN FLETCHER. *The Woman Hater*. STC 1693. UMI 982: 13.

In addition to the allusion noted by Boswell & Holton (No. 752), there is another in this comedy "lately acted by the Children of Paules" (title page). In the third scene of act four, Beaumont and Fletcher echo a line from *The Manciple's Prologue*: "Sires, what! Dun is in the myre!" (line 5). Pandar says:

Dun's ith' myre, get out againe how a can . . . . (sig. H1r)

Another edition in 1607, STC 1693, same pagination.
    Other editions: B1618 (1648), sig. D3v; B1619 (1649), sig. D3v.

77.   C., R., trans. *A World of Wonders*. STC 10553. UMI 342: 4 and 787: 3 (as STC 10554).

In addition to the reference noted by Spurgeon (3: 4.60) and Boswell & Holton (No. 759), there is another. In translating *Apologie pour Hérodote* by Henri Estienne (1531–1598), R. C. echoes a line from *The Merchant's Tale*: "Old fish, and young flesh woll I haue full faine" (line 1418). R.C. translates:

For considering the common saying in every mans mouth, *Yong flesh, and old fish* . . . . (235).

An issue: STC 10554 (1608), same pagination.

78.   DEKKER, THOMAS, and WEBSTER, JOHN. *West-ward Hoe.* STC 6540. UMI 881: 18.

In addition to the allusion noted by Boswell & Holton (No. 757), there is another in this comedy "divers times acted by the Children of Paules." Dekker and Webster echo a line from *The Manciple's Prologue*: "Sires, what! Dun is in the myre!" (line 5). A character called Parentheses says: "I see i'me borne still to draw Dun out ath mire for you." (sig. D3r).

1608

79.   DAY, JOHN. *Humour Out of Breath.* STC 6411. UMI 880: 12.

In this comedy "divers times latelie acted, by the Children of the Kings Revells" (title page), there is an echo of a line from *The Manciple's Prologue*: "Sires, what! Dun is in the myre!" (line 5). Near the end of the first act, Page says, "I must play dun, and draw them all out o'th mire." (sig. C2r).

80.   WEST, RICHARD. *Wits A.B.C: or, A Centurie of Epigrams.* STC 25262. UMI 725: 12.

Epigram No. 68 is headed "In Pisonem," and West (*fl.* 1606–1619) echoes a line in *The Reeve's Prologue*: "For in oure wyl ther striketh evere a nayl, | To have an hoor heed and a grene tayl, | As hath a leek" (3876–78). He writes:

> One foote already's placed in the grave,
> And yet he will a female fellow have,
> > Wherefore I thinke (a thing but seldome seene)
> > Although his head be gray, his tayle is greene. (sig. L2r)

1609

81.   DAVIES, JOHN. *Humours Heav'n on Earth.* STC 6332. UMI 1376: 4.

In a section headed "The Second Tale: Containing, the Civile Warres of Death and Fortune," John Davies of Hereford (1565?–1618) echoes a line from *The Reeve's Tale*: "The gretteste clerkes been noght wisest men" (line 4054). In a passage about supposedly faithful servants who feather their own nests and who climb highest in their own conceit, in a shoulder note for stanza 62, he writes:

> [They are] Men lerned, without jugement, whome the Proverbe, The greatest Clarkes are not the wisest men, concerneth. (204)

1610

82.   CAMDEN, WILLIAM. *Britain: or, A Chorographicall Description of the Most Flourishing Kingdomes, England, Scotland, and Ireland, and the Ilands Adjoyning.* STC 4509. UMI 919: 1.

In addition to the references noted by Boswell & Holton (No. 811), there is another. Under the running heading "Degrees of States in England," in a section about Vavasors, Camden quotes modernized lines from *The General Prologue of The Canterbury Tales* that describe the Franklin: "A shirreve hadde he been, and a contour. | Was nowher swich a worthy vavasour" (lines 359–60). He writes:

> *Vavasors* or *Valvasors* in old time, stood in the next ranke after Barons. . . . in Chaucers time it was not great, seeing that of his Franklin a good yeoman or Freeholder, he writeth but thus:
>   *A Sheriffe had he beene and a Contour,*
>   *Was no where such a worthy Vavasour.* (170)

Other editions: STC 4510 (1637), 170; C359 (1695), clxxviii.

1612

83.   DABORNE, ROBERT. *A Christian Turn'd Turke: or, The Tragicall Lives and Deaths of the Two Famous Pyrates, Ward and Dansiker.* STC 6184. UMI 830: 13.

In this play, Daborne (d. 1628) echoes a line from *The Manciple's Prologue*: "Sires, what! Dun is in the myre!" (line 5). In "scena ultima," a character called Rabshake says, "Is *Dunne* in the mire? for old acquaintance sake wee'l dragge you out sir: you are in travell, I am the sonne of a Midwife, Il'e helpe to deliver you" (sig. H4v).

84.   GREENHAM, RICHARD. *The Workes of Richard Greenham, Minister and Preacher.* STC 12318. UMI 1174: 5.

In "A Profitable Treatise Containing a Direction for the Reading and Understanding of the Holy Scriptures," Greenham echoes a line from *The Reeve's Tale*: "The gretteste clerkes been noght wisest men" (line 4054). In a passage about those with "a heart prepared to learne," he writes:

> They that want this, how much soever they have heard or read, yet shall they never have sound and settled judgement. And this is one cause why it is said, *that the greatest Clerkes are not the wisest men.* (175)

In an essay headed "Of the power and priviledges of Gods word," in a passage about the importance of meditation, Greenham again echoes a line from *The Reeve's Tale*:

> [M]editation is the life of learning, the want where of causeth, that the greatest Clerkes are not the wisest men. (858)

85.   WILSON, THOMAS. *A Christian Dictionarie.* STC 25786. UMI 816: 2.

Wilson (1563–1622) is identified on the title page as "minister of the Word, at Saint Georges in Canterbury." In a little poem headed "The Dictionary to the Readers," Wilson appears to echo a line from *Troilus and Criseyde*, "Unknowe, unkist, and lost, that is unsought" (1: 809). He writes:

> *Unkened, unkist, (saith Proverbe olde)*
> *Love springs ftrom knowledge, thus we hold:* [Etc.] (sig. ¶5r)

As Spurgeon (1: 142) notes, the line was also echoed in E. K.'s prefatory epistle to Spenser's *Shepheardes Calendar* (1579); see SPENSER, Boswell & Holton No. 384.

Other editions: STC 25787 (1616), sig. ¶5r; STC 25788 (1622), sig. A8v; STC 25789 (ca. 1635), sig. A8v; W2940 (1647), UMI 2163: 8, sig. A4v; W2940A (1648), sig. A4v.

Another edition with a different title: *A Complete Christian Dictionary*, W2942 (1654), no surviving copy known.

1613

86.   BROWNE, WILLIAM. *Britannia's Pastorals.* STC 3914. UMI 1725: 8.

In addition to allusions to Chaucer noted by Spurgeon (3: 4.62) and to *The Nun's Priest's Tale* noted by Boswell & Holton (No. 863), there may be an allusion to *The Merchant's Tale*. In book 1, "Song 2," in a passage about mismatched mates, Browne (1590–ca. 1645) writes:

> How many Shepherds daughters, who in dutie
> To griping fathers have inthral'd their beautie,
> To wait upon the *Gout*, to walke when pleases
> Old *January* halt. (34)

Other editions: STC 3915 (1616), 43 (really 34); STC 3916 (1625), 45.

87.   NICCOLS, RICHARD. *The Three Sisters Teares Shed at the Late Solemne Funerals of the Royall Deceased Henry, Prince of Wales.* STC 18525. UMI 1321: 10.

In this elegy for the late, lamented Prince Henry, Niccols (1584–1616) echoes the title of *The House of Fame.* He writes:

> I came to that great house of F A M E ,
> That sacred Temple built by K I N G s of yore,
> Th' admired workmanship of whose faire frame
> Excels all others that have beene before. (sig. C1r)

88.   NIXON, ANTHONY. *Great Brittaines Generall Joyes. Londons Glorious Triumphs.* STC 18587. UMI 1282: 22.

A different version of this work was previously published; see PEELE (1593). To save readers the trouble of flipping back and forth, new as well as old references are recorded here.

The title page advises readers that the poems published herein were "Dedicated to the Immortall memorie of the joyfull Marriage of the two famous and illustrious Princes, Fredericke and Elizabeth. Celebrated the 14. of Februarie, being S. Valentines day. With the Installment of the sayd potent Prince Fredericke at Windsore, the 7. of Februarie aforesaid." The newly-weds were Frederick of Bohemia and Elizabeth, "The Winter Queen."

Under the heading "Prince Frederick created Knight of the Garter, and instald at Windsor the 7 day of February 1612," Nixon echoes the title of *The House of Fame*:

> At last I found King *Edward* was the man,
> Accompanide with Kings & Conquerours,
> That from the spatious Aerie house of fame,
> Set forward royall to sollemnize,
> Th'installment of some new created knights. (sig. C3r)
> . . . .
> At last me thought, King Edward thus bespake,
> . . . .
> . . . . in honor of my Knights
> Before this day created, and instal'd,
> But specially in honor of this Knight,
> That at this day this honor hath receav'd
> Under King James, great Brittaines Soveraigne
> With princely traines, I from the house of fame
> Doe resalute thee heere, and gratulate
> To this new Knight, created by a King

Peerles for wisdome and for majesty,
The honor of the Garter . . . . (sig. C4r)

89.   PAGE, S. *The Love of Amos and Laura.* STC 4275. UMI 1197: 4.

The work at hand is printed with I. C.'s *Alcilia Philoparthens* (see Boswell &
Holton No. 864). In a verse epistle, "The Author to His Booke," Page may echo
Chaucer's line, "Go, litel bok, go litel myn tragedye" (*Troilus and Criseyde* 5: 1786):

Go little booke into the largest world,
And blase the chastnes of thy maiden Muse [etc.]
  (no sig., verso of title page, inserted between sigs. K3–4)

90.   PARROTT, HENRY. *Laquei ridiculosi: or, Springes for Woodcocks.* STC
19332. UMI 660: 8.

In an epigram headed "Quod laudamus amamus," Parrott echoes a line from
The Reeve's Tale: "The gretteste clerkes been noght wisest men" (line 4054). He
writes:

Marcus maintaines it boldly with his pen,
And will approve it by Philosophy,
That greatest Clarkes are not the wisest men,
(And therein shewes you many reasons why:)
Amongst the rest not least considerate,
Brings his defence from *Tom the Coryate.* (sig. C2v)

1614

91.   MOSSE, MILES. *Justifying and Saving Faith Distinguished from the Faith
of the Devils.* STC 18209. UMI 1249: 12.

Mosse is identified on the title page as "pastor of the church of God at Combes
in Suffolke, and Doctor of Divinitie." In this sermon preached at Paul's Cross in
London on 9 May 1613, Mosse refers to Chaucer and echoes a line from *Troilus
and Criseyde*, "Unknowe, unkist, and lost, that is unsought" (1: 809). In a passage
about "faith of special mercie," he writes of those theologians who argue to the
contrary:

[T]hey are uncooth, and let them be unkissed: to use olde *Chaucers*
phrase. (79)

As Spurgeon (1: 142) notes, the line was also echoed in E. K.'s prefatory epistle to
Spenser's *Shepheardes Calendar* (1579); see SPENSER, Boswell & Holton No. 384.

92.   SAUL, ARTHUR. *The Famous Game of Chesse-Play.* STC 21772. UMI 859: 1.

In a poem headed "To his Booke," Saul (d. 1617) may echo Chaucer's line, "Go, litel bok, go litel myn tragedye" (*Troilus and Criseyde* 5: 1786):

> *Goe forth my little Booke,*
> *Thou art no longer mine:*
> *Each man may on thee looke,*
> *The shame or praise is thine.*
> . . . .
> *Hadst thou remain'd with me,*
> *Thou shouldst have had no blame,*
> *Since thou abroad wouldst be,*
> *Go forth and seeke thy fame.* (sig. A4r)

Other editions: STC 21773 (1618), sig. A5v–6r; STC 21774 (1640), sig. A5v–6r; S729A (1652), sig. A5v–6r; S730 (1672), sig. A5v–6r; S730A (1673), sig. A5v–6r.

93.   SYLVESTER, JOSHUA. *The Parliament of Vertues Royal.* STC 23581. UMI 861: 5.

In this translation by Sylvester (1563–1618) of Jean Bertaut's *Panarète*, Sylvester echoes the title of *The House of Fame*.

> Shee seem'd like *Pallas* . . . she thus replyde:
>   Celestiall Herald, While th'heroick Prince
> Whose gentle Yoak his *Celticks* so contents,
> Carv'd with his Sword a Statue to my Name,
> To stand triumphant in the House of *Fame*,
> Nothing could hold me from his steps, a part . . . . (6–7)

Also found in *All the Small Works of That Famous Poet Josuah Silvester* (1620), STC 23575, same pagination.

1615

94.   WITHER. GEORGE. *Fidelia.* STC 25905. UMI 1564: 5.

Wither (1588–1667) is not named on the title page, but in the second edition he is identified as "G. W. of Lincolnes Inne, Gentleman." In a passage about avaricious parents who force their children into loveless marriages, Wither may allude to *The Merchant's Tale.* He writes:

For these respectlesse of all care, do marry
Hot youthfull *May* to cold old *January*.
Those for some greedy end doe basely tie
The sweetest faire to foule deformitie. (sig. B10v)

Other editions: STC 25906 (1617), sig. B8r; STC 25907 (1619), sig. C2v.

Also collected in *The Workes of Master George Wither* (1620), STC 25890, sig. X5v.

1616

95.   HAKEWILL, GEORGE. *An Answere to a Treatise Written by Dr. Carier.* STC 12610. UMI 1069: 20.

Hakewill (1578–1649) is identified on the title page as "Doctour of Divinity, and chapleine to the Prince his Highness." The "Treatise" mentioned in the title was "a letter to his Majestie wherein he layth downe sundry politike considerations; by which hee pretendeth himselfe was moved, and endevoureth to move other to be reconciled to the Church of Rome, and imbrace that religion, which he calleth catholike" (title page). The work is laid out with quotations from Carier and Hakewill's response. In section 45, Hakewill compares the Church of Rome to a grasping stepmother and cites Chaucer and alludes to *The Summoner's Tale*. He writes:

[W]e cannot in common reason entertaine union with her, much lesse acknowledge subjection unto her. . . . The Frier in *Chaucer* would have nothing be killed for his sake, only he desired the liver of the capon, and the braine of the pig: So the *Pope* would be contented there should bee no innovation in *England*, upon condition his *Supremacie* and the *Masse* . . . were readmitted. . . . (293)

96.   NIXON, ANTHONY. *The Foot-Post of Dover with His Packet Stuft Full of Strange and Merry Petitions.* STC 18591A. UMI 1606: 27.

In a passage describing a harlot, the narrator of this work says that this "peart one . . . as ready to give the welcome to her customers, as a boy in a barre" would never give him the time of day. But "Opinion" disagrees and compares the harlot to "Cresida," an allusion to *Troilus and Criseyde*. Nixon writes:

This is one (said Opinion) whose face is a painted Sepulcher . . . and her love, like the passage of a Serpent over a stone, which once past, can never be seene. She will promise mountaines, and perform Molehils. She will say she loves with Dido, and yet faine with Cresida . . . . (sig. B3r)

In this passage Nixon plagiarizes *Greenes Mourning Garment* (1593), q.v.

1617

97.   GREENE, ROBERT. *Alcida. Greenes Metamorphosis.* STC 12216. UMI 1173: 18.

In addition to the reference to Chaucer noted by Franklin B. Williams, Jr., and by Boswell & Holton (No. 940), there is another. In Alcida's "first Historie," she mentions Troilus and "Cresida" and perhaps alludes to *Troilus and Crisedye.* Greene writes:

> Your late passionate speech . . . makes me think that Venus is your chiefe goddesse, and that love is the lord, whose livery you weare: if it be so, neighbour take heede (for fancie is a Shrew) . . . and Troilus may stand long enough on the walls before Cresida wave her glove for a salve. (sig. D1r)

1618

98.   HUTTON, HENRY. *Follie's Anatomie: or, Satyres and Satyricall Epigrams.* STC 14028. UMI 963: 12.

In this collection of epigrams, Hutton echoes a line in *The Manciple's Prologue*: "Sires, what! Dun is in the myre!" (line 5). His "Epilogus" ends:

> I doe referre my Muse, unto such eyes,
> Which truely can their judgements equalize:
>   Such, will be meanes, to save her from the fire
>   And if neede stand, to draw *Dun* out ith' mire. (sig. D2v)

1619

99.   NORTH, SIR EDWARD, trans. Guevera's Αρχοντορολογιον [Archontorologion]: *or, The Dial of Princes.* STC 12430. UMI 1102: 12.

In this translation by Sir Edward North of a Spanish edition of Bishop Antonio de Guevara's *Libro llamado Relox de principes*, there appears to be an echo of the Wife of Bath's claim that "Women desiren have sovereyntee" (*The Wife of Bath's Tale*, line 1038). Near the end of the volume, in chapter 11, in a letter addressed to "the Ladie Macrine," North translates:

I know ye women desire one thing greatly: that is, to have soverainty of
us . . . . (762)

100. WITHER. GEORGE. *Fidelia. Newly Corrected and Augemented.* STC
25907. UMI 1401: 14.

Wither (1588–1667) is identified on the title page as a gentleman of Lincoln's
Inn. In a passage about avaricious parents who force their children into loveless
marriages, Wither may allude to *The Merchant's Tale.* He writes:

For these respectlesse of all care, do marry
Hot youthfull *May* to cold old *January.*
Those for some greedy end doe basely tie
The sweetest faire to foule deformitie. (sig. C2v)

Other editions: STC 25905 (1615), sig. B11v; STC 25906 (1617), sig. B11v; STC
25907 (1619), sig. C2v.
  Also found in *The Workes* (1620), STC 25890, sig. X5v.
  Also collected in *Juvenilia* (1622), STC 25911, sig. Pp4v; STC 25911a
(1626), sig. Pp4v; STC 25912 (1633), 471.

1623

101. TAYLOR, JOHN. *The Praise and Vertue of a Jayle and Jaylers.* STC 23785.
UMI 1157: 19.

Under the heading "The Vertue of a Jayle, and necessitie of Hanging," Taylor
(1580–1653), well known as "the water poet," echoes the title of *The House of
Fame* as he writes of role of the Tower of London as a prison:

For though the Tower be a Castle Royall,
Yet ther's a Prison in't for men disloyall:
Though for defence a Campe may there be fitted,
Yet for offence, men thither are committed.
It is a house of fame, and there is in't
A Palace for a Prince, a Royall Mint, [etc.] (sig. B3v)

Also found in *All the Workes of John Taylor the Water-Poet* (1630), STC 23725
(UMI 977: 11), 130 (sig. Mm1v).

1624

102.   CHAPMAN, GEORGE. Dedicatory poem in *The Crown of All Homers Workes Batrachomyomachia: or, The Battaile of Frogs and Mise.* STC 13628. UMI 667: 8.

In his dedicatory poem addressed "To my ever most-worthie-to-be-most honor'd lord, the Earle of Somerset, &c.," Chapman (1559/60–1634) echoes the title of *The House of Fame.* In a passage in praise of General Norris, he writes:

> And as our *English Generall,* (whose Name
> Shall equall interest finde in T'House of Fame,
> With all Earths great'st Commanders) in Retreate
> To *Belgian Gant,* stood all *Spaines* Armies heate [etc.] (sig. &2v)

103.   FEATLEY, DANIEL. *The Romish Fisher Caught and Held in His Owne Net.* STC 10738. UMI 793: 4.

Featley (1582–1645) is identified on the title page as "Doctor in Divinity." In addition to the reference noted by Boswell & Holton (No. 1061), there is also an echo from *The Manciple's Prologue*: "Sires, what! Dun is in the myre!" (line 5). Featley writes:

> Hold hooke and line, and the *Fisher* shall catch a Gudgeon. I grant, a Similitude needeth not . . . runne upon foure feet . . . and therefore cannot draw *Dunne* out of the mire. (125)

An issue in 1624: STC 10738.3, same pagination.

104.   MONTAGU, RICHARD. *Immediate Addresse unto God Alone.* STC 18039. UMI 1146: 11.

In a sermon originally delivered before "his majesty" at Windsor but "now revised and enlarged," Montagu (1577–1641) defends himself against "a false imputation of M. Antonius De Dominis" and in the process echoes a line from *Troilus and Criseyde*, "Unknowe, unkist, and lost, that is unsought" (1: 809). In a passage about the Roman Catholic custom of having "simple men invoke Saints as they doe God" (118), Montagu writes:

> It is flat and egregious foolerie at the best . . . nor all Saint-invocators in the World can proove it so: I would gladly see and know, by what warrant I on earth so uncouth and therefore unkist, so unknowne unto them altogether, for ought can bee proved . . . . (119)

As Spurgeon (1: 142) notes, the line was also echoed in E. K.'s prefatory epistle to Spenser's *Shepheardes Calendar* (1579); see SPENSER, Boswell & Holton No. 384.

1625

105.   *Grammaire angloise.* STC 12173.3. UMI 1878: 11.

In this French-printed guide to English usage, the author uses a proverb that echoes a line from *The Merchant's Tale*: "Old fish, and young flesh woll I haue full faine" (line 1418). In a passage headed "For Marchauntes to But [*sic*, i.e., buy] and sell," Mason (*fl.* 1620) writes:

> And they say in our parish that yong phisitions make the churchardes [*sic*] crooked, and old attorneies sutes to go awry: but to the contrary yong atturneies and olde phisitions, yong flesh, and olde fish be the best. (135)

106.   PURCHAS, SAMUEL. *Purchas His Pilgrimes.* STC 20509. UMI 972: 1.

In the first book, chapter 1, §VIII, "Of Ophir," Purchas (1577?–1626) echoes a line from *The Reeve's Tale*: "The gretteste clerkes been noght wisest men" (line 4054). He writes:

> So necessary to Humane and Divine knowledge is Geographie and History, the two *Eyes* with which wee see the World, without which our greatest Clerkes are not the wisest men, but in this part blind and *not able to see farre off.* (30)

In book 9, chapter 12, §V, in a passage about the Bijag kingdom of West Africa, Purchas appears to allude to a line from *Troilus and Criseyde*, "Unknowe, unkist, and lost, that is unsought" (1: 809). He writes:

> These Ilands are rich and fertile, pleasant with Trees and Rivers . . . stored with Cattell great and small, Ivorie, Fish, Rice, Waxe, Iron, and on the shoare Ambergrise, but them *uncouth* and *unkissed* . . . . (1560)

As Spurgeon (1: 142) notes, the line was also echoed in E. K.'s prefatory epistle to Spenser's *Shepheardes Calendar* (1579); see SPENSER, Boswell & Holton No. 384.
    Also found in the second edition, STC 20506 (1614), UMI 1461: 2. Boswell & Holton No. 888.

107.   WEBSTER, WILLIAM. *A Plaine and Most Necessary Booke of Tables for Simple Interest.* STC 25182.5. No UMI. (Copy at Yale, Sterling)

A commendatory poem headed "The Authour to his Book" begins with a faint echo of Chaucer's line, "Go, litel bok, go litel myn tragedye" (*Troilus and Criseyde* 5: 1786). Webster (*fl.* 1625–1634) writes:

> Goe booke abroad, and see that thou unpartially decide
> Cases of Interest, where thou find'st such causes to be tride.
> Such is the world, that in the world thou need'st not idle be:
> A common use, is taking use, so use enough for thee. . . .

Other editions: STC 25183 (1629), sig. *A*3v; STC 25183.5 (1634), sig. *A*3v; STC 25184 (1639), sig. A4v; W1233 (1647), sig. A4v.

1627

108.   HAWKINS, WILLIAM. *Apollo Shroving.* STC 12963. UMI 1105: 4.

This drama was "composed for the schollars of the free-schoole of Hadleigh in Suffolke. And acted by them on Shrovetuesday, being the sixt of February, 1626" (title page). Therein Hawkins (d. 1637) echoes a line from *Troilus and Criseyde*, "Unknowe, unkist, and lost, that is unsought" (1: 809). The second scene of the third act features a character called Complement and Implement, his page. Complement asks, "But how if Sir *Orgolio* say then hee'le come thither too, and be my shadow there, and play the under-Marshall at my becke?" Implement responds: "He cannot be so uncivill, as to intrude, unbid, uncouth, unkist" (44).

As Spurgeon (1: 142) notes, the line was also echoed in E. K.'s prefatory epistle to Spenser's *Shepheardes Calendar* (1579); see SPENSER, Boswell & Holton No. 384.

109.   TAYLOR, JOHN. *An Armado, or Navy, of 103. Ships & Other Vessels.* STC 23726a. UMI 1717: 9.

Taylor, known far and wide as "the water poet," seems to echo a line from *The Manciple's Prologue*: "Sires, what! Dun is in the myre!" (line 5). In "The Footman-Ship, with her Regiment," in a passage about sailors singing and dancing as they work, he writes:

> [T]his Ship sails a Trot, her light-footed, nimble-heeel'd Mariners (like so many dancers) capring in the *Pumpes* and vanities of this sinfull world . . . to the *Dune of Dusty my deere, Dirty come thou to me, Dun out of the mire, or I wayle in woe and plunge in paine* . . . . (sig. C1v)

Another edition: STC 23727 (1635), sigs. C1v–D1r.
Also found in Taylor's *Workes* (1630), STC 23725, 86.

1628

110.   HAYMAN, ROBERT. *Quodlibets Lately Come Over from New Britaniola, Old Newfound-land.* STC 12974. UMI 926: 7.

In addition to the references noted in Boswell & Holton No. 1119, there is another. In "The Third Booke of Quodlibets," Hayman (1578/79–1631?) echoes a line from *The Reeve's Prologue*: "For in oure wyl ther striketh evere a nayl, | To have an hoor heed and a grene tayl, | As hath a leek" (3876–78). In No. 57, "To sir Senix Fornicator," he writes:

> Winter hath seaz'd upon thy beard, and head,
> Yet for all this, thy wilde Oates are not shed.
> Me thinkes when Hills are overspred with Snow,
> It should not wantonly be hot below.
> But thou most like unto a *Leeke* dost seeme:
> For though thy head be *white*, thy tayle is *green*. (47)

111.   JACKSON, JOHN. *Ecclesiastes. The Worthy Church-man: or, The Faithfull Minister.* STC 14297. UMI 991: 22.

Jackson (1600–1648) is identified on the title page as "parson of Marske in Richmond-shire." In the first section, under the heading "The Vertue," he echoes a line from *The Reeve's Tale*: "The gretteste clerkes been noght wisest men" (line 4054). Jackson writes:

> It hath beene long said, *Greatest Clerks are not alwaies wisest men*; so as it seemes Schollers must be glad to take simplicity to themselves by tradition. (3)

112.   KNEVET, RALPH. Στρατιωτικον [Stratiotikon]*: or, A Discourse of Militarie Discipline.* STC 15037. UMI 1385: 2.

In a dedicatory poem addressed "To Sir Roger Townsend," Knevet (1600–1671) echoes the title of *The House of Fame*. He writes:

> I Sent my Muse unto the house of fame
> Of her to enquire out some Honourd name
> Worthy of my Verse, and shee commends to mee
> A *Townsend*, then I quickly thought of thee [etc.] (sig. B1v–2r)

113.   SANDYS, GEORGE, trans. *Ovid's Metamorphosis.* STC 18965. UMI 897: 5.

Although Ovid writes of *Rumor*'s dwelling place, George Sandys (1578–1644) echoes the title of *The House of Fame* in this translation. In book 12, in a passage about the "blew scal'd Dragon," he writes:

> Amid the world, 'twixt Aire, Earth, *Neptunes* brine,
> A place there is; the triple Worlds confine.
> Where all that's done, though far remov'd, appeare:
> And every whisper penetrates the eare.
> The House of *Fame*: who in the highest towre
> Her lodging takes. (318)

Other editions: STC 18966 (1632), 400; STC 18967 (1638), 232; STC 18968 (1640), 221; O684 (1656), 232; O686 (1664), 232; O687 (1669), 232; O688 (1678), 232; O688A (1690), 232.

1629

114.   *An Inconstant Female. With a Reward of Her Disdaine in Equalitie.* STC 25230. UMI 1046: 8.

This broadside ballad was written to be sung "To an excellent new Tune." In a passage about "false dissembling love," the writer appears to allude to *Troilus and Criseyde*:

> Now a Troylus
> I still must live, yet joylesse
>   of Cresida:
> Loves mistaken,
> And I forsaken
>   and left for aye: [Etc.]

115.   LIGHTFOOT, JOHN. *Erubhin: or, Miscellanies Christian and Judiacall.* STC 15593. UMI 843: 14.

Lightfoot (1602–1675) is identified on the title page as "Master in Arts, sometimes of Christs Colledge in Cambridge." In chapter 6, "Of Jewish Learning," he cites Chaucer and quotes a modernized line from *The Reeve's Tale*: "The gretteste clerkes been noght wisest men" (line 4054). He writes:

> But as in *Chaucer the greatest Clarkes are not the wisest men*, so among them, these that are so great textualists, are not best at the text. (21)

1631

116.   CHAPMAN, GEORGE. *Caesar and Pompey a Roman Tragedy.* STC 4883. UMI 1198: 11.

In the second act, in a scene featuring a character called Ophioneus, Chapman (1559?–1634) echoes a line from *The Reeve's Tale*: "The gretteste clerkes been noght wisest men" (line 4054). He writes:

No Clerke? what then?
The greatest Clerks are not the wisest men. (sig. C4v)

A variant edition in 1631: STC 4993, sig. C4v.
   Other editions: C1946 (1652), sig. C4v; C1947 (1653), sig. C4v.

117.   LENTON, FRANCIS. *Characterismi: or, Lentons Leasures Expressed in Essayes and Characters.* STC 15463. UMI 842: 08.

Lenton (*fl.* 1630–1640) is identified in later editions as "Her Majesties poet" and "a person of quality." In his character "A True Friend," Lenton echoes a line in *The Manciple's Prologue*: "Sires, what! Dun is in the myre!" (line 5). He writes:

[H]ee is not compos'd of words, but actions, alwayes ready at a dead lift, to draw Dun out of the myre. (sig. H1v)

Other editions with different titles: *A Piece of the World, Painted in Proper Colours,* STC 15464.5 (1640), sig. H1v; *Characters: or, Wit and the World in Their Proper Colors,* L1095 (1663), sig. H1v.

1632

118.   B., E. "The Life and Death of Mr. Bolton" in *Mr. Bolton's Last and Learned Worke of the Foure Last Things.* STC 3242. UMI 1128: 5.

In a biographical essay about Robert Bolton, E. B. (Edward Bagshaw?) echoes a line in *The Reeve's Tale*: "The gretteste clerkes been noght wisest men" (line 4054). He writes:

He . . . [had] a very strong memory. . . . For, (as Philosophers observe) that memory tends to admiration, being of a quite differing temperature from the understanding, inclines rather to folly, and becomes the ground of that Proverbe, *The greatest Clerkes are not alwaies the wisest men.* (sig. a8v)

Other editions: STC 3243 (1633), sig. a8v; STC 3244 (1635), sig. a8v; STC 3245 (1639), sig. a8v; B3512 (1641), sig. a8v.

119.   FLETCHER, PHINEAS. *The Way to Blessedness*. STC 11085. UMI 836: 20.

Fletcher (1582–1650) is identified on the title page as "B. in D. and minister of Gods Word at Hilgay, in Norfolke." He echoes Chaucer's description of the poor Parson, "Ne maked him a spiced conscience" (*The General Prologue*, line 526) and *The Wife of Bath's Prologue*, "Ye sholde been al pacient and meke, | And han a sweete spiced conscience" (lines 434–35). Fletcher writes:

> What? Thinke you that none but such strait-laced creatures can enter into *Gods* Kingdome? Doe you not see your Father, a wise man, this, or that scholler, such, or such a Minister use no such spiced conscience, and yet make no doubt but to do as well as you, and come to heaven before you. (23)

120.   TOWNSHEND, AURELIAN. *Albions Triumph. Personated in a Maske at Court*. STC 24155. UMI 978: 15.

In a masque performed by the king and his lords on Twelfth Night 1631, i.e., 1632, Townshend (*fl.* 1601–1643) echoes the title of *The House of Fame*. Under the heading "The second Song," he writes:

> *From fayre ALBIPOLIS shall soone proceed*
> *A Triumph: Mighty, as the Man design'd*
> *To weare those Bayes; Heroicke, as his mind;*
> *Just, as his actions; Glorious, as his Reigne.*
> *And like his Vertues, Infinite in Treyne.*
> *Th' Immortall Swannes, contending for his Name,*
> *Shall beare it singing, to the House of Fame.* (5–6)

1633

121.   DOWNE, JOHN. *Certaine Treatises*. STC 7125. UMI 1200: 18.

Downe (1570?–1631) is identified on the title page as "the late reverend and learned divine . . . rector of the church of Instow in Devonshire, Bachelour of Divinity, and sometimes fellow of Emanuell Colledge in Cambridge." In a section headed "A Defence of the Lawfulnesse of Lots in Gaming Against the Arguments of N. N.," he asserts that one of N. N.'s points is pointless and echoes a line from *Troilus and Criseyde*, "Unknowe, unkist, and lost, that is unsought" (1: 809) Downe writes:

[N]either knowe I nor care I, seeing it nothing belongs unto the question. And so leaving it unkith [*sic*] unkist, I passe unto the second testimonie. (9)

As Spurgeon (1: 142) notes, the line was also echoed in E. K.'s prefatory epistle to Spenser's *Shepheardes Calendar* (1579); see SPENSER, Boswell & Holton No. 384.

1636

122. SLATER, MASTER. *The New-Yeeres Gift Presented at Court, from the Lady Parvula to the Lord Minimus, (commonly called Little Jefferie) Her Majesties Servant, with a Letter as It Was Penned in Short-hand: Wherein Is Proved Little Things Are Better Then Great. Written by Microphilus.* STC 22631. UMI 1008: 8.

By way of proving that little things are to be preferred to large ones, the author echoes a line from *The Reeve's Tale*: "The gretteste clerkes been noght wisest men" (line 4054). He writes:

[H]ow *little* knowledge is better then *Great*, may bee thus demonstrated, the *Greatest-Clerkes are not the wisest men*. (96)

Other editions: STC 22632 (1638), same pagination.

1637

123. BRIAN, THOMAS. *The Pisse-Prophet: or, Certaine Pisse-Pot Lectures.* STC 3723. UMI 656: 10.

Brian is identified on the title page as "M.P. lately in the citie of London, and now in Colchester in Essex." Near the end of chapter 3, Brian echoes a line in *The Manciple's Prologue*: "Sires, what! Dun is in the myre!" (line 5). He writes: "I hope you well perceive my fetches, which helpe me out, or else Dun might have stucke full fast in the mire" (27).

Other editions: STC B4437 (1655), 47; STC B4438 (1679), 46.

124. PRYNNE, WILLIAM (?). *A Catalogue of Such Testimonies in All Ages.* STC 4788. UMI 222:17.

This work was originally published in 1637 and reissued twice in the 1640s; subsequent seventeenth-century editions have had their dates altered in ink. Boswell & Holton mistakenly assumed that the 1637 date was a misprint.

As Dobbins notes (*MLQ*), Prynne (1600–1669) names his sources in a sort of appendix: "These Testimonies I shall Marshal into 5 distinct *Squadrons*, for order sake. . . . The 5. Squadron is compacted and made up of our owne dome-sticke writers, Martyrs, Authors, aswell ancient as Modern, which I shall here digest into a Chonological order" (1–7). For the year 1380, he cites: "Geofry Chancer [*sic*] the Ploughmans tale part, 1, 2" (8, col. 1; sig. B2v).

In his list of errata, Prynne corrects line 26 on page 8 to read "Chaucer."

1638

125.   CLARKE, JOHN. *Phraseologia puerilis, Anglo-Latina, in usum tirocinii scholastici: or, Selected Latine and English Phrases.* STC 5361. UMI 1093: 13.

Clarke (b. in or before 1596, d. 1658) is identified on the title page as "B.D. and Master of the Free Schoole in Lincolne." In this schoolbook for youngsters "to initiate them in speaking and writing elegantly in both languages," Clarke echoes a line from *The Manciple's Prologue*: "Sires, what! Dun is in the myre!" (line 5). He translates "Hæremus in vado, quis nos expediet?" as *"Who will helpe Dunne out of the Mire?"* (sig. B6r–v).

Other editions: C4473 (1650), sig. B1v; C4474 (1655), no UMI; C4474A (1670), 100.

1639

126.   BANCROFT, THOMAS. *Two Bookes of Epigrammes and Epitaphs.* STC 1354. UMI 823: 8.

In the first book of epigrams, Bancroft (*fl.* 1633–1658) echoes a line from *The Reeve's Tale*: "The gretteste clerkes been noght wisest men" (line 4054). The title of epigram 182 is "The greatest Clerkes, not the wisest men" (sig. E3r).

127.   CLARKE, JOHN. *Parœmiologia Anglo-Latina un usum scholarum concinnata: or, Proverbs English and Latine.* STC 5360. UMI 953: 1.

In "Imprudentiæ," Clarke (1596?–1658) echoes a line from *The Reeve's Tale*: "The gretteste clerkes been noght wisest men" (line 4054). He writes:

> *The wisest man may be over-seene.*
> *He that stands by, sees more than he that playes the game.*
> *'Tis a good horse that never Stumbleth.*
> *The greatest clerkes are not alway [sic] the wisest men.*
> *A mere schollar is a mere ass.* (151)

Another edition: C4472A (1646), UMI 2605: 4

1640

128. *A Certain Relation of the Hog-Faced Gentlewoman Called Mistris Tanna-kin Skinker.* STC 22627. UMI 1008: 06.

The anonymous author of this *Relation* echoes the Wife of Bath's claim that "Women desiren have sovereyntee" (*The Wife of Bath's Tale*, line 1038). In spite of her unfortunate disfigurement, the protagonist of this tale found true love and she says to her beloved: "*Now Sir, you have given me that which all women most desire, my Will, and Soveraignty*" (sig. B4v).

129.   MILL, HUMPHREY. *A Nights Search. Discovering the Nature and Condition of All Sorts of Night-Walkers.* STC 17921. UMI 1028: 6.

Section 39 is headed "Of a company of Roysters comming to a Stews, and chaffering with the Bawd for the Whores, as men doe for Jades in Smithfield, &c.," Mill ironically echoes the title of *The House of Fame*, for the house is really a house of ill-fame. Mill (*fl.* 1646) writes of a trio of "Proud Pluto's Captains":

Black damme *Jack*, bold *Dick*, and high-way Ned,
(They were no scoundrels, they were better bred)
Came to a house of fame, they would have bought
They knew not what . . . [etc.] (193)

130.   SHIRLEY, JAMES. *The Humorous Courtier.* STC 22447. UMI 939: 4.

In addition to a reference noted by Boswell & Holton (No. 1370), there may be another in this comedy that was "presented with good applause at the private house in Drury-Lane" (title page). In a scene featuring a character called Comachio, Shirley (1596–1666) echoes the title of *The House of Fame.* He writes:

Behold (quoth she) I neede no
Marble house for my fame to dwell in . . . (sig. B4v)

131.   SHIRLEY, JAMES. *St. Patrick for Ireland.* STC 22455. UMI

In the third act, in a song sung by a character called Bard, Shirley (1596–1666) echoes a line from *The Manciple's Prologue*: "Sires, what! Dun is in the myre!" (line 5). He writes:

Love is a bog, a deep bog, a wide bog.
Love is a clog, a great clog, a close clog.
'Tis a wildernesse to loose our selves,
A halter 'tis to noose our selves.
Then draw Dun out o'th mire:
And throw the clog into the fire. (sig. D3r)

Also collected in *Two Playes* (1657).

> Queene *Katherine* . . . seemed neither to Mistris *Anne Bullen*, nor the
> King to carry any sparke of discontent, or displeasure, but accepted
> all things in good part, and with great wisdome, and much patience,
> dissembled the same, having Mistris *Anne Bullen* in more estimation for
> the Kings sake, then when she was with her before, declaring herselfe
> indeed to be a very patient *Grissell*, as by her long patience in all her
> troubles shall hereafter more plainly appeare. (27)

Another edition in 1641: C1619, same pagination.
   Other editions: C1619A (1650?), 22–23; and *The Life and Death of Thomas
Woolsey, Cardinal*, C1618 (1667), 34–35.

STC Books Cited in this Work

Entries are arranged in alphabetical order by author or title (if author is unknown). Numbers refer to the entry number. Some titles have been shortened, and occasionally spelling has been modified.

A

A., J. "Commendatory Poem" in *T. Lucretius Carus. The Epicurean Philosopher*, 1997, 2379, 2396

———. Verses in John Batchiler's *Christian Queries to Quaking-Christians*, 1660

Addison, Joseph. "An Account of the Greatest English Poets" in *The Annual Miscellany for the year 1694*, 2255

Aggas, Edward. *An Answeare to the Supplication against Him*, A54

Aicken, Joseph. *The English Grammar*, 2236

Alsop, George. *A Character of the Province of Mary-land*, 1710

Alsop, Vincent. *Anti-sozzo: sive, Sherlocismus enervates*, 1862, 1877

Ashmole, Elias. *The Institutions, Laws & Ceremonies of the Most Noble Order of the Garter*, 1792, 2220

———. *Theatrum chemicum Britannicum*, 1478

The Athenian Mercury, 2171, 2172, 2198, 2221

Atkins, James. "Commendatory Poem" in Sir John Mennes's *Wit Restor'd*, 1576

Atkinson, William. *A Full Devoute and Gostely Treatyse of the Imytacyon and Folowynge the Blessed Lyfe of Our Moste Mercyfull Savyour*, A5

Atwell, George. *The Faithfull Surveyor*, 1577, 1642, 1696

Aubrey, John. *Miscellanies*, 2314

Austin, Samuel. Commendatory poem in Thomas Flatman's *Naps upon Parnassus*, 1578

Axe, Thomas. *A Catalogue of English Books*, 2315

B

B. *The Arraignment of Co-Ordinate-Power*, 1998

B., E. "The Life and Death of Mr. Bolton" in *The Workes of the Learned Robert Bolton*, 1380, A118

B., R. "On Our English Poetry" in Nahum Tate's *Panacea: A Poem upon Tea*, 2397

B., T. "A Dedication" in Michael Drayton's *England's Heroical Epistles*, 2143, 2285, 2336

Baker, R. Commendatory poem in Guido Bentivoglio's *The Compleat History of the Warrs of Flanders*, 1503

Baker, Richard. *An Abridgement of S'. Richard Bakers Chronicle of the Kings of England*, 2021

———. *A Chronicle of the Kings of England*, 1402, 1490, 1610, 1697, 1757, 1840, 1922, 2022, 2316

———. *Theatrum redivivivum: or, The Theatre Vindicated*, 1643, 1758

———. *Theatrum Triumphans*, 1643

Baldwin, William. *A Myrrour for Magistrates*, A17

Bale, John. *The Apology of Johan Bale agaynste a Ranke Papyst*, A14

Bancroft, Thomas. *Two Bookes of Epigrammes and Epitaphs*, A126

Barnard, John. *Theologo-Historicus: or, The True Life of Peter Heylyn*, 1999

Barnard, John Augustine, and Edmund Bohun. *A Geographical Dictionary*, 2222, 2286

Barnes, Joshua. *The History of that Most Victorious Monarch Edward III^d*, 2124

Baron, William. *A Just Defence of the Royal Martyr*, 2380

Barrow, Henry. *A Brief Discoverie of the False Church*, A55

Basset, Thomas. "Catalogue" in Hugo Grotius, *Christ's Passion. The Second Edition*, 2091

Batchiler, John. *Christian Queries to Quaking-Christians*, 1660

Bateman, Christopher. *A Catalogue of the Library of a Person of Honour*, 2256

Baxter, Richard. *Which Is the True Church?*, 1923

Beaumont, Francis, and John Fletcher. *The Woman Hater*, 1438, 1453, A76

Behn, Aphra. Interpolation in Bernard Le Bovier de Fontenelle's *History of Oracles, and the Cheats of the Pagan Priests*, 2125, 2381

———. *Love Letters Between a Noble-Man and his Sister*, 2248

Bentivoglio, Guido. *The Compleat History of the Warrs of Flanders*, 1503

Bernard, Francis, M. D. *A Catalogue of the Library*, 2360

Beverley, Peter. *The Historie of Ariodanto and Jenevra*, A27

Bibliotheca Anglicana: or, A Collection of Choice English Books, 2070

Bibliotheca Baconia, 2071, 2126

Bibliotheca Curiosa: or, A Choice Collection of Books, 2337

Bibliotheca Digbeiana, 1944

Bibliotheca insignis: or, A Catalogue of Excellent . . . Books, 2223

Bibliotheca realis & instructissima, sive catalogus variorum librorum, 2158

Bibliotheca selecta, 2127

Billingsley, H. Annotation in *The Elements of Geometrie of Euclide*, A21

Birckbeck, Simon. *The Protestants Evidence*, 1561

Blague, Daniel. *A Catalogue of Latine Greek & English Books*, 2173

Blome, Richard. *The Art of Heraldry*, 2050, 2224

———. *An Essay to Heraldry*, 2023

Blount, Thomas. *The Academie of Eloquence*, 1504, 1534, 1661, 1679, 1759, 2000

———. *Glossographia: or, A Dictionary*, 1535, 1593, 1624, 1760, 1841, 1960

————. Νομο-λεξικον [nomo-lexikon]: *A Law-Dictionary*, 1761

————. Νομο-λεξικον [nomo-lexikon]: *A Law-Dictionary. The Second Edition*, 2174

Blount, Thomas Pope. *Censura celebriorum authorem*, 2159

————. *De re poetica: or, Remarks upon Poetry*, 2257

Boethius. *Of the Consolation of Philosophy*, 2307

Bohun, Edmund, in Louis Moréri's *Great Historical, Geographical, and Poetical Dictionary*, 2258

Boileau-Despréaux, Nicholas. *The Art of Poetry*, 2019

Bold, Henry. *Latine Songs with Their English, and Poems*, 2051

————. *Poems Lyrique Macaronique Heroique, &c.*, 1680

Bolton, Edmund. *The Cities Great Concern*, 1842

Bowman, Thomas. *Catalogus librorum*, 2092

Bradstreet, Ann. *The Tenth Muse*, 1467

————. *Several Poems.*, 1921

Bramhall, John. *A Just Vindication of the Church of England*, 1505, 1625

————. *The Right Way to Safety after Ship-Wrack*, 1626

————. *The Serpent Salve*, 1403

————. *The Works*, 1878, 1893

Brathwaite, Richard. *A Comment upon the Two Tales of Chaucer*, 1698

————. *Times Treasury*, 1479

Brian, Thomas. *The Pisse-Prophet: or, Certaine Pisse-Pot Lectures*, 1518, 1924, A123

Bridges, John. *A Defence of the Government Established in the Church of Englande for Ecclesiastical Matters*, A44

Britaine, William de. *Humane Prudence*, 2072, 2144, 2225, 2338, 2398

Brome, James. "The Life of Mr. Somner" in William Somner's *A Treatise of the Roman Ports and Forts in Kent*, 2226

Brome, Alexander. *A Canterbury Tale, Translated out of Chaucers Old English into Our Now Usuall Language. Whereunto Is Added the Scots Pedler*, 1382

Brown, Thomas. *A Description of Mr. D[ryde]n's Funeral. A Poem*, 2399

————. *The Late Converts Exposed: or, The Reasons of Mr. Bays's Changing His Religion*, 2160

Browne, William. *Britannia's Pastorals*, A86

Bryskett, Lodowick. *A Discourse of Civill Life*, A75

Buchler, Johann. *Sacrarum prosanarumque phrasium poeticarum thesarurus*, 1750, 1770, 1939

Bullinger, Heinrich. *Fiftie Godlie and Learned Sermons*, A29

Bullord, John. *Bibliotheca Belwoodiana*, 2259

————. *Bibliotheca curiosa*, 2161

————. *Bibliotheca Littletoniana*, 2287

————. *Bibliotheca realis & instructissima*, 2162

————. *A Catalogue of Books in Folio*, 2178

———. *A Catalogue of Books of Two Eminent Mathematicians*, 2175
———. *A Catalogue of Excellent Greek, Latine and English Books*, 2176
———. *A Catalogue of Extraordinary Greek and Latin Books*, 2199
———. *A Catalogue of Latin and English Books*, 2177
———. *A Catalogue of the Libraries of S* Andrew Henley and an Eminent Clergy-man*, 2400
———. *A Catalogue of the Library of Ralph Hough, Esq.*, 2401
———. *A Catalogue of Theological, Philosophical, Historical, Philological, Medicinal & Chymical Books*, 2339
———. *Catalogus libris exquisitissimis rarissimisque*, 2402
———. *A Curious Collection of Books*, 2288
———. *An Excellent Collection of Books*, 2260
———. *The Library of Mr. Tho. Britton, Smallcoal-man*, 2261
———. *The Library of the Right Reverend Robert, late Lord Bishop of Chichester*, 2340
Bullokar, John. *An English Expositor*, 1512, 1554, 1673, 1727, 1787, 1891, 1956, 2043, 2139, 2309, 2373
Bunyan, John. *The Pilgrim's Progress. The Second Part*, 2024, 2073, 2093, 2163, 2227, 2317
Burel, John. "An Application Concerning Our Kings Majesties Persoun" in *To the Richt High, Lodwik Duke of Lenox*, A62
Burgh, Benedict. Interpolation in Cato's *Paruus*, A1
———. *The Godly Adverstisement or Good Counsell of the Famous Orator Isocrates. Whereunto Is Annexed Cato in Olde Englysh Meter*, A1
Burnet, Gilbert. *A Relation of a Conference Held about Religion at London*, 1879, 1925, 2094
Burnyeat, John. *The Truth Exalted*, 2188

C

C., D. Commendatory poem in *A Present for Youth*, 2001
C., H. *The Plain Englishman's Historian*, 1926
C., R., trans. *A World of Wonders*, A77
Camden, William. *Britain: or, A Chorographicall Description*, A82
Carter, Matthew. *Honor Rediviuus [sic]: or, An Analysis of Honor and Armory*, 1519, 1611, 1817, 2200
Cartwright, William. *Comedies Tragi-Comedies, with Other Poems*, 1470
———. *The Lady-Errant*, 1468
———. *The Ordinary*, 1469
The Case of Ministring at the Communion-Table, 2002
Catalogi librorum manuscriptorum Angliæ et Hiberniæ in unum collecti, cum indice alphabetico, 2341
A Catalogue Containing Variety of English Books, 2074

A Catalogue of Books of the Several Libraries of the Honorable Sir William Coventry, and the Honorable Mr. Henry Coventry, 2095

A Catalogue of Books to be Sold by Auction, 2201

A Catalogue of Choice Books, 2096

A Catalogue of Choice English Books, 2097, 2098

A Catalogue of Excellent Books, in Greek, Latin and English, 2262

A Catalogue of Latin and English Books, Both Antient [sic] and Modern, 2342

A Catalogue of Latin, French, and English Books, 2099

A Catalogue of the Libraries of Mr. Jer. Copping . . . and Anscel Beaumont, 2100

A Catalogue of Valuable and Choice Books, 2382

A Catalogue of Very Good English and Latin Books, 2145

Catalogus variorum in pluriis facultatibus variisq[ue] linguis insignium librorum, 2128

Catalogus variorum librorum, 1945, 2025, 2075

Cavendish, George. *The Life and Death of Thomas Woolsey, Cardinal*, 1716

———. *The Negotiations of Thomas Woolsey, the Great Cardinal of England*, 1383, 1457

The Censure of the Rota upon Mr. Milton's Book, 1612

A Certain Relation of the Hog-Faced Gentlewoman Called Mistris Tannakin Skinker, A128

Chapman, George. *Caesar and Pompey*, 1480, 1491, A116

———. Dedicatory poem in *The Crown of All Homers Workes Batrachomyomachia*, A102

Character of the Rump, 1613

Charles I, King of England. Βασιλικα [Basilika]. *The Works of King Charles the Martyr*, 1644, 2101

———. *The Papers Which Passed Betwixt His Majestie and Mr Alex: Henderson*, 1454

Charleton, Walter. *The Cimmerian Matron, a Pleasant Novel*, 2025a.

———. *The Ephesian and Cimmerian Matrons*, 1731

Chaucer, Geoffrey. *The Works of Our Ancient, Learned, & Excellent English Poet, Jeffrey Chaucer*, 2102

"Chaucer Junior." *Canterbury Tales: Composed for the Entertainment of All Ingenious Young Men and Maids at Their Merry Meetings*, 2103

"A Character" in James Strong's *Joanereidos: or, Feminine Valour*, 1417, 1843

Chaucer's Ghoast, or, A Piece of Antiquity, 1793

Chetwood, Knightly. "To the Earl of Roscommon" in Wentworth Dillon's *An Essay on Translated Verse*, 2026, 2052

Chiswell, Richard. *Bibliotheca Smithiana*, 1978

Choyce Drollery: Songs & Sonnets, 1538

The Cities Warning Peece, 1404

Clarke, John. *Parœmiologia Anglo-Latina un usum scholarum concinnata: or, Proverbs English and Latine*, A127

———. *Phraseologia puerilis*, 1458, 1762, A125

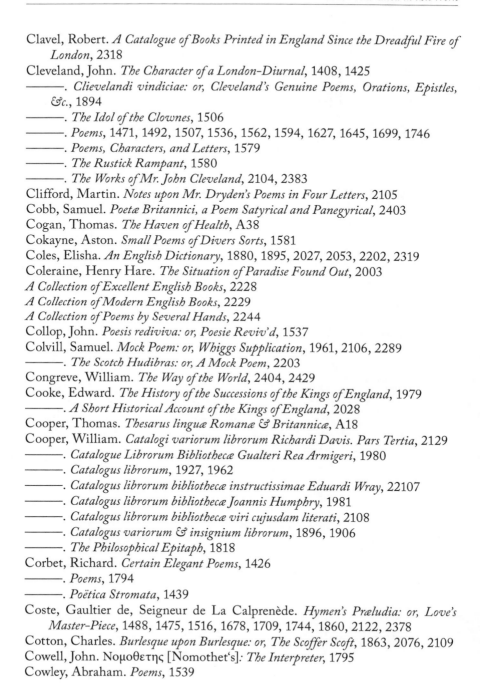

Clavel, Robert. *A Catalogue of Books Printed in England Since the Dreadful Fire of London*, 2318

Cleveland, John. *The Character of a London-Diurnal*, 1408, 1425

——. *Clievelandi vindiciae: or, Cleveland's Genuine Poems, Orations, Epistles, &c.*, 1894

——. *The Idol of the Clownes*, 1506

——. *Poems*, 1471, 1492, 1507, 1536, 1562, 1594, 1627, 1645, 1699, 1746

——. *Poems, Characters, and Letters*, 1579

——. *The Rustick Rampant*, 1580

——. *The Works of Mr. John Cleveland*, 2104, 2383

Clifford, Martin. *Notes upon Mr. Dryden's Poems in Four Letters*, 2105

Cobb, Samuel. *Poetæ Britannici, a Poem Satyrical and Panegyrical*, 2403

Cogan, Thomas. *The Haven of Health*, A38

Cokayne, Aston. *Small Poems of Divers Sorts*, 1581

Coles, Elisha. *An English Dictionary*, 1880, 1895, 2027, 2053, 2202, 2319

Coleraine, Henry Hare. *The Situation of Paradise Found Out*, 2003

A Collection of Excellent English Books, 2228

A Collection of Modern English Books, 2229

A Collection of Poems by Several Hands, 2244

Collop, John. *Poesis rediviva: or, Poesie Reviv'd*, 1537

Colvill, Samuel. *Mock Poem: or, Whiggs Supplication*, 1961, 2106, 2289

——. *The Scotch Hudibras: or, A Mock Poem*, 2203

Congreve, William. *The Way of the World*, 2404, 2429

Cooke, Edward. *The History of the Successions of the Kings of England*, 1979

——. *A Short Historical Account of the Kings of England*, 2028

Cooper, Thomas. *Thesarus linguæ Romanæ & Britannicæ*, A18

Cooper, William. *Catalogi variorum librorum Richardi Davis. Pars Tertia*, 2129

——. *Catalogue Librorum Bibliothecæ Gualteri Rea Armigeri*, 1980

——. *Catalogus librorum*, 1927, 1962

——. *Catalogus librorum bibliothecæ instructissimae Eduardi Wray*, 22107

——. *Catalogus librorum bibliothecæ Joannis Humphry*, 1981

——. *Catalogus librorum bibliothecæ viri cujusdam literati*, 2108

——. *Catalogus variorum & insignium librorum*, 1896, 1906

——. *The Philosophical Epitaph*, 1818

Corbet, Richard. *Certain Elegant Poems*, 1426

——. *Poems*, 1794

——. *Poëtica Stromata*, 1439

Coste, Gaultier de, Seigneur de La Calprenède. *Hymen's Præludia: or, Love's Master-Piece*, 1488, 1475, 1516, 1678, 1709, 1744, 1860, 2122, 2378

Cotton, Charles. *Burlesque upon Burlesque: or, The Scoffer Scoft*, 1863, 2076, 2109

Cowell, John. Νομοθετης [Nomothet's]: *The Interpreter*, 1795

Cowley, Abraham. *Poems*, 1539

————. *The Works of Mr. Abraham Cowley*, 1732, 1742, 1747, 1796, 1844, 1907, 1946, 1963, 2029, 2130, 2230, 2405

Croft, Herbert. *The Legacy of the Right Reverend Father in God, Herbert, Lord Bishop of Hereford*, 1928

Crompton, Hugh. *Poems*, 1563

Crosse, Henry. *The Schoole of Pollicie*, A72

————. *Vertues Common-wealth: or, The High-way to Honour*, A72

Crouch, Nathaniel. *Martyrs in Flames: or, Popery (in Its True Colours) Displayed*, 2231

The Crown of All Homers Workes Batrachomyomachia: or, The Battaile of Frogs and Mise, A102

Culpeper, Thomas. *Essayes or Moral Discourses and Essayes on Several Subjects*, 1776

D

Daborne, Robert. *A Christian Turn'd Turke*, A83

Dare, Josiah. *Counsellor Manners, His Last Legacy to His Son*, 1819, 1881, 2263, 2361, 2384

Davenport, Robert. *King John and Matilda*, 1520, 1646

Davies, John (of Hereford). *Humours Heav'n on Earth*, A81

Davies, John. *A Memorial for the Learned*, 2077

Davies, John, trans. Voiture's *Letters of Affaires, Love, and Courtship*, 1564

Davies, Sir John. *Epigrammes*, A67

Day, John. *Humour Out of Breath*, A79

Defoe, Daniel. *The Compleat Mendicant or Unhappy Beggar*, 2385

Dekker, Thomas. *Satiro-Mastix: or, The Untrussing of the Humorous Poet*, A70

Dekker, Thomas, and John Webster. *West-ward Hoe*, A78

De Laune, Thomas. *Angliæ metropolis: or, The Present State of London*, 2164

————. *The Present State of London: or, Memorials*, 1964

Deloney, Thomas. *The Garland of Good-Will*, 1595, 1908, 2004, 2054, 2131, 2320

Denham, John. *On Mr. Abraham Cowley His Death and Burial amongst the Ancient Poets*, 1717

————. *Poems and Translations*, 1733, 1777, 2030

Dennis, John. *The Usefulness of the Stage to the Happiness of Mankind, to Government and to Religion*, 2362

Des Périers, Bonaventure. *The Mirrour of Mirth and Pleasant Conceits*, A37

Dillon, Wentworth. *An Essay on Translated Verse*, 2026, 2052

A Discourse of Artificial Beauty, 1647

Done, John. *A Miscellania of Morall, Theologicall, and Philosophicall Sentences*, 1459

Doomes-Day: or, The Great Day of the Lords Judgement, 1427

Dowland, John. *The Third and Last Booke of Songs and Aires*, A73

Downe, John. *Certaine Treatises*, A121

Drayton, Michael. *England's Heroical Epistles*, 2143, 2285

————. *Idea. The Shepheards Garland*, A56

Dring, Peter. "Catalogue" in George Alsop's *A Character of the Province of Mary-land*, 1710

Drummond, William. *Polemo-middmia. Carmen macaronicum*, 2182

Dryden, John. *Amphitryon: or, The Two Socia's*, 2165, 2179

———. "Dedicatory Epistle" in *The Satires of Decimus Junius Juvenalis*, 2232, 2343

———. "Dedicatory Epistle" in *The Works of Virgil*, 2344, 2363

———. *Fables Ancient and Modern*, 2406

———. *The Hind and the Panther*, 2110

———. *Troilus and Cressida*, 1929, 2204, 2290

———. *The Works of Mr. John Dryden*, 2180, 2233, 2264, 2291

Du Bosc, Jacques. *The Accomplish'd Woman*, 1540, 1778

Dugdale, William. *Origines juridiciales: or, Historical Memorials of the English Laws*, 1712, 1779, 1947

Dunmore, John. *Bibliotheca Bissaeana: sive catalogus librorum*, 1930

———. *Catalogus librorum*, 1965

———, and Richard Chiswell. *Catalogus librorum in quavis lingua*, 1909

Dunton, John. *The Informer's Doom*, 2005

———. *The Young-Student's-Library*, 2205

D'Urfey, Thomas. *The Campaigners: or, The Pleasant Adventures at Brussels*, 2364

———. *Pendragon: or, The Carpet Knight His Kalendar*, 2365

———. *The Progress of Honesty*, 1966

———. *The Virtuous Wife*, 1948

Dutton, John. *John Dutton's, Alias Prince Dutton's Farewel to Temple-Bar*, 2265

The Dyaloge Bytwene Julius the Second, Genius, and Saynt Peter, A9

E

E., A. B. C. D. *Novembris monstrum: or, Rome Brought to Bed in England*, 1384

Edwards, John. *A Discourse Concerning the Authority, Stile, and Perfection of the Books of the Old and New-Testament*, 2234, 2266, 2321

Elyot, Thomas. *The Dictionary of Syr Thomas Eliot Knyght*, A10

———. *The Image of Governance*, A11

Enchridion legume, 1820

England's New-yeares Gift, 1440

The English Part of the Library of the Late Duke of Lauderdale, 2181

An Epistle to S.r Richard Blackmore, Occasion'd by the New Session of the Poets, 2407

Evelyn, John. "The Immortality of Poesie" in *Poems by Several Hands*, 2055

———. *Numismata. A Discourse of Medals, Antient and Modern*, 2345

———. *Publick Employment and an Active Life Prefer'd to Solitude*, 1718

———. *Sylva: or, A Discourse of Forest-Trees*, 1681, 1763, 1931

Examen poeticum: Being the Third Part of Miscellany Poems, 2254

F

A Fair Character of the Presbyterian Reformling's Just and Sober Vindication, 2292

Familiar and Courtly Letters, 2408

Fanshawe, Richard, trans. *Il pastor fido: The Faithful Shepherd*, 1428, 1441

Faria y Sousa, Manuel de. *The Portugues Asia*, 2293

Featley, Daniel. *The Romish Fisher Caught and Held in His Owne Net*, A103

Fell, John. *The Life of the Most Learned, Reverend and Pious D' H. Hammond*, 1628, 1648

Ferguson, Robert. *A View of an Ecclesiastick in His Socks & Buskins*, 2366

Finch, Charles. "Bellositum" in *Musarum Anglicanarum analecta*, 2206, 2386

Fisher, Payne. *The Catalogue of Most of the Memorable Tombes*, 1734

———. *The Tombes, Monuments, and Sepulchral Inscriptions, Lately Visible in St. Pauls Cathedral*, 2031

———. *Veni; vidi; vici. The Triumph of the Most Excellent & Illustrious Oliver Cromwell*, 1481

Flatman, Thomas. *Naps upon Parnassus*, 1578

Flavel, John. *Husbandry Spiritualized*, 1748, 1780, 1845, 1910, 2235, 2409

———. *Pneumatologia*, 2068

Flecknoe, Richard. *The Diarium*, 1541

———. *Miscellanea: or, Poems*, 1493

———. *Seventy Eight Characters*, 1897

Fletcher, Phineas. *The Way to Blessedness*, A119

Fletcher, Robert. Epistle in *An Introduction to the Loove of God*, A34

The Flying Post: or, The Post-Master, 2410

Ford, Simon. *The Conflagration of London Poetically Delineated*, 1719

Forde, Thomas. Αυτοκατακριτος [Autokatakritos]: *or, The Sinner Condemned of Himself*, 1735

———. *Virtus rediviva: or, A Panegyrick for our Late King Charls [sic] the I*, 1614, 1629

Foulis, Henry. *The History of the Wicked Plots and Conspiracies of Our Pretended Saints*, 1649, 1846

A Fraction in the Assembly, 1442

Fraunce, Abraham. *The Lawiers Logike*, A47

Freake, Edmund. "Epistle to the Reader" in *An Introduction to the Love of God*, A24

A Friend of the Author. "Commentary" in Walter Pope's *The Salsbury-Ballad*, 1882

Friendly Advice to the Correctour of the English Press at Oxford, 1982

Fuller, Thomas. *The Church-History of Britain*, 1521, 1542

———. *History of the Worthies of England*, 1650

G

G., E. "To the Author" in Martin Llewellyn's *Men Miracles*, 1422, 1543, 1630, 1932

G., R. *Ludus scacchia. A Satyr with Other Poems*, 1864, 1883

Gadbury, John. Εφημερις [Ephemeris]: or, A Diary Astrological, Astronomical, Meteorological, 2146, 2267, 2294
———. Obsequium rationabile: or, A Reasonable Service, 1865
Garencieres, Theophilus de. Epistle in The True Prophecies or Prognostications of Michael Nostradamus, 1797, 2056
Gascoigne, George. A Hundreth Sundrie Flowres, A22
———. The Pleasauntest Workes, A22
———. The Posies, A22
———. The Whole Woorkes, A22
Gataker, Thomas. Vindication of the Annotations, 1494
Gayton, Edmund. The Art of Longevity: or, A Diæteticall Instition, 1596
———. Pleasant Notes upon Don Quixot, 1508
———. The Religion of a Physician, 1662
Gearing, William. The History of the Church of Great Britain, 1847, 1866
A General Collection of Discourses of the Virtuosi of France, 1682
Gibbon, John. Introductio ad Latinam blasoniam, 1983
Gibson, Edmund. Camden's Britannia, Newly Translated, 2295
———. "Notes" in William Drummond's Polemo-middmia. Carmen macaroni-cum, 2182
Gildon, Charles. The Post-Boy Rob'd of His Mail, 2207
The Golden Age: or, The Reign of Saturn Review'd, 2367
Gower, John. Confessio amantis: That Is to Say in Englysshe, The Confessyon of the Lover, A2
Gower, John. The Cow-ragious Castle-combat, 1413
Gracián y Morales, Baltasar. The Heroe of Lorenzo, 1482
Grammaire angloise, A105
Grange, John. The Golden Aphroditis, A30
Greene, Robert. Alcida. Greenes Metamorphosis, A97
———. Arbasto. The Anatomie of Fortune, A39
———. Ciceronis amor. Tullies Love, A48
———. Greenes Mourning Garment, A57
———. Greenes Never Too Late: or, A Powder of Experience, A52
———. Euphues His Censure to Philautus, A45
———. The History of Arbasto King of Denmarke, A39
———. The Historie of Orlando Furioso, A60
———. The Scottish Historie of James the Fourth, Slaine at Flodden, A66
Greenham, Richard. The Workes of Richard Greenham, Minister and Preacher, A84
Greenwood, William. Απογ ϛογης [Apograph' storg's]: or, A Description of the Passion of Love, 1565
Greville, Fulke. The Life of the Renowned Sr Philip Sidney, 1472
Grotius, Hugo. Christ's Passion. The Second Edition, 2091
Gry., Hu. "Upon the Authors Muse," in Sinetes Passion uppon His Fortunes, A64
Guild, William. An Answer to a Popish Pamphlet, 1544

—————. *Anti-Christ Pointed and Painted Out in His True Colours*, 1522

Guillim, John. *A Display of Heraldry*, 1615, 1683, 1713, 1933

H

H., N. "[In obitum celeberrimi Joannis Dryden]" in *Luctus Britannici: or, The Tears of the British Muses*, 2411

—————. *The Ladies Dictionary*, 2268

H., S. "To his Ingenious Friend," in Joseph Aicken's *The English Grammar*, 2236

Hacket, John. *Scrinia reserata: A Memorial Offer'd to the Great Deservings of John Williams*, 2237

Hacon, Joseph. *A Vindication of the Review*, 1651

Hakewill, George. *An Answere to a Treatise Written by Dr. Carier*, A95

Hall, George. *The Triumphs of Rome over Despised Protestancie*, 1523, 1720

Hall, Henry. "To the Memory of John Dryden, Esq." in *Luctus Britannici: or, The Tears of the British Muses*, 2412

Hall, Joseph. *Contemplations upon the Remarkable Passages in the Life of the Holy Jesus*, 1934

—————. *A Modest Confutation of a Slanderous and Scurrilous Libell*, 1399

Hardyng, John. *The Chronicle*, A12

Harington, James. *The Commonwealth of Oceana*, 1545, 1582

—————. "The Introduction," in Anthony à Wood's *Athenæ Oxonienses*, 2208

—————. *The Oceana of James Harrington, and His Other Works*, 2413

Harrington, James, the elder. *Politicaster: or, A Comical Discourse*, 1597

Harrington, John. *A Briefe View of the State of the Church of England*, 1495

Harris, John. *The Divine Physician*, 1884

Hartley, John. *Catalogus universalis librorum*, 2387

Hartley, John, and George Huddleston. *A Catalogue of the Library of the Reverend and Learned Dr. Scattergood, Deceas'd*, 2346

Hawkins, William. *Apollo Shroving*, A108

Hayman, Robert. *Quodlibets Lately Come Over from New Britaniola, Old New-found-land*, A110

Head, Richard. *The Floating Island: or, A New Discovery*, 1821

Head, Richard, and Francis Kirkman. *The English Rogue. The Third Part*, 1781, 1848

Heale, William. *The Great Advocate and Oratour for Women*, 1984

Heath, Robert. *Paradoxical Assertions and Philosophical*, 1598, 1684

Heraclitus Ridens: At a Diaglogue between Jest and Earnest, 1967

Herodian's History of the Roman Emperors, 2368

Heylyn, Peter. *Certamen epistolare: or, The Letter-Combate*, 1599

—————. *Extraneus vapulans: or, The Observator Rescued*, 1546

Heywood, John. *A Dialogue*, A13

—————. *Two Hundred Epigrammes, upon Two Hundred Proverbs with a Thyrde Hundred Newely Added*, A16

J

J., W. "Preface" in Renè Le Bossu's *Treatise of the Epick Poem*, 2298

Jackson, John. *Ecclesiastes. The Worthy Church-man: or, The Faithfull Minister*, A111

Jackson, Thomas. Μαραν αθα [Maran atha]*: or, Dominus veniet*, 1567

———. *The Works*, 1824

Jevon, Thomas. *The Devil of a Wife*, 2078, 2240, 2299

Johnson, Edmund, commendatory poem in John Gower's *The Cow-ragious Castle-combat*, 1413

Johnson, Richard. *The Famous History of the Seven Champions of Christendom. The Third Part*, 2079, 2323

Jones, Bassett. *Herm'ælogium: or, An Essay on the Rationality of the Art of Speaking. Offered*, 1601

Jonson, Benjamin. *The Sad Shepherd: or, A Tale of Robin-Hood*, 1386

———. *Sejanus His Fall*, A74

———. *The Works of Ben Jonson*, 2211, A74

Jordan, Thomas. *The Debtors Apologie*, 1409

———. *Tricks of Youth*, 1664

———. *The Walks of Islington and Hogsdon*, 1568

K

Keepe, Henry. *Monumenta Westmonasteriensia*, 1986, 2007

Kennett, White. *Parochial Antiquities*, 2300

The Kingdom's Weekly Intelligencer, 1429

Knevet, Ralph. Στρατιωτικον [Stratiotikon]*: or, A Discourse of Militarie Discipline*, A112

Knox, John. *A Historie of the Reformation of the Church of Scotland*, 1410, A46

Kynaston, Francis, *Leoline and Sydanis*, 1400, 1418

L

Lacy, John. *The Dumb Lady*, 1798

———. *Sir Hercules Buffoon*, 2032

The Ladies Losse at the Adventures of Five Hours, 1665

Lady Alimony: or, The Alimony Lady, 1602

Lane, John. *Alarum to Poets*, 1443

Langbaine, Gerard, the younger. *An Account of the English Dramatick Poets*, 2184, 2389

Le Bossu, Renè. *Treatise of the Epick Poem*, 2298

Le Bovier de Fontenelle, Bernard. *History of Oracles, and the Cheats of the Pagan Priests*, 2125, 2381

Le Fèvre, Raoul. *The Destruction of Troy*, 1460, 1764, 1885, 1949, 2033

Leigh, Edward. *Analecta Caesarum Romanorum: or, Select Observations*, 1430, 1569, 1685

———. *Choice Observations of All the Kings of England*, 1631

———. *England Described*, 1603

———. *Fœlix Consortium*, 1666

———. *Poems, upon Several Occasions, and, to Several Persons*, 2112

———. *Select and Choice Observations*, 1667, 1765

———. *A Treatise of Religion & Learning*, 1548

Lenton, Francis. *Characterismi: or, Lentons Leasures Expressed in Essayes and Characters*, A117

———. *Characters: or, Wit and the World in Their Proper Colors*, 1668

Le Sylvain, Alexandre. *The Orator*, A63

Lewkenor, Lewis. Interpolation in *The Resolved Gentleman*, A61

Lightfoot, John. *Erubhin: or, Miscellanies Christian and Judiacall*, A115

———. *The Works of the Reverend and Learned John Lightfoot*, 2034

Lindsay, David. *The Workes*, 1444, 1549, 1700, 1766, 1799, 2008, 2080, 2324

Littlebury, Robert. *Catalogus bibliothecæ illustrissimi domini Gulielmi Ducie Vicecomitis Duni*, 1950

Llewellyn, Martin. *Men Miracles*, 1422, 1543, 1630, 1933

Lloyd, David. *The Legend of Captain Jones*, 1445, 1550, 1604, 1782

———. *Memoires*, 1736, 1898

———. *The States-men and Favourites of England*, 1701

———. *State-worthies*, 1767

Locke, Matthew. *The Present Practice of Musick Vindicated*, 1825

Lodge, Thomas. *Rosalynde. Euphues Golden Legacie*, A53

Look to It London, 1446

Loveday, Robert. *Loveday's Letters Domestick and Forrein*, 1605, 1653, 1669, 1749, 1826, 1899, 2035

Lort, Roger. *Epigrammatum*, 1423

Lucretius His Six Books of Epicurian Philosophy, 2396

Luctus Britannici: or, The Tears of the British Muses for the Death of John Dryden, 2411, 2412, 2414, 2415, 2431

Lupton, Donald. *England's Command on the Seas*, 1496

Lydgate, John. *The Boke Calledde John Bochas Descrivinge the Falle of Princis, Princessis, [and] Other Nobles*, A3

———. *The Cronycle of all the Kynges That Have Reygned in Englande*, A15

———. *The Glorious Lyfe of Seint Albon Prothomartyr of Englande*, A7

———. *The Proverbes of Lydgate*, A6

———. *The Siege of Thebes*, A4

Lyly, John. *Euphues and His England*, A32

———. *Euphues the Anatomy of Wit*, A32

M

Maimbourg, Louis. *The History of the League*, 2036

Marmion, Shakerley. *The Antiquary*, 1387

Marvell, Andrew. *The Last Instructions to a Painter*, 1722

———. *Miscellaneous Poems*, 1969

———. *The Rehearsal Transposed*, 1800

Mason, John. *Mentis humanae metamorphosis: sive conversio, The History of the Young Converted Gallant*, 1886

Mason, Margery, pseud. *The Tickler Tickled*, 1937

Massinger, Philip. *The City-Madam*, 1584, 1606

———. *Three New Playes*, 1525

Massinger, Philip, Thomas Middleton, and William Rowley. *The Old Law*, 1551

Match Me These Two: or, The Conviction and Arraignment of Britannicus and Lilburne, 1431

Mede, Joseph, *The Apostasy of the Latter Times*, 1389, 1401, 1411, 1514, 1532

Medwall, Henry. *Nature. A Goodly Interlude*, A8

Miege, Guy. *The New State of England under Their Majesties K. William and Q. Mary*, 2185, 2241, 2270, 2390

Mennes, John. *Musarum deliciæ: or, the Muses Recreation*, 1526

———. *Recreation for Ingenious Head-peeces*, 1414, 1461, 1509, 1670, 1702, 1723, 2009

———. *Wits Recreations*, 1390

———. *Wit Restor'd*, 1576

———. *Wit Restor'd in Several Select Poems Not Formerly Publish't*, 1585, 1591

Mercurius Britanicus, 1419

Meriton, Luke. *Pecuniae obediunt omnia. Money Masters All Things: or, Satyrical Poems*, 2369

Middleton, Thomas. *No Wit, [and No] Help Like a Womans*, 1570

———. *Two New Playes*, 1571

Mill, Henry. *A Funeral Elegy*, 1420

Mill, Humphrey. *A Nights Search. Discovering the Nature and Condition of All Sorts of Night-Walkers*, A129

Millington, Edward. *Bibliotheca Ashmoliana*, 2271

———. *Bibliotheca Bassetiana*, 2347

———. *Bibliotheca Carteriana*, 2149

———. *Bibliotheca Castelliana*, 2081

———. *Bibliotheca Cogiana*, 2272

———. *Bibliotheca Jacombiana*, 2113

———. *Bibliotheca Levinziana*, 2370

———. *Bibliotheca Lloydiana*, 2010

———. *Bibliotheca Massoviana*, 2134

———. *Bibliotheca Maynardiana*, 2114

———. *Bibliothecæ nobilissimæ pars tertia & ultima*, 2301

———. *Bibliotheca Prestoniana*, 2325

———. *Bibliotheca selectissima: sive, catalogus variorum librorum antiquorum & recentiorum*, 2348

————. *Playes*, 1654
————. *Poems and Phancies*, 1687, 1737
Newcastle, William Cavendish. "On Her Book of Poems" in Margaret Cavendish's *Poems and Phancies*, 1687, 1737
A New Dialogue betwixt Heraclitus & Towzer, 1971
A New Song of the Misfortunes of an Old Whore and Her Brats, 2136
The New Wife of Beath [sic], *Much Better Reformed*, 2417
Niccols, Richard. *The Three Sisters Teares Shed*, A87
Nicholson, John. *A Catalogue of Excellent Books*, 2304
Nicholson, Samuel. *A Sermon, Called Gods New Yeeres-Guift Sent unto England*, A71
Nicolson, William. *The English Historical Library*, 2329
————. *The English Historical Library, Part III*, 2391
Nixon, Anthony. *The Foot-Post of Dover with His Packet Stuft Full of Strange and Merry Petitions*, A96
————. *Great Brittaines Generall Joyes. Londons Glorious Triumphs*, A88
North, Sir Edward, trans. Guevera's Αρχοντοροδογιον [Archontorologion]: *or, The Dial of Princes*, A99

O

Ogilby, John, trans. *The Fables of Æsop Paraphras'd in Verse*, 1473, 1703, 1738, 1828, 1867
Oldham, John. "A Pastoral" in the Earl of Rochester's *Poems, &c. On Several Occasions*, 2187, 2330
————. *Poems, and Translations*, 2011
————. *Some New Pieces Never Before Publisht*, 1972, 2038
————. *The Works of Mr. John Oldham*, 2083, 2212, 2305, 2371
Oldys, Alexander. *An Ode, By Way of Elegy, on the Death of the Incomparable Mr. Dryden*, 2418
"On John Burnyeat's Book" in Burnyeat's *The Truth Exalted*, 2188
Orrery, Charles Boyle. *Dr. Bentley's Dissertations on the Epistles of Phalaris, and the Fables of Aesop Examin'd*, 2372
Osborne, Francis. *Historical Memoires on the Reigns of Queen Elizabeth and King James*, 1586
————. *The Works of Francis* Osborn, 1829, 1987, 2152, 2419
Ovid's elegies: Three Books by C. M. Epigrames by J. D., A67
Ovid's Metamorphosis, trans. Sandys, A113
Owen, John. Θεολογουμενα παντοδαπα [theologoumena pantodapa]: *sive, De natura*, 1634

P

P., G. "The Praise of Chastitie" in *The Phœnix Nest*, A58
P., H. *A Looking-Glass for Children*, 1830
P., L. *Two Essays Sent in a Letter from Oxford*, 2306

————. *Wit and Drollery. Joviall Poems*, 1635

Philipps, Thomas. *Bibliotheca Angleseiana*, 2084

The Phœnix Nest, A58

Pierce, Thomas. *The Law and Equity of the Gospel*, 2085

The Pindar of Wakefield, 1406

Pix, Mary. *To the Right Honourable Earl of Kent . . . This Poem*, 2422

Plattes, Gabriel. "A Caveat for Alchymists" in *Chymical, Medicial, and Chyrurgical Addresses*, 1527

Playford, Henry. "Advertisement" in *The Postboy*, 2423

The Pleasant and Sweet History of Patient Grissel, 2086

Plot, Robert. *De origine fontium*, 2063

————. *The Natural History of Oxford-Shire*, 1900

————. *The Natural History of Stafford-shire*, 2087

A Poem on the Coronation of King William and Queen Mary, 2153

Poems on Affairs of State from the Time of Oliver Cromwell, 2350

The Politicks of Malecontents, 2039

Polsted, Ezekiel. Καλᾶς Τελωνήσανται [Kalos Telonesantai]: *or, The Excise Man*, 2351

Poole, Josua. *The English Parnassus: or, A Helpe to English Poesie*, 1572, 1901, 1913

Poor Robin . . . An Almanack After a New Fashion, 1688, 1704, 1715, 1725, 1739, 1751, 1771, 1786, 1801, 1833, 1852, 1870, 1887, 1902, 1914, 1939, 1954, 1973, 1988, 2012, 2040, 2064, 2088, 2117, 2138, 2154, 2167

Poor Robins Intelligence, 1888, 1903

Pope, Walter. *The Salsbury-Ballad*, 1882

The Post Boy, 2423, 2425

The Post Man, 2426

Preston, Richard Graham. *Angliae speculum morale*, 1772, 2275

————. Epistle in Boethius's *Of the Consolation of Philosophy*, 2308

Prideaux, Mathias. *An Easy and Compendious Introduction for Reading All Sorts of Histories*, 1448, 1462, 1510, 1528, 1689, 1802, 1834, 1989

Prince, Vincent. *The Protestant Almanack*, 2155, 2189

Prynne, William. *A Catalogue of Such Testimonies in All Ages as Plainly Evidence Bishops and Presbyters to Be Both One, Equall and the Same*, 1388

————. *The Antipathie of the English Lordly Prelacie, Both to Regall Monarchy and Civill Unity*, 1394

————. *A Catalogue of Such Testimonies in All Ages*, 1394

————. *Canterburies Doome*, 1421

————. *The Substance of a Speech Made in the House of Commons*, 1455

Prynne, William (?). *A Catalogue of Such Testimonies in All Ages*, A124

————. ed. Jan Hus's *A Seasonable Vindication of the Authority of Christian Kings, Lords, Parliaments*, 1620, 1740

Purchas, Samuel. *Purchas His Pilgrimes*, A106

————. *Theatre of Politicall Flying-Insects*, 1573

R

Rabelais, François. *Pantagruel's Voyage to the Oracle*, 2276

Rainolds, John, and John Hart. *The Summe of the Conference*, A41

Ramesey, William. *The Gentlemans Companion*, 1803

Ramsay, William. *Conjugium conjurgium: or, Some Serious Considerations on Marriage*, 1835, 1853, 1871, 1889, 2041, 2277

Rapin, René. *Reflections on Aristotle's Treatise of Poesie*, 1855

Ray, John. *A Collection of English Proverbs*, 1773, 1915

———. *A Collection of English Words Not Generally Used*, 1854, 2190

———. *The Wisdom of God Manifested in the Works of the Creation*, 2191, 2213

The Resolved Gentleman, A61

Rich, Barnabe. *A Right Exelent [sic] and Pleasaunt Dialogue*, A25

Robinson, Richard. *A Golden Mirrour*, A50

———. *The Rewarde of Wickedness*, A26

Rochester, John Wilmont, earl of. *Poems, &c. On Several Occasions*, 2187

Rogers, George. *The Horn Exalted: or, Roome for Cuckolds*, 1636, 1638

Rogers, John. *Sagrir: or, Doomes-day Drawing Nigh.* 1511

R[ogers], T[homas]. *A Posie for Lovers: or, The Terrestrial Venus Unmaskt*, 2278

Rolls, Nathaniel. *Bibliotheca ornatissima: or, A Catalogue of Excellent Books*, 2214

Rookes, Thomas. *The Late Conflagration*, 1726

Rowlands, Richard. *See* Verstegen

Rymer, Thomas. "Preface of the Translator" in René Rapin's *Reflections on Aristotle's Treatise of Poesie*, 1855, 2279

———. *A Short View of Tragedy*, 2243

———. *The Tragedies of the Last Age*, 1916, 2215

Ryves, Bruno. *Mercurius Rusticus: or, The Countries Complaint*, 2065

S

S., G. *Anglorum speculum: or, The Worthies of England, in Church and State*, 2042

S., J. *The Case of the Quakers Relating to Oaths Stated*, 1856, 2332

———. *The Present State of England*, 2013

S., R. *Ludus ludi literarii: or, School-boys Exercises and Divertisements*, 1804

S., W., in John Bullokar's *An English Expositor*, 1512, 1554, 1673, 1727, 1787, 1890, 1955, 2043, 2139, 2309, 2373

Saker, Austin. *Narbonus. The Laberynth of Libertie*, A33

Sadler, John. *Rights of the Kingdom*, 1456, 1990

Salmon, Thomas. *A Vindication of an Essay to the Advancement of Musick*, 1805

Sanderson, William. *A Compleat History of the Life and Raigne of King Charles*, 1589

Sandys, George, trans. *Ovid's Metamorphosis*, A113

Sandys, George, trans. *Ovid's Metamorphosis Englished*, 1555, 1690, 1752, 1917, 2168

Sanford, Francis. *A Genealogical History of the Kings of England*, 1904, 2014

The Satires of Decimus Junius Juvenalis, 2232

Simpson, John. *Catalogus Bibliotheca Collegii Sionii*, 1463

Sinetes Passion uppon His Fortunes, A64

Skinner, Stephen. *Etymologicon linguæ anglicanæ*, 1788

———. *An Etymologicon of the English Tongue*, 1753

Slater, Master. *The New-Yeeres Gift Presented at Court, from the Lady Parvula to the Lord Minimus*, A122

Smallwood, Matthew. *Catalogus librorum*, 2044

Smith, James. "The Preface to Penelope and Ulysses" in *Wit Restored*, 1556, 1591, 1637, 1993

Smith, John. *The Mysterie of Rhetorique Unvail'd*, 1557, 1707, 1837, 2018, 2141

Smith, Richard. Commendatory poem in Richard Robinson's *The Rewarde of Wickedness*, A26

Smith, Thomas. *Catalogus librorum manuscriptorum bibliothecæ Cottonianæ*, 2334

Soames, William, and John Dryden. An interpolation in Nicholas Boileau-Despréaux's *The Art of Poetry*, 2019

Some Modest Remarks on Dr. Sherlocks New Book, 2193

Somner, William. *Dictionarium Saxonico-Latino-Anglicum*, 1607

———. *A Treatise of the Roman Ports and Forts in Kent*, 2226

South, Robert. *Twelve Sermons Preached upon Several Occasions*, 2281, 2352

Sparrow, Anthony. *A Rationale upon the Book of Common Prayer*, 1741, 1809, 1892, 2045

Speed, Samuel. *Fragmenta carceris: or, The Kings-Bench Scuffle*, 1857, 1873

Spelman, Henry. *Glossarium archaiologicum*, 1692, 2120

———. *Reliquiae Spelmaniae. The Posthumous Works Relating to the Laws and Antiquities of England*, 2374

Spencer Redivivus Containing the First Book of the Fairy Queen, 2121

Spencer, John. Καινα και παλαια [Kaina kai palaia]. *Things New and Old*, 1590

Spenser, Edmund. *The Shepheardes Calender*, A31

———. *The Works of That Famous English Poet*, 1940

Sprat, Thomas. "An Account" in *The Works of Mr. Abraham Cowley*, 1742

———. *History of the Royal Society of London*, 1729

State-Poems; Continued From the Time of O. Cromwel, 2353

Staveley, Thomas. *The Romish Horseleech*, 1858

Stevenson, Matthew. *The Twelve Moneths: or, A Pleasant and Profitable Discourse of Every Action*, 1638

Stillingfleet, Edward. *An Answer to Mr. Cressy's Epistle*, 1874

———. *The Grand Question*, 1957

Stone, Nicholas. *Enchiridion of Fortification*, 1416, 1754

S'too Him Bayes: or, Some Observations upon the Humour of Writing Rehearsals Transpros'd, 1838

Stow, John. *A Survey of London*, 1379

Strong, James. *Joanereidos: or, Feminine Valour*, 1417

Ware, James. *A Catalogue of Books*, 2377

———. *A Catalogue of Books in Several Faculties & Languages*, 2395

———. *Librorum manuscriptorum*. 1450

Warner, William. *Albions England*, A51

Waterhouse, Edward. *An Humble Apologie for Learning and Learned Men*, 1501

———. *Fortescutus illustratus: or, A Commentary*, 1677

Watkyns [or Watkins], Rowland. *Flamma sine fumo: or, Poems Without Fictions*, 1659

Webb, John. *An Historical Essay*, 1755, 1921

Webster, William. *A Plaine and Most Necessary Booke of Tables for Simple Interest*, A107

———. *Webster's Tables*, 1435

The Weekly Pacquet of Advice from Rome, 1995

Weever, John. *The Mirror of Martyrs: or, The Life and Death of Sir John Old-Castle*, A69

Wesley, Samuel. *An Epistle to a Friend Concerning Poetry*, 2435

———. *The Life of our Blessed Lord & Saviour Jesus Christ*, 2251, 2284, 2357

———. *Maggots: or, Poems on Several Subjects*, 2069

West, Richard. *Wits A.B.C: or, A Centurie of Epigrams*, A80

Westminster-Drollery, 1789, 1811

Westmorland, Mildmay Fane. *Otia sacra optima fides*, 1451

Wharton, George. "To my Very Honoured Friend," in Gaultier de Coste, Seigneur de La Calprenède's *Hymen's Præludia: or, Love's Master-Piece*, 1488, 1475, 1516, 1678, 1709, 1744, 1860, 2122, 2378

Whitehead, George. *The Case of the Quakers Concerning Oaths Defended as Evangelical*, 1861, 1876

Whitlocke, Bulstrode. *Memorials of the English Affairs*, 1877, 1996

A Wife for a Husband, and a Husband for a Wife, 1942

Williams, Roger. *The Bloody Tenent yet More Bloody*, 1489

Willis, John. *The Art of Stenography*, 1412, 1436

Wilson, John. *The Cheats*, 1695, 1790, 2047, 2252

———. *The Projectors*, 1710

Wilson, Thomas. *A Christian Dictionarie*, 1437, 1452, 1515, A85

———. *A Complete Christian Dictionary*, A85

Windsor-Drollery. Collected by a Person of Quality, 1813

Winstanley, William. *Englands Worthies*, 1623, 2048

———. *The Lives of the Most Famous English Poets: or, The Honour of Parnassus*, 2123

———. *The New Help to Discourse*, 1745, 1814, 1958, 2049, 2335

———. *The Protestant Almanack*, 1959, 2218, 2436

Winstanley, William, compiler. *Poor Robin's Jests: or, The Compleat Jester*, 1756

Wit and Drollery, 1556, 1560

Wit and Mirth: or, Pills to Purge Melancholy, 2441

INDEX OF CHAUCER'S WORKS

Index of Chaucer's Life
and Literary Reputation

General Index

This index includes names of authors, translators, and editors of STC books; names of modern critics; names of mythological, pastoral, and biblical characters; and names included in the text of individual entries. The index does not include references to Spurgeon, Boswell, and Holton, whose names appear frequently in the text.

Barnes, Julian, 1880
Baron, William, 2380
Bartas, *see* Saluste, Guillaume de,
    Seigneur du Bartas
Basset, Thomas, 2091
Basset, William, 2347
Batchiler, John, 1660
Baxter, Richard, 1923
Beaumont, Anscel, 2100
Beaumont, Francis, 1438, 1453, 1548,
    1588, 1803, 1832, 2048, 2185, 2205,
    2216, 2418
Becket, Thomas, 1745, 1992, 2042
Behn, Aphra, 2058, 2125, 2205, 2248,
    2381, 2418
Benedict, Saint, 1469
Bentivoglio, Guido, 1503
Bentley, Richard, 2372
Berengar of Tours, 1396
Bernard, Edward, 2341
Bernard, Francis, 2341, 2360
Birckbeck, Simon, 1561
Blackmore, Richard, 2407
Blague, Daniel, 2173
Blome, Richard 2023, 2050, 2224
Blount, Thomas, 1504, 1534, 1535, 1593,
    1624, 1661, 1679, 1759, 1760, 1761,
    1795, 1841, 1960, 2000, 2174, 2257
Blount, Thomas Pope, 2159
Boccaccio, Giovanni, 1623, 1643, 1670,
    1702, 1723, 1929, 2009, 2067, 2161, 2201,
    2243, 2257, 2306, 2313, 2406, 2429
    The Falle of Princes, 1390
Bodley, Thomas, 2341
Boethius, 1521, 1607, 1636, 1906, 1919,
    2308
Bohun, Edmund, 2222, 2258, 2286
Boileau-Despréaux, Nicholas, 2019
Bold, Henry, 1680, 2051
Boleyn, Anne, 1383
Bolton, Edmund, 1842
Bolton, Robert, 1380
Bond, Richmond P., 1586, 1721, 1789,
    1961, 2345, 2365
Bowman, Thomas, 2092
Boyle, Charles, *see* Orrery
Boyle, Francis, *see* Shannon

Bradford, John, 2075
Bradstreet, Ann, 1467, 1920
Bradwardine, Thomas, 1521, 2159
Bramhall, John, 1403, 1505, 1625, 1626,
    1878, 1893
Brandon, Charles, Duke of Suffolk, 1588
Brathwait, Richard, 1381, 1479, 1698,
    1711, 1970
Brian, Thomas, 1518, 1924
Brigham, Nicholas, 1478, 1623, 1986,
    2197, 2257
Brigham, Rachel, 1986
Briseis, 1440
Britaine, William de, 2072, 2144, 2225,
    2338, 2398
Brome, Alexander, 1382
Brome, James, 2226
Brown, Thomas, 2160, 2399
Bruce, Robert, *see* Ailesbury
Buchanan, George, 1803, 2205
Buchler, Johann, 1750, 1770, 1938
Buckingham, George Villiers, 2418
Buckley, Mr., 1623
Bullokar, John, 1512, 1554, 1673, 1727,
    1787, 1890, 1955, 2043, 2139, 2309,
    2373
Bullord, John, 2161, 2162, 2175, 2176,
    2177, 2199, 2259, 2260, 2261 2287,
    2288, 2339, 2340, 2400, 2401, 2402
Bunyan, John, 2024, 2073, 2093, 2153,
    2163, 2227, 2317
Burgsersoe, John, 1623
Burnet, Gilbert, 1879, 1925, 2094
Burnyeat, John, 2188
Burscough, Robert, 2341
Burwash, J., 2042
Butler, Samuel
    Hudibras, 1494n, 1803, 1961, 2138,
    2154, 2265
Button, Ralph, 1970
Byblis, 1399
Bysshe, Edward, 1930

C., D., 2001
C., H., 1926
Cæsar, Augustus, 1654
Cæsar, Julius, 1654, 1755

Maynard, Edward, 2114
Mearnes, Charles, 2116
Mede, Joseph, 1389, 1401, 1411, 1514, 1532
Medusa, 1563
Melpomene, 1526
Mena, Johannes, 1623
Menander, 1832
Mennes, John, 1390, 1414, 1461, 1509,
    1526, 1576, 1585, 1670, 1702, 1723,
    2009
Mercurius Melancholicus, 1447
Mercury, 1467, 1526, 2165
Meriton, Luke, 2369
Merlin, 1385, 1494, 1521, 1529
Merton, Walter de, 1521
Meun, Jean de, 1535, 1869, 1982
Middleton, Thomas, 1551, 1570, 1571
Miege, Guy, 2185, 2241, 2270, 2390
Mill, Henry, 1420
Millington, Edward, 1951, 1952, 1970,
    2010, 2037, 2057, 2081, 2082, 2113,
    2114, 2115, 2116, 2134, 2135, 2149,
    2150, 2151, 2242, 2271, 2272, 2273,
    2301, 2302, 2325, 2326, 2347, 2348,
    2370, 2416
Milton, John, 1391, 1392, 1399, 1415,
    1612, 1827, 1943, 1951, 1972, 1997,
    2232, 2248, 2249, 2251, 2297, 2303,
    2327, 2349, 2406
Mohammed, 2234
Molière (Jean-Baptiste Poquelin), 1798,
    2165, 2253
Monro, Alexander, 2327
Montague, Walter, 1540
Montaigne, Michel de, 2060
Montecute, Thomas, *see* Salisbury
Moone, John, 1402
More, John, 2341
More, Thomas, 1623, 1842, 2140
    Utopia, 1448, 2003, 2005
Morgan, Sylvanus, 1632, 1714
Morley, George, 1633
Moses, 1392
Motteux, Peter Anthony, 2238, 2276
Murford, Nicholas, 1464
Musgrave, John, 1708

N., J., 2186
Nabbes, Thomas, 1953
Nedham, Marchamont, 1431, 1484
Nevil, Cecily, 1904
Newcastle, Margaret Cavendish, 1552,
    1654, 1686, 1687, 1737, 1783, 2092
Newcastle, William Cavendish, 1687,
    1737
Nero, Roman emperor, 1654
Nicholas of Lynn, 1464, 1650, 2042
Nicolson, William, 2329, 2391
Norton, Sampson, 1478
Norton, Thomas, 1818
Nostradamus, Michael, 1797, 2056

Odysseus, *see* Ulysses
Ogilby, John, 1473, 1703, 1738, 1828, 1867
Oldham, John, 1972, 2011, 2038, 2083,
    2153, 2187, 2212, 2305, 2330, 2371
Oldmixon, John, 1882
Oldys, Alexander, 2418
Olivarez, count of, 1546
Oliver, Elizabeth, 2151
Oppian, 2372
Orinda, *see* Katherine Philips
Orrery, Charles Boyle, 2372, 2418
Osborne, Francis, 1586, 1829, 1987, 2152,
    2419
Otway, Thomas, 2205
Outram, William, 1962
Ovid, 1555, 1599, 1619, 1652, 1690, 1752,
    1793, 1803, 1917, 2059, 2168, 2185,
    2205, 2374, 2406, 2429
Owen, John, 1634

P., H., 1830
Packer, Philip, 1681
Parker, Derek, 1494*n*
Parker, Martin, 1393, 1618
Parker, Samuel, 1784
Parkhurst, Thomas, 2061
Parsons, Robert, 2137
Partridge, James, 2307
Partridge, John, 1497
Paschall, Andrew, 1915
Patrick, Simon, 1768